SAUNDERS
Fundamentals for Nursing Assistants

ARLENE POLASKI, MSN, RN
Faculty
Charlotte-Mecklenburg Hospital Authority
School of Nursing
Charlotte, North Carolina

JUDITH P. WARNER, BSN, RN
Director of Nursing
Integrated Health Services of Erie at Bayside
Erie, Pennsylvania

W.B. SAUNDERS COMPANY
A Division of Harcourt Brace & Company
Philadelphia · London · Toronto · Montreal · Sydney · Tokyo

W.B. SAUNDERS COMPANY
A *Division of Harcourt Brace & Company*

The Curtis Center
Independence Square West
Philadelphia, Pennsylvania 19106

Polaski, Arlene.
    Saunders fundamentals for nursing assistants / Arlene Polaski,
Judith P. Warner.
        p.   cm.
    ISBN 0-7216-3608-X
    1. Nurses' aides.   2. Care of the sick.   I. Warner, Judith P.
II. Title.
    [DNLM: 1. Nurses' Aides.   WY 193 P762s 1994]
RT84.P65   1994
610.73'06'98—dc20
DNLM/DLC   93-26105

Saunders Fundamentals for Nursing Assistants   ISBN 0-7216-3608-X

Printed in the United States of America.

Last digit is the print number: 9   8   7   6   5   4   3   2   1

To future nursing assistants and to the many nursing assistants who through their example have taught others about caring.

Preface

Nursing assistants serve an important role in giving care to others. They are with patients for many hours each day and work hard to show their caring qualities and commitment to giving good basic care.

Our purpose in writing this textbook is to welcome and prepare nursing assistants as new care givers who are members of the health care profession. Nursing assistants must learn a lot of information in order to make patients safe and comfortable. They need to learn how to act legally and ethically and how to communicate positively with patients, families, and staff. They need to know how to give care in various settings, including the home, the nursing home, and the hospital.

Saunders Fundamentals for Nursing Assistants is written in an easy-to-read format that is intended to help the nursing assistant learn to give proper care. The textbook is divided into eight units that progress from introductory concepts of health care to the actual practice of giving care to people in need of help. The textbook includes many unique topics and features such as:

Communication—Because verbal as well as nonverbal communication is important in the role of care giver, many important communication techniques are discussed.

Hiring—A discussion of hiring practices is presented to help the future nursing assistant search out and apply for positions in health care. Knowledge of the hiring process and how one should act during this process are valuable tools for the nursing assistant seeking a certified nursing assistant position when the nursing assistant course and the certification examination are completed.

Rationales—Rationales are presented for actions that are often taken when performing procedures. We believe rationales help the students understand why an action is taken.

Definitions—Definitions for new vocabulary words are included in the margins the first time they appear to help students comprehend the information as they read. These definitions are also included in a glossary at the end of the book.

Activity Corner—Activities designed to help the student grasp major concepts discussed in the chapter and explore their own feelings as well as patients' feelings are included at the end of each chapter. The activity corners are intended to help the student apply learning.

Caring Comments—These are bits of information interspersed throughout the chapters to provide nursing assistants with helpful hints and precautions regarding patient care.

To assist instructors with course development, there is an instructor's manual, a student workbook, and a slide set, which includes all illustrations and photos from the textbook. The instructor's manual contains a listing of objectives, an outline of the important points of the chapter, current resources, learning activities, the answers to the student workbook activities, a test bank of multiple choice questions and check-off sheets for procedures included in the textbook.

The student workbook contains a variety of worksheets for the learner. Students are given the opportunity to test learning through various exercises, including fill-in-the-blank, matching, crossword puzzles, and true and false statements. Check-off sheets for procedural skills are also included.

To all nursing assistant students—We hope you enjoy your nursing assistant course and find *Saunders Fundamentals for Nursing Assistants* and the student workbook helpful. We hope they provide a solid base of knowledge as you begin your career as a nursing assistant.

ARLENE POLASKI
JUDITH P. WARNER

Acknowledgments

We would like to acknowledge our families, who offered support and understanding from start to finish. To Don Polaski and Rod Warner, thanks. No words can express how much their strong presence meant to us during the long hours of writing and rewriting.

Special thanks go to Mary McClimans, who helped with her nursing and teaching expertise; to Tom Zilonka who led us through the first steps in the brave new world of the computer; and to Margaret Klan, who checked and rechecked and typed the manuscript.

Thanks also to all family, friends, students, and former students who served as models—Èleonore Lacey; Edward Gould; Mary, Laura, and Daniel McClimans; Donna Bessetti; Beth, Elise, Steven, and Garrett Weigant; Julia, Rachel, and Matthew Reichard; Brenda Gore; Kim DiTullio; Patty Russell; Naomi Rawlings; Mary Degnan and children; Gina Edwards; Thang Tran; Missy Wirotratana; Sister Phyllis McCracken; Kaye Peters; and Leonard Wroblewski. Thanks also to the many persons, though unnamed, who assisted and supported this project.

Thank you to our local agencies that supported us—Saint Mary's Home of Erie, Pennsylvania, and Woman's Christian Association Hospital in Jamestown, New York. Our colleagues and the administration of Jamestown Community College deserve special thanks and recognition for their support.

Thanks to our photographer, Barb Proud, and her assistant, Allison, who produced the many fine photographs that appear in the text.

Reviewers deserve special thanks. Their constructive comments and criticisms of the manuscript and art program during development of this text contributed greatly to the final product. Their insightful suggestions are very much appreciated.

We are grateful for the assistance and support of the many personnel at W. B. Saunders Company who worked on this project. In particular, we wish to express thanks to Margaret M. Biblis, Senior Acquisitions Editor, and Shirley A. Kuhn, Senior Developmental Editor, who supported us from the beginning and provided many valuable suggestions along the way.

ARLENE POLASKI
JUDITH P. WARNER

List of Procedures

Contents

Beginning a Career
in Health Care

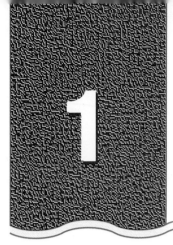

Learning About Health Care

Objectives

AFTER YOU COMPLETE THIS
CHAPTER, YOU WILL BE ABLE TO:

Define health.
Define illness.
List five types of health care
facilities.
Identify the purposes of health
care facilities.
Describe the roles of the health
care team members.
Identify the nursing assistant's
role in patient care.

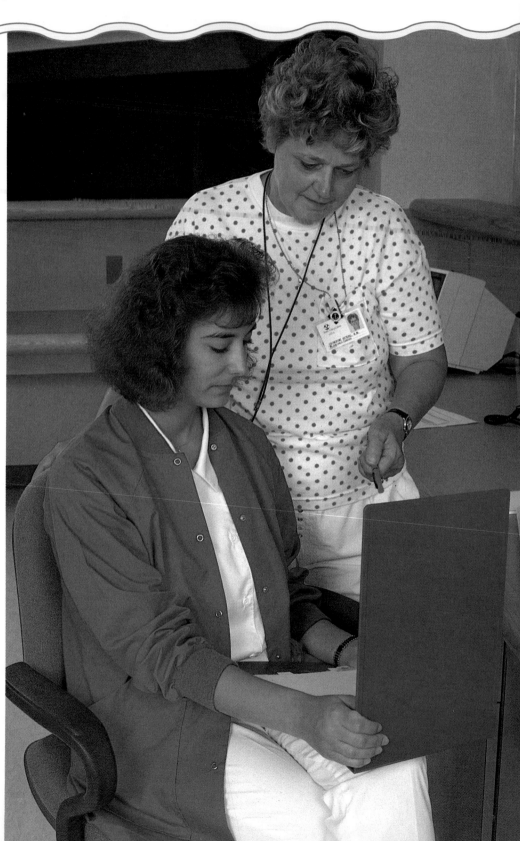

Overview Every individual should experience a healthy sense of well-being. Individuals describe health in their own way. Good health may be threatened by permanent or temporary illness. At some time in their lives, most people experience illness.

A person who is not healthy has certain expectations about care. Family members are the most frequent care givers. When family and friends cannot help, an individual turns to health care providers for care. There is a health care institution for almost any kind of patient need, for example, short- or long-term care, care for the young or the elderly, and care for disabled or disadvantaged persons.

As a nursing assistant, you will be a member of the health care team. Along with other team members at the health care institution, you will provide care to help individuals regain and keep good health. You will give nursing care under the direct supervision of the registered nurse. You will be in a position to offer care, compassion, and concern to patients.

WHAT DO YOU KNOW ABOUT HEALTH?

Here are seven statements about health. Consider them to test your current ideas about health. If you think the statement is true, circle the T; if you think the statement is false, circle the F. Change the false statements to make them true.

1. T F Individuals describe health in their own way.
2. T F Health is not threatened by temporary illness.
3. T F Patient rights apply only to persons in the health care institution.
4. T F Long-term health care institutions (such as nursing homes) admit only elderly patients.
5. T F Nursing assistants give care under the direction of a registered nurse.
6. T F A nursing assistant is a member of the health care team.
7. T F A hospice provides care to terminally ill patients and their families.

ANSWERS

1. **True.** Individuals' feelings and ideas about health are distinctly their own.
2. **False.** Any illness weakens the body and can threaten the person's concept of health.

3. **False.** Each person is entitled to patient rights. The person who is ill at home is entitled to patient rights.

4. **False.** Certain health care institutions admit only adults (age 18 and older). Others care for children from birth to age 18.

5. **True.** The registered nurse has ultimate responsibility for the care of the patient. Nursing assistants provide care under the direction of the registered nurse.

6. **True.** A nursing assistant is a member of the health care team who has duties and responsibilities unique to the position.

7. **True.** Care givers who work in a hospice are specially trained to attend to the needs of terminally ill patients and their families.

HEALTH AND ILLNESS

HEALTH

HEALTH

any state of physical, emotional, and social well-being felt by an individual

WELL-BEING

a healthy, happy life; living a full life

Health is any state of physical, emotional, and social well-being felt by an individual. Individuals describe health in their own way.

Individuals function according to their needs for physical, emotional, and social well-being. **Well-being** is the state of being healthy and happy and living a full life. How individuals might describe their feelings about physical, emotional, and social well-being is shown in the box; write your own description of physical, emotional, and social well-being in the third column.

EXAMPLES OF HOW PEOPLE MIGHT DESCRIBE WELL-BEING		
Type of Well-Being	**Example of Description**	**Your Description**
Health	"I am usually pretty healthy—I never miss work because I'm sick."	
Energy	"I have enough energy to do the things I should do every day."	
Comfort	"I can eat a variety of foods without having stomach problems." "Headaches never seem to bother me." "Eight hours of sleep is plenty for me."	
Emotional	"Everyone says I'm a healthy, cheerful person." "I'm even-tempered, but certain things make me a little anxious."	
Social	"Playing on the softball team helps me make a lot of friends."	

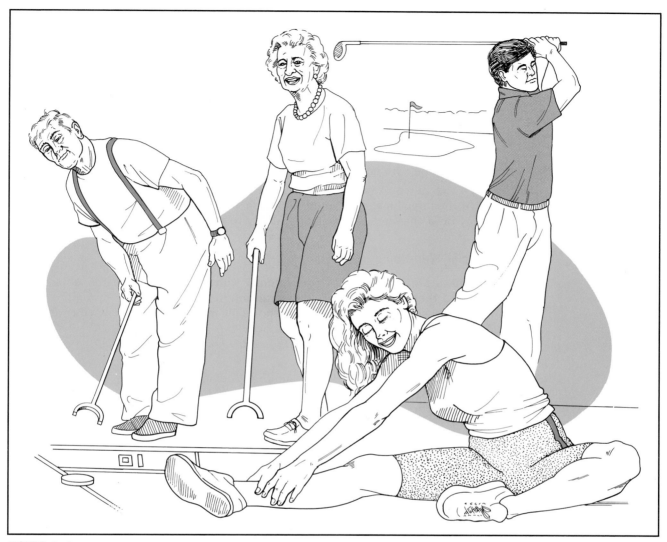

FIGURE 1–1
The way a person functions is a reflection of the person's physical health and well-being.

Physical Well-Being

When the body functions without problems, a person is considered to be in good physical health (Figure 1–1). Body functions include

- Eating and digesting food and eliminating urine and feces
- Using the senses to see, hear, smell, taste, and touch
- Breathing and circulating oxygen in the blood
- Thinking and feeling
- Walking and moving
- Sleeping and resting
- Protecting itself against disease
- Keeping itself safe

A problem or disruption in any body function may cause a change in the person's state of physical health and well-being. People respond differently to changes caused by problems or disruptions in their body functions.

Emotional Well-Being

When a person's emotional status is well balanced, the person is even-tempered and cheerful and can adapt easily to changes. Stress and anxiety are caused by problems or pressures in a person's life. The person might not feel good about himself or herself. The person who has good emotional health shows the ability to

- Use a problem-solving process to make acceptable decisions
- Respond to life with an even temper
- Keep a cheerful disposition
- Cope with stress and anxiety

The person with good emotional health responds to challenges in a positive, healthful manner. When a person has poor emotional health, the result may be a change in the person's ability to respond to challenging situations.

Social Well-Being

Humans are social beings who interact with others and with the environment around them. Disease and illness can interfere with a person's ability to interact as a social being. A person who is ill may no longer have the ability to begin or keep up with many social activities. People whose social well-being is disrupted may become withdrawn, sad, unhappy, or depressed. People with social well-being are able to

- Start a conversation with another person or persons
- Make friends
- Participate in activities that involve other people
- Meet the social expectations of their family, friends, and employers
- Live comfortably within their means

Social well-being is important to physical and emotional health. A problem or disruption in physical health, emotional health, or social well-being may affect one or both of the others (Figure 1–2). Humans function best when there is a balance in healthy behaviors.

ILLNESS

ILLNESS

sickness; a condition different from the normal health state; any change, temporary or long-lasting, in a person's emotional health and well-being

Illness is any change, temporary or long-lasting, in a person's physical and emotional health and social well-being. An illness may be

Acute
Chronic
Terminal

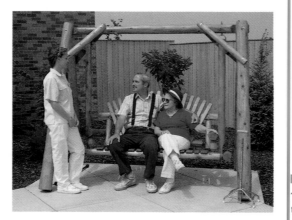

FIGURE 1–2

Taking time to relax is important to emotional well-being.

An **acute illness** is one in which the patient has symptoms that may be severe but do not last very long. A person who has appendicitis (inflammation of the appendix) has an acute illness. After removal of the appendix during surgery, the patient is well again.

A **chronic illness** is one in which the patient has symptoms over a long period of time. Many body functions may be affected. The person who has arthritis (inflammation of the joint) has a chronic illness. The pain, swelling, and stiffness associated with arthritis can be treated with medications to make the person comfortable.

Terminal illness is an illness in which the end result is death; the patient's life expectancy must be 6 months or less. A patient with lung cancer may have a terminal illness, because most types of lung cancer have no cure.

Illness is also a role a person assumes during a change in health status. Because individuals view illness in different ways, they also behave in their own particular ways when they are ill. As shown in the chart, individuals may demonstrate any combination of positive and negative behaviors when they assume the role of an ill person.

ACUTE ILLNESS
illness in which the symptoms may be severe but do not last very long

CHRONIC ILLNESS
illness in which the symptoms last a long time

TERMINAL ILLNESS
illness in which the end result is death; the patient's life expectancy must be 6 months or less

EXAMPLES OF BEHAVIORS PEOPLE MAY DEMONSTRATE WHEN THEY ARE ILL

Positive Behaviors	Negative Behaviors
Smiling cheerfully	Acting sad, quiet, irritable, or restless
Mentioning their illness to other people when appropriate	Mentioning their ill health to anyone who will listen
Participating in daily activities as usual	Not participating in daily activities

CARING COMMENTS

Illness can make persons feel helpless and defenseless. They may be genuinely unable to do anything for themselves, even though they want to. Think about a time you were very ill and someone took care of you. You wanted someone to make you comfortable. As a nursing assistant, you should respond to your patient's need for comfort and safety. A back rub or an extra blanket can make your patient more comfortable; be sure side rails are raised for any patient who is weak or unconscious.

The person who is not healthy has patient rights, expects and deserves competent care, and may choose to assume the sick **role.**

ROLE
a socially accepted behavior pattern

HEALTH–ILLNESS CONTINUUM

The **health–illness continuum** is a way to measure the state of health or wellness of an individual. The health–illness continuum ranges from the state of feeling very healthy and well to a state of feeling near death (Figure 1–3). Because health means something different to every person and can change on a day-to-day basis, people may place themselves at different places on the continuum (Figure 1–4).

HEALTH–ILLNESS CONTINUUM
a way to show how you feel about your own state of health or illness

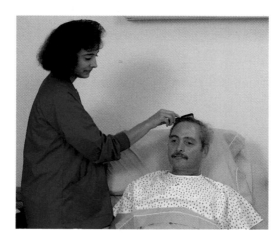

FIGURE 1–3

Patients may feel helpless when they are too weak or ill to care for themselves.

CARING COMMENT

To find out how your patients feel about their health, you can ask, "On a scale of one to ten, how do you feel today?"

HEALTH CARE INSTITUTIONS

Health care institutions are facilities that are designed to care for people who are ill. A health care facility may be owned by a private organization or by a government. An individual may receive either acute or long-term health care or both in a health care facility. Some facilities care for only people of a certain age (for example, only the elderly) or only patients with a certain illness (such as burns). There is a health care institution to meet the needs of patients of all ages and types of illness.

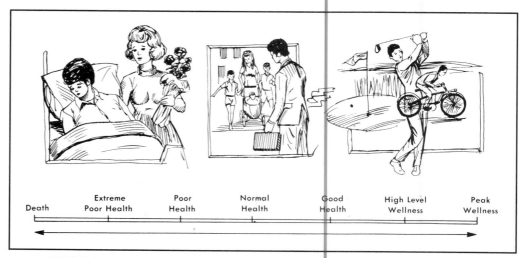

| Death | Extreme Poor Health | Poor Health | Normal Health | Good Health | High Level Wellness | Peak Wellness |

FIGURE 1–4

The health–illness continuum. (From DuGas BW: Introduction to Patient Care: A Comprehensive Approach to Nursing, 4th ed. Philadelphia, W. B. Saunders Company, 1983.)

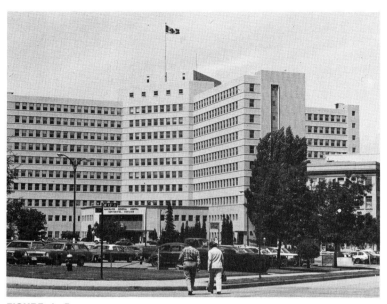

FIGURE 1-5

A hospital provides many health care services to the people in a community and its surrounding areas. (From DuGas BW: Introduction to Patient Care: A Comprehensive Approach to Nursing, 4th ed. Philadelphia, W. B. Saunders Company, 1983.)

ACUTE CARE FACILITIES

A **hospital** is an acute care facility. It offers health care for people who are acutely ill. A variety of services are provided by an acute care facility, including care for critically ill or injured patients, sophisticated diagnostic testing, and specialized medical care and surgeries. People who are injured in accidents or become severely ill receive care in acute care health facilities (Figure 1-5). Another name for this type of facility may be "health care center" or "medical center." An acute care facility may offer other health care services such as one-day surgery, rehabilitation, maternity care, and mental health care.

HOSPITAL
an institution for the care and treatment of the acutely ill and injured

LONG-TERM CARE FACILITIES

Long-term care facilities provide services for people who need care over long periods of time. The period of time may range from several weeks to many years. Individuals of any age may reside in a long-term care institution. The most well-known age group to make use of long-term care is the elderly (Figure 1-6). Other groups include infants, children, mentally disadvantaged individuals, and people of any age who have physical disabilities.

OTHER TYPES OF HEALTH CARE INSTITUTIONS

Hospice

A **hospice** is a place for the care of persons (and their families) who are in the last stages of life. Hospice care is a special kind of care designed for the person who is very ill and knows death is approaching. It is provided for people who are terminally ill. Hospice care does not necessarily have to be given in a hospice; it may be given in the patient's home. The care giving often

HOSPICE
a place for the care of persons (and their families) in the last stages of life

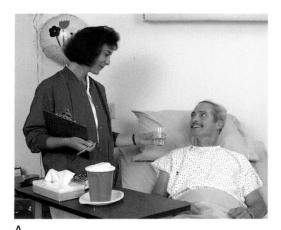

A

CONDITIONS THAT MAY REQUIRE LONG-TERM CARE

Chronic pain
Parkinson's disease
Alzheimer's disease
Stroke (if weak or paralyzed)
Complications following major trauma
Postoperative complications (paralysis, coma, etc.)

Such patients may need help with
    Walking
    Transferring
    Socializing
    Activities of daily living such as eating, bathing, dressing,
      and toileting
    Maintaining a safe environment
    Taking medications

B

FIGURE 1–6

A, A nursing home or other long-term care facility may offer specialized care for people with particular problems. B, List of conditions that may require long-term care.

involves family members and friends. Hospice care is designed to make terminally ill individuals comfortable and secure during their last days.

Rehabilitation Center

REHABILITATION

a program that helps a patient to return to as normal a life as possible

Rehabilitation care is provided for individuals who need supportive care and teaching in order to be able to care for themselves once again. A rehabilitation center may accept a variety of patients or may specialize and accept patients who have suffered a specific disease. A rehabilitation center may accept only patients with head trauma or only patients who have had a stroke. Rehabilitation services may include medications, physical therapy, occupational therapy, and any other service that will help patients reach the goal of self-care to the best of their abilities.

Mental Health Care Facilities

In another type of specialty care institution, care is given to young and old persons who are mentally ill. Drug and alcohol treatment centers are examples of mental health care facilities. Treatment may be long or short term. Short-term treatment is given in local hospital treatment centers and includes in-patient care and outpatient care in the community. The length of time necessary for treatment varies according to the needs of the patient. Long-term mental health care may be provided in an institution that offers such long-term care. What is considered a long period of time ranges from 4–6 weeks to a lifetime. A person who needs mental health care may be placed in a group home in the community. A group home offers a secure and supportive environment for the follow-up care of the mental health patient who lives in the community.

Home Health Care Agency

Home health care is a service (run by a hospital or another public or private agency) that allows individuals to remain in their home and receive help from care givers. The care giver may give the patient a bath; prepare meals and feed the patient; assist the patient in and out of bed; and assist with walking, toileting, and dressing. If a patient needs help with housework and shopping, these services may also be provided (see Chapter 32).

HOME HEALTH CARE
nursing care and personal services (housekeeping, shopping, etc.) provided for patients who live at home and cannot perform activities of daily living for themselves

PURPOSES OF HEALTH CARE INSTITUTIONS IN ADDITION TO PROVIDING CARE

Health care institutions offer other services in addition to caring for patients. They also serve the community by educating people about health promotion and disease prevention.

There may or may not be a charge for community educational services. Education about health and health care may also be directed to patients in the institution. The physician may recommend a certain education program to a patient. Some programs are designed for patients and the family members who are involved in their care.

Health care institutions also take steps to educate their employees about health promotion and disease prevention. Employees may be required to attend continuing education programs and are encouraged to attend other programs that will benefit them and their patients.

Individuals' physical and emotional health and social well-being are enhanced when they take advantage of the health services and educational programs offered by a variety of health care institutions.

Health Promotion

Health promotion is the attempt to improve the quality of life by informing people of behaviors that promote health. Health promotion can be done in acute and long-term care institutions, doctors' offices, the school, the workplace, and residences. Examples of health-promoting actions are given in the following chart. Each of these activities is necessary to promote healthy body functions as well as a healthy outlook on life.

HEALTH-PROMOTING ACTIVITIES

- Eating 3 well-balanced meals each day
- Exercising at least 3 or 4 times each week
- Drinking 6–8 glasses of water every day
- Sleeping about 8 hours every night
- Relaxing when stressed

Disease Prevention Programs

Disease prevention programs are an attempt to improve the quality of life by helping persons to act to prevent the occurrence of disease and illness. People who practice disease prevention feel better and have lower medical costs. In the future, health care institutions will stress the importance of preventing disease. **Immunization** shots against measles in children and against influenza (the flu) in the elderly are examples of the prevention of disease. Guidelines to help prevent disease are listed in the following chart.

DISEASE PREVENTION
actions taken to prevent disease

IMMUNIZATION
a procedure that helps the body develop cells (antibodies) against a specific harmful microorganism

---

DISEASE-PREVENTING ACTIVITIES

- Participating in health screening programs (blood pressure measurement, sickle cell anemia testing, cholesterol screening, etc.) offered by the community
- Receiving (and seeing that one's children receive) immunization against any disease that can be prevented in one's age group
- Seeking information on measures that prevent disease (how to quit smoking, how to lose weight, etc.)
- Scheduling a physical examination on a routine basis

THE ORGANIZATION OF A HEALTH CARE INSTITUTION

Health care institutions provide care for individuals in need. An institution may choose to offer care only to a particular group of people, such as handicapped children or patients who have suffered head injuries. Specialty units such as the cardiac care unit and intensive care unit are areas in the institution in which a specially trained care giver meets the needs of special patients. The institution itself is organized into departments that coordinate and function to provide patient care services (Figure 1–7). The following chart shows an example of how departments function as part of an organization.

DEPARTMENTS OF A HEALTH CARE INSTITUTION

Department	Function
Administration	Directs the operation and services of the institution
Patient services	Plan and give care to those who are sick or injured
Support services	Help create and maintain a healthy environment

Administration

The administration division of the health care institution is made up of individuals who direct the institution in the fulfillment of its stated mission and goals.

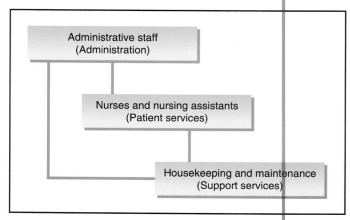

FIGURE 1–7

Relationship of the three main departments in a health care institution.

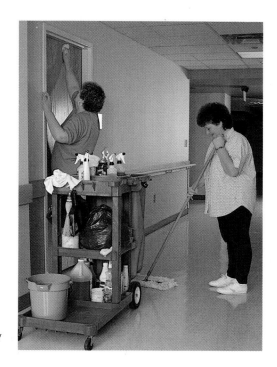

FIGURE 1–8
A clean environment is made possible by members of the support staff.

The administrative staff consists of the officers of the institution as well as the board of directors. As a group, these individuals plan for future changes in health care. Financial responsibilities belong to the administrative personnel as well. The heads of departments (or divisions) are also part of the administration.

Patient Services

The members of the health care team are the individuals who are directly involved with patient care. Nurses and their assistants are directly involved with the hands-on care of patients 24 hours a day. Many support personnel help with patient care in indirect ways, such as preparing meals and cleaning patients' rooms. Other care givers, such as x-ray and laboratory technicians, beauticians and barbers, and transport personnel, may be involved directly or indirectly with services provided to patients while they are in the health care institution.

Support Services

Support services from many other departments of the health care institution contribute to making each patient's stay comfortable and safe. The personnel of the buildings and grounds, including the engineers, housekeepers, maintenance staff, and other support service staff, all contribute to create an environment that will help make the patient's stay in the hospital or nursing home more comfortable and accident-free (Figure 1–8).

THE HEALTH CARE TEAM

The **health care team** is the group of care givers involved in providing care to patients (Figure 1–9). The members of the health care team may include the

    Physician
    Registered nurse

HEALTH CARE TEAM
a group of people who have the education necessary to provide care to patients

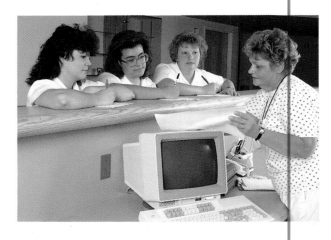

FIGURE 1–9
The health care team plans patient care at the beginning of the shift.

Licensed practical/vocational nurse
Nursing assistant (also called nurse's aide or orderly)

Personnel who work in other departments also give care to patients. These include personnel from

Physical therapy
Recreational therapy
Occupational therapy
Speech and hearing therapy
Nutrition and diet therapy
Social services
Chaplain or spiritual services

The chart gives examples of health care team members and their roles.

MEMBERS OF THE HEALTH CARE TEAM AND THEIR ROLES	
Member	**Role**
Physician	Diagnoses disease
	Orders and evaluates treatment
Registered nurse	Assesses, plans, intervenes in, and evaluates patient care
	Coordinates and manages patient care
	Teaches patients health promotion and illness prevention
	Supervises and educates personnel who care for patients (Figure 1–10)
Licensed practical/vocational nurse	Gives direct care to patients, performs treatments, and administers medication under the supervision of a registered nurse
Nursing assistant (also called a nurse's aide, nurse technician, or orderly)	Gives patient care under the supervision of the registered or licensed practical or vocational nurse
	Observes the patient and reports to the registered nurse

Unit secretary (also called a ward clerk or health unit coordinator)	Transcribes the physician's orders for patient care Performs receptionist duties
Physical therapist	Provides therapy that regains/maintains the patient's mobility
Recreational therapist	Provides activities that help patients socialize and interact
Occupational therapist	Assists patients in applying talents used in a previous or new occupation
Speech and hearing therapist	Assists patients to overcome speech and hearing difficulties
Nutrition (dietary) therapist	Provides education about special diets Determines patient's likes and dislikes in food and fluids
Social worker	Determines and secures supportive services such as home health care and financial referral
Chaplain, spiritual services	Ministers to the spiritual needs of the patient

THE EDUCATION OF THE HEALTH CARE TEAM MEMBERS

Patient care is provided by care givers who have been educated as health care providers. Each care giver is educated to give care at a certain level of responsibility. Educational programs range in duration from a few months to several years, depending on regulatory requirements and the level of care a person desires to give.

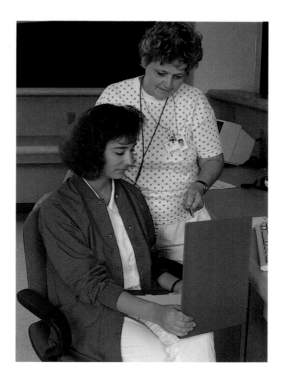

FIGURE 1–10

The registered nurse shows a nursing assistant important information about her patient.

Physician

PHYSICIAN

a medical doctor or doctor of osteopathy

Patient care and specific treatments are ordered by the physician who is in charge of a patient. The **physician** is a graduate of a medical college; medical college is attended after graduation from a 4-year college. After graduation from medical or osteopathic college, the person is designated a medical doctor (MD) or a doctor of osteopathy (DO). The following is a list of the specialties for which physicians receive extra training after graduating from medical or osteopathic college.

MEDICAL SPECIALTIES

Title	Specialty Service
Surgeon	Performs surgical procedures
Family practitioner	Provides medical care for all members of the family
Neurologist	Specializes in diseases of the nervous system
Ophthalmologist	Specializes in diseases of the eyes and disorders of visual function
Cardiologist	Specializes in diseases of the heart and blood vessels
Pulmonary specialist	Specializes in diseases that affect breathing function
Gynecologist	Specializes in diseases that occur in women only
Endocrinologist	Specializes in diseases of the glands that secrete hormones
Gastroenterologist	Specializes in diseases that affect the stomach and intestines
Nephrologist	Specializes in diseases of the kidneys
Urologist	Specializes in diseases of the urinary tract
Proctologist	Specializes in diseases that affect the anus, rectum, and/or sigmoid colon
Orthopedic specialist	Specializes in disorders of joint and skeletal function
Oncologist	Specializes in diseases that affect cell growth, that is, tumors
Rheumatologist	Specializes in rheumatic (joint and muscle) diseases
Dermatologist	Specializes in skin diseases
Allergist	Specializes in treating allergic conditions
Radiologist	Specializes in the use of x-rays to diagnose and treat diseases
Pediatrician	Specializes in the care of well and ill children (from birth to the beginning of adulthood)
Obstetrician	Specializes in the care of women during pregnancy, labor, and the period following birth
Gerontologist	Specializes in caring for persons with diseases and changes associated with aging
Psychiatrist	Specializes in caring for patients affected with mental, behavioral, and/or emotional disorders
Physiatrist	Specializes in the use of physical therapy to treat and prevent bodily disorders

Registered Nurse

There are 2-, 3-, and 4-year **nursing** programs that prepare a graduate nurse. After passing the examination provided by the state board of nursing, the graduate nurse is designated a **registered nurse (RN)**.

TWO-YEAR NURSING PROGRAM A 2-year nursing program may be offered by a community college, a college, or a university. A graduate of a 2-year program earns college credit for courses such as anatomy and physiology, psychology, and nutrition as well as the nursing courses. The graduate of the 2-year program earns an **associate degree in nursing (ADN)**.

THREE-YEAR NURSING PROGRAM A 3-year nursing program is usually offered by a hospital's school of nursing. Some hospitals' school of nursing programs are designed to be completed in less than 3 years. A hospital's school of nursing may offer college credit for courses such as anatomy and physiology and psychology. Credit for such courses may be transferred to a college if the graduate desires to earn a 4-year college nursing degree, a **bachelor of science degree in nursing (BSN)**. The credit for nursing courses is usually not transferable to a college nursing program. The graduate of a hospital school of nursing earns a diploma in nursing.

FOUR-YEAR NURSING PROGRAM A 4-year nursing program is offered by a college or university. The opportunity to learn about management, research, and leadership is included in the 4-year program. All courses earn credit toward a BSN.

Licensed Practical/Vocational Nurse

The 1- to 2-year nursing program leads to licensing in practical or vocational nursing. Nursing programs may be offered by a hospital's school of nursing, a local school district, or a community college. After passing the examination of the state board of nursing, the graduate is called a **licensed practical/vocational nurse (LPN/LVN)**.

Certified Nursing Assistant

Nursing assistants must attend an approved program of learning and earn a certificate that allows them to give patient care under the direction of a registered or licensed practical/vocational nurse. The programs range from about 3–8 weeks to 3–6 months. When the examination is passed, the person is called a **certified nursing assistant (CNA)**. A nursing assistant may be employed as a nurse's aide, orderly, or patient care technician. A nursing assistant must be certified to work in a long-term care facility; certification is not necessarily required to work in a hospital or for a home health care service.

Further Education

After graduation from any of the health care programs of learning, a health care worker may decide to go on to the next step by seeking further education. For example, a certified nursing assistant may decide to become a licensed practical or vocational nurse. After becoming a licensed practical or vocational nurse, the next step would be to enter a program that offers registered nursing. An individual might seek still further education and continue up the career ladder in the care-giving profession (Figure 1–11).

Care givers may also decide to specialize in an area of care. Further education in specialties such as pediatrics, geriatrics, cardiac care, orthopedic care, and so on is available at different levels for the person who desires to take advantage of the opportunity. The following chart shows how two individu-

NURSING
the art and science of caring for others

REGISTERED NURSE
a graduate nurse registered and licensed to practice by a state authority

LICENSED PRACTICAL/VOCATIONAL NURSE
a graduate of a school of practical or vocational nursing who is licensed by a state authority and practices under the supervision of a registered nurse

CERTIFIED NURSING ASSISTANT
a person who is certified to give care to patients under the direct supervision of a registered or a licensed practical/vocational nurse

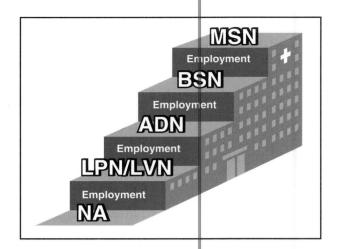

FIGURE 1–11
Sample career ladder for nursing health care givers. NA, nursing assistant; LPN, licensed practical nurse; LVN, licensed vocational nurse; ADN, associate degree in nursing; BSN, bachelor of science in nursing; MSN, master of science in nursing.

als who chose the nursing profession used educational opportunities to advance in the profession.

SAMPLE CAREER PATHS OF TWO HEALTH CARE GIVERS	
Care Giver 1	**Care Giver 2**
1975 Graduated from an LPN/LVN program.	**1985** Graduated from high school where CNA certification was earned.
1975–1979 Employed as an LVN in a small community hospital.	**1985–1990** Studied in a 4-year nursing program. Employed part-time as a CNA in a children's home.
1980–1983 Studied full-time and graduated from a 2-year program to become an RN. Employed part-time nights in a nursing home.	**1990 to present** Graduated from college and passed the state board of nursing examination. Employed as a staff member (RN) in the emergency department of the local hospital. Studying part-time in a program leading to a master of science degree in nursing.
1983–1990 Employed full-time as an RN in the cardiac care unit of a large hospital. Studied part-time to earn a bachelor's degree in nursing at the local university.	
1990 to present Employed as a cardiac nurse specialist and enrolled in a program to earn a master's degree in nursing.	

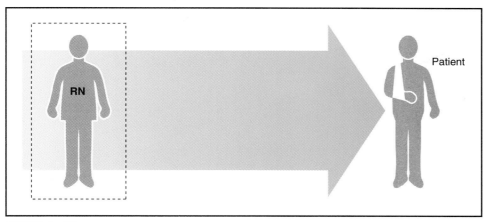

FIGURE 1–12

Primary Nursing: The RN is directly responsible to the patient during the patient's entire stay in the health care institution.

ORGANIZATION OF NURSING CARE

Over the years, nurses have developed different approaches to providing care for patients. The approaches are known as

Primary nursing (Figure 1–12)
Team nursing (Figure 1–13)
Functional nursing (Figure 1–14)

Primary Nursing

The current approach to nursing care is the system known as "primary care." **Primary nursing** gives a registered nurse 24-hour responsibility and **accountability** for a patient's care until the patient is discharged. The primary nurse is also responsible for the assessment and planning of care. Nursing orders are developed by the primary nurse, and other care givers follow them for total care of the patient. In addition, the primary nurse is responsible for the teaching and discharge planning of the patient.

PRIMARY NURSING
the nurse's 24-hour accountability
for the patient's care
ACCOUNTABILITY
taking responsibility for your actions

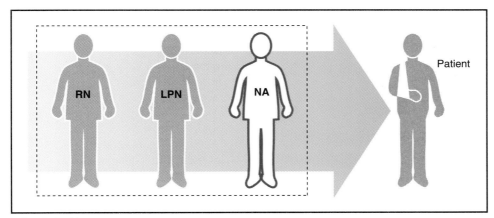

FIGURE 1–13

Team Nursing: During each shift, a different RN leads a team of care givers in providing care for the patient.

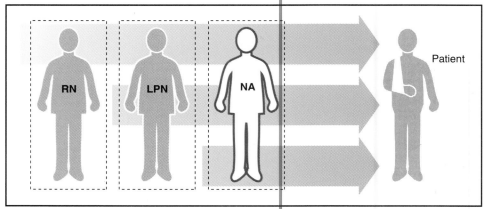

FIGURE 1-14

Functional Nursing: A different task is assigned to each care giver. No single care giver is responsible for the entire care of a patient during the shift.

Team Nursing

TEAM NURSING
a team of care givers caring for a group of patients

Another approach to patient care is called "team nursing." **Team nursing** is directed by a team leader, either a registered nurse or a licensed practical/vocational nurse, for each shift in the health care institution. A team of care givers cares for a group of patients according to the level of education of each care giver and the special needs of the patient.

Functional Nursing

FUNCTIONAL NURSING
the type of nursing wherein patient care is divided into certain functions (for example, one nursing assistant might be assigned to weigh patients)

Lastly, another approach called "functional nursing" may be used. In **functional nursing,** care is accomplished by assigning specific tasks, rather than patients, to a variety of care givers. One care giver may be assigned to measure all the vital signs of all patients on the nursing unit, and another may be assigned to only bathe or feed patients. Nurses experiment with each of these approaches and may adapt or combine them to provide the best care for the particular type of patients in their care.

THE NURSING ASSISTANT'S ROLE IN PATIENT CARE

The nursing assistant's role is to help in the care of patients. When giving care, the nursing assistant should display the following traits:

Caring   Dependability
Honesty   Empathy
Accuracy   Responsibility

CARING

CARING
an attitude of interest in and concern about helping others

Nursing is caring. **Caring** is an attitude of interest and concern about helping others. The caring person seeks to attend to others' needs. Caring is reflected in the way you interact with patients and staff. It is reflected in the little, often unnoticed things you do for others (Figure 1–15). Checking the patient's identification bracelet before performing a nursing procedure is extremely important. A simple act like offering to help a patient sit up shows you care. Giving a back rub at bedtime shows you care enough about patients to help them relax and fall asleep easier. Listening to the patient or family members shows your care

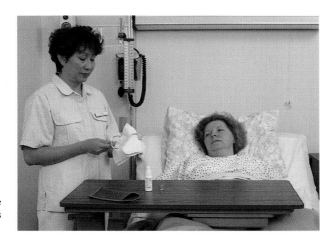

FIGURE 1–15
Caring is something felt inside and shown outwardly by actions taken to help others.

and concern about their feelings and needs. Helping other care givers on the unit shows your interest in and concern about others and motivates other care givers to help you when you need help with the care of your patients.

HONESTY

Honesty is living up to a sense of fairness. An honest person does not lie or cheat. You need to be honest when giving patient care because being honest helps your patients, as well as others on the health care team, develop a sense of trust in you.

ACCURACY

Strive to be as accurate and correct as possible. In certain situations accuracy is critical. For example, the results of vital sign measurements you report must be accurate because important decisions may be based on your measurements. Whenever you are uncertain of results, it is your responsibility to seek help from the nurse. You will be considered responsible and honest when your goal is to be as accurate as possible.

DEPENDABILITY

Being **dependable** means reporting to work on time, keeping absences to a minimum, keeping your promises to patients, doing assigned tasks to the best of your ability, and performing routine tasks without having to be told each time. Being dependable means that your patients and co-workers can rely on you.

DEPENDABLE
reliable; when people know they can count on you

EMPATHY

Empathy is understanding or being aware of another person's feelings, thoughts, or experiences. Showing empathy means being able to put yourself in another person's place and see things as that person sees them. When people are ill or injured, they usually behave differently than when they are healthy. A patient may act angry, hostile, or abusive, but if you realize the reason behind the behavior you will not take it personally because you will have empathy for the patient.

EMPATHY
understanding or being aware of another person's feelings, thoughts, or experiences

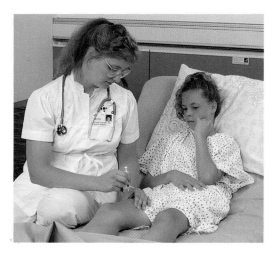

FIGURE 1–16
The care giver who explains a procedure before starting builds trust with the patient.

RESPONSIBILITY

When you accept the responsibility of patient care, you are held accountable for your behavior or conduct. You are responsible for giving patient care under the supervision of the registered nurse or licensed practical/vocational nurse. While you are giving care, you are responsible for observing the patient and reporting your observations to the nurse. You are responsible for giving the best care you can to the patient. Always act in a responsible manner to build trust with your patients and with other care givers (Figure 1–16).

Responsibility to Your Patients

The nursing assistant is responsible for a great variety of patient-associated activities. When you are given a patient assignment, you are responsible for

- Giving or assisting with proper patient care (Figure 1–17)
- Keeping the patient safe
- Communicating with the patient and family
- Communicating with other care givers
- Completing the assignment in a timely manner

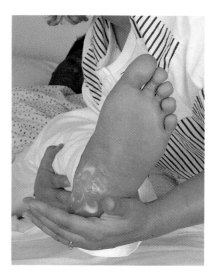

FIGURE 1–17
Note how the nursing assistant supports the patient's lower extremity while massaging the foot with lotion.

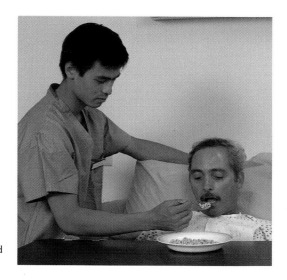

FIGURE 1-18

There are many responsibilities associated with feeding a patient.

Being responsible means you can be held accountable for your actions. If you are asked to do something, you follow through and complete the assignment as best you can. You accept responsibility for your own work. For example, if you are asked to feed a patient, you are responsible for (Figure 1–18)

- Checking for the correct kind of diet order (regular, liquid, etc.)
- Washing your hands
- Checking the patient's identification bracelet
- Positioning the patient
- Protecting clothing and linens
- Cutting and preparing the food on the tray
- Asking the patient what food is desired
- Feeding the patient
- Allowing enough time for the patient to chew and swallow each bite
- Making the patient clean and comfortable after the meal is over
- Cleaning up after the patient is fed
- Recording the input on the intake and output record if the patient is on an input and output (I&O) order
- Reporting to the nurse how much the patient was able to eat and drink
- Performing any other duties that help make eating an enjoyable experience for the patient

Each assignment is made up of a series of steps. You are responsible for following through on each step. Giving a patient a bed bath, transferring a patient, and giving an enema to your patient are common assignments that are completed by following a series of steps.

CARING COMMENT

When you are feeding a patient, you are expected to perform a series of steps to complete the procedure. If you feed the patient so quickly that the patient is not able to swallow in-between bites and as a result chokes on the food during the feeding, you would accept the responsibility for your actions (feeding the patient too fast) and the result (the choking episode).

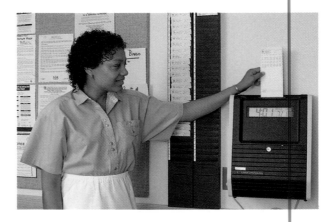

FIGURE 1-19
The nursing assistant arrives on time and is dressed appropriately.

Responsibiity to Your Employer

In addition to your responsibility to your patients and their families, you are responsible to your employer for your actions. The employer has the right to expect that you will

- Perform assignments as you have been taught
- Communicate courteously with others in the health care setting
- Arrive on the unit at the time scheduled (Figure 1-19)
- Arrive well groomed and dressed neatly according to the dress code of the health care institution
- Follow other rules and regulations as listed in the employee handbook and the institution's job description of the nursing assistant position

CARING COMMENT

A patient or family member may try to reward you with a gift or money. This is called tipping. You should gently explain to the patient or family member that your services do not require a tip. Your refusal of a tip may hurt a patient's feelings; you should be gentle, yet firm, when you refuse a tip. If the patient or family member offers you a small token of appreciation, such as a piece of fruit or candy, you may choose to accept and thank the patient.

CHAPTER WRAP-UP

- Health is a concern of every individual.
- Individuals need to consider the state of their physical, emotional, and social well-being.
- The health care you give helps ill or injured individuals regain their former state of well-being.
- A great variety of institutions offer health care services:
  Acute care facilities
  Long-term care facilities
  Hospices
  Mental health care facilities
  Home health care services
  Rehabilitation centers

- Health care team members include the
    Physician
    Registered nurse
    Licensed practical or vocational nurse
    Nursing assistant or orderly
    Registered dietician
    Chaplain
    Other specialized health care personnel
- A health care institution is organized into departments that are responsible for
    Administration
    Patient services
    Support services
- The health care team includes those who give direct patient care:
    Physician
    Registered nurse
    Licensed practical/vocational nurse
    Nursing assistant
- Personnel from other departments may give direct or indirect care to patients.
- There are specific programs of education for each level of health care provider. A program may be as short as 6 weeks or longer than 12 years.
- There are three different approaches to nursing care:
    Primary nursing
    Team nursing
    Functional nursing
- Always strive to be a caring, responsible, honest, and accurate nursing assistant, because your contributions to the care of patients are valued.

REVIEW QUESTIONS

1. Describe a healthy person. Tell what happens when a person is ill. How does illness affect a person's physical, emotional, and social well-being?

2. Name three different kinds of health care institution in your community. What services do these health care institutions offer?

3. List members of the health care team who give patient care. What responsibilities does each member have?

ACTIVITY CORNER

Write down how you feel when you are healthy and when you are ill.

Feelings When Healthy	**Feelings When Ill**
_____	_____
_____	_____
_____	_____
_____	_____

Compare your feelings. What kind of help do you want when you are feeling ill?

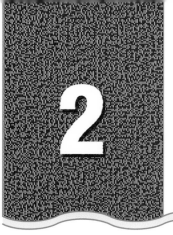

2 Finding a Job

Objectives

AFTER YOU COMPLETE THIS
CHAPTER, YOU WILL BE ABLE TO:

Make a list of your job-related
needs before you seek
employment.

State how to read an
advertisement for a job.

Practice filling out an application
form.

Demonstrate how to act during
an interview.

Describe what behaviors will
help you keep your job.

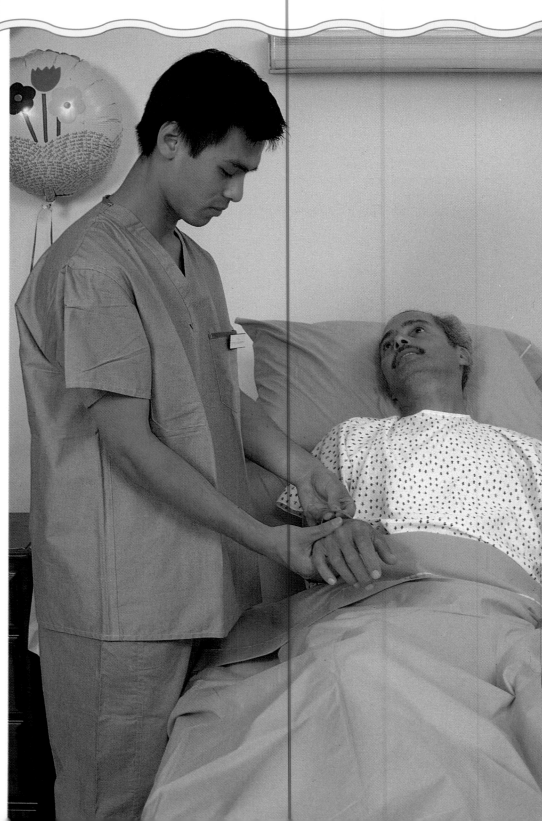

Overview Finding a job involves a number of things. You need to know how the hiring process works. Being prepared to fill out an application and knowing how to act in an interview are important. When you complete your nursing assistant course, you are ready to look for employment.

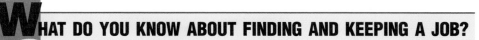

WHAT DO YOU KNOW ABOUT FINDING AND KEEPING A JOB?

Here are four statements about finding and keeping a job. Consider them to test your current ideas about employment. If you think the statement is true, circle the T; if you think the statement is false, circle the F. Change the false statements to make them true.

1. T F The classified advertisement section of your local newspaper is the only source of job information.
2. T F Filling out an application is the first step of the hiring process.
3. T F You should dress in a clean pair of blue jeans and blouse or shirt for a job interview.
4. T F Orientation is the time during which you learn about the job.

ANSWERS

1. **False.** Classified ads are a valuable source, but they are not the only source. You might hear about jobs by word of mouth, for example, from friends and family members. Employment agencies run by your state or by a private company also have information about available jobs. In some areas, health care institutions welcome calls from individuals asking about jobs.

2. **True.** The application gives the hiring health care institutions valuable information about you and your ability to do the job.

3. **False.** Wearing blue jeans is not appropriate for a job interview. Wear a cleaned, pressed pair of slacks or skirt with a clean shirt or top for a good first impression.

4. **True.** Orientation gives you a chance to learn all about the institution. It gives you the chance to ask questions and find out what is expected of you.

THE HIRING PROCESS

When you complete the training requirements of your nursing assistant program, you will take an examination (test) to become a certified nursing assistant. This means the employer can expect certain care-giving behaviors from you. Once you are certified, you may want to seek **employment** at a health care institution.

EMPLOYMENT
an activity usually done for pay

SEEKING EMPLOYMENT

When you are ready to seek employment, you should make a list of your needs:

- Type of institution you want to work at (acute care hospital, long-term care institution, or home health care)
- Location of the institution (near home or accessible via public transportation)
- Availability of child care, if this is a consideration
- Shift you want to work (day, evening, or night)
- Whether you want full- or part-time employment
- Date you will be ready to start work
- Desired wages

When the list is complete, you can start your search for employment. Keep your needs in mind when you start reading the **classified advertisements** and telling your friends that you are job hunting.

CLASSIFIED
divided into sections

ADVERTISEMENTS
public notices, usually placed in a newspaper

The classified advertisements in the "Employment" section of your newspaper may have a listing for "Health Care Personnel" or "Medical Help." Read the advertisements under this heading and make a list of institutions that are advertising for certified nursing assistants or nursing assistants. Match the list of these institutions to your list of needs.

An advertisement will usually tell you

- What qualifications are desired (for example, certification)
- Where the health care institution is located
- How soon you may need to start
- Whether the opening is for the day, evening, or night shift or rotation from one shift to another (for example, you may be required to work 2 weeks of days and 2 weeks of nights)
- Whether the position is full-time or part-time
- How to contact the health care institution (most advertisements will give you the address of the institution and indicate a time that you should come to apply)
- The starting wage

When your list of health care institutions is complete, you are ready to go to each facility and fill out an application for employment.

FILLING OUT AN EMPLOYMENT APPLICATION

APPLICATION
a form used to request something, such as employment

Each health care institution has an employment office or a personnel office. Find this office and ask for an **application** for employment. The application will request information about you and your education and employment histories (Figure 2–1). At most institutions, you will be asked to fill out an application in the office.

When you go to pick up an application or interview for a position, dress neatly and cleanly. You want to create a good first impression. Blue jeans and

United Health, Inc.
Unicare Health Facilities

This company does not discriminate in hiring or employment on the basis of race, color, religious creed, national origin, sex, age, handicap, marital status, veteran status or sexual preference.

EMPLOYMENT APPLICATION

DO NOT WRITE IN THIS BOX		
FACILITY/DIVISION		
DEPARTMENT		
JOB TITLE		
SALARY: HR. MO. YR.		
STARTING DATE		

GENERAL INFORMATION

Please **PRINT** the following information.

LAST NAME	FIRST NAME	MIDDLE NAME	DATE OF APPLICATION
PRESENT ADDRESS	HOME PHONE	BUSINESS PHONE	SOCIAL SECURITY NO.

CITY	STATE	ZIP	TO ASSIST US IN CHECKING YOUR WORK, SCHOOL, OR OTHER RECORDS, PLEASE INDICATE IF YOU HAVE EVER BEEN KNOWN BY ANY OTHER NAME:

POSITION APPLIED FOR	WHAT OTHER JOBS WOULD YOU CONSIDER?	MINIMUM SALARY/WAGE EXPECTED $	DATE AVAILABLE FOR WORK

ARE YOU SEEKING	ARE YOU ABLE TO ROTATE SHIFTS? (complete only if applicable to job)	SHIFT DESIRED
☐ FULL TIME WORK ☐ PART TIME WORK ☐ SEASONAL	☐ YES ☐ NO	☐ EVE. SHIFT ☐ DAY SHIFT ☐ NIGHT SHIFT ☐ ANY SHIFT

ARE YOU WILLING TO WORK OVERTIME? ☐ YES ☐ NO	HOW WERE YOU REFERRED TO US?	ARE YOU WILLING TO TRAVEL? ☐ YES ☐ NO	ARE YOU WILLING TO RE-LOCATE? ☐ YES ☐ NO

Are you over 17 years of age?   ☐ YES   ☐ NO

Are you legally able to work in the United States under the immigration laws of the United States?
☐ YES   ☐ NO

Have you been convicted of a felony within the last seven years?
☐ YES   ☐ NO
If yes, give details.
_____
_____
_____

Have you ever filed an application with this company?
☐ YES   ☐ NO   If yes, when?_____

Do you have any friends or relatives employed here?
☐ YES   ☐ NO   If yes, give names:
_____
_____
Company policy prohibits close relatives working in a reporting relationship.

List professional organizations/associations you belong to:
_____
_____

Registry or Professional license no.
_____ State _____
_____ State _____

EDUCATION

	CITY, STATE	MAJOR COURSE	CIRCLE LAST YEAR COMPLETED	TYPE OF DEGREE
GRADE SCHOOL				
HIGH SCHOOL			1 2 3 4	
COLLEGE/UNIVERSITY			1 2 3 4	
TECHNICAL/BUSINESS			1 2 3 4 1 2 3 4	

CLERICAL EXPERIENCE

☐ Typing (Speed WPM)	☐ Dictaphone	☐ Data Entry Terminal	☐ Bookkeeping Experience
☐ Shorthand (Speed WPM)	☐ Calculator	☐ Word Processing Equipment	☐ Other_____

WORK EXPERIENCE

LICENSED NURSES	☐ HOSPITAL	☐ NURSING HOME	☐ MENTAL HEALTH	☐ OTHER
NURSING ASSISTANTS	☐ HOSPITAL	☐ NURSING HOME	☐ MENTAL HEALTH	☐ OTHER
SPECIAL SERVICES	☐ THERAPY	☐ DIETARY	☐ SOCIAL WORK	☐ OTHER
OTHER	☐ HOSPITAL	☐ NURSING HOME	☐ MENTAL HEALTH	

FIGURE 2–1

A sample application form used by an employer. You can use this form to practice filling in a job application. (Courtesy of United Health, Inc., Unicare Health Facilities.)

Illustration continued on following page

EMPLOYMENT INFORMATION

Starting with PRESENT or MOST RECENT, list all previous employers in the last ten years. Include self-employment, summer and part-time jobs, military service. Use separate sheet, if necessary.

Employer _____ Telephone _____

From		To	
Mo.	Yr.	Mo.	Yr.

Job title _____ Supervisor _____

Street Address _____

SALARY OR WAGE

City _____ State _____ Zip _____

Describe your Duties _____

_____

Reason For Leaving _____

Employer _____ Telephone _____

From		To	
Mo.	Yr.	Mo.	Yr.

Job title _____ Supervisor _____

Street Address _____

SALARY OR WAGE

City _____ State _____ Zip _____

Describe your Duties _____

_____

Reason For Leaving _____

Employer _____ Telephone _____

From		To	
Mo.	Yr.	Mo.	Yr.

Job title _____ Supervisor _____

Street Address _____

SALARY OR WAGE

City _____ State _____ Zip _____

Describe your Duties _____

_____

Reason For Leaving _____

Employer _____ Telephone _____

From		To	
Mo.	Yr.	Mo.	Yr.

Job title _____ Supervisor _____

Street Address _____

SALARY OR WAGE

City _____ State _____ Zip _____

Describe your Duties _____

_____

Reason For Leaving _____

PLEASE READ BEFORE SIGNING:

I certify that the answers given in this application and in the employment interview(s) are true and complete to the best of my knowledge.

I authorize investigation of all statements contained in this application and further authorize my former employers, government agencies, schools, and personal references to provide any information they have regarding me. I hereby release all employers, government agencies, schools, and references from any liability for providing information concerning me.

In the event of employment, I understand that false or misleading information given in my application or interview may result in discharge and that my employment here is contingent upon a physical exam, if required. I understand also that the immigration and Reform Control Act of 1986 requires that employers hire only U.S. citizens and aliens authorized to work in the United States and that all persons hired will be required to submit documents for verification to establish identity and employment authorization.

In consideration of my employment, I agree to conform to the rules and regulations of my employer and that my employment and compensation can be terminated with or without cause and with or without notice at any time at the option of either my employer or myself. I understand that no company representative other than the president has any authority to enter into any agreement for employment for any specified period of time, or make any agreement contrary to the foregoing.

I certify that I am not currently employed, other than as may be shown on this application. I further certify that in applying for employment I am not acting on behalf or in the interest of any other person, organization or entity, but I am simply seeking gainful employment for my own behalf. If employed, I agree to inform the company if I obtain any other employment while working for the company.

I hereby acknowledge that I have read and understand the above statements.

Date _____ Signature of Applicant _____

ATTACH RESUME IF AVAILABLE

FIGURE 2–1

Continued

_____
(Company Name)

_____   Date _____
(Address)

_____
(City, State, Zip)

Attention: _____ or Current Employment Officer

The person named below, who has applied to this company for employment, states that he/she was in your employ

from _____ to _____ at _____
(Location)

_____ Social Security No. _____
(Last Name)   (First Name)   (Maiden Name)

Kindly furnish the information requested below. Such information will be held in strict confidence and not divulged to the applicant. Your reply by return mail will be greatly appreciated.

Sincerely yours,

Signed _____
Title
Facility
Address
City, State, Zip

Are the above employment dates correct?_____If not, please show correct dates from _____ to _____

Position held _____ (Check here if part time worker ☐)

Please discuss fully and frankly the reason for separation: _____
_____

If not against company policy, would you re-employ?   ☐ Yes   ☐ No

Please check the box that describes, as closely as possible, the applicant's work performance.

	Excellent	Good	Fair	Poor
Quality of work	☐	☐	☐	☐
Quantity	☐	☐	☐	☐
Working relationship with other employees	☐	☐	☐	☐
Attendance record	☐	☐	☐	☐
Working relationship with clients	☐	☐	☐	☐

Has the applicant had any difficulty regarding the following:

Handling company money or property   ☐ Yes   ☐ No

Drinking   ☐ Yes   ☐ No

Did applicant have any worker's compensation claims or any history of poor health, back problems, hernia or any other problems that could affect job performance?   ☐ Yes   ☐ No

Other comments _____
_____
_____

Signed _____

Date _____   Title _____

I hereby consent to and authorize the above named employer to release the information requested within this form. And I hereby hold harmless and release said employer from any liability in furnishing this information.

Date_____   Applicant's Signature_____

UHF 800 10/83 (Standard Reference Letter)

FIGURE 2-1

Continued

REFERENCES
people you name on an employment application as being able to provide a statement of your qualifications

sweat shirts are not considered appropriate clothes to wear when you seek a position as a care giver.

You should prepare ahead of time by writing out important information on a piece of paper to take with you. This information could include the names, addresses, and phone numbers of **references.** These should include people you know or worked for. Be sure you first get the permission of anyone whom you plan to name as a reference. Such a step will make you less anxious while you are filling out the application form.

If you are unsure about any requested information, ask the employment office representative so that you are clear about the information the institution wants. Print or write neatly and legibly. Be acccurate and truthful with any information you include on the application. Once you have filled out the application, the next step is the interview.

INTERVIEWING FOR A JOB

An **interview** may be granted when you finish filling out the application for employment, or it may be scheduled at a future date (Figure 2–2). If the interview is scheduled for a later date, be sure to arrive at the scheduled time. This shows that you are prompt and responsible. You should answer questions honestly and to the best of your ability. The institution's interviewer might ask you questions like the following:

- Is there any particular reason you chose to become a nursing assistant?
- Why do you want to work for us as a nursing assistant?
- Have you done any work with patients in the past?
- What times of the day are you available?
- When can you start to work?

The person who interviews you for a position will usually signal the end of the interview by saying, "Do you have any questions you would like to ask?" The Questions To Ask During an Interview chart offers some questions you can ask during a job interview.

INTERVIEW
a formal meeting to obtain information

QUESTIONS TO ASK DURING AN INTERVIEW

- What kinds of patients will I give care to?
- What kind of orientation program do you offer new employees?
- Is a special uniform required for the position?
- Are there openings on the day (or evening or night) shift?
- Do you have full- or part-time positions available?
- How long will my application remain active?

If the interviewer does not offer information about **wages** and **benefits,** you may ask for this information near the end of the interview:

- What is the starting wage?
- What benefits do you offer (for example, health and dental insurance, vacation, and education)?

WAGES
payment for services
BENEFIT
something extra, such as a service, provided by an employer

The interviewer may tell you that a position is available and ask you to return for another interview with the nurse or supervisor of the unit to

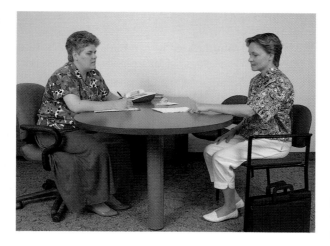

FIGURE 2-2
The interview is an important part of the hiring process.

which you would be assigned. After all required interviews are completed, if the interviewer feels you have the **qualifications** for an open position, you may be hired. If a position is not available, you will be informed of this also. It is permissible to ask the interviewer if you can check back in a certain amount of time to see whether your application is still in the active file. It is best to check back in person. However, you may possibly be asked to telephone the personnel office for this information. You should clarify this before you leave the interview.

Following the interview, you should send a brief thank-you note to any persons who interviewed you. The note should be handwritten. Figure 2–3 is a sample of an appropriate thank-you note.

When the interviewer or other representative of the health care institution tells you that you are hired, you will be asked to complete a health examination. In most cases, the institution arranges for an examination by a physician who is paid by the institution.

QUALIFICATIONS
special abilities or skills

Dear Ms. (or Mr.) Smith:
    Thank you for the interview for the job of certified nursing assistant. I am a good worker and believe I am qualified to give care to patients in your facility.

    I am looking forward to hearing from you soon.

                Sincerely,
                Jane Jones
                Jane Jones

FIGURE 2-3
Sample of a thank-you note to someone who interviewed you.

PHYSICAL EXAMINATION

PHYSICAL EXAMINATION
an examination of a person's state
of health by a physician

A **physical examination** determines the state of your health. It is conducted by a physician. The physical examination usually consists of

- Questions about your past medical history, especially your history of childhood communicable diseases and immunizations
- Measurement of your height and weight
- Measurement of your body temperature, pulse, respirations, and blood pressure
- Questions about medications you are taking
- Examination of your eyes, ears, nose, and throat
- A pelvic examination (for women)
- A rectal examination
- Blood and urine **specimens** for examination by a laboratory

SPECIMEN
sample; a small piece of body tissue
or a secretion used for examination

The results of the physical examination give you and the health care institution an indication of the state of your health at that particular moment in time.

YOUR FIRST DAY ON THE JOB

ORIENTATION
special time set aside to tell you
about something, such as a new job

The first day of work consists of **orientation** to the organization. You are told the institution's rules and regulations and expectations for employee behavior. You may receive an employee handbook that lists the rules and regulations as well as the benefits for which you are eligible.

You learn about many important behaviors during orientation, for example, the procedure for calling in when you are ill or injured and the smoking policies for patients as well as employees. Fire safety and infection control are also important parts of orientation.

During the orientation, you are also informed of the benefits of working in the health care institution. Keep your employee handbook in a safe place and refer to it when you need specific information about your benefits.

DEDUCTION
taking something away

You are asked to sign forms for insurance coverage and for federal, state, and local tax **deductions.** Read all papers carefully before you sign. Be sure to ask questions about any information you do not understand.

Finally, you are given a schedule of your work hours and informed of the length of the probationary period of your employment.

KEEPING YOUR JOB

When you enter the work force, it is important to adhere to certain policies that will help you keep your job. The following guidelines will help you do good work and secure your job:

- Report to work on time
- If you will be late, follow the rules for calling in to notify your supervisor when to expect you
- If you are ill or injured, follow the rules for calling your supervisor

DRESS CODE
guidelines for dressing

- Dress according to the **dress code** that was discussed during your orientation and is written in your employee handbook
- Be sure to keep your patients comfortable and safe
- Treat all people you meet with kindness and courtesy

JOB DESCRIPTION
a statement of the behaviors
expected of a person who performs
a specific job

- Know what is written in your **job description** and act accordingly
- Complete all of your job assignments on time
- Complete only the tasks for which you have been trained
- Ask questions whenever you are unsure what you should do
- Work as a member of the health care team

- Follow the rules and regulations of the health care institution
- Accept responsibility for your actions

PERFORMANCE EVALUATION

Your job **performance** is evaluated after a period of time specified by the institution. **Evaluation** may occur at 30 days, 90 days, and/or 6 months and once a year thereafter. If you follow the preceding guidelines and work within your job description (Figure 2–4), you are likely to earn a favorable evaluation.

PERFORMANCE
an action; how you do something
EVALUATION
a critical assessment of value, worth, character, or effectiveness

---

JOB DESCRIPTION

TITLE: Certified Nursing Assistant
REPORTS TO: Unit Nurse Manager
DEPARTMENT: Nursing Service

I. SUMMARY OF POSITION:
Performs resident care activities and related nursing services necessary in caring for the personal needs, safety, and comfort of residents as assigned. Assists in providing a physical, social and psychological environment which will allow the resident to achieve the highest level of functioning. Performs duties in accordance with established nursing objectives, standards, facility policies and procedures, and residents' rights.

II. MAJOR RESPONSIBILITIES:
A. Essential Functions
1. Personal Care. (Provide personal care for residents by assisting as needed or performing entire procedure when necessary.)
   a. Bathe residents in bed, shower or tub. Must be able to operate whirlpools or other types of specialty tubs. Clean tubs after each use.
   b. Shampoo residents' hair in bed, shower or tub. Groom resident's hair as resident desires in a becoming style. Assist women with makeup as needed.
   c. Shave residents as needed using either a safety or electric razor.
   d. Brush teeth of residents daily, including partial or full dentures.
   e. Clean and cut fingernails as required. Clean toenails as necessary.
   f. Dress residents in clean and appropriate dress, including underwear, stockings/socks and shoes for daytime and night.
2. Admission, Discharge, Transfer
   a. Assist in the implementation of admission, discharge and transfer of residents according to facility procedure.
3. Resident Rights
   a. Know the residents' rights. Help the residents exercise and/or protect their rights.
   b. Become knowledgeable of residents' choices and follow those choices accordingly.
   c. Report residents' complaints to the nurse manager.
   d. Maintain confidentiality of resident information.
   e. Provide psychological support for all residents to help them adjust to their disabilities.
   f. Preserve the dignity and comfort of the dying.
4. Resident Independence
   a. Assist and encourage residents to be independent in areas of activities of daily living.
   b. Assist and encourage residents to be active and out of bed for reasonable periods of time as permitted.

FIGURE 2–4

Sample job description. (Currently being revised. Courtesy of United Health, Inc., Unicare Health Facilities.)

Illustration continued on following page

    c. Promote resident mobility through proper transfer techniques to/from bed, wheelchair, stretcher.

    d. Assist and encourage residents in rehabilitation programs to maximize their independence.

    e. Assist with daily range of motion exercises. Assist with ambulation as needed.

    f. Maintain good body alignment and proper positioning of residents.

    g. Assist and encourage bed residents to change position at least every two hours.

    h. Transport residents from one place to another via wheelchair, stretcher.

5. Elimination. (Monitor elimination status of residents.)

    a. Offer and remove bedpans and urinals.

    b. Assist residents to use commode.

    c. Instruct and assist with bowel and bladder training program.

    d. Check, change and clean incontinent residents as instructed.

    e. Give enemas as directed.

    f. Document and report bowel and bladder patterns.

    g. Collect urine and stool specimens as requested.

    h. Give catheter care; measure and record intake and output.

6. Mealtimes. (Assist at mealtimes.)

    a. Prepare residents for meals. Assist to dining room as necessary.

    b. Distribute and collect trays.

    c. Feed or assist residents.

    d. Instruct residents in use of self-help devices.

    e. Serve nourishments.

    f. Keep fresh drinking water at bedside and encourage fluid intake as instructed.

    g. Observe residents for difficulties in chewing or swallowing while eating.

    h. Report and document nutritional and fluid intake.

7. Vital Signs

    a. Take, record and report vital signs and weights using a variety of sphygmomanometers, thermometers and scales.

8. Infection Control. (Utilize proper infection control procedures.)

    a. Practice proper handwashing technique.

    b. Handle clean and dirty linens properly, without contamination.

    c. Follow universal precautions procedures: use protective equipment and properly dispose of contaminated wastes.

9. Environment and Safety. (Assure a safe, clean and comfortable environment for the resident.)

    a. Place call lights within reach of residents and answer call lights promptly.

    b. Follow procedures for the restraint proper program; make frequent observation of residents.

    c. Know and implement facility safety rules.

    d. Demonstrate proper use of equipment. Report equipment needs or repairs.

    e. Clean equipment and utility areas as assigned.

    f. Assure adherence to smoking policy.

    g. Observe proper ventilation, temperature, light and noise level for day and night activities.

    h. Report any incidents or accidents to the unit nurse manager.

    i. Keep the resident living area neat and orderly; personal care items stored properly; clothing hung in closets or placed in soiled bins as appropriate.

    j. Assist in fire control and resident evacuation during fire or disaster emergencies.

10. CPR

    a. After receiving CPR training, must be able to be a first responder in a medical emergency; e.g., initiate and continue CPR until emergency help arrives.

11. Observations and Reporting

    a. Attend shift report at beginning and end of each tour of duty.

FIGURE 2–4

Continued

      b. Perform and document resident care activities according to written and verbal instruction from the charge nurse.

      c. Coordinate work assignment with other resident activities such as therapy, doctors' appointments, etc.

      d. Observe residents for changes in behavior or condition and report all pertinent information to the unit nurse manager.

12. Care Plans

      a. Participate in the development and implementation of resident care plans according to facility policy and procedure. Keep informed of revisions in care plans through participation in mini-conferences.

13. Hospitality

      a. Maintain a friendly, helpful attitude toward residents, their families, staff, volunteers and visitors.

14. Attendance

      a. Maintain a consistent attendance record to ensure proper resident care.

15. Orientation and Inservice

      a. Participate in required orientation and inservice programs and attend staff meetings as requested.

B. Other Duties

1. Report needs for personal belongings to appropriate persons.
2. Assist and encourage residents to participate in activity programs and special therapies as directed by the nurse manager and prescribed by the physician.
3. Care for and apply prosthetic devices as instructed.
4. Complete ancillary charge tickets for nursing supplies used.
5. Perform other duties as assigned and consistent with level of preparation and experience.

III. QUALIFICATIONS

A. Required:

1. Completion of a nursing assistant certification program or proof of valid certification.
2. Ability to read, write, speak and understand English.
3. Ability to relate positively, effectively and appropriately with residents, families, community members, volunteers and other facility staff.
4. Possess special interest in and a positive attitude about working with long-term care residents and the elderly.
5. Acceptable references.
6. Physical Requirements:

      a. Free of communicable disease.

      b. Meet facility policies and procedures regarding necessary physical health.

      c. Meet the following criteria:

      Criteria = 0—Not at all
                    1—Occasionally (1%–33%)
                    2—Frequently (34%–66%)
                    3—Continuously (67%–100%)

      Bending/stooping = 3
      Reaching above shoulder = 2
      Pushing/pulling = 2
      Standing/walking = 3
      Sitting = 1
      Lifting: 10–35 lbs. = 3
                 36–70 lbs. = 2
                 71–100 lbs. = 2

The criteria for bending/stooping, standing/walking and lifting must be met to be employed because they are essential functions and elements of the job.

Signature   Date

FIGURE 2–4
Continued

ANECDOTAL
a brief story about something that happened

Your performance is evaluated by your supervisor. Your supervisor will be observing you and your work and making notes about your progress. Such notes are called **anecdotal** notes, and your supervisor will consult them when writing the evaluation. In some institutions, problem activities as well as appropriate behaviors are recognized in a written anecdotal note.

The evaluation indicates your strengths and weaknesses and may also include suggestions on how you can improve your performance. You can respond with a smile and a thank you and the good feeling inside that goes along with doing a job well. If problems arise, respond to any discussion of the situation with a calm, accepting manner. You must be able to accept responsibility for your actions. Telling your supervisor how you will correct a problem is a mature and appropriate response. You should try to follow your supervisor's suggestions, because they are designed to help you become a better nursing assistant.

CARING COMMENTS

DEPENDABLE
reliable; when people know they can count on you

Strive to be on time for work. This shows you are a reliable, **dependable** person. The history of your attendance at a previous job is also important.

The evaluation of your job performance is based on the institution's job description for the nursing assistant position.

CHAPTER WRAP-UP

- The hiring process includes
    Filling out an application
    Completing an interview
    Passing a health examination
- An interview is a formal meeting during which information is exchanged.
- Orientation to a job is a special time during which you learn what is expected of you.
- Follow the rules and regulations of the health care institution where you are employed.
- The institution's job description of the nursing assistant position is the guideline used for evaluating how well you are doing your job.

REVIEW QUESTIONS

1. Describe the hiring process.
2. What information is needed to fill out an application for the position of nursing assistant?
3. List the behaviors that are important in keeping a job.
4. Explain why a job description is important.

ACTIVITY CORNER

Complete the following checklist. It can be used when you read the advertisements for your first job as a nursing assistant.

Type of Agency You'd Like to Work For:

_____ Nursing home

_____ Hospital

_____ Home health care

_____ Other

Location Desired:

_____ Within walking distance

_____ Within driving distance

_____ Close to subway

_____ Close to bus stop

Number of Hours Desired:

_____ Full-time (40 hours)

_____ Part-time (less than 40 hours)

Type of Shift Desired:

_____ Day   (7:00 A.M.–3:30 P.M.)

_____ Evening   (3:00 P.M.–11:30 P.M.)

_____ Night   (11:00 P.M.–7:30 A.M.)

_____ Rotate   (rotating between two or all three shifts)

Prepare for a job search:

1. Ask people who know you to provide a reference for you. You can ask a former employer, teacher, or minister to give you a reference.
2. Write down the name, title, address, and phone number for each reference.

Reference #1

Name: _____

Title: _____

Address: _____

_____

Phone number: _____

Reference #2

Name: _____

Title: _____

Address: _____

_____

Phone number: _____

Reference #3

Name: _____

Title: _____

Address: _____

_____

Phone number: _____

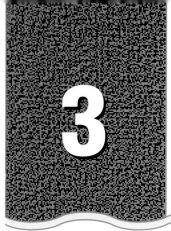

3

Understanding the Law and Ethics of Nursing Care

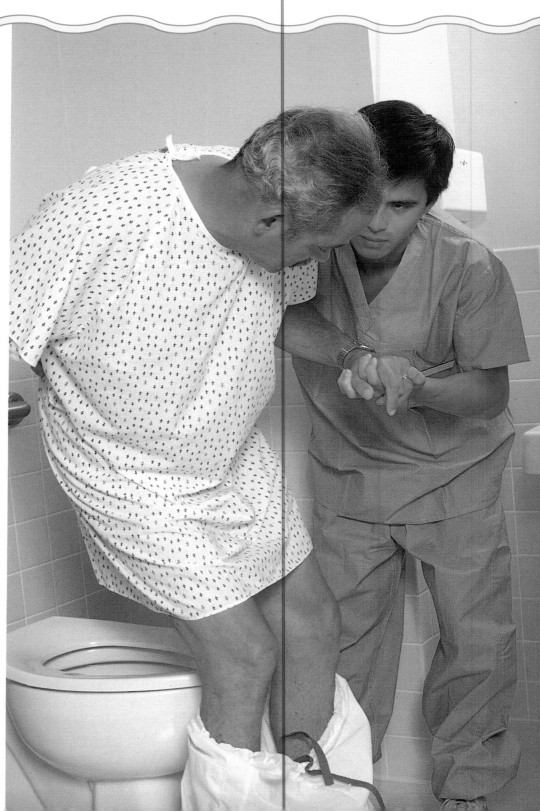

Objectives

AFTER YOU COMPLETE THIS CHAPTER, YOU WILL BE ABLE TO:

Define ethics and legal considerations.

Explain a code of ethics.

Outline the legal responsibilities of the nursing assistant.

Discuss the Patient's Bill of Rights.

Discuss the need for patient confidentiality and privacy.

Identify the desirable characteristics of a nursing assistant.

Overview Patients are entitled to certain rights and expectations. The Patient's Bill of Rights is a document that tells patients about their rights when they are receiving care. The nursing assistant must provide care within the guidelines set by the Patient's Bill of Rights.

WHAT DO YOU KNOW ABOUT LAW AND ETHICS?

Here are nine statements about legal and ethical situations. Consider them to test your current ideas about the law and ethics. If you think the statement is true, circle the T; if you think the statement is false, circle the F. Change the false statements to make them true.

1. **T** F Ethics deals with what is good and bad in terms of duty and behavior.
2. T **F** Only physicians and registered nurses follow a code of ethics.
3. T **F** Civil law protects us from crimes such as murder and robbery.
4. T **F** Slander occurs when you harm a person's reputation by the words you write.
5. **T** F False imprisonment is the act of restraining another person without the person's consent.
6. **T** F Malpractice occurs when you fail to give services for which you were trained.
7. **T** F A patient has the right to refuse treatment and to be informed of the consequences of the refusal.
8. **T** F A nursing assistant is a care giver who responds to patient needs.
9. **T** F Each nursing assistant should be familiar with the job description written by the employer.

ANSWERS

1. **True.** Responsible persons act within a code of ethics.
2. **False.** Physicians and nurses follow a professional code of ethics. In addition, each individual follows a personal code of ethics in relationships with others.
3. **False.** Civil law involves relationships with other people. Criminal law protects us from crimes such as murder and robbery.
4. **False.** Slander occurs when you harm another's reputation by the words you say about the person. Libel occurs when you harm the reputation of another person by the words you write.

5. **True.** Placing a person in protective devices without obtaining the person's consent is an act of false imprisonment.

6. **True.** You are responsible for completing assigned activities in the manner in which you were taught in school.

7. **True.** The right to refuse treatment cannot be denied to any person, unless they are judged mentally incompetent, insane, or a threat to themselves or others.

8. **True.** Responding to patient needs in a caring manner is expected of a nursing assistant.

9. **True.** The job description is the employer's written statement of the functions expected of the nursing assistant who is hired.

LAWS AND LEGAL CONSIDERATIONS

LAWS

rules or regulations; the binding customs or practices of a community; rules of conduct that are formally recognized

CONDUCT

to act or behave in a particular way

Laws are rules of **conduct** that guide people to live as good citizens. Laws allow people to live together in peace, harmony, and safety. When you fail to obey the law you may be fined or sent to prison. Government bodies on the national, state, and local levels make and pass laws to protect all citizens. Each person is responsible for acting within the law; thus individuals are liable for their own actions. In your role as a nursing assistant, you are responsible for your actions. Following the guidelines in the chart will help you obey the laws that should be upheld when you care for patients.

GUIDELINES FOR OBEYING LAWS

- Work under the supervision of the registered nurse or licensed practical or vocational nurse (Figure 3–1)
- Display an attitude of caring and concern for others

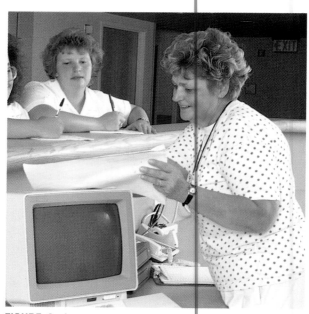

FIGURE 3–1

Getting instructions from the nurse before you begin care is essential.

- Perform only the tasks for which you have been trained
- Accept **responsibility** for your own actions
- Clarify with your supervisor any information you do not understand about the patient care for which you are responsible
- Follow the guidelines listed in your job description
- Attend classes scheduled for your continuing education so that you are up to date on your skills
- Practice the Golden Rule—treat others as you would like them to treat you

RESPONSIBILITY
reliability; trustworthiness

THE TWO TYPES OF LAW: CRIMINAL AND CIVIL

When a law is disobeyed, a crime is committed. A **crime** is a wrong committed against a person or a person's property. A crime may result in a prison term, a fine, or a short jail sentence to punish the wrongdoer. The patient–care giver relationship is governed by **civil law.** Civil law involves relationships between people. Your relationship with your patient is protected by civil law. A patient may seek to right a personal wrong in court. Other crimes are considered under criminal law. Criminal law is broken when a person commits murder or robbery.

CRIME
a wrong committed against a person or a person's property; the wrong may be a crime under criminal law or civil law

CIVIL LAW
the law governing relationships between people

Breaking Criminal Law

THEFT   Theft is the act of stealing. Taking another person's property is stealing. It does not matter whether the stolen item is large or small or of great or little value. Taking an apple from a patient's fruit basket when the patient did not give permission is stealing. Telling an accomplice (partner) that a patient will be leaving the room and there is money in the drawer is called "aiding and abetting." You would be an accomplice to the crime of robbery. A person accused of theft or of being an accomplice to the crime is prosecuted under criminal law and subject to imprisonment (Figure 3–2).

Breaking Civil Law

A crime in which a civil law is broken is called a **tort.** A tort may result in a civil trial in which compensation for damages to the injured party may be awarded. A tort can be intentional or unintentional.

TORT
a crime that breaks a civil law

INTENTIONAL TORTS

Intentional torts include defamation, assault, battery, false imprisonment, and discrimination. These are intentional actions that harm a person or a person's reputation.

DEFAMATION   **Defamation** occurs when you harm a person's reputation by words you write (libel) or say (slander) about the person. Saying that a co-worker took a patient's money when this is untrue is defamation by slander. Writing a letter that accuses another person of breaking into a locker at work when this is untrue is defamation by libel. Be certain that what you write and say about others is honest and accurate.

ASSAULT AND BATTERY   **Assault** is the intentional *attempt or threat* to touch another person's body without that person's consent. Reaching out to move a patient after the patient has said "Don't touch me" is assault.

    Battery is the *act* of touching another person's body without consent. Battery occurs if you touch the body of a person who has already told you not to.

DEFAMATION
harming the reputation of another by words you write (libel) and say (slander) about another individual

ASSAULT
the intentional attempt to touch or threat to touch another person's body without that person's consent

BATTERY
the act of touching another person's body without consent

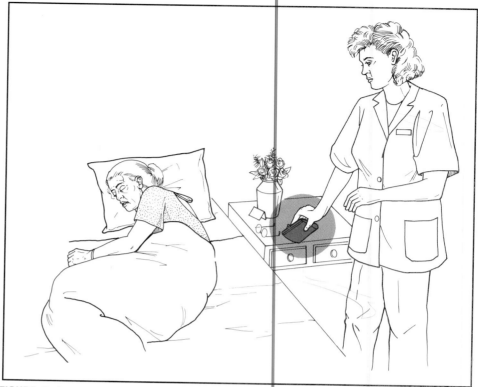

FIGURE 3-2

Stealing anything that belongs to a patient is a crime and reason for immediate dismissal from your job.

Always tell patients what you are going to do and ask whether they understand the procedure or treatment. N*ever* proceed with any procedure or treatment when the patient has refused. Report any situation of patient refusal to the supervisor or nurse, who will take responsibility for the next action.

Patients in the health care setting permit care givers to give care within the scope of their training. This is called **informed consent.** Patients should be informed of and agree to any procedure or treatment planned for them. Patients can withdraw their consent for care or treatment at any time. For example, a patient may withdraw consent by refusing to participate in a treatment. When this happens, do not attempt to do the treatment or threaten to force the treatment on the patient. If you do so, you may be guilty of assault or assault and battery.

FALSE IMPRISONMENT False imprisonment is the act of restraining another person without that person's consent. Patients have the right to leave a health care institution if they wish (unless they are restrained by court order). They do not need the permission of another person. Patients also have the right to move about freely. False imprisonment occurs if you restrain patients so that they cannot get out of bed or a chair. A physician may order protective or safety devices (previously called "restraints") for patients who are in danger of causing harm to themselves or others. The physician must specify the kind of protective device and when it should be used. Never make the decision to apply protective devices, because it is not within the scope of your training. Follow the guidelines in Chapter 12 for the care of patients in protective devices.

DISCRIMINATION Discrimination is the act of treating people differently because

INFORMED CONSENT

when a person is informed of (told about) a procedure or treatment and agrees (gives consent) to having the procedure or treatment done

of their skin color, religious beliefs, culture, age, or sex. The act of discrimination violates civil law. Not answering a patient's call signal because the patient's skin is not the same color as yours is discrimination. Not allowing a person to listen to a favorite television evangelist because the patient's religion is different from yours is discrimination. Be certain to treat all patients alike and not judge other people on the basis of color, creed, culture, age, or sex.

UNINTENTIONAL TORTS

Unintentional torts result in harm to the person even though harm was not intended. Negligence and malpractice are unintentional torts. Figures 3–3 to 3–6 portray examples of negligence and malpractice. Can you identify which ones represent neglect and which ones represent malpractice?

NEGLIGENCE **Negligence** is unintentional harm caused to a person or a person's property by your actions. You can unintentionally injure a patient by not performing care as you were taught. If your patient is in bed receiving a bed bath, you usually place the bed in a higher position so it is easier for you to reach. If you need to leave the room for supplies and leave the bed in the high position and the side rails in the down position, the patient may be harmed by falling even though you had no intention of causing injury to the patient.

MALPRACTICE When you fail to give a service for which you were trained, **malpractice** can result. You might be assigned to a patient who is scheduled to be turned and positioned every 2 hours. The patient may develop skin breakdown (decubitus ulcers) if you do not turn and position the patient when you should have. A person who stays in one position for long periods of time can suffer many complications associated with the decrease of blood circulation to

NEGLIGENCE

an unintentional act that results when your actions harm a person or his or her property

MALPRACTICE

failure to give a service for which one is trained

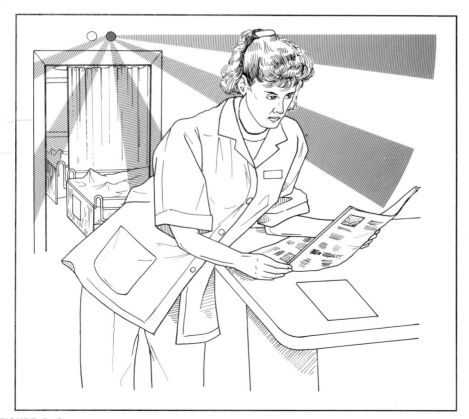

FIGURE 3–3
An example of negligence is not answering a patient's call signal.

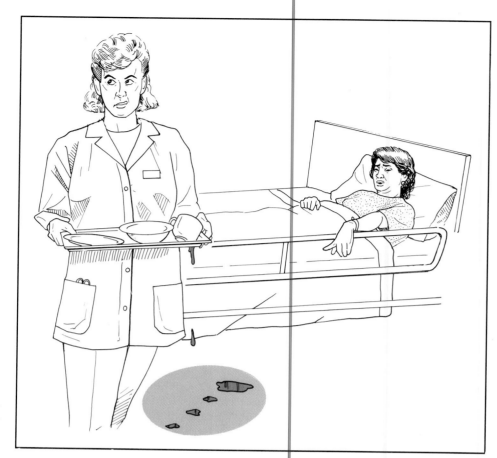

FIGURE 3-4

An example of negligence is failing to wipe up a spill or call the attention of a member of the housekeeping staff to it.

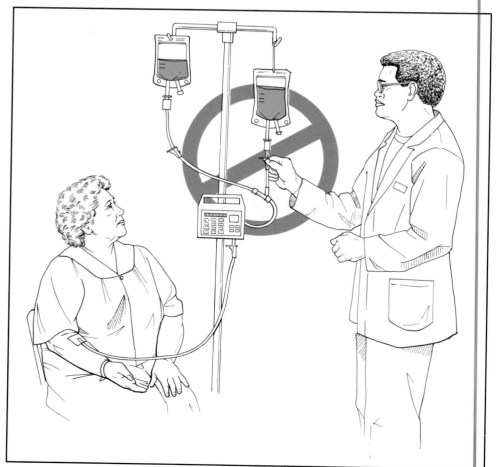

FIGURE 3-5

An example of malpractice is regulating an IV, which a nursing assistant is not permitted to do.

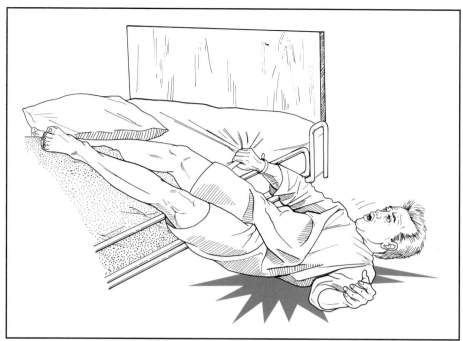

FIGURE 3-6
An example of malpractice is leaving the side rails down when you are trained to raise them for a patient's safety.

certain body parts. The patient has the **right** to expect that you will give care within the scope of your training.

LIABILITY

When you give patient care, you are liable for your actions. To be liable is to be legally responsible. You are responsible and accountable for your actions within the patient–care giver interaction. The **Patient's Bill of Rights** was created to help ensure that each patient receives effective care and satisfaction (Figure 3–7). Certain of these rights are directly related to the care you give as a nursing assistant.

CONSIDERATE AND RESPECTFUL CARE

Patients have the right to expect considerate and respectful care from you. As a nursing assistant, you should show consideration and respect for your patients. Consider patients' needs when you provide care. When patients who feed themselves soil their gown, the need for a clean garment is demonstrated. You show consideration by cleaning the patients and changing their gowns as part of your care.

Treat people with respect by addressing them by the proper title (for example, Mrs., Ms., or Mr.) and their last name. Patients who prefer to be on a first-name basis will tell you to call them by their first name.

The patients have the right not to be **abused. Patient abuse** may be

Verbal
Physical
Psychologic

RIGHT
something to which a person has a just claim

LIABILITY
the state of being liable (responsible by law)

PATIENT'S BILL OF RIGHTS
a statement written of the rights patients are entitled to when receiving health care

PATIENT ABUSE
verbal, emotional, or physical mistreatment of a patient

A PATIENT'S BILL OF RIGHTS

Management Advisory

Patient and Community Relations

Introduction

Effective health care requires collaboration between patients and physicians and other health care professionals. Open and honest communication, respect for personal and professional values, and sensitivity to differences are integral to optimal patient care. As the setting for the provision of health services, hospitals must provide a foundation for understanding and respecting the rights and responsibilities of patients, their families, physicians, and other caregivers. Hospitals must ensure a health care ethic that respects the role of patients in decision making about treatment choices and other aspects of their care. Hospitals must be sensitive to cultural, racial, linguistic, religious, age, gender, and other differences as well as the needs of persons with disabilities.

The American Hospital Association presents A *Patient's Bill of Rights* with the expectation that it will contribute to more effective patient care and be supported by the hospital on behalf of the institution, its medical staff, employees, and patients. The American Hospital Association encourages health care institutions to tailor this bill of rights to their patient community by translating and/or simplifying the language of this bill of rights as may be necessary to ensure that patients and their families understand their rights and responsibilities.

Bill of Rights*

1. The patient has the right to considerate and respectful care.

2. The patient has the right to and is encouraged to obtain from physicians and other direct caregivers relevant, current, and understandable information concerning diagnosis, treatment, and prognosis.

   Except in emergencies when the patient lacks decision-making capacity and the need for treatment is urgent, the patient is entitled to the opportunity to discuss and request information related to the specific procedures and/or treatments, the risks involved, the possible length of recuperation, and the medically reasonable alternatives and their accompanying risks and benefits.

   Patients have the right to know the identity of physicians, nurses, and others involved in their care, as well as when those involved are students, residents, or other trainees. The patient also has the right to know the immediate and long-term financial implications of treatment choices, insofar as they are known.

3. The patient has the right to make decisions about the plan of care prior to and during the course of treatment and to refuse a recommended treatment or plan of care to the extent permitted by law and hospital policy and to be informed of the medical consequences of

this action. In case of such refusal, the patient is entitled to other appropriate care and services that the hospital provides or transfer to another hospital. The hospital should notify patients of any policy that might affect patient choice within the institution.

4. The patient has the right to have an advance directive (such as a living will, health care proxy, or durable power of attorney for health care) concerning treatment or designating a surrogate decision maker with the expectation that the hospital will honor the intent of that directive to the extent permitted by law and hospital policy.

   Health care institutions must advise patients of their rights under state law and hospital policy to make informed medical choices, ask if the patient has an advance directive, and include that information in patient records. The patient has the right to timely information about hospital policy that may limit its ability to implement fully a legally valid advance directive.

5. The patient has the right to every consideration of privacy. Case discussion, consultation, examination, and treatment should be conducted so as to protect each patient's privacy.

These rights can be exercised on the patient's behalf by a designated surrogate or proxy decision maker if the patient lacks decision-making capacity, is legally incompetent, or is a minor.

FIGURE 3–7

Patient's Bill of Rights. (Reprinted with permission of the American Hospital Association, copyright 1992.)

6. The patient has the right to expect that all communications and records pertaining to his/her care will be treated as confidential by the hospital, except in cases such as suspected abuse and public health hazards when reporting is permitted or required by law. The patient has the right to expect that the hospital will emphasize the confidentiality of this information when it releases it to any other parties entitled to review information in these records.

7. The patient has the right to review the records pertaining to his/her medical care and to have the information explained or interpreted as necessary, except when restricted by law.

8. The patient has the right to expect that, within its capacity and policies, a hospital will make reasonable response to the request of a patient for appropriate and medically indicated care and services. The hospital must provide evauation, service, and/or referral as indicated by the urgency of the case. When medically appropriate and legally permissible, or when a patient has so requested, a patient may be transferred to another facility. The institution to which the patient is to be transferred must first have accepted the patient for transfer. The patient must also have the benefit of complete information and explanation concerning the need for, risks, benefits, and alternatives to such a transfer.

9. The patient has the right to ask and be informed of the existence of business relationships among the hospital, educational institutions, other health care providers, or payers that may influence the patient's treatment and care.

10. The patient has the right to consent to or decline to participate in proposed research studies or human experimentation affecting care and treatment or requiring direct patient involvement, and to have those studies fully explained prior to consent. A patient who declines to participate in research or experimentation is entitled to the most effective care that the hospital can otherwise provide.

11. The patient has the right to expect reasonable continuity of care when appropriate and to be informed by physicians and other caregivers of available and realistic patient care options when hospital care is no longer appropriate.

12. The patient has the right to be informed of hospital policies and practices that relate to patient care, treatment, and responsibilities. The patient has the right to be informed of available resources for resolving disputes, grievances, and conflicts, such as ethics committees, patient representatives, or other mechanisms available in the institution. The patient has the right to be informed of the hospital's charges for services and available payment methods.

The collaborative nature of health care requires that patients, or their families/surrogates, participate in their care. The effectiveness of care and patient satisfaction with the course of treatment depend, in part, on the patient fulfilling certain responsibilities. Patients are responsible for providing information about past illnesses, hospitalizations, medications, and other matters related to health status. To participate effectively in decision making, patients must be encouraged to take responsibility for requesting additional information or clarification about their health status or treatment when they do not fully understand information and instructions. Patients are also responsible for ensuring that the health care institution has a copy of their written advance directive if they have one. Patients are responsible for informing their physicians and other caregivers if they anticipate problems in following prescribed treatment.

Patients should also be aware of the hospital's obligation to be reasonably efficient and equitable in providing care to other patients and the community. The hospital's rules and regulations are designed to help the hospital meet this obligation. Patients and their families are responsible for making reasonable accommodations to the needs of the hospital, other patients, medical staff, and hospital employees. Patients are responsible for providing necessary information for insurance claims and for working with the hospital to make payment arrangements, when necessary.

A person's health depends on much more than health care services. Patients are responsible for recognizing the impact of their lifestyle on their personal health.

Conclusion

Hospitals have many functions to perform, including the enhancement of health status, health promotion, and the prevention and treatment of injury and disease; the immediate and ongoing care and rehabilitation of patients; the education of health professionals, patients, and the community; and research. All these activities must be conducted with an overriding concern for the values and dignity of patients.

FIGURE 3-7 *Continued*

ABUSE

Verbal Abuse

VERBAL ABUSE

any use of words that are not considerate and respectful of the patient's rights

Verbal abuse is any use of words that are not considerate and respectful of the patient's rights. Verbal abuse occurs when a care giver screams or shouts at a patient. Using inappropriate words (swearing) or inappropriate language (baby talk to an adult) and teasing or making jokes about the patient are forms of verbal abuse.

Physical Abuse

PHYSICAL ABUSE

mistreatment that causes harm to the body

Physical abuse occurs when the patient is physically harmed. The harm may or may not be intended. Hitting or pinching a patient constitutes physical abuse. Not following through on assigned procedures and treatments may result in bodily harm. For example, neglecting to do range of motion exercises for the patient may result in stiff, painful joints of the arms and legs. The patient may lose the ability to use an arm or a leg as a result. Each of these is a form of physical abuse because the result is harmful to the patient.

Psychologic Abuse

PSYCHOLOGIC ABUSE

mistreatment that causes a person to feel threatened

Psychologic abuse occurs when the patient feels threatened by your actions. Never threaten a patient in an attempt to gain cooperation for a procedure. Never threaten harm to a patient. Never tease, make fun of, or belittle a patient. Patients who are ill may not be able to cope in their usual way and might feel psychologically weak and threatened.

Reporting Abuse

ADVOCATE

to speak or act for persons who are unable to speak or act for themselves

Just as you should never abuse a patient in any way you should not allow patient abuse by another care giver to go unnoticed. The care giver's role includes that of patient advocate. The **advocate** speaks for patients who cannot speak for themselves and are therefore unable to report abuse. If you see another care giver abuse a patient, report clearly the situation you observed to the supervisor or the nurse. In most health care institutions, a care giver who abuses patients is usually discharged from duties (fired) immediately.

INFORMED CONSENT

Patients have the right to informed consent. When admitted to a health care institution, a person is asked to sign a series of papers. The admitting personnel explain each document to the person or the person's guardian (a parent or someone appointed by a court). After the explanation, the person's signature is requested. This is a "blanket" type of informed consent because the patient (or the patient's representative) agrees to the usual procedures and treatments that are recognized as part of patient care and treatment. This informed consent also implies (means) that you are allowed to touch the patient when you perform procedures.

This blanket informed consent obtained at admission does not include permission for any surgical or experimental procedure that may be needed (see Chapter 25). A separate consent form is signed later when the surgical procedure or experiment is explained to the patient. At the same time, the physician or nurse explains the complications that may occur as a result of the procedure as listed on the consent form. Surgical procedures or experiments cannot be started until the patient signs the specific written consent form.

THE RIGHT TO REFUSE CARE

Patients have the right to refuse care and treatment from any member of the health care team. They also have the right to be informed of what could happen to them as a result of refusing care. The physician is obligated to explain what can happen as a result of the refusal. Some patients may choose to refuse care or treatment even when they are aware of the consequences (Figure 3–8).

As a care giver, it may be difficult for you to accept a patient's decision to refuse care or treatment. Because you care, your own expectation is that patients should receive all help available to save their life. When a patient refuses treatment, the best course of action is to be supportive of the patient and family. You can be supportive by listening, making the patient comfortable, and providing for the patient's daily needs such as bathing, dressing, and eating. The simple act of listening is valuable in case the patient or family wishes to talk about their choices. Report to the nurse the feelings the patient is expressing about the choice to refuse care or treatment. You can make the patient as comfortable as possible by giving back rubs, helping with position changes, and keeping the patient warm. When the patient needs a bath, help with dressing and toileting, or assistance with eating, you can help the patient or complete the task.

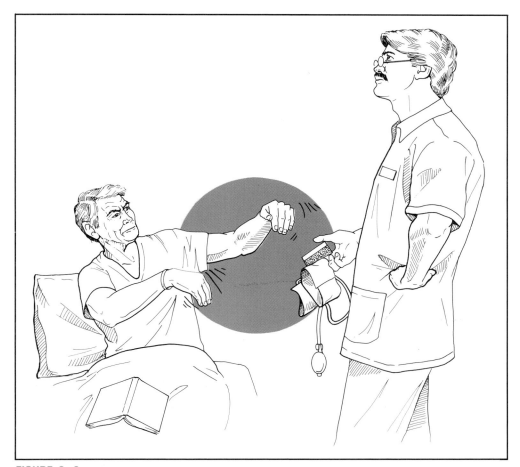

FIGURE 3–8
The patient has the right to refuse care.

CARING COMMENT

Your feelings about a patient's decision either to refuse or to accept treatment can affect how you respond to that patient or the family. You should be supportive of the decision and not pass judgment on the patient's choice of health care.

RESPECT FOR PRIVACY

Patients have the right to expect that their privacy will be protected. The person admitted to a health care institution becomes a "patient." Patients lose control over the activities of daily living. As a result, many daily activities they previously performed according to their own time schedule are changed or not done at all. Very ill patients may need help with hygiene or toileting needs. You should make every effort to provide privacy during any procedure you do for these patients (Figure 3–9). Always close the curtains around the bed, close the window drapes, and close the door. Keep the patient covered so that body parts are not exposed. If a patient is unable to keep a blanket or sheet in place, put pajama bottoms on the patient. Robes may be available if the patient needs to get out of bed. If the patient is seated in a chair or wheelchair, fold a blanket or sheet and place it across the knees to provide a cover and warmth.

CONFIDENTIALITY

CONFIDENTIALITY
the act of keeping information private

Patients have the right to expect that all communications and records about their care will be treated as confidential. All information (verbal and written) about patients is confidential. **Confidentiality** means that you keep the information to yourself. As a nursing assistant, you will be given certain information

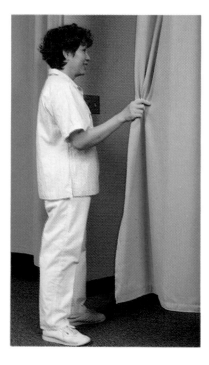

FIGURE 3–9
Always pull the curtain when the patient has the need for privacy.

to help you in your care of patients. The guidelines in the chart below will help you keep the things you hear about patients and their care to yourself.

GUIDELINES FOR CONFIDENTIALITY

- Never repeat information given to you in your role as a nursing assistant.
- Restrict your sharing of information to the reports of observations you give to the nurse.
- If anyone (a family member or visitor) asks about the patient, refer all such questions to the supervisor or nurse.
- Never discuss the patient or anything about the patient in the public places of the institution, such as the hallway, elevator, or cafeteria.
- Never bring such information into discussions outside the health care institution.
- The best action is to keep silent about any information you see or hear.

CARING COMMENT

You may overhear discussions about patients, their illnesses and reactions to them, and care givers' feelings about patients. Remember that anything you hear or read about a patient is confidential information.

RESPONSE TO SERVICES

Patients have the right to expect a reasonable response when they ask a care giver for services. You represent the health care institution when the patient has certain needs. You are responsible for responding to services for which you are trained. Giving a bath, helping with toileting and grooming, lifting and transferring patients, answering call bells or lights, and many other ways of responding to patient needs are expected from nursing assistants. For example, you might assist patients to the bathroom and help them sit on the toilet (Figure 3–10). When patients ring the call signal, they have the right to expect that you will respond to help them clean up and go back to bed. You are responsible for telling the supervisor or nurse when

- You have not been taught a procedure
- You feel you need more training

CARING COMMENT

Your supervisors at the health care institution expect you to tell them if you have not been taught something. Be courteous when you are asked to explain what you have been taught. Follow through *only* on the activities you have learned in your nursing assistant program or in an orientation or continuing education program.

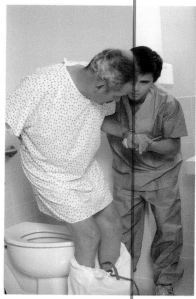

FIGURE 3–10
Assisting a patient to the bathroom is an important responsibility of the care giver.

ETHICS
rules that govern right conduct (see code of ethics)

ETHICAL
acting or behaving within the rules of good and moral conduct

CODE OF ETHICS
a system of principles and rules that a group or person follows as a guide for what is good and bad and morally obligated

ETHICS

Ethics are rules that govern right conduct. A code of ethics provides a guide for what is good and bad and morally obligated. Health care givers as well as other professionals practice under a code of ethics. **Ethical** behavior means that a person behaves according to a code of ethics. A **code of ethics** is developed and accepted by members of a profession. The code is published, and all members of the profession should behave within the principles and rules of their code. The code is also available for public review.

CARING COMMENT

A patient's well-being relies on the care giver's responsibility for accuracy and honesty in giving care.

VALUES

VALUE
something or someone of worth or importance

A **value** is something or someone of worth or importance. Individuals develop values as they use moral law to direct their behavior in everyday life. For example, the person who values relationships with others will do whatever is necessary to keep lines of communication open. People's actions reflect what they value. Individuals develop their own value system and use it to make decisions and act. Each person's value system is unique. Your values about such issues as health, education, or relationships may differ from a patient's. It is important that you learn to understand and accept the right of others to have value systems different from your own. As a professional, you must not let your personal opinion influence the quality of care you provide.

THE NURSING ASSISTANT

CHARACTERISTICS OF NURSING ASSISTANTS

Nursing assistants are **caring** individuals who have a genuine desire to help other people. They are sensitive to other people's needs and treat all persons with respect. They perform their duties and procedures thoroughly and as learned during training. They behave in a truthful and reliable manner.

Many characteristics are valued in the individuals who decide to become nursing assistants. The characteristics are important in the care of patients of all ages. They are important and necessary to work in a people-oriented profession like health care. Characteristics include

Caring
Desire to help others
Sensitivity and gentleness
Empathy
Respect
Honesty

Caring

Caring has been associated with the profession of nursing for as long as people have been ill. It is a respect for people and a regard for their well-being and needs. It is a response to another individual whether that individual is healthy or ill.

Desire to Help Others

The desire to help others, whether they are healthy or ill, results from a deep caring **attitude** about others' welfare. Helping others results in a feeling of satisfaction in one's actions. The feeling of satisfaction comes from your ability to help other people meet their physical and emotional needs.

Sensitivity and Gentleness

Sensitivity is an awareness of others' physical and emotional needs. A gentle nature is appreciated by others and is reflected in the way care givers respond to the needs of others. A gentle nature and a kind touch are a comfort to the patients in your care (Figure 3–11).

Empathy

The care giver who "feels," that is, tries to imagine and understand what the patient is feeling, is an empathetic person. Remember that **empathy** is not the same as sympathy. **Sympathy** is showing pity for another person. Most people are uncomfortable knowing someone pities them.

Respect

Respect is an important quality in the care giver. Care given with respect for the patient's rights can help the patient's self-esteem.

Honesty

The person who is honest is truthful and trustworthy. Always report and record your observations truthfully. If you find an item in a patient's room that is not

CARING
an attitude of interest in and concern about helping others

ATTITUDE
a pattern of mental views based on previous experience that was gathered over time

SENSITIVITY
awareness of others' physical and emotional needs

EMPATHY
understanding or being aware of another person's feelings, thoughts, or experiences
SYMPATHY
feeling pity for another person

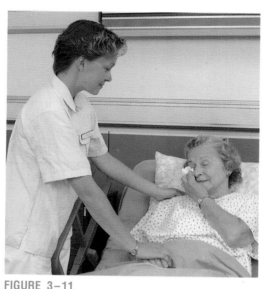

FIGURE 3-11
Touch is one way to communicate that you care about your patient.

claimed by a patient, follow your institution's procedure for lost and found objects. When an item is missing from a patient's belongings, report this information to the nurse or supervisor.

CARING COMMENT

The persons in a health care institution include patients, visitors, and staff. The opportunity for stealing may arise. If you see a theft occur or are a victim of theft, it is important that you report the incident to the nurse or supervisor. The nurse or supervisor will follow the course of action as stated in the policy of the health care institution.

CHAPTER WRAP-UP

- Laws are passed and enforced to protect all citizens.
- Civil law involves relationships between people.
- A crime in which a civil law is broken is called a tort.
- Torts can be intentional or unintentional.
- Intentional torts include defamation, assault, battery, and false imprisonment.
- Negligence and malpractice are unintentional torts.
- The Patient's Bill of Rights is a statement of the rights patients have when they receive care from you and other employees of the health care institution.
- A code of ethics is a series of statements about what is good and morally obligated for you to follow when you give care.
- A code of ethics helps the care giver to select choices that are ethically and morally acceptable.
- Keep legal considerations and ethical behavior in mind when you care for patients. Function according to the principles you learned as a student nursing assistant.

- You are responsible and accountable for your own actions.
- Always give care under the supervision of a registered nurse or a licensed practical or vocational nurse.

REVIEW QUESTIONS

1. What is a tort? Give one example of each intentional tort and one example of each unintentional tort.
2. What is the Patient's Bill of Rights? Why is it important?
3. What personal qualities do you bring to the helping profession?

ACTIVITY CORNER

When you read your newspaper or listen to the news on television or radio, watch for these terms and fill in examples from everyday life:

Abuse _____

Assault _____

Battery _____

Assault and battery _____

Malpractice _____

Ask yourself if people think they are breaking the law when they commit these acts.

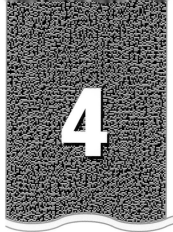

4

Understanding the Nursing Process

Objectives

AFTER YOU COMPLETE THIS
CHAPTER, YOU WILL BE ABLE TO:

Explain the problem-solving
    technique.
Describe the nursing process.
Identify the nursing assistant's
    role in the nursing process.
List observations that a nursing
    assistant can make.
Use the problem-solving
    technique to make decisions
    in your professional and
    personal life.

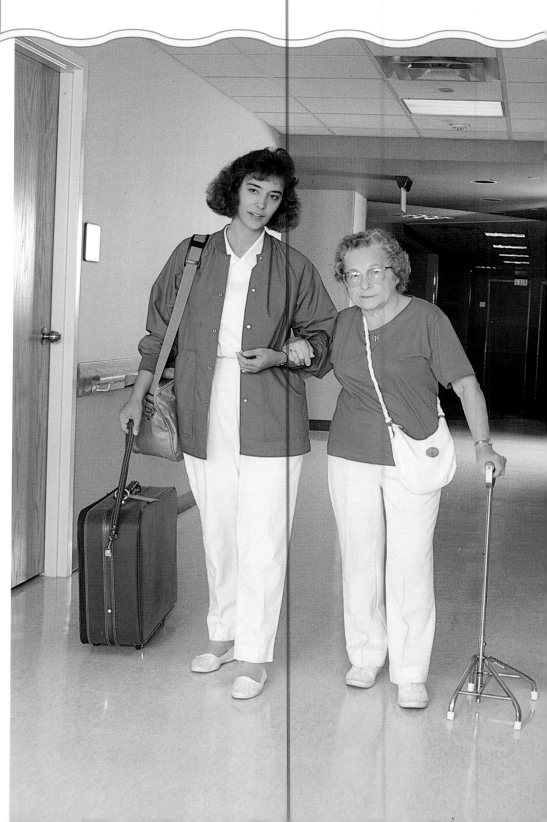

Overview As a nursing assistant, you perform your job responsibilities under the supervision of a registered nurse. You work closely with the nurse to follow a specific course of action.

You can successfully help with patient care by learning how to make important observations about your patients, how to solve problems, and how to help the nurse evaluate and improve patient care.

WHAT DO YOU KNOW ABOUT THE NURSING PROCESS?

Here are eight statements about the nursing process. Consider them to test your current ideas about the nursing process and your role as a nursing assistant. If you think the statement is true, circle the T; if you think the statement is false, circle the F. Change the false statements to make them true.

1. T F The nursing process is a problem-solving technique.

2. T F Nurses plan the patient's care on the basis of a nursing diagnosis.

3. T F The nursing assistant can use the problem-solving technique.

4. T F Nursing interventions (actions) are carried out by registered nurses only.

5. T F Observation is an important part of the problem-solving process.

6. T F Subjective observations are the pieces of information you get through seeing and hearing.

7. T F The problem-solving technique should never be used in the home.

8. T F A statement made by a patient is an objective observation.

ANSWERS

1. **True.** The steps of the nursing process are very similar to the steps of the problem-solving technique.

2. **True.** Planning is the second step of the nursing process. It begins only after information is gathered and analyzed.

3. **True.** The problem-solving technique is a system that can help a person make decisions.

4. **False.** Nursing interventions can be carried out by members of the health care team under the supervision of a registered nurse.

5. **True.** Accurate observation is the basic step of the nursing process and the problem-solving technique. In the nursing process, it is called assessment.

6. **False.** Subjective observations include the patient's or the patient's family members' statements to you.

7. **False.** When you learn to use the problem-solving technique, you will find it extremely helpful in making wise decisions in your personal as well as professional life.

8. **False.** Objective observations are those you can see, hear, touch, taste, and smell.

THE NURSING PROCESS

The **nursing process** is a systematic problem-solving method used by registered nurses to

- Assess the patient and analyze information to identify a nursing diagnosis
- Plan for the patient's care
- Intervene (carry out that care) and direct others' care of the patient
- Evaluate patient care

The word *process* means "a series of actions that lead to an end." An easy way to understand the nursing process is to notice that nurses take a series of steps each time there is a nurse–patient interaction. In this way, nursing care is based on a systematic series of steps that result in good patient care. There are four steps in the nursing process:

1. Assessment (Figure 4–1)
2. Planning (Figure 4–2)
3. Intervention (Figure 4–3)
4. Evaluation (Figure 4–4)

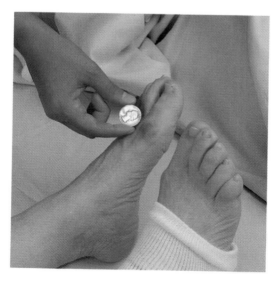

FIGURE 4–1

Steps of the nursing process. Observe skin breakdown.

PATIENT PLAN OF CARE						
DATE	PROBLEM	GOAL	INTERVENTION	SIGN	REVIEW	SIGN
11/1/93	Changes in skin integrity	Patient's skin will stay intact while in long-term care.	Turn and position q 2 h — schedule is posted in room. Check pressure points at q. position change. Give 240 cc of fluids q/h while awake. —Likes water, lemonade, tea.	M. Murray, RN		

FIGURE 4–2
Plan for treatment.

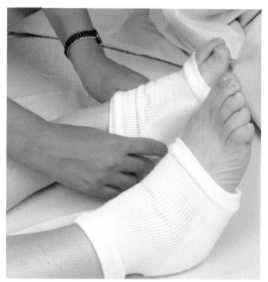

FIGURE 4–3
Apply a special device to reduce pressure on the heel.

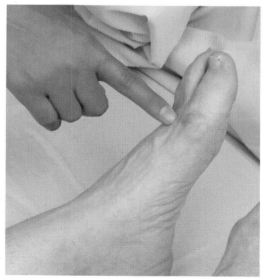

FIGURE 4–4
Evaluate the area of skin breakdown.

CARING COMMENT

Notice that the first letter of each step of the nursing process spells APIE. APIE is an easy way to remember the steps of the nursing process in the correct order.

A̲ssessment
P̲lanning
I̲ntervention
E̲valuation

ASSESSMENT

ASSESSMENT

gathering information through the use of subjective and objective observations

Assessment is the first step of the nursing process. It is an ongoing function in which the nurse looks at and evaluates the patient and the health care environment (e.g., room temperature, amount of light, cleanliness). To gather information during assessment, the nurse uses subjective and objective observations. A more detailed discussion of subjective and objective observations is found in Chapter 6. However, a brief explanation of these two ways of observing follows.

Subjective Observations

SUBJECTIVE OBSERVATION

information gathered through another person's statements, for example, "I am cold"

Subjective observations are statements made by the patient or the patient's family. A statement like "I have pain" is subjective because the patient gives you the information. There is no way to know whether the patient really is experiencing pain. Only patients can describe their own feelings and experiences (Figure 4–5). The patient's statement is a subjective observation.

CARING COMMENT

To get a better idea about what kind of statements are subjective observations, read the following sentences. The ones in italics are subjective observations.

"I'm thirsty for a drink of water."

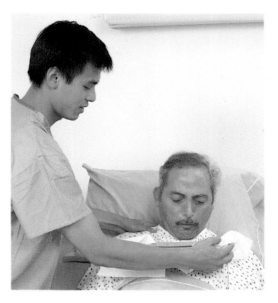

FIGURE 4–5
A patient who told the nursing assistant, "I feel nauseated."

"The patient stopped breathing."
"Blood was pouring from the wound."
"My fingers and toes feel numb."
"It's hard to describe how anxious I am."

Objective Observations

Objective observations are also used by the nurse during assessment. The five senses—sight, hearing, smell, taste, and touch—are used to gather objective observations. After you gather objective information, another person can observe the same person or situation and present information similar to yours (Figure 4–6).

- By using the sense of sight, you can determine whether a person has eaten an entire meal.
- When you serve the meal, your sense of smell is activated and you can smell the food you are serving.
- The patient might ask you for another serving; thus your sense of hearing is stimulated.
- If you move a bowl of hot soup, you activate your sense of touch.
- Your sense of taste is activated when you go on break and bite into an apple.

OBJECTIVE OBSERVATION
information gathered by using the five senses: sight, hearing, smell, taste, and touch (for example, sight: a quarter-sized rash on the left arm)

CARING COMMENT

Keep in mind the difference between what you sense and what the patient tells you. The objective observations in the following statements appear in italics.

"The patient said the soup was too hot."
"The patient will not move his right arm."
"The drainage from the open wound is green."
"I feel dizzy when I sit up."
"The patient fell in the bathroom."

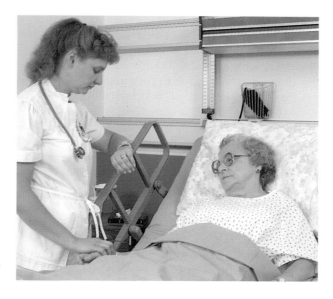

FIGURE 4–6
Counting a pulse (heart beat) is an objective observation.

NURSING DIAGNOSIS
a description of actual or potential health changes that a nurse is legally allowed and professionally prepared to treat

MEDICAL DIAGNOSIS
the physician's decision about what illness a patient has; the diagnosis is based on information gained through a physical examination, an interview with the patient or the patient's family, a medical history of the patient, and results of laboratory and radiologic testing

ARTHRITIS
inflammation of a joint

Nursing Diagnosis

After making subjective and objective observations about a patient, the nurse analyzes all the observations to develop a nursing diagnosis. A **nursing diagnosis** is a description of actual and potential health problems that change a person's life processes or functions and is clearly different from a medical diagnosis. A **medical diagnosis** is made by the physician, on the basis of information gathered through a physical examination of the patient, an interview with the patient or the patient's family, a medical history of the patient, and results of laboratory and radiologic testing. Heart attack and **arthritis** are examples of medical diagnoses.

When a nurse writes that a patient has a "potential for injury related to a history of falls," a nursing diagnosis is being made. The registered nurse is professionally prepared and legally allowed to treat patients on the basis of the nursing diagnosis identified. The nursing diagnosis completes the first step of the nursing process.

CARING COMMENT

The nursing diagnosis is based on both subjective and objective observations. When a nursing diagnosis states that the patient, for example, an elderly man, has the potential to fall, it could be based on the fact that

- The patient's daughter reported that her father fell twice in the last week
- A nursing assistant saw the patient struggling to keep his balance while walking near the handrail
- The patient is taking medication that can make him dizzy

It would *not* be part of the nursing diagnosis to write "The patient's hip pain means he could have arthritis."

PLANNING

PLANNING
a step in the nursing process that is a blueprint for action

GOAL
aim

CARE PLAN
a written tool developed by a registered nurse to communicate and document a plan of care for an individual patient

The second step of the nursing process is planning. **Planning** is the development of a course of action. It is always based on the nursing diagnosis. The registered nurse and the patient plan care to maintain or restore the patient's well-being (Figure 4–7). The registered nurse, members of the care plan team from other disciplines, and the patient may also plan care for the patient in a long-term care or rehabilitation setting. A patient **goal** is identified as part of the plan. Then actions are designed to help the patient reach the goal.

As many actions as needed are planned. The plan is recorded in the patient's records. It is a communication tool used by health care team members (dietician, nurses, nursing assistants, etc.) to give the patient consistent care. The **care plan** for each patient in a facility is also available in a holder called a "Kardex." It is a metal holder that provides quick access to the planned actions for the care of a patient. The care plan may also be found in the patient's chart or in a special binder at the nurses' station. In some institutions, the patient care plan is available to nursing assistants; if this is the case at your institution, you should read each patient's care plan daily to keep current with the patient's status. You can suggest changes in the care plan as the patient's condition changes (improves or worsens).

An example of a goal is, "The patient will lose 5 pounds in the next 2 months." One action that can help the patient reach that goal is to teach the patient about fats and carbohydrates in the diet. Another action might be to

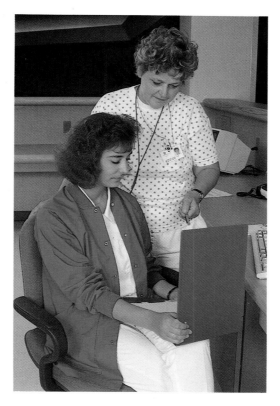

FIGURE 4-7

The Kardex holds a written plan of care for each patient. To keep current, the nursing assistant needs to read the Kardex care plan about an assigned patient every day.

help the patient plan menus that include the five food groups. Helping the patient establish new thinking patterns regarding food may also be helpful. One of the best ways to lose weight is to exercise. Teaching the patient about exercise and its benefits is another action (intervention) the nurse might use.

INTERVENTION

Intervention is the carrying out of the planned action (Figure 4–8). Interventions can be carried out by a variety of care givers. When each care giver

INTERVENTION

carrying out the patient's plan of care

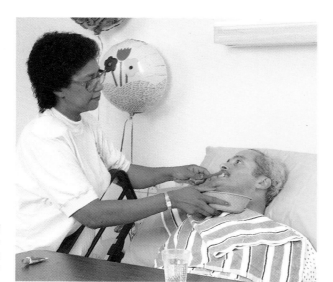

FIGURE 4-8

Helping a patient with care of the mouth and teeth is an intervention that helps prevent breakdown of the mucous membranes of the mouth.

follows the same care plan, the interventions are consistent. Patient confusion results when each person is doing something different, especially if a procedure is complex and time consuming. The nurse shares the care plan with you to direct your actions. Seek out the nurse anytime you are not clear about what action to take.

EVALUATION

EVALUATION

the step in the nursing process in which the total plan of care is assessed and any necessary changes are made

In **evaluation,** the last step in the nursing process, the effectiveness of the care plan is critically assessed. The nurse and the care plan team evaluate whether the patient goal has been met. The following questions can be asked during evaluation:

- Has the patient goal been met within the time frame suggested?
- Was any part of the goal not met? If so, should the plan be continued or revised to help the patient meet the goal?
- Is the plan of action still valid, or can it be discontinued?

The nurse uses as much information as possible to make an accurate evaluation of the patient's goal (Figure 4–9). Nurses are responsible for the evaluation of the patient goal and any revision or addition to the care plan. It is important for you to realize that the registered nurse uses the nursing process as part of the professional practice of nursing.

THE PROBLEM-SOLVING TECHNIQUE

The problem-solving technique is a method similar to the nursing process. It is used to solve problems in a systematic way. Many people use the problem-solving technique without realizing it. You can learn to use the problem-solving technique (Figure 4–10). The steps are as follows:

1. Observe and gather data
2. Review all information
3. Identify the problem
4. Plan a course of action
5. Follow the planned action
6. Evaluate the results

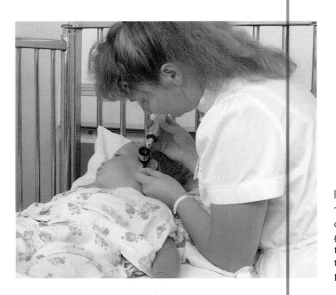

FIGURE 4–9

The registered nurse evaluates a child's response to medication given for an ear infection after the nursing assistant reported that the child had said he had pain in the ear.

Observe and gather data

The nurse says Mrs. Lee cannot move her arms very well and she needs to be fed her lunch. You note Mrs. Lee does not move her right arm at all and can move her left arm only if you help her. Mrs. Lee can respond to questions with a yes or no. She can sit up in bed with no changes in her breathing. She opens her mouth when you ask her to do so.

Review all information

The information indicates Mrs. Lee can cooperate by opening her mouth to receive food but cannot use any utensil to feed herself.

Identify the problem

Mrs. Lee's need for nutrition.

Plan a course of action

Plan to make time for feeding Mrs. Lee in a relaxed, calm environment, to feed her warm foods first, to feed her what she indicates she likes, and to report to the nurse how the feeding progressed.

Follow the planned action

Feed Mrs. Lee her lunch as planned.

Evaluate the results

Did Mrs. Lee eat the food on her tray? How much was eaten (25%, 50%, 75%, or 100%)? Was extra food given that was not on the tray? Did Mrs. Lee express dislike for any food? Report the information to the nurse.

FIGURE 4–10

An example of the problem-solving process.

The first letters of the following sentence spell out the steps of the problem-solving technique:

Oscar Runs In Place For Ever
Observe and gather data
Review all information
Identify the problem
Plan a course of action
Follow the planned action
Evaluate the results

COMPARISON OF THE STEPS OF THE NURSING PROCESS AND THE PROBLEM-SOLVING TECHNIQUE

Nursing Process	Problem-Solving Technique
Assessment	
Observing and analyzing data and identifying nursing diagnoses	Observing and gathering data Reviewing all information Identifying the problem
Plan	
etting the patient goal and the planned action	Planning a course of action
Intervention	
Carrying out the action as planned	Following the planned action
Evaluation	
Assessing the plan for effectiveness; determining whether the patient goal was met	Evaluating the results

The following is an example of how the problem-solving technique might work for you on the job.

EXAMPLE

At work you observe a patient trying to climb over the side rails of a bed. Other information you gather is that the patient is 65 years old and is sleepy because she has just returned from the operating room. A review of your observations tells you the patient is in danger of falling. You have just identified the problem—the danger of falling out of bed. The patient can be injured if she falls out of bed.

Your planned action is as follows:

1. Ease the patient back into bed, make her comfortable, and show her how to use the call signal.
2. Stay with her until she relaxes.
3. Make sure the bed is in the lowest position and all side rails are raised.
4. Follow the plan you have thought out. When the patient is safely positioned in her bed, evaluate the results and report your actions to the nurse.

THE NURSING ASSISTANT AND OBSERVATIONS

The keen observations you make become important information for the nurse to use to plan patient care. Subjective observations are statements the patient

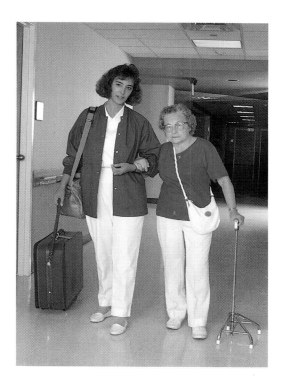

FIGURE 4-11

Begin to observe the patient as soon as the patient is admitted to the unit. The patient may be able to walk when admitted to a long-term care institution. The patient may be in a wheelchair or on a stretcher when admitted to a hospital.

makes directly to you. Not all patient statements are important. Statements about a television program or the weather do not affect the patient's care. Be alert for statements that describe feelings or changes patients notice in their body functions. You should report them to the nurse using the patients' own words as closely as you can. The nurse then plans care on the basis of the observations you have reported.

Admission and daily observations may be part of your nursing assistant responsibilities (Figure 4-11). The nurse tells you what observations you are responsible for making.

CARING COMMENT

Learn to observe for the usual and expected as well as any unusual observations that might signal that a patient has a problem. Any time you observe something out of the ordinary, report the observation to the nurse, who takes the responsibility for making a decision.

CHAPTER WRAP-UP

- The nursing process is a problem-solving technique used by registered nurses.
- The four steps of the nursing process are
  Assessment
  Planning
  Intervention
  Evaluation

- You are expected to make observations and report them accurately to the nurse.
- The many observations you report are useful when nursing care activities and interventions are being planned.
- The problem-solving technique is a method of solving problems that you can use to make your patient care safe and effective.
- The steps of the problem-solving process are as follows:
    Observe and gather data
    Review all information
    Identify the problem
    Plan a course of action
    Follow the planned action
    Evaluate the results
- When you use the problem-solving technique, you make decisions by gathering information and thinking it through first.

REVIEW QUESTIONS

1. What are the steps of the nursing process?
2. Give examples of observations a nursing assistant might make.
3. What does a nursing diagnosis describe?
4. Describe the problem-solving technique. Give one example of how the problem-solving technique can help you make a wise decision.

ACTIVITY CORNER

The problem-solving technique can be used when you

- Oversleep and make yourself late for important appointments, work, or school
- Feel you do not have enough time to study

Check each step as you use the problem-solving technique.

Oversleeping

1. Observe the time you awoke. _____
2. Review how much time you overslept. _____
3. Identify oversleeping as the problem. _____
4. Decide how you can avoid oversleeping. Actions might include going to bed earlier or getting a reliable alarm clock. _____
5. Follow through. _____
6. Evaluate. Did you avoid oversleeping? _____

Lack of study time

1. Gather data on extra time you have when activities such as cooking, doing laundry, and grocery shopping are done. _____
2. Review information for unscheduled times. _____
3. Identify the problem as lack of study time. _____
4. Plan time in your schedule for studying. _____
5. Follow through and study at the scheduled times. _____
6. Evaluate. Do you have enough time to study? _____

Name a personal problem situation in which you might use the problem-solving process.

_____

_____

Plan a solution to your problem.

1. _____

2. _____

3. _____

4. _____

5. _____

6. _____

UNIT TWO

Ways of Communicating

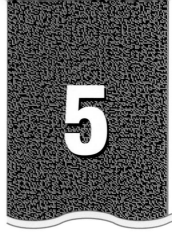

5

Communicating with People

Objectives

AFTER YOU COMPLETE THIS
CHAPTER, YOU WILL BE ABLE TO:

Explain how communication
  occurs.
Describe verbal communication.
Describe nonverbal
  communication.
Give examples of verbal and
  nonverbal communications.
Explain the importance of
  feedback.
Identify ways to communicate
  with patients whose sight or
  hearing is impaired.
Give examples of
  communication helpers.
Give examples of
  communication barriers.

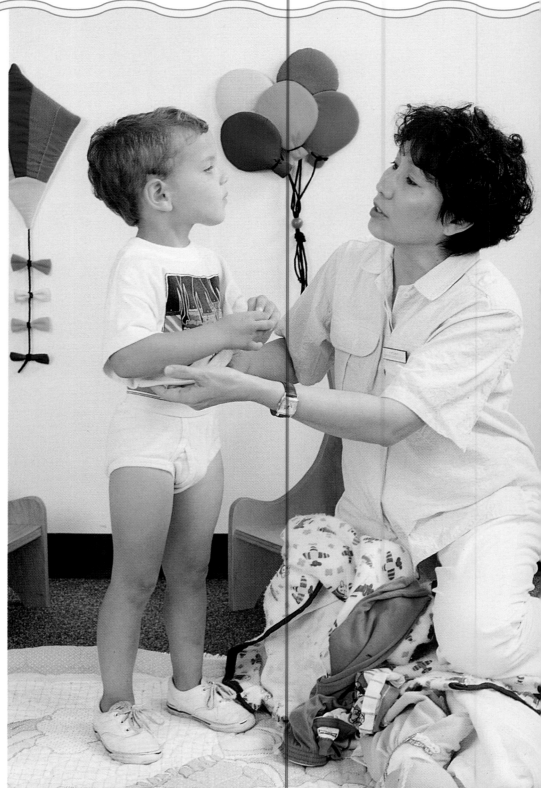

Overview Communication is the exchange of information between two or more people. In the health care setting, good communication is absolutely necessary for quality patient care. Also, by learning good communication skills, you can avoid many unnecessary problems and misunderstandings with your patients and co-workers.

For example, imagine that you dash into the hospital room of an elderly man who has some difficulty hearing. He is sitting in a wheelchair. You explain in a few fast sentences, without looking at him, that you are taking him down to the x-ray department.

The patient, who hasn't understood a word you have said, suddenly finds himself rolling along a strange corridor, into an elevator, and down a gray underground hallway. He doesn't know why. He doesn't know what's about to happen to him. He's afraid.

Later, still upset, he calls his son to complain. His son rushes to the hospital, ready to talk to everyone there, from the parking lot attendant to the head administrator.

When things settle down, you are left with a nurse who is angry with you and a patient and his family who are unnecessarily frightened and enraged. You may also have created a poor image of yourself as a health care provider.

In this imaginary scene, all the trouble could easily have been avoided if you had just taken a few moments to clearly communicate with the patient so he understood what was about to happen.

Patients and their families rely on your communication skills. Other health care team members depend on you to accurately communicate information about patients too. By learning and practicing good communication skills you will be able to fulfill these expectations.

WHAT DO YOU KNOW ABOUT COMMUNICATING?

Here are eight statements about communication. Consider them to test your current ideas about communication. If you think the statement is true, circle the T; if you think the statement is false, circle the F. Change the false statements to make them true.

1. T F Communication is a two-way interaction.

2. T F A statement like "You'll feel fine later" is the correct way to reassure a patient.

3. T F When you remain silent, no communication occurs.

4. T F Communicating is the act of using words.

5. T F A person's words and body language should match.

6. T   F   Body language is more accurate than the spoken word.
7. T   F   People tend to raise their voices when speaking to a blind person.
8. T   F   The hands and the mouth are communication tools.

ANSWERS

1. **True.** Even when you are not speaking with words, your body language speaks for you.
2. **False.** "You'll feel fine later" is a cliché that you say automatically.
3. **False.** Remaining silent is a behavior that tells something through your body language.
4. **False.** Although words are the major form of communication, touch, sign language, and music are also forms of communication.
5. **True.** Because people's body language reflects their true feelings, words should match body language.
6. **True.** We are unaware of our body language. Because the body speaks for us, it reflects our true feelings.
7. **True.** Unfortunately, people assume that a patient who has one handicap automatically has others. This is not necessarily so.
8. **True.** The hands and mouth, along with facial expression and other movements, give expression and animation to our communication efforts.

THE ART OF COMMUNICATING

When we communicate with others we express our problems, interests, worries, hopes, joys, and needs. We also learn more about the people with whom we live and work as well as those in our care. The words, sounds, gestures, facial expressions, and posture we use all express our thoughts and feelings. When you communicate using respect and honesty, others develop a sense of trust and openness in their interactions with you.

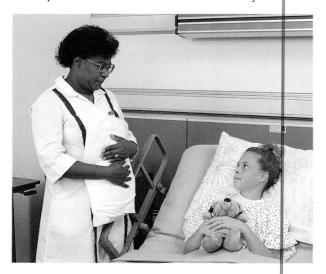

FIGURE 5-1

Effective body language. There is eye contact, each person has a serious facial expression, and bodies are turned toward each other. Notice how the care giver is imitating the patient.

CARING COMMENTS

Your gestures and expressions give the listener as much information as your words. The patient and others receive an accurate picture of your feelings when your body language matches what you say (Figure 5–1).

You will be more successful using your new communication skills when you have a positive, willing attitude.

THE ESSENTIAL PARTS OF COMMUNICATION

Communication is an exchange of information. When information is exchanged between people, an **interaction** occurs. Each interaction is based on three important points:

- **Knowledge base**—The knowledge we acquire while growing and maturing is called a **knowledge base.** We use our knowledge base to create questions, find answers, and make decisions. We bring our personal knowledge base to every interaction we have with another person.
- **Feelings**—The feelings of the people involved in any interaction color the messages and responses they use. Feelings give personal identity to any interaction. Most times, we are not aware of how much our feelings contribute to an interaction.
- **Past experiences**—Past experience helps us learn to handle events realistically. Any experience, whether positive or negative, helps shape our future interactions with others.

In order for communication to occur, the following four essential parts are necessary:

Sender
Message
Receiver
Feedback

These four parts occur in a series of events called the **communication process** (Figure 5–2). The exchange of information occurs when all parts of the communication process are completed. The process is repeated many times in the course of an interaction. The act of communicating involves at least two people, a sender and a receiver.

COMMUNICATION
an exchange of information
INTERACTION
communication between two or more people
KNOWLEDGE BASE
the basis of one's information and understanding

COMMUNICATION PROCESS
a method of communicating that uses a sender of a message and a receiver who responds with feedback

THE SENDER

The sender is the person who begins or continues an interaction by "sending" information to another person. The sender uses the spoken or written word and body language (e.g., nodding the head or making a fist) to give the information.

As an example, imagine two housemates, Sarah and Kate. Sarah comes into the kitchen in the morning and begins to speak. Sarah is the sender.

THE MESSAGE

The information that the sender expresses is the message. It may be a question or a statement. The message is sent through sound (for example, words or music) or body language (Figure 5–3).

Sarah's message is "I'll be home late tonight."

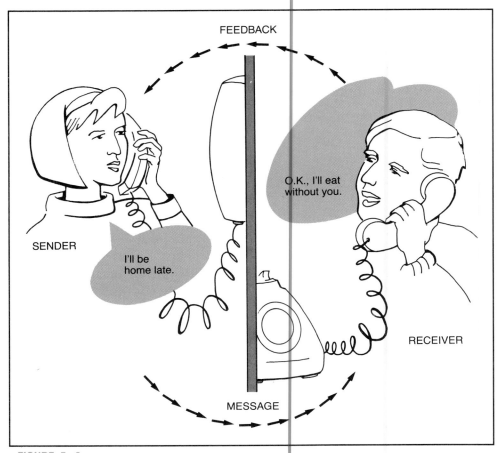

FIGURE 5-2
The communication process.

THE RECEIVER

The receiver is the person who "gets" (hears and sees) the message from the sender. A receiver pays attention and is a good listener.

The receiver of Sarah's message is her housemate, Kate.

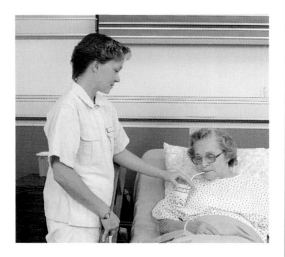

FIGURE 5-3
A clean, well-fitting uniform and good grooming help communicate to your patients that you are a caring and competent person.

FEEDBACK

The receiver listens to the message and understands it. The receiver then repeats the sender's message or otherwise acknowledges it to make sure it was understood correctly.

In the kitchen, Kate gives Sarah **feedback** by saying, "O.K., if you're going to be late, I won't bother waiting, I'll go on and eat without you."

VERBAL COMMUNICATION

Verbal communication, the most common way people communicate, involves the use of words or sounds. To take part in verbal communication, a person must possess the ability to send and receive messages. Speaking and writing are two ways most people learn to send messages. The spoken word is effective only when the receiver of the message can hear and the sender can speak. A speech therapist is someone who is trained to help people who have difficulty speaking. The written word is effective only for receivers who can see or have someone read the message to them. Most of your communications with patients are verbal. Express all messages to patients as clearly as possible and listen carefully to their feedback. Always introduce yourself when you first care for a patient. Because so many different care givers contact the patient during a shift, you may need to reintroduce yourself several times.

COMMUNICATION HELPERS

Communication helpers are ways to make the communication process better so that the message is more likely to be understood. Pay attention to what the patient says. You should look at patients when they speak to you. Not all words have the same meaning to every person, so observation of the patient's body language is necessary.

Listening

Paying attention tells patients you are interested in their message. Most patients send a clear message that you, as the receiver, will understand. Remember that some people find it difficult to express their feelings and needs in words. **Listening** is an important part of communication.

A General Lead

A general lead helps patients expand on a statement they have made. By simply saying "Oh?" or "Go on" or "Hmm," you are telling patients that you are an attentive listener and wish to continue the communication. For example, a patient, during a bath, might say to you, "My daughter called this morning and told me she's having problems in school." You could say, "Go on." The patient might reply, "She knows she has to go to school, but she misses me and I feel she is not doing well because I'm sick." By using a general lead, you might learn information that will help the nurse in planning the patient's care.

A Broad Opening Statement

When you wish to encourage patients to introduce a particular topic of concern or interest to them, use a broad opening statement. This allows patients to choose the direction of the interaction. You are allowing patients to select the topics they wish to discuss. For example, you might notice that a patient is

FEEDBACK
when the receiver in the communication process repeats the information the sender sent (or otherwise acknowledges it) to make sure the message is clear and well understood

VERBAL COMMUNICATION
the use of words or other sounds such as music or groans to exchange information

LISTENING
paying attention; hearing a message with thoughtful attention

especially quiet today. You could say, "You seem quiet today. Is there something you would like to talk about?" Another example would be to pick up on something the patient mentioned earlier in the shift. Perhaps the patient told you several times of feeling angry. You could say, "You seem to be angry about what is happening to you. Let's take this time to talk about your feelings."

Reflection

When you feel the need to explore information with your patients, try a technique called reflection. Use key words your patients say to reflect a main idea back to them. Reflection allows patients to expand on their original statement and helps communication about a topic important to them. When a person says, "I'm feeling really sad today," you can respond, "You're feeling sad?" Avoid using *only* reflection, however, because, if it is used too often, patients may ask if you are listening to them.

Silence

Silence is a useful helper. A few moments of silence can help patients gather their thoughts so they can state what they need. Be careful not to remain silent for extended periods of time though. When you remain silent for short periods of time, patients are supported by your presence and become more trusting. It becomes easier for them to exchange information when they sense you truly care. You may feel comfortable with silence in your own home but find it difficult to use effectively with patients. Keep trying. When you have become comfortable with using silence, your role as a helping care giver is enhanced.

Clarification

Ask patients to clarify (make more clear) any message you do not understand. Always make sure the message is what the patients intend. When you are not sure of the message, you are responsible for asking patients to help you understand. If a person tells you, "I have pain when I bend my arm," you can clarify by using a statement like, "Bend your arm and point to where the pain is."

The chart below gives more examples of communication helpers.

COMMUNICATION HELPERS

Communication Helper	Example	
General lead	Patient:	"I'm so angry!"
	Care giver:	"Oh?"
Broad opening statement	Patient:	"We were in a bad accident yesterday."
	Care giver:	"You mentioned something about your accident earlier today. There's time to talk about it now."
Reflection	Patient:	"I'm worried about my two children."
	Care giver:	"You're worried about your children?"
Silence	Patient:	"It's really nice of you to sit here for a moment."
	Care giver:	(Silence)
Clarification	Patient:	"I still don't feel so good."
	Care giver:	"Are you still nauseated?"

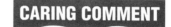

Communication helpers become easier to use with practice. Try to use them in all of your interactions. Remember, if you are unsure of what a patient is trying to communicate to you, it is okay to ask.

COMMUNICATION BARRIERS

Communication barriers are ways of speaking that block the exchange of messages. You should work extra hard to avoid the use of **barriers** when you communicate with others. Learn to recognize communication barriers and replace them with communication helpers.

BARRIER
a way of blocking something; an obstruction

Clichés

Avoid all-purpose answers, or **clichés.** Clichés are used without thought. They are used because they are comfortable and not threatening. "Don't worry" is an example of a cliché; it makes patients feel as if you do not really care about them and their problem. For example, when patients are scheduled for an extremely painful test, they might say, "I'm afraid! They say the pain is awful and I don't think I can take it." If you respond by saying, "Don't worry, most patients say it's not too bad. You'll be fine," patients may feel you are not treating them as an individual. You would help the patient as an individual by responding with a communication helper such as, "Your worried about having pain during the test?" Such a response would encourage patients to talk more about their feelings and concerns.

CLICHÉ
a very familiar phrase people use automatically without thinking about what they are saying

CARING COMMENT

Make a conscious effort to avoid using clichés. Begin by promising yourself not to use one common cliché, such as "Don't worry," that you find you use frequently during the day. Any time you feel the need to use that cliché, replace it with a communication helper. After several weeks of practice, repeat the same process with other clichés you use.

"Why" Questions

"Why" questions make a person defensive. "Why?" demands an explanation. When people respond to such a question, they may not answer honestly because they may feel threatened by the question. For example, if you and a friend had planned a vacation trip to Florida and the friend changed the destination to Texas, your first thought would be to ask, "Why did you do that?" Try to use a statement like "What are your reasons?" This approach provides a relaxed atmosphere that allows the person to talk openly, without becoming defensive.

Say you bring a lunch tray into a patient's room and the patient tells you, "I don't want to eat." If you respond with a "Why not?" the patient may become angry and not answer. You would help more by responding, "You don't want to eat?" The patient may then tell you why the meal is not wanted.

CARING COMMENT

Whenever you find yourself ready to use a "why" question, stop and think. Instead of always asking "why," try saying, "Was there a reason?" or "Let's talk about that."

Opinion or Advice

Avoid giving your opinion or advice because your opinion or advice may not be the message the doctor or other health team member intended. "If I were you, I would . . ." is one way people offer their advice.

At times, patients and their family members may experience difficulty in making a decision. They may ask you directly, "What would you do?" Because you may not have all the information about the situation, it is best to ask the nurse or your supervisor to address the situation.

For example, if the patient needs to make a decision about a surgical procedure and asks you, "Do you think I should have surgery?" You would respond *incorrectly* by saying, "My mother had the same kind of surgery and she did very well." Your response should be, "You seem to have some questions about the surgery; the nurse can answer them for you."

Changing the Subject

Allow the patient to take the lead in an interaction. When you change the subject, it indicates that you are unwilling to discuss something that the patient would like to talk about. Or perhaps the topic is painful to you. If patients change the subject, it may be because the topic they had been discussing became painful to them. As an example of how a care giver changes the topic, consider the following situation: Mary Jean Smith is an older woman who lives alone in an apartment. She is admitted to the hospital for lower back pain, and the doctor is planning to run tests to identify the cause of the pain. She mentions her pain each time the care giver is in the room. The care giver never takes the time to talk with Ms. Smith about her pain and usually makes a comment such as, "Do you like to go shopping?" or "Would you like a snack?" The helping response should have been, "Tell me a little more about your pain."

CARING COMMENT

Learn to recognize what topics cause you to change the subject. It will prepare you to use communication helpers instead of this particular barrier.

Yes or No Responses

When you ask a question in which a patient can only answer yes or no, it tends to end the communication. When you are seeking direct information, it is acceptable to use a question that requires a yes or no response. For example, when you ask the question, "Do you have any allergies?" you probably want a yes or no answer.

However, if you suspect your patient has a problem or a concern, asking "Is something bothering you?" invites a yes or no response and ends the communication. Instead, a statement like "Let's talk about what's bothering you" or "It appears that something is bothering you" encourages patients to open up and talk freely about their feelings and concerns.

The following chart shows communication barriers you should avoid.

COMMUNICATION BARRIERS TO AVOID		
Communication Barrier	**Example**	
Cliché	Patient:	"I'm worried about having the test done."
	Care giver:	"You'll do fine!"
"Why" questions	Care giver:	"Why don't you want a bath today?"
	Patient:	"Who said I don't want a bath today?"
Opinion or advice	Patient:	"I have such awful menstrual cramps. What should I do?"
	Care giver:	"A heating pad on your stomach will help you."
Changing the subject	Patient:	"The pain seems to be getting worse."
	Care giver:	"Did you fill out your menu?"
Yes or no responses	Care giver:	"Do you have a headache?"
	Patient:	"No."

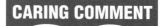

CARING COMMENT

Make sure you report new or important information to the nurse or your supervisor so that any changes in care can be accomplished.

NONVERBAL COMMUNICATION

Nonverbal communication occurs when a message is sent without the use of words. We use body language to send positive and negative messages. Many experts believe that nonverbal communication is the most accurate way of communicating. Messages are most accurate when the verbal and the nonverbal communications match, as in the case of someone smiling while warmly greeting another person. Remember that positive body language is a communication helper, whereas negative body language is a barrier to communication. Below are examples of positive and negative nonverbal messages and possible interpretations.

NONVERBAL COMMUNICATION the exchange of information without using words, for example, shrugging the shoulders to express "I don't know"

POSITIVE NONVERBAL COMMUNICATION	
Nonverbal Message	**Possible Interpretation**
Nodding your head while keeping a pleasant smile on your face	Encourages the patient to keep talking
Using appropriate eye contact and leaning toward the patient	Shows you are attentive
Sitting close and using gentle touch	Encourages the patient to talk freely
Sitting quietly with the patient	Shows your support

NEGATIVE NONVERBAL COMMUNICATION	
Nonverbal Message	**Possible Interpretation**
Pursed lips and flared nostrils	Anger
Fake smile	Displeasure
Downcast eyes and mouth	Sadness
Sloppy, messy appearance	Neglect
Unpleasant body odor	Poor grooming

BODY LANGUAGE
the posture, gestures, and facial expressions that a person uses in communicating with others

Body language refers to physical movements that send messages. When senders of a message shake their head up and down, you as the receiver understand that their message is yes. Your brain interprets body language accurately even though you are not always aware of receiving a nonverbal message. The people sending the message are not always aware of their body language, as in the case of people saying "I'm fine" while there is a frown on their face. Body language is expressed in posture, gestures, and facial expressions (Figure 5–4). These three components of body language combine to give a total effect to the communication.

BEHAVIOR
the manner of conducting oneself

The body uses certain **behaviors** to express happiness, sadness, anger, and pain. One can observe only the body language (behaviors) because no one can actually see happiness, sadness, anger, pain, and other such qualities (Figure 5–5).

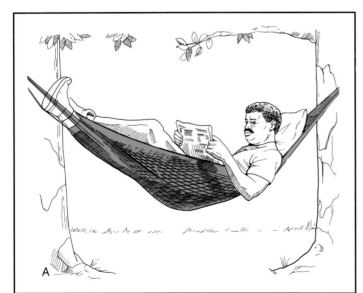

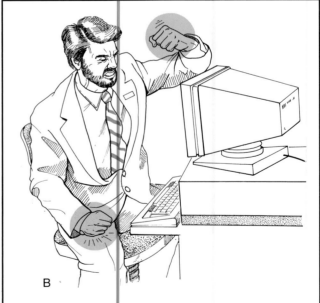

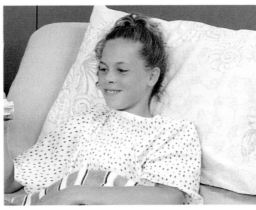

FIGURE 5–4

Body language. A, A message of rest and relaxation is communicated by body language. B, This gesture sends a clear message of anger or frustration. C, This facial expression communicates happiness and cheerfulness.

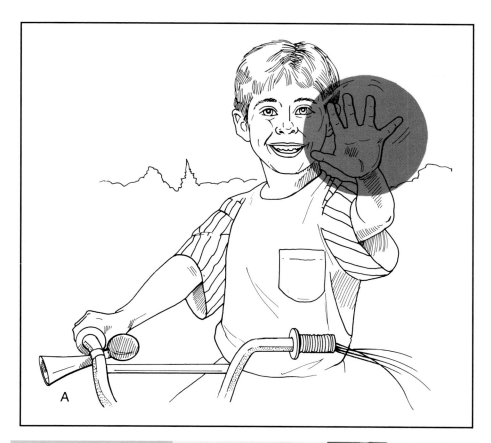

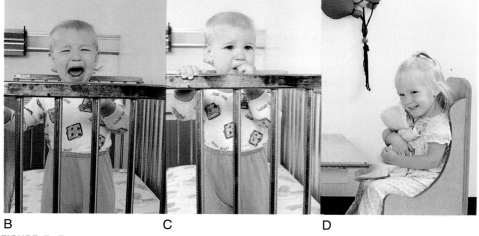

B　　　　　　　C　　　　　　　D

FIGURE 5-5

Common nonverbal messages. A, This person is waving good-bye. B, Tears may communicate a sad or unhappy person. C, A downcast face sends a message of unhappiness. D, A hug offers a message of security and love.

POSTURE

Posture is the way we sit or stand when we communicate. If someone is sitting relaxed in a reclining chair and saying "Come on in and check out this football game on TV," the words and posture match. If the same friendly words are said while the person is standing stiffly, blocking the doorway to the house, then the verbal and nonverbal messages do not match, and you receive a mixed message. Posture is more difficult to observe consciously. Because gestures and facial expressions are more animated, people are more aware of them.

POSTURE

the natural and comfortable bearing of the body in healthy persons

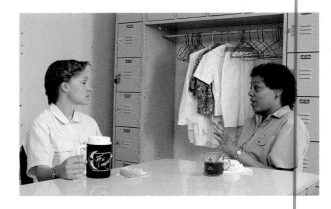

FIGURE 5-6

Gestures add meaning to an interaction.

GESTURES

GESTURE

motioning of the limbs or body as a means of expression

The movement of a body part to give emphasis to what is said is called a **gesture** (Figure 5–6). People pound their fist on the table to make an important point. When you point your finger and shake your hand, the gesture tells others that you are emphasizing a particular point. Infants and toddlers make very effective use of gestures to communicate their needs and wants to others. Sometimes people tap their fingers or a foot when they are annoyed or upset. Think about positive and negative gestures you use to tell others how you are feeling.

FACIAL EXPRESSION

Another way people send messages nonverbally is through facial expressions. Facial expression is a wonderful feature of the art of communicating. People's eyes and the structures around them, their nose, cheeks, and forehead as well as the lips and mouth area, combine to give individuality to nonverbal expression. A person who smiles sends a happy message, while the person with downcast eyes and mouth sends a sad message.

CARING COMMENT

Nonverbal messages are sent automatically; therefore, they are the most accurate. If you receive a mixed message from a patient or co-worker, it is your responsibility to be sure you understand the message correctly. Remember that you also send messages that are both nonverbal (body language) and verbal (words). Be certain the message you send is what you mean to express.

OTHER WAYS TO COMMUNICATE

WRITTEN COMMUNICATION

No matter what form of communication is used, there is always a message that is sent, received, and interpreted between at least two people (Figure 5–7). The written word (the message) is a common form of communication. Written communication is used to record patient information (see Chapter 6). You also use the written word to interact with those who cannot communicate verbally.

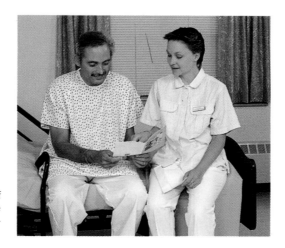

FIGURE 5–7

Cards and letters are an important form of communication. Receiving a mail message is an example of the communication process.

Before using written communications with patients, you must make sure they can read and write. The writer is the sender, the written word is the message, and the reader is the receiver who gives feedback. Patients who have a broken jaw or a tube in their throat to help them breathe cannot talk. If these patients are alert and aware, paper and pencil, along with body language, are their communication link to the outside world. They can write answers and requests to care givers.

COMMUNICATION BOARDS

Patients who cannot speak may use a **communication board** to help them express their needs by pointing at specific words. Special cards with preprinted words are also available for this purpose. When preprinted forms are not available, try writing simple words on cardboard with a felt-tip pen. Remember to use common, everyday words if a communication board is needed. A communication board is a useful tool when the patient can only communicate by pointing at words. For patients who do not understand words (for example, certain stroke patients), the communication board is not effective. In this case, a picture board is substituted.

COMMUNICATION BOARD
a board that helps persons express their needs by pointing at specific words that are printed on it

PICTURE BOARDS

On a picture board, pictures are used instead of words to help patients communicate their needs and wants (Figure 5–8). Patients can point, nod their head, or blink their eyes at the picture message of their choice. If picture request cards are not available, try a simple drawing with a felt-tip pen. A cup, a straw, and a television set, for example, are easy to draw. If you are not artistic, pictures cut from magazines are acceptable. This helpful communication tool is used with certain stroke patients. It can also work for people who do not speak the same language and for children to make their needs and wants known.

INTERPRETER

People use language to pronounce words and make sentences so that everyone who understands that particular language can communicate. A primary language is the language that most members of a certain community or country use to

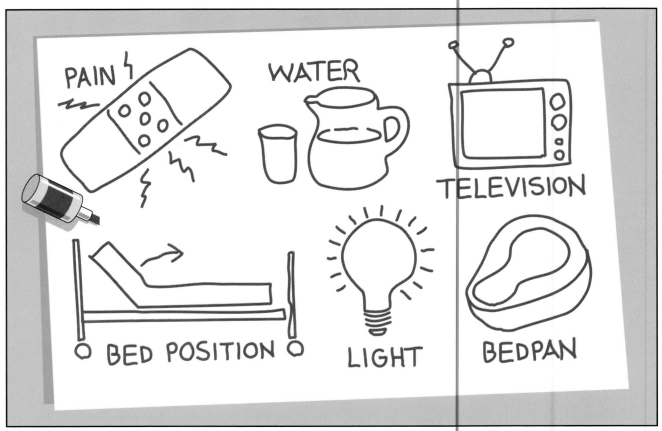

FIGURE 5-8
A sample picture board.

communicate. English is the primary language of most Americans. However, some Americans who weren't born in America use the language they learned as a child as their primary language. When they learn English and use it at all times, it becomes their primary language. An interpreter or family member may be helpful for patients who do not have English as their primary language. Patients have the right to an interpreter. Your nurse or supervisor will contact an interpreter when one is needed. Most health care institutions keep a list of volunteer interpreters who have agreed to help when needed.

SIGN LANGUAGE

SIGN LANGUAGE
a formal language that uses hand and matching mouth gestures to communicate words and meanings to people who cannot hear

Sign language is a formal language in which hand and matching mouth and lip gestures are used to communicate words and meanings to people who cannot hear. The sign becomes the message that is sent and received by the hearing-impaired person (Figure 5-9). Many hearing-impaired people are able to read lips. This helps them to interpret sign language. The hearing-impaired person who is born without the ability to hear usually learns to sign and use the mouth

FIGURE 5-9

A, Sign language is used to express common needs and feelings. B, Sign language alphabet. (B, redrawn from Bragonier R Jr, Fisher D: What's What: A Visual Glossary of the Physical World. Maplewood, NJ, Hammond, 1990.)

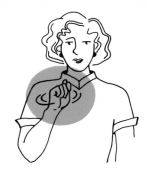

TOILET, BATHROOM
Shake the "t" hand, palm facing outward, in front of the chest, left to right, several times.

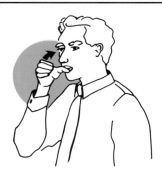

DRINK, BEVERAGE
Hold a "c" hand in front of the mouth, palm facing body and thumb touching the bottom lip. Keeping the thumb in place, pivot hand upward toward the nose.

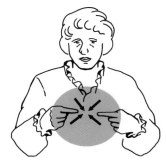

HURT, PAIN, ACHE, SORE
Jab the extended index fingertips toward each other in front of the body several times without letting them touch, palms facing chest. Note: Can be signed near the point of pain.

A

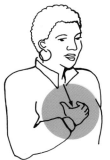

HUNGRY, STARVED
Bring the fingertips and thumb of the "c" hand, palm toward chest and knuckles pointing left, downward from near the throat to the chest.

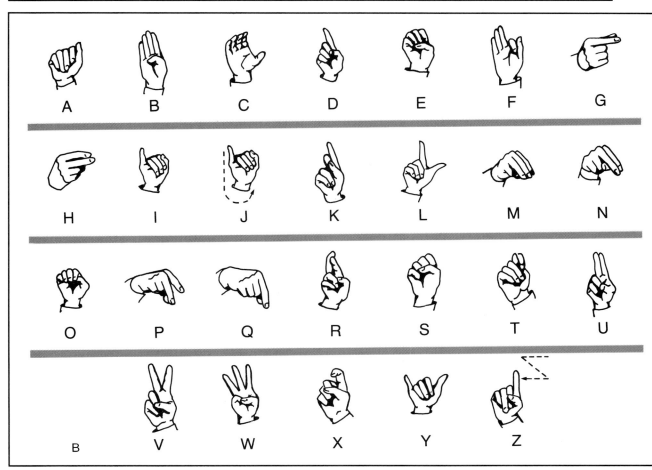

B

FIGURE 5-9 *See legend on opposite page*

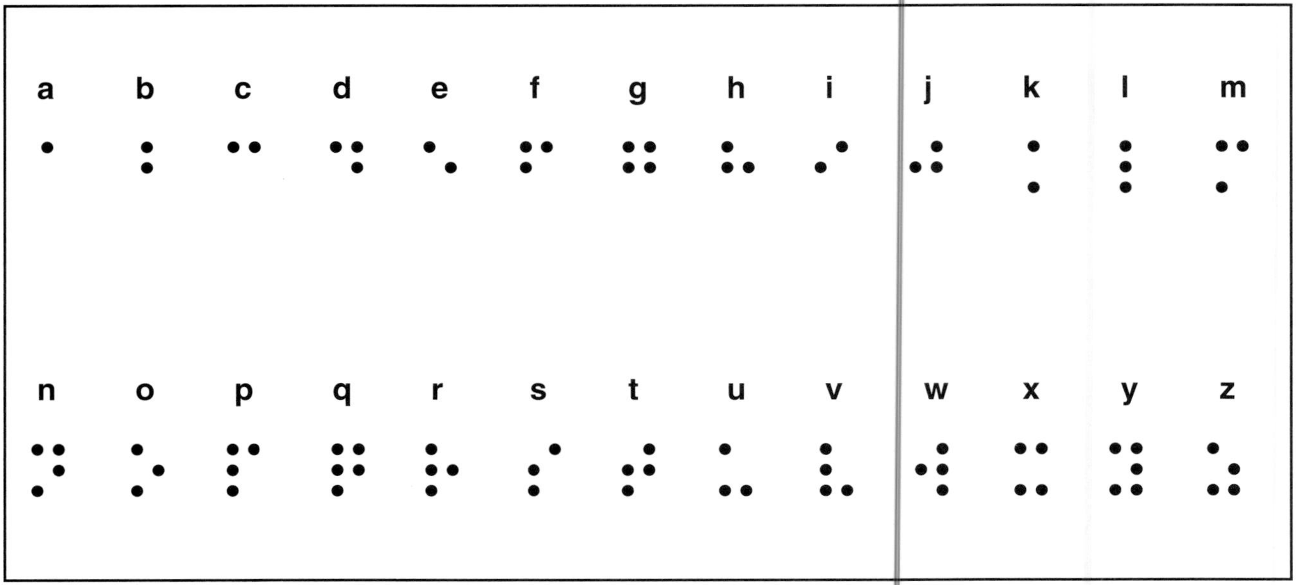

a	b	c	d	e	f	g	h	i	j	k	l	m

n	o	p	q	r	s	t	u	v	w	x	y	z

FIGURE 5–10
Braille—a blind person's language.

to form words. Any person can learn to use signing as a form of communication with hearing-impaired individuals.

Health care institutions provide interpreters who are proficient in the use of sign language. Family members who interpret ("sign") may withhold information because they think it is in the patient's best interest.

BRAILLE

BRAILLE

a system of writing/reading used by persons who are blind

Braille serves as the written word for blind people. It helps persons who are blind communicate through the use of touch. A series of raised dots on special paper are messages that are read by the blind person's fingertips and interpreted in the brain (Figure 5–10).

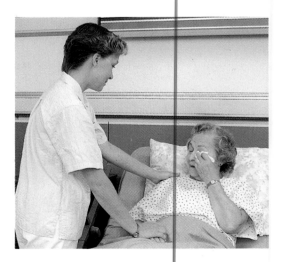

FIGURE 5–11
Use touch to show you care about and accept the patient.

TOUCH

The use of touch is important in the care of patients (Figure 5–11). A gentle, kind touch sends a caring message to the patient. Rough, hurried actions that disregard the patient's comfort are not acceptable. These actions can cause injury or discomfort to the patient. Such actions on the care giver's part are abusive toward the patient and result in disciplinary action by the employer.

MUSIC

Music is a universal language. Words are not necessary to understand the message in music. A lively beat sends an upbeat message to the receiver. A slow, calm melody produces a relaxing effect.

CARING COMMENT

Your goal is to communicate well with all patients. Be sensitive to your patients' needs, and be creative with the many ways that are available to communicate. For example, with a deaf patient, you might use a combination of a communication board, picture board, and sign language. A blind patient might prefer listening to an audiotape of music or a book being read to hearing a TV show.

OTHER FORMS OF COMMUNICATION IN THE HEALTH CARE INSTITUTION

The following are the communication tools used to exchange messages in the health care institution:

  Call signal
  Intercom
  Telephone
  Computer

These communication tools help care givers respond more effectively to patients' needs.

CALL SIGNAL

The **call signal** is a communication tool used by patients who must remain in bed or in a chair (Figure 5–12A). When a call signal, also known as a call bell, is activated by the patient, a message of "need" is sent, and you as the care giver respond when you receive the message. The patient is taught how to use the call signal at the time of admission and is reminded as necessary. You should respond quickly and courteously when the patient rings the call signal (Figure 5–12B).

  In responding, you enter the room and ask the patient, "What can I do for you?" or "How can I help you?" Then turn off the call signal by pressing the cancel button. When the call signal has been cancelled, all care givers on the unit know that someone has responded to the patient's call. Try to accommodate the patient by doing whatever you can within your training and legal limits. When the patient asks you to do something that is outside your limits, ask the nurse or your supervisor for direction or assistance.

CALL SIGNAL
a communication tool used by patients who must remain in bed or in a chair; also called a call light or call bell

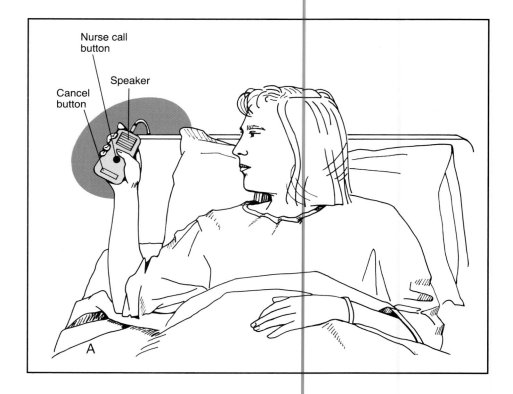

Nurse call button

Speaker

Cancel button

A

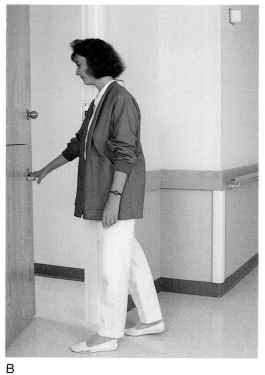

B

FIGURE 5–12

A, The call signal is used by the patient to call the care giver to attend to a patient need. Secure the call signal within the patient's reach. B, The nurse assistant should respond to the call signal as soon as possible.

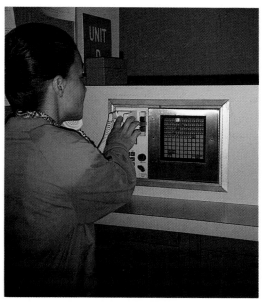

FIGURE 5-13

The intercom enables quick communication between the patient and care giver.

INTERCOM

An intercom is a communication tool frequently used in health care institutions to alert a person of a special need or request (Figure 5-13). Two-way speakers in each patient room are connected to a main terminal. When in the room, a patient can make a request to the care giver at the main terminal. The main terminal is located at the nursing station because of its central location. A loudspeaker is part of the equipment and is used to communicate with care givers who are on the unit. In the hospital or nursing home, intercoms are used by care givers to respond quickly to patient needs and requests. Young or confused patients respond better to a personal appearance from you, however, because they may not know where the voice is coming from.

TELEPHONE

The telephone is a common way to communicate. This method saves time and allows people to communicate across distances. Patients use the telephone to keep in touch with loved ones while they are hospitalized (Figure 5-14). When you answer the phone on the unit, follow this procedure:

1. Announce the unit name and location.
2. Give your name and title.
3. Ask "How can I assist you?"
4. Do *not* offer any information or take doctor's orders or special reports.
5. Find the person to whom the call is directed.

COMPUTERS

Computers communicate through electronics. A message can be sent over telephone lines from one computer to another. The world of business uses com-

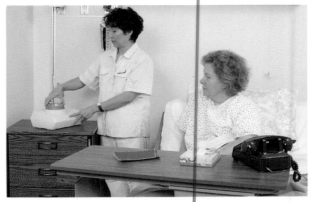

FIGURE 5–14
Keep a telephone near the patient so the patient can stay in touch with family and friends.

puters to store information and communicate. Computers in the health care institution are used to store and communicate information about patients. For example, a patient care plan might be stored in the computer and printed out for each care giver at the beginning of each shift. Another example of computerized communication in the health care setting is the communication between the diagnostic laboratory and the patient's unit. When laboratory testing is completed, results may be stored in the laboratory's computer. The information is sent to the unit's computer, the information is then printed out on the unit, and the paper copy is placed in the patient's chart. In the future, more health care institutions will use the computer to communicate quickly and conveniently and to store and retrieve patient information quickly (Figure 5–15).

SUCCESSFUL COMMUNICATION IN SPECIAL SITUATIONS

The ability to communicate successfully takes hard work and effort. Learn to use positive communication helpers and body language to interact with patients, patients' family members, and other care team members. The failure to

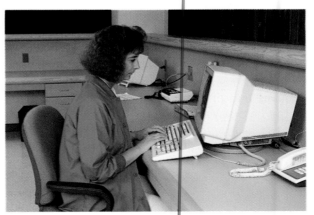

FIGURE 5–15
Many care givers learn to use a computer in the health care institution.

follow appropriate communication can be a violation of patients' rights to considerate and respectful care.

GUIDELINES FOR SUCCESSFUL COMMUNICATION

Correct Action	Wrong Action
Paying attention	Acting like you are in a hurry may show you do not care about the patient
Sitting near the patient	Standing far away gives the impression you are in command and do not have time for the patient
Leaning forward	Folding your arms across your chest puts distance between you and the patient and looks like a nonverbal barrier
Approaching the bedside	Talking from the bathroom or the doorway shows disinterest on your part
Speaking in a low, pleasant voice	A loud voice can irritate an ill person and whispering or mumbling around patients can make them feel uncomfortable
Using clear English	Slang and curse words are discourteous and abusive
Using simple, ordinary terms	Medical terms and abbreviations are confusing and open to misinterpretation by others
Asking patients if they need anything or have any questions	Hurrying away shows disinterest and lack of concern
Finding the person who can give correct answers to the patient's question	Answering incorrectly is a disservice to the patient
Responding to patients' requests	Ignoring a request reflects laziness or lack of concern as well as neglectful behavior
Speaking to patients who are semi-conscious or unconscious, because they are often aware of their surroundings and can hear	Silence or talking about patients in their presence is not courteous

Not all people interact in the same manner. Remember that messages are sent and received in many different ways. You are responsible for learning how to communicate so that messages are understandable and helpful to the patient. Various circumstances require special methods of communication.

CHILDREN

Children, especially very young children, may be difficult to understand. They may not be able to communicate their needs accurately to you. Parents can

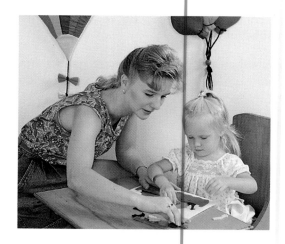

FIGURE 5-16

Parents play an important role in communicating for toddlers who cannot always communicate for themselves.

help communicate a child's needs to you (Figure 5-16). This results in less frustration for the child and you. Because infants and toddlers do not always communicate with words, pay attention and respond to their body language. Most hospitals encourage parents to visit often and even remain overnight with their children. Parents serve as an important communication link as well as a support system for their children.

THE ELDERLY

Elderly adults may be affected by disease or the normal aging processes that interfere with their communication efforts. For example, a person who has suffered a stroke may have difficulty pronouncing words or may be unable to use the correct word to express a need. Be sure to give the patient enough time to respond.

The vision-impaired person may hear quite well. Speak clearly and do not shout. The hearing-impaired person may or may not use a hearing aid. At times, you must speak loudly and use a low tone of voice. A higher pitch (high tone of voice) is more difficult to hear; it can occur when a person gets excited and screams. In some cases, paper-and-pencil communication works best for the patient.

OTHER CIRCUMSTANCES

As discussed earlier, when English is not the patient's primary language, you must rely on others to help you communicate with the patient. A family member or an interpreter can help make a patient's specific needs known to care givers.

The term *handicapped* does not mean vision or hearing impairment. For example, a handicapped person may be a person who uses a wheelchair because he or she cannot walk. Handicapped persons are often able to see and hear and have average or above-average intelligence. You must not talk down to handicapped patients. Communicate as you always do, and make adjustments, if necessary, as you go along. Some handicapped persons prefer the term "disadvantaged" or "disabled" to the term "handicapped." In some areas, the term "physically challenged" is used.

Remember that family members and friends are hurting as much as their loved one. Often, they need someone with whom they can talk and share their feelings and concerns. Always let the family know you will inform the head nurse or supervisor of any problems.

Visitors may ask for directions to other areas of the health care institution. Give courteous instructions on how to find a place to eat, a public restroom, a visitors lounge, a telephone, and other service areas of the institution.

CARING COMMENT

Do not talk down to any person regardless of the person's age or condition.

CHAPTER WRAP-UP

- Communication is an exchange of information. It consists of using verbal and nonverbal skills to
   send,
   receive,
   interpret,
   and feedback messages.
- Giving feedback can avoid misunderstanding or misrepresentation of
   thoughts and ideas,
   wants and needs,
   requests.
- Communication helpers make verbal messages clear and understandable. Examples of communication helpers are
   General lead—helps the conversation to continue
   Broad opening statement—helps introduce a topic of concern
   Reflection (stating key words back to the person)—encourages the person to continue
   Silence—gives the person time to gather thoughts and continue
   Clarification—helps make a message more clear to the listener
- The use of communication barriers gives a message that is unclear and open to misinterpretation. Examples of communication barriers are
   Cliché (an all-purpose answer)—does not help a person feel special
   "Why" question—makes people feel they must give an explanation
   Opinion or advice—gives information that may be incorrect or confusing to the person
   Changing the subject—forces the person to talk about what you want to talk about
   Yes or no question—ends communication
- Verbal communication is the most common form of exchanging messages.
- Nonverbal communication in the form of body language is the most accurate way of sending a message.
- Each situation is a unique communication experience. Successful communication can be helped by
   Paying attention
   Sitting near the person at eye level
   Leaning forward
   Using eye contact

Using a pleasant tone of voice
Using clear English and speaking in simple, ordinary terms
Asking if there are questions or needs
Responding to requests

REVIEW QUESTIONS

1. What are the four essential parts of communication?
2. Give three examples of communication helpers. Tell how communication helpers benefit the patient and the health care team member.
3. Give three examples of communication barriers. Tell how the communication barriers can be corrected by the communication helpers.
4. How will you communicate with the visually impaired patient? the hearing impaired patient? the handicapped patient? children? the elderly?

ACTIVITY CORNER

Look for shortcomings in your communication skills. Work to improve your communication abilities at work; at home; and when you're doing such everyday things as shopping, entertaining friends, or making arrangements for a trip.

Plan a special communication practice time with someone you know. Choose two communication helpers and practice using them. A general lead and reflection are easy ones to start with. Answer the following questions about your communication efforts:

- Were you successful in using at least two communication helpers?
  Yes _____ No _____
- Did the person know you were using communication helpers?
  Yes _____ No _____
- Did you use any communication barriers?   Yes _____ No _____
- Can you think of ways to change the barriers to helpers?   Yes _____
  No _____
- Do you feel you were successful in using communication techniques?
  Yes _____ No _____
- Do you feel you can use communication helpers with patients?
  Yes _____ No _____

Watch out for communication barriers! Count the number of times someone else uses communication barriers when talking to you. List the number of times. _____

Pick two of the communication barriers and decide which communication helpers you would have used instead.

1. First communication barrier you identified:

   _____

   How would you change the barrier into a helper?

   _____

2. Second communication barrier you identified:

   _____

   How would you change the barrier into a helper?

   _____

Observe body language. Watch three people for 3–5 minutes each. You can watch them while they are talking with you or with someone else. List what the persons are saying with their bodies in the first column (include facial expressions as well as body movements). Write down a possible interpretation of body language in the second column.

Person Number 1:   **Possible Interpretation:**

_____   _____

_____   _____

_____   _____

Person Number 2:   **Possible Interpretation:**

_____   _____

_____   _____

_____   _____

Person Number 3:   **Possible Interpretation:**

_____   _____

_____   _____

_____   _____

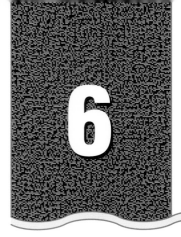

6

Reporting and Recording

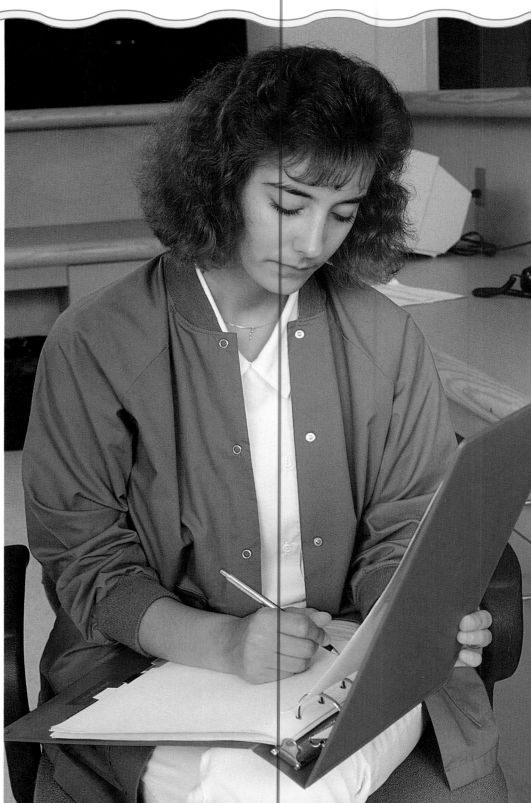

Objectives

Describe an observation.

Explain the difference between a subjective observation and an objective observation.

Describe an oral report.

Discuss the importance of reporting patient status.

Discuss the importance of objective reporting.

List three reasons for a change of shift report.

Use observational skills whenever you communicate with or care for patients.

Overview As a nursing assistant, you are responsible for reporting and recording information about patients. Some health care institutions also require you to give written reports of your observations. By reporting and recording information honestly and accurately, you will be able to fulfill your legal and ethical responsibilities.

WHAT DO YOU KNOW ABOUT REPORTING AND RECORDING?

Here are six statements about reporting and recording. Consider them to test your current ideas about the process of reporting and recording. If you think the statement is true, circle the T; if you think the statement is false, circle the F. Change the false statements to make them true.

1. T F The patient record is also known as the patient chart.
2. T F A flow sheet is used to record measurements made at frequent intervals.
3. T F The patient record is discarded after the patient leaves the hospital.
4. T F Objective observations are the things patients tell you about themselves.
5. T F Noticing a patient's cool, clammy skin is an example of the care giver's use of the sense of smell.
6. T F Observation of the patient is continuous.

ANSWERS

1. **True.** The patient record is commonly called the patient chart.
2. **True.** Vital signs measured every 15 minutes after surgery are recorded on a flow sheet.
3. **False.** The patient record is maintained permanently by the health care institution.
4. **False.** Objective observations are the things you see, hear, taste, touch, and smell.
5. **False.** Cool, clammy skin is a tactile (touching) observation. The olfactory organs are used to smell.
6. **True.** You observe patients each time you come in contact with them.

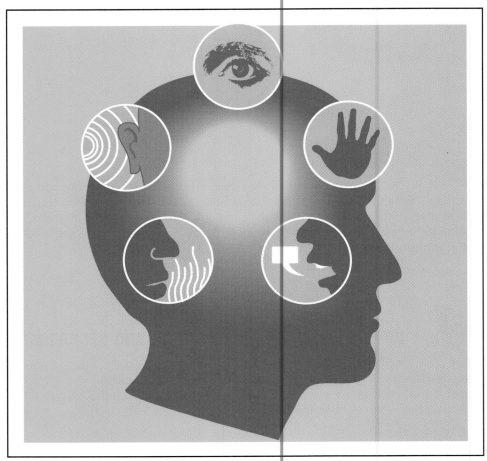

FIGURE 6–1
Use the senses to observe the patient's condition.

HEALTH CARE TEAM
the group of members involved in providing care to patients

ASSESSMENT
gathering information through the use of subjective and objective observations

PLANNING
developing a program of how to go about doing something

The registered nurse relies on information from *all* members of the **health care team** to plan care and make decisions about patients. Health care personnel share information about patients' status (condition) and what they did for patients. They contribute information about patients' needs and what kind of care patients require. As a nursing assistant, you contribute by sharing your observations about your patients. You use all of your senses to observe (Figure 6–1). Normal observations as well as any unusual observations about the patient are reported. This is part of your responsibility and contribution to the **assessment** and **planning** phases of patient care.

INFORMATION

PATIENT RECORD
patient chart; a document that contains information about a patient and the patient's condition

Health care team members must be knowledgeable about their patients. To plan and make decisions about a patient's care, they use information they have gathered about the patient. Information must be easily available in a central location, such as the nursing station. Remember that information may be verbal as well as written. Written information about a patient is found in a document called the **patient record.**

PATIENT RECORD

The patient record, also called the patient chart, contains all the following daily information about a patient:

Health status
Treatment
Response to treatment and care

It is a permanent record that provides information as part of the patient's health history.

The health care institution is responsible for the permanent storage of the patient record. It is also responsible for providing the patient record to a physician or a court of law when requested to do so. For a patient with a history of many admissions, the court may ask the institution to provide the patient records for all of the patient's previous admissions. A physician may also ask for all the patient records for a patient's previous admissions. Old admission records provide background information about the patient.

The patient record contains information about the patient from various departments in the health care institution (Figure 6–2). It is divided into sections so that information may be located easily. The forms used to document information about the patient are stamped with the patient's name, room number, and other information required by the institution. All written information is dated and signed by the person responsible for communicating the information. The title (for example NA, RN, or MD) is included after the name. Another title for nursing assistant is certified nursing assistant (CNA). Black pen is usually required by most health care institutions to record patient information because it photocopies better.

What Is Included on the Patient Record

The information available in the patient record includes

- admission record

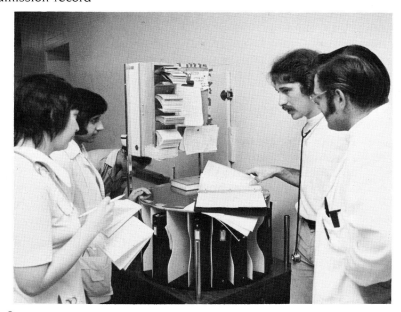

FIGURE 6–2

A nursing assistant checks a chart for information about a patient. (From DuGas BW: Introduction to Patient Care: A Comprehensive Approach to Nursing, 4th ed. Philadelphia, W. B. Saunders Company, 1983.)

- doctor's progress notes and orders for treatment
- results of the history and physical examination performed by the physician
- results of any diagnostic tests that are ordered
- nursing history and assessment
- nurses' notes
- informed consent sheets

Information documented by other members of the health care team is recorded on specialized forms. These forms are designed to provide information about the care and status of the patient whenever other departments (emergency room care, x-ray department) or services provide care. In some institutions, the same style of form is used by health team members from other departments to document their observations on the patient's chart. When a patient is scheduled for surgery, many specialized forms are added. These include

Surgical consent forms
Anesthesia reports
Reports of the progress of surgery
Postanesthesia reports
Nurses' notes

These specialized forms document the care and status of a patient while in the surgical department (see Chapter 26).

ADMISSION RECORD   The admission sheet is a record of the admitting process. It contains practical information required by the institution for **admission.** By having the information on file the patient does not have to repeat it later on. The admission record contains the following information:

- date and time of admission
- patient number
- name, address, and telephone number
- date of birth, age, and race
- social security number
- diagnosis
- physician's name
- history of **allergies**
- next of kin (nearest relative) and telephone number
- place of employment and occupation
- insurance coverage
- church or religious affiliation
- **advance directives**

Advance directives are required by law. They describe patients' wishes about life-sustaining measures. They may state whether patients' have a **Living Will** or requests that no cardiopulmonary resuscitation be used if their heart and lungs stop functioning.

GRAPHIC SHEET   The **graphic** sheet is a special document that provides information for quick, easy reference (Figure 6–3). It is designed to provide a record of **measurements** or observations, made over a period of time, of the patient's

- vital signs (blood pressure, body temperature, pulse, and respiration measurements)
- height and weight
- number and times of bowel movements
- intake and output total
- appetite at each meal

Graphic sheet recording is done on a 24-hour basis, and there are usually 5 or 6 days on each sheet. Entries can be made more than once in a day and are recorded in the appropriate time column. Any person who reviews the chart can

ADMISSION

the process by which the patient enters the health care system

ALLERGY

an abnormal response caused by exposure to an allergen (for example, dust or food); hypersensitivity

ADVANCE DIRECTIVE

a notice of the patient's wishes about what should be done if the patient's heart and lungs stop functioning

LIVING WILL

a form patients sign when they do not wish to have their life prolonged by any means

GRAPHIC

the use of drawings or words to make information more clear and understandable

MEASUREMENT

an extent or amount determined by measuring

9/91 W.C.A. HOSPITAL **VITAL SIGNS GRAPH/FLUID BALANCE SUMMARY**	

DATE																															
HOSPITAL DAY																															
POST-OP DAY																															

TIME		04	08	12	16	20	24	04	08	12	16	20	24	04	08	12	16	20	24	04	08	12	16	20	24	04	08	12	16	20	24
T	104																														
E																															
M	103																														
P	102																														
E																															
R	101																														
A	100																														
T																															
U	99																														
	98⁶	–	–	–	–	–	–	–	–	–	–	–	–	–	–	–	–	–	–	–	–	–	–	–	–	–	–	–	–	–	–
R	98																														
E	97																														
• - Oral	97																														
• - Rectal																															
A - Axillary	96																														

	04	08	12	16	20	24	04	08	12	16	20	24	04	08	12	16	20	24	04	08	12	16	20	24	04	08	12	16	20	24
Pulse																														
Resp																														
BP																														
Weight																														

	0600	1400	2200	0600	1400	2200	0600	1400	2200	0600	1400	2200	0600	1400	2200
Total 8 hr. Intake															
Total 8 hr. Intake															
24 Hour Intake															
24 Hour Output															
24 Hour Fluid Balance	+ –			+ –			+ –			+ –			+ –		
Stool															

FIGURE 6-3

Vital signs graphic sheet combined with intake and output summary. The nursing assistant is able to record information on the graphic sheet. (Courtesy of Woman's Christian Association Hospital, Jamestown, NY.)

POSTOPERATIVE VITAL SIGNS FLOW SHEET

Time	Blood Pressure	Temperature	Pulse	Respirations	Initials
1000	160/100	99²	80	14	JR
1015	158/100	99²	80	16	JR
1030	150/90	99²	82	16	JR
1045	150/92	99⁴	84	16	MK
1100					

Initials	Signature	Initials	Signature
JR	John Ray NA		
MK	Margarit Klan, LPN		

Patient Stamp

FIGURE 6–4

Postoperative vital signs flow sheet. The nurse and the nursing assistant can record information on the postoperative flow sheet.

easily see if the patient's status has changed or remains the same. You may be required to record any important information that you measure and observe about your patient on the graphic sheet (see Figure 6–3).

FLOW SHEET A **flow sheet** is a record of a series of measurements and observations made at frequent time intervals (Figure 6–4). These intervals may be as often as every 5 minutes. A nursing assistant can record information on a patient's postoperative flow sheet (see Figure 26–6). Another type of flow sheet is the intake and output record which may be kept in the patient's room (see Chapter 19).

FLOW SHEET

a record of a series of measurements and observations made at frequent intervals during a specific time period

9/91

W.C.A. HOSPITAL

NURSING HISTORY & ASSESSMENT

Addressograph

Physician: _____ Date of Admission: _____ Time: _____

VITAL SIGNS: T_____ AP_____ R _____ BP_____ (R)_____ (L)_____ WT_____ HT _____

ADMITTED FROM: Admissions _____ E.R._____ Direct Admit _____ O.R. _____
MODE: Ambulatory _____ W/C_____ Walker _____ Stretcher_____

HISTORY/INFORMATION OBTAINED FROM: _____ RELATIONSHIP: _____

PRESENT COMPLAINT: _____

　Location:_____ Onset: _____ Frequency: _____
　Precipitating Factors: _____
　Duration: _____ Relief Achieved by: _____

DNR: ( ) Yes ( ) No　　Health Care Proxy: ( ) Yes ( ) No

ALLERGIES

DRUGS/FOODS/OTHER	REACTION

PRESENT DIET: (List Restrictions): _____
Present Appetite vs. Usual Appetite: ( )SAME ( )BETTER ( )WORSE
Difficulty Swallowing: ( )YES ( )NO COMMENTS:_____
Difficulty Chewing: ( )YES ( )NO COMMENTS:_____

IMMUNIZATIONS: (14–18 years old) Up-to-date: ( )Yes ( )No

MEDICAL HISTORY　　**KEY:** M=Mother F=Father S=Sister B=Brother

Medical History	Self	Onset	Treatment	Family Member
Heart Disease				
Hypertension				
Diabetes				
Kidney Disease				
Arthritis				
Seizures				
Sleep Disorders				
CVA				
Respiratory Disease				
Cancer				
Emotional Illness				
Congenital Anomalies/Handicap				
Other Serious Illnesses				

SURGERIES (List/Date): _____
_____
_____

SMOKING: ( )No ( )Yes Amount_____ # Years _____　Quit Smoking: ( )Yes How Long Ago:_____
ALCOHOL: ( )Never ( )Occasionally ( )Regularly　What do you drink: _____
DRUGS: Type/Frequency: _____　Type/Frequency: _____

FIGURE 6–5

The nursing history and assessment form is filled in by the nurse when a patient is admitted. (Courtesy of Woman's Christian Association Hospital, Jamestown, NY.)

Illustration continued on following page

W.C.A. HOSPITAL

NURSING HISTORY & ASSESSMENT

– Page 2 –

PRESENT MEDICATIONS (Prescription and Over-The-Counter)

*CODE: A=Sent Home,   B=Not Brought In,   C=Kept on Unit

Name	Dosage	Times	Last Dose	Purpose (Pt. Perception)	*Code

SOCIAL: Living Alone _____ Spouse _____ Children _____ (Ages _____)   Other: _____

Do you take care of anyone else? No_____ Spouse _____ Children _____   Other: _____

Who manages their care while you are unable? _____

HOME PHYSICAL LAYOUT: (   ) 1 Floor (   ) 2 Floors   Location of BR _____ Location of Bedroom _____

MEDICAL EQUIPMENT IN HOME: (   ) None (   ) Crutches (   ) Cane   (   ) Walker (   ) Wheelchair (   ) Hospital Bed

(   ) Commode   (   ) O$_2$ (   ) Lifeline   (   ) Other: _____

PREADMISSION HOME SERVICES NOW IN USE: (   ) None   (   ) Nursing   (   ) Homemaker   (   ) Personal Care Aide

(   ) P.T.   (   ) Meals on Wheels (   ) Hospice   Agency: _____

NEW NEEDS: (   ) Nursing   (   ) Personal Care Aide   (   ) Meal Preparation   (   ) Transportation   (   ) Placement

(   ) Other: _____

In the event that I need help in planning for my hospital discharge, please contact:

_____

Name	(Relationship)	Address	Phone

HAS THE PATEINT BEEN ORIENTED TO: **WAS FAMILY NOTIFIED OF ADMISSION?**   ( ) Y ( ) N

Patient Bill of Rights ( ) Y   ( ) N   No Smoking Policy ( ) Y   ( ) N   Bed Operation ( ) Y   ( ) N   Television ( ) Y   ( ) N

Intercom   ( ) Y   ( ) N   Menu   ( ) Y   ( ) N   Roommate   ( ) Y   ( ) N   Siderails   ( ) Y   ( ) N

Visiting   ( ) Y   ( ) N   Call Bell   ( ) Y   ( ) N   Telephone   ( ) Y   ( ) N   Bathroom ( ) Y   ( ) N

Chaplaincy Program ( ) Y   ( ) N

NAME AND PHONE NUMBER OTHER THAN THOSE LISTED ON FRONT SHEET: _____

_____

PROPERTY/VALUABLES/JEWELRY

(   ) Dentures–(   ) Full/ (   ) Partial   (   ) Glasses   (   ) Contacts   (   ) Hearing Aide–(   ) Right/ (   ) Left

(   ) Electric Razor   (   ) Money: $_____ (Bedside _____ Safety Deposit Receipt _____)   (   ) Watch _____

(   ) Rings _____ (How Many?___)   Other: _____

(   ) Clothing (Describe: _____)

(   ) Other: _____

"Do you understand that we are not responsible for any clothing or personal effects that you will keep in your hospital room, or for any articles that might be sent or brought to you during your hospital stay?

Yes (   ) _____

_____

Signature of Patient or Relative   (Relationship)

History taken by: _____ Signature/Title

FIGURE 6–5

Continued

NURSING HISTORY AND ASSESSMENT   When a patient is admitted to the unit, the nurse takes a nursing history and does a nursing assessment so that care planning can begin (Figure 6–5). The nursing history and assessment give a picture of the patient's condition at admission.

NURSES' NOTES   Nurses' notes are a written record of the care given to a patient (Figure 6–6). The nurse makes continuous observations (subjective and objective) while giving care. Important observations are then described in the nurses' notes. When the nurse performs a treatment (for example, changing a dressing or giving a foot soak), the treatment and the patient's response to it are recorded. The nurse records all medication given to the patient and the patient's response to the medication. Because the nurse's role includes teaching and counseling, these events, and the patient's response to them, are also written down.

Because nurses' notes are a legal document, subjective and objective observations are written as clearly and concisely as possible. When a health care institution grants you permission to read a patient's chart, you will find helpful background information about your patient. The health care institution may require you to write down the care you give the patient and the observations you are trained to make.

DATE	TIME	NURSES' NOTES
10/1/92	0730	Awake and alert. To BR c̄ 1 assist. Voided 275 cc. clear yellow urine. Assisted to chair.
		Ate all of soft diet/ breakfast. Completed all of bath except legs & back assist. ————
		A. Mohraine NA ————
	1000	Ambulated 100 ft. in hallway c̄ — assistance of one. Used hand rail for support.
		Resting in bed c̄ all side rails ↑. A. Mohraine NA ————

Patient

FIGURE 6–6

Nurses' notes.

CARING COMMENT

Your observations about every patient are confidential. Share your information only with the nurse or supervisor.

OBSERVATION

OBSERVATION

noting a fact or occurrence about something or someone

An **observation** is the act of recognizing a fact or occurrence about your patient. A major responsibility of nursing assistants is to accurately report observations about the patients in their care. The observations you report to the registered nurse help the nurse plan the patient's care. Two kinds of observations are important for you to know and practice:

- objective observations (what actually happened; what you observed)
- subjective observations (what the patient told you and your opinion or what you thought had happened)

Use the Guide for Patient Observations to help you gather the subjective and objective information you are seeking about your patients.

GUIDE FOR PATIENT OBSERVATIONS
Functioning of the Senses and Alertness

Senses

- Can patients see you? Can they see well enough to read or watch television?
- Are glasses, contacts, or artificial eye(s) used? Did patients bring them, or are they at home?
- Can patients hear a normal tone of voice?
- Is a hearing aid used? Did patients bring it? Is the battery still functioning? Is a supply of batteries available?
- Can patients tell you whether they smell pungent odors (such as alcohol and disinfectant)?
- If you touch patients' toes, can patients tell you they feel your fingers?
- Are patients sensitive to hot or cold and to sharp or dull objects?

Awareness

- Are patients awake and alert or drowsy?
- Are patients aware of people, place, and time?
- Do patients sleep at night, or do they arouse easily?
- For patients who are infants or children, is a parent encouraged to stay?
- Do infants or children respond in a way appropriate to their age?
- Do patients respond to stimuli (for example, their name being called or loud noises)?

Vital Signs Functioning
Temperature

* Are **temperature** measurements within patients' normal range?
* Is the skin warm, red, and flushed or pale, cool and clammy?

Respirations

* What is the breathing rate? Is it regular or irregular?
* Is coughing or sputum (mucous secretion from the respiratory system that is ejected through the mouth) present?
* If sputum is present, is it clear, white, yellow, green, or rusty in color? Is it thick or thin?
* If oxygen has been ordered for patients, is it being administered? At what rate? By which method?

Pulse

* At what rate is the heart beating? Is it a regular or an irregular rate? Was an apical pulse (pulse heard through a stethoscope placed over the patient's chest) counted?
* Is it a bounding pulse? (In a bounding pulse, you cannot make the pulse disappear when you apply pressure to the artery.)
* Is it a thready pulse? (A thready pulse disappears when you apply pressure to the artery.)

Blood Pressure

* What is the **blood pressure** measurement?
* What is patients' usual range of blood pressure measurements?

Comfort

When patients tell you they are in **pain**, you might ask them the following:

* Where is the pain located?
* Describe the pain: Sharp, dull, throbbing, cramping, or intermittent?
* How long have you had the pain? Have you had this kind of pain before? What makes it better? How long does it last?
* (For young children) Can you show me where the pain is on this doll? (A young child may only be able to say, "It hurts all over.")
* Are there any objective observations of pain, such as moaning, crying, grimacing, or holding a limb?

Sleep and Rest

* Do patients **sleep** through the night without awakening? Are patients easily aroused when you call them by name?
* Does fatigue (tiredness) occur during the day? Do you notice dozing and yawning? Are patients able to **rest** during the day?
* Do patients follow a sleep routine at bedtime at home? Can they follow the same routine in the health care institution? What sleep aids do they use (such as music, reading, or drinking warm milk)?

Box continued on following page

TEMPERATURE
the degree of heat or cold, expressed in terms of a specific scale

CIRCULATION
the movement of blood through the body by the pumping action of the heart

RESPIRATIONS
the exchange of oxygen and carbon dioxide between the atmosphere and the body's cells

PULSE
the beat of the heart as felt through the walls of the arteries

BLOOD PRESSURE
the pressure of the circulating blood against the blood vessels

PAIN
a feeling of discomfort, suffering, or agony

SLEEP
the natural periodic suspension of consciousness during which the powers of the body are restored

REST
freedom from activity and labor

NUTRITION

the study of food's relationship to health; the act of providing food to nourish the body

ELIMINATION

the way the body rids itself of unusable food and fluid; the discharge of the waste products created by the body's metabolism

BOWEL

the intestine

BLADDER

the elastic muscular sac that collects urine before it leaves the body

URINE

fluid that contains water and the waste products of the body

GUIDE FOR PATIENT OBSERVATIONS *Continued*

Sleep and Rest *Continued*

- What is patients' physical appearance when their sleep and rest are disturbed? Are there pale dark circles under their eyes? Are their eyes puffy? Red?
- In children is there a reluctance to go to sleep?
- Do children awaken frequently during the night? Is a parent able to stay with children during the night?

Nutrition

- Do patients eat all meals (breakfast, lunch, and dinner)? How much of the meal did they eat?
- How are patients' appetite for food? Are they on a special diet?
- What are patients' food likes and dislikes?
- If present, are dentures loose or well fitting?
- Are patients permitted to eat food or drink fluids?
- Are patients nauseated or vomiting? Is there a history of choking? Do patients have difficulty swallowing? Is part of their throat paralyzed?
- Do infant or toddler patients suck on a nipple well enough to empty a bottle of formula?
- Are infant or toddler patients held while being fed a bottle?
- Can patients feed themselves?

Elimination

Bowel

- How often do patients pass a stool (have a **bowel** movement)? What is their daily pattern? Is there a history of diarrhea or constipation?
- Are patients able to control their bowels or is incontinence (loss of bowel or **bladder** control) present?
- Is the stool watery, soft, formed, or hard? Do patients feel pain when the bowels move?
- Is the color a normal brown? Or is it greenish, black (tarry), tan, clay-colored, or a dark brown resembling coffee grounds?
- Is a red color or mucus present in the stool?

Bladder

- How often do patients void (empty the bladder)?
- Is a sufficient quantity of urine voided? Is intake and output being measured?
- Are patients continent or incontinent? Does incontinence occur all the time or only at night?
- Is a urinary catheter present? Is it indwelling (inserted into the bladder) or applied externally (males)?
- Is the **urine** clear or cloudy? Does the color range from a light, straw-colored yellow to a dark amber? Is it red? Is mucus present?
- Does the urine have an odor? Is it a fruity or foul odor?

- Do patients tell you there is pain or burning when they void?
- For patients who are incontinent of bowel and/or bladder, are diapers (children) or incontinent pants (adults) checked and changed every 2 hours or as often as necessary?

Activity and Mobility (Ability to Move)

- Do patients have full range of motion? Do they move all four extremities? How often?
- Have passive range of motion exercises been ordered? To which extremity? How often?
- Can patients turn themselves in bed, or do they need assistance?
- Are patients independent in moving in and out of bed?
- Do patients need a cane, crutches, braces, or wheelchair to get around?
- Have patients had a limb amputated? If so, do they use hand, arm, or leg prostheses (artificial substitutes for missing body parts)?
- Do patients perform activities of daily living (ADLs) independently, or do they need some assistance? (ADLs include dressing, eating, toileting, and grooming.)
- Do patients tell you they have pain in the joints or pain when they move? Can they make a fist, bend the knee, or move about without pain?
- Do patients need assistance to ambulate? If so, how many people usually assist?
- How independent are toddlers or young patients?

Protection

Skin

- What is the condition of patients' **skin**, teeth, hair, and nails?
- Is patients' skin dry, moist, pink, or pale? Are reddened areas present over the bony prominences (areas that stick out)? Are any areas open or swollen?
- Is skin in the perineal area (the area around the scrotum and anus in males and the vulva and anus in females) cleansed whenever patients are incontinent?
- Are patients' teeth brushed regularly? Are dentures clean?
- Is hair clean and combed?
- Are fingernails and toenails clean and trimmed?
- Does the patient need assistance with hygiene?

Safety

- Do patients have a history of dizziness upon standing?
- Are patients strong enough to stand and walk without help? Are they aware of their weakened state?
- Can patients call for help by using the call signal?
- Do patients wear nonslip slippers or shoes?
- Are all side rails kept in a raised position when patients are weak, confused, sedated, or unsure of where they are?

SKIN
the protective outer covering of the body

Box continued on following page

GUIDE FOR PATIENT OBSERVATIONS *Continued*
Protection (Safety) *Continued*
• Does the health care institution require raised side rails for patients of a certain age? • Are crib rails for infants and young children kept in a raised position? • What do patients know about wheelchair safety? • Have **protective devices** been ordered? If applied, are they checked and released at 2-hour intervals? Is the condition of the skin observed at 2-hour intervals? Is toileting offered at 2-hour intervals?
Psychologic, Social, and Cultural Functions
• Do patients have a supportive family or friends? • Are patients able to cope with their situation in the health care institution? • Are infants and children comforted when their parents are not present? • Is religious support available?

PROTECTIVE DEVICE
a piece of equipment designed to prevent patients from harming themselves or others; formerly called a restraint

OBJECTIVE OBSERVATION

OBJECTIVE OBSERVATION
information gathered by using the five senses: sight, hearing, smell, taste, and touch

NAUSEA
an unpleasant, uncomfortable feeling in the stomach; may be experienced with vomiting

VOMITUS
results of vomiting; material ejected from the stomach through the mouth

An **objective observation** is an observation that you actually see, hear, touch, or smell (Figure 6–7). These are the kinds of observations that another person can observe the same as you. For example, think about patients who have **nausea** and pain. You might

- *see* them clenching their fists and making facial grimaces
- *see* **vomitus** (results of vomiting) if it occurs
- *hear* them moaning or catching their breath when moving
- *touch* their cool, clammy (damp) skin
- possibly *smell* the presence of vomitus when it occurs

These kinds of observations can be noted in patients of all ages. All objective observations should be reported to the nurse.

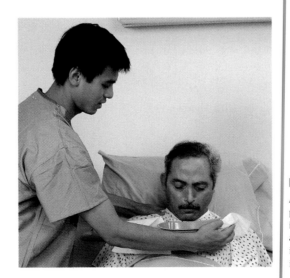

FIGURE 6–7
All five senses are used to observe the patient who is vomiting. Charting should include the time vomiting occurred; the amount, color, and consistency of the vomitus; and how the patient felt after vomiting.

OBJECTIVE OBSERVATIONS

Observation	Objective Description
Functioning of the Senses and Awareness	Pupils dilated
	Patient responds when called by name
Senses	Patient wearing glasses while watching television
	Patient responds to loud noises
	Foul odor present
Temperature	Skin is warm and dry
	Extra blankets on the patient's bed
	Patient sleeping with windows open
Functioning of the Circulation	
Respirations	Noisy, congested breathing
	Cough that produces thick yellow sputum
	10 respirations per minute
Pulse	Pulse full and bounding
	Pulse regular at 80 beats per minute
	Pulse below 60 or over 90
	Apical pulse, irregular at 50 beats per minute
Blood pressure	150/110, sitting
	162/116, standing
Comfort and Rest	Moaning, crying out
	Refusal to move
	Both fists clenched
	Infant awake all night
Nutrition	Ate 50% of breakfast
	Drank 3 ounces of formula
	Fed himself lunch
Elimination	
Bowel	Two bowel movements a day
	Clay-colored, soft stool
	Unable to move bowels while on the bedpan
Bladder	Voided 250 cc of clear, yellow urine
	Urine specimen sent to laboratory
	Red-tinged urine
Activity and Mobility	Walks unassisted
	Unable to comb own hair
	Turned and positioned every 2 hours
Protection	
Skin	Bathed self in tub
	Brushed dentures at bedtime
	Refused foot soak
Safety	Smoking in bed
	All side rails raised
	Call signal in place
Psychologic, Social, and Cultural Functions	Smiling
	Initiates conversation
	Establishes eye-to-eye contact

SUBJECTIVE OBSERVATION

SUBJECTIVE OBSERVATION
information gathered through the statements of another person, for example, "I am cold"

A **subjective observation** is anything patients *tell* you about themselves. When patients tell you, "I have pain," it is a subjective observation because they tell you about it—you cannot see, hear, touch, or smell patients' pain. When you report and record subjective observations, use the same words patients used.

CARING COMMENTS

Subjective observations are particularly difficult to obtain from infants and toddlers who cannot speak. Therefore, you must rely on your skills in obtaining objective observations of young patients. If an older patient is unable to communicate in words, use writing, sign language, or a communication board to get subjective information.

It is not appropriate to include your opinion or what you thought happened as subjective observations in the patient's chart.

SUBJECTIVE OBSERVATIONS	
Observation	**Subjective Statement**
Functioning of the Senses and Awareness	
Senses	"I've been in the hospital for three days."
	"I can't see much without my glasses."
	"I need a hearing aid to hear better."
	"I can't smell anything since this cold started."
Temperature	"I feel hot."
	"Give me a blanket for these chills."
	"Is it hot in this room?"
Functioning of the Circulation	
Respirations	"It's hard for me to breathe."
	"I feel like some oxygen would help me."
	"My nose is so stuffed up that I have to breathe through my mouth."
Pulse	"I can feel my heart racing."
	"My head throbs with every beat of my heart."
Blood pressure	"My high blood pressure causes some awful headaches."
	"When I get angry, I can feel my blood pressure go up."
Comfort and Sleep	"It feels like someone is standing on my chest."
	"It hurts all over."
	"My hands are sore when it's cold outside."
	"I didn't get any sleep last night."
Nutrition	"I love to eat."

	"These oranges have vitamin C in them."
	"I seem to have lost my appetite."
Elimination	
Bowel	"I always go to the bathroom after my morning coffee."
	"I'm regular as a clock."
	"I feel constipated today."
Bladder	"Sometimes I hesitate when I try to empty my bladder."
	"My urine never burns."
	"The catheter makes me feel like I need to go all the time."
Activity and Mobility	"I can't move around like I used to."
	"Look, I can jump!"
	"I can move my arms and legs very well."
Protection	
Skin	"My skin feels dry after I shower."
	"I need help wringing out the washcloth."
	"No, I don't care to take a bath every day."
Safety	"I thought I could walk by myself."
	"I don't have any slippers."
	"I'm fine; I don't need the side rails up."
Psychologic, Social, and Cultural Functions	"I feel as sad as I look."
	"My crying is under control."
	"Sunny days make me feel happy."

OBSERVATION IS AN ONGOING PROCESS

Observation is a continuous process. Learn to use all of your senses all of the time to make observations. Observe your patients during each contact with them. Patient contact occurs most frequently while you are bathing them, dressing them, assisting them with a bedpan or to the toilet, feeding them, or helping them ambulate (walk). Observe as much as you can about your patients, such as

- the condition and temperature of patients' skin
- patients' ability to move all extremities (arms, hands, legs, and feet)
- patients' ability to correctly identify people, time, and place
- patients' ability to answer questions correctly
- changes in patients' **behavior** or how they communicate

Remember to report all observations accurately and promptly.

BEHAVIOR
the manner of conducting oneself

REPORTING OBSERVATIONS

Reporting your observations helps other health care team members stay up to date on patients' conditions. Your observations are used by the nurse and the

REPORTING
giving a verbal account of a patient or an occurrence

TERMINOLOGY
a group of special terms

health care team to help make decisions about patients' nursing care. Reporting is a form of verbal communication that can be done quickly, and it allows a degree of expression that cannot be captured by the written word. Using appropriate **terminology** when reporting observations helps everyone understand and respond to patients' needs. The use of both objective and subjective reporting gives the most accurate picture of patient behaviors. For example, when a patient has vomited, the objective observations you would report would be the vomiting as well as vital sign measurements, amount of vomitus, a description of the vomitus, and whether the patient is sweating. An example of a subjective observation that you would report would be that the patient told you, "I feel so dizzy and nauseated."

ORAL REPORTING

Oral reporting is the quickest and simplest way to communicate facts about your patients. For each patient, care givers need to hear an oral report before they begin nursing care. When giving an oral report, you must be accurate and honest. A small pocket-size notebook in which you can make short notes can help you remember what you need to include in your report. When you receive an oral report from another care giver, be certain to clarify any information that you do not understand. Jotting down notes on a notepad helps you remember

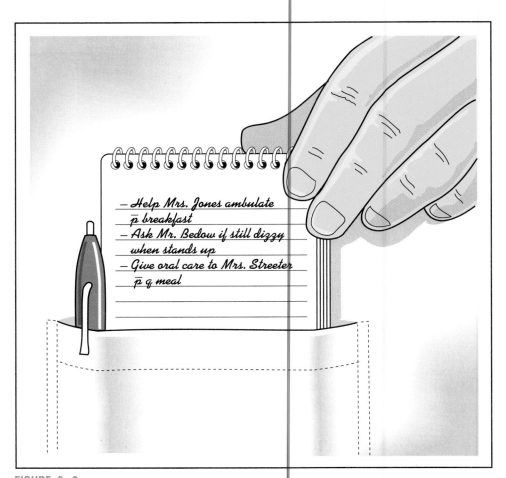

FIGURE 6-8

Write down information about your patients on a small notebook that fits in your pocket.

important facts when you write down the plan for the nursing care you are responsible for giving (Figure 6–8).

CHANGE OF SHIFT REPORT

The **change of shift report** is an oral report given by the registered nurse to care givers at the beginning and end of each shift. It is given for the following reasons:

- The patient's status is communicated to the incoming shift of health team workers.
- The nurse needs your observations to help give a complete report about your patients' activities and behaviors during your shift.
- The health care workers who receive the change of shift report use the information to help them understand patients and their condition better and to give nursing care according to patients' needs.

Some health care institutions encourage nursing assistants to do "walking rounds." During this time, the care givers going off shift and the care givers coming on shift communicate and coordinate their patient care.

CHANGE OF SHIFT REPORT
a report of a patient's condition and needs, given when care givers change shift, to ensure continuity of care

PATIENT CARE PLANS

The **care plan** is a tool developed by the registered nurse and the health care team (Figure 6–9). It is used to communicate to care givers the nursing care each patient needs. Each institution designs its own care plans, and the information is updated as often as necessary. It is often referred to as a "Kardex" (Kardex is a trade name) care plan because all written care plans are kept together in a special file for easy access.

CARE PLAN
a written tool developed by a registered nurse to communicate and document a plan of care for an individual patient

CARING COMMENT

When you need quick up-to-date information about your patient's care, check the patient's care plan.

RECORDING OBSERVATIONS

When you record observations, you are producing a written record of your patients' statements and behaviors. **Recording** observations is known as "charting." **Narrative charting** is a description of information you observe and the statements patients tell you about themselves. Narrative charting is like writing a small story about patients and their concerns.

SAMPLE: For an 8:00 a.m. entry, you might write: States "I had a good night's sleep." BP 120/80, T 98.6, P 72, R 16. Awake, alert, responds to questions appropriately. Transfers OOB with assistance of one. Ate 100% of soft diet for breakfast. Voided 350 cc clear yellow urine in bedside commode. (You end with your signature and title.)

Chronologic charting is a method used to record events as they happen in time. For example, your first entry at 8:00 a.m. might state that the patient was awake, sitting in bed, and taking nothing by mouth. The next entry at 10:00 a.m. might note that the patient took in 300 ml of apple juice. Each entry is timed,

RECORDING
writing down information about a patient or an occurrence

NARRATIVE CHARTING
a written description of information observed and patients' statements about themselves

CHRONOLOGIC CHARTING
a method of charting in which events are recorded according to the sequence in which they happened

PLAN OF CARE FOR RESIDENT

Patient's Name _____

1. BEHAVIOR - check behaviors as per assessment and write Freq.

- ☐ AGITATION
- ☐ DEPRESSION
- ☐ FORGETFULNESS
- ☐ ANGER
- ☐ DISRUPTIVE
- ☐ CONFUSION

DISORIENTATION TO:
- ☐ Time
- ☐ Person
- ☐ Place

- ☐ COMBATIVE
- ☐ HOSTILE
- ☐ WANDERER

DANGEROUS TO:
- ☐ Self
- ☐ Others
- ☐ Manipulative
- ☐ Verbally Abusive
- ☐ Withdrawn
- ☐ Antisocial
- ☐ Other _____ (Describe inside)

Describe behavior to be modified &/or controlled: _____

Intervention:
- ☐ R/O (Describe inside)
- ☐ Reassurance (Describe inside)
- ☐ Positive reinforcement of appropriate behavior
- ☐ Physical Restraint for ☐ safety and/or ☐ behavior management is ordered.
  - A.☐ Pelvic   B.☐ Mitt   E.☐ Chest/Vest G.☐ Roll Belt
  - B.☐ Wrist   D.☐ Gerichair F.☐ Waist   H.☐

Needed due to _____
- Will be released q 2h for 10-20 min per nursing staff and need will be reassessed.
- Resident checked q ½h while in restraint.   Freq. _____
- ☐ Behavior medication is used: Refer to med sheet.
- ☐ Side rails up while in bed. Freq.☐ _____ PRN ☐ _____ HS ☐ _____ CONT. ☐

2. PERSONAL HYGIENE

SERVICE	DESCRIBE WHAT IS DONE BY NURSING STAFF	FREQ.

COMPLETE BATH
- ☐ TUB
- ☐ BED
- ☐ SHOWER
- ☐ INDEPENDENT
  - ☐ N.A. will wash and dry entire body
  - ☐ N.A. will wash & dry
  - ☐ N.A. will assist by ☐ helping in/out tub/shower
  - ☐ preparing H₂O ☐ getting soap & linens x _____ weekly
  - ☐ N.A. will supervise

PARTIAL BATH
- ☐ N.A. will wash and dry ☐ face ☐ hands ☐ underarms qd
- ☐ N.A. will prepare H₂O, soap, washcloth & towel & PRN
- ☐ INDEPENDENT ☐ N.A. will ☐ supervise ☐ assist

PERI CARE
- ☐ N.A. will wash, rinse, and dry perineal area. qd
- ☐ N.A. will prepare H₂O, soap, washcloth & towel. & PRN
- ☐ INDEPENDENT ☐ N.A. will ☐ supervise ☐ assist

ORAL CARE ☐ IND.
- ☐ N.A. will ☐ prepare articles for resident to do qd
  - own oral care and/or will ☐ supervise ☐ assist & PRN
- ☐ No Teeth ☐ N.A. will clean with toothbrush, toothpaste and rinse
- ☐ Dentures ☐ N.A. will clean inside mouth and rinse
- ☐ upper ☐ lower ☐ N.A. will clean with denture cleanser and rinse
- ☐ Special mouth care _____

HAIR CARE ☐ IND.
- ☐ N.A. will wash & dry hair q _____
- ☐ S ☐ A ☐ N.A. will comb hair q _____
- ☐ Beautician will wash & dry hair q _____

SHAVING ☐ IND.
- ☐ not applicable
  - ☐ N.A. will assemble shaving articles
  - ☐ and shave face and/or will ☐ supervise ☐ assist q _____

NAIL CARE ☐ IND.
- ☐ N.A. will clean and/or trim fingernails q _____
  - after assembling equipment. & PRN
- ☐ Podiatrist visits q _____

THERAPY
- ☐ Therapist ☐ Rehabaide Freq. _____
  - (see POT & IHP)

DRESSING ☐ IND.

- ☐ N.A. will completely dress q AM

UNDRESSING ☐ IND.
- ☐ N.A. will completely undress q PM
- ☐ N.A. will ☐ put in/take out dentures ☐ put on/take off glasses ☐ put in/out hearing aid
- ☐ N.A. will ☐ zip/unzip ☐ button/unbutton clothes
- ☐ place arms into/out of clothing ☐ put on/take off shoes and/or stockings
- ☐ tie/untie gown ☐ supervise ☐ choose clothing
- ☐ remove dirty clothes

3. EATING

Diet: _____
- ☐ Nourishments: Type _____ Freq. _____
- ☐ INDEPENDENT
- ☐ N.A. will supervise as resident feeds self and will assist
  Due to _____
  - ☐ cut meat ☐ butter bread ☐ open packages
  - ☐ pour liquids ☐ place utensils within reach
  - ☐ Adaptive device is used. ☐ Nursing Staff applies
    Due to _____
- ☐ N.A. will spoon feed resident due to _____ Freq. _____

☐ TUBE FEEDING will be given per nurse. This will be documented on Treatment Sheet
- Freq. _____ TUBE SIZE: _____
- TYPE ☐ Nasogastric ☐ Gastrostomy ☐ J-Tube
- DATE OF INITIAL INSERTION _____

4. MOBILITY

Wt Bearing Capability
- ☐ Full R L ☐ Partial R L ☐ Non R L
- ☐ Resident walks independently - no staff intervention.

The following ambulatory device is used.
- ☐ W/C ☐ Walker ☐ Cane ☐ Prosthesis ☐ Special shoes
- ☐ Crutches ☐ Brace ☐ Splint ☐ Gerichair ☐ Quad Cane
- FREQ. _____
- ☐ Needs nursing staff assist in use of equipment in order to ambulate. Freq. _____
- ☐ Nursing staff will assist by:
  - ☐ Assisting to get out of bed/chair. Freq. _____
  - ☐ Supporting resident to stand. Freq. _____
  - ☐ Balancing and guiding resident. Freq. _____
  - ☐ Nursing staff will walk resident Freq. _____
- ☐ Resident is capable of ambulation but refuses due to mental status.
- ☐ Resident is unable to ambulate due to:
  - ☐ N.A. will pivot from bed to chair Freq. _____ and return.
  - ☐ N.A. will lift from bed to chair Freq. _____ and return.
  - ☐ Hoyer Lift is used by nursing staff. Freq. _____
- ☐ Range of motion Active/Passive Exercise will be given per nursing staff to prevent
  - ☐ Contractures ☐ Loss of muscle tone To: _____ Freq. _____
  - ☐ Loss of joint range of motion Freq. q2h
- ☐ Turn in bed and position per N.A. will be done
- ☐ INDEPENDENT TURN ☐ Reposition q2h in chair.

5. APPLIANCES

- ( ) Sheepskin chair/bed
- ( ) Water mattress/cushion
- ( ) Air mattress chair/bed
- ( ) Elastic hose
- ( ) Prosthesis
- ( ) Elbow/heel pad
- ( ) Headgear/splint/cast/brace to _____
- ( ) Other _____

Gerichair for positioning ★
Waist restraint for positioning ★
Posey vest for positioning ★
OTHER _____

Above appliance is needed due to _____
★ ☐ Will be released q2h for 10 min. per nursing staff and need will be reassessed.
Resident checked q½ hr while in restraint.

SPEECH
- ☐ Normal
- ☐ Impaired due to _____

VISION
- ☐ Normal
- ☐ Glasses
- ☐ Blind Left _____ Right _____
- ☐ Other
- ☐ Impaired

HEARING
- ☐ Normal ☐ Impaired Right _____ Left _____
- ☐ Hearing Aid Right _____ Left _____
- ☐ Other

SENSATION
(Paralysis? Indicate where) _____

6. DRESSING/NON-ROUTINE SKIN CARE — See tx sheet.

All care will be given by nurse.

7. INCONTINENCE/CATHETERS

Resident is continent of ☐ Bladder ☐ Bowels
- ☐ Resident is independent in toileting
- ☐ External ☐ SUPRA PUBIC ☐ Indwelling catheter
  - Size # _____ Date of insert _____
- Is needed due to _____
- Change: _____
- ☐ Irrigations will be done by nurse Freq. _____ Type _____ Amt. _____
- ☐ Catheter care will be done by nursing staff. Freq. _____
- ☐ ✓ color, consistency, patency, volume of urine, ☐ wash with soap & H₂O.
- ☐ Swab Meatus c̄ Betadine ☐ Other _____ Freq. _____ ☐ Only at noc.

Resident is incontinent of ☐ Bladder Freq. _____
  ☐ Bowels Freq. _____
- ☐ Peri care will be given after each incontinency with cleansing of perineal area per N.A.
- ☐ Toilet in advance of need per N.A. q _____ as resident cannot state need to use the bedpan or bathroom due to:
  - ☐ Decreased cognition of bodily functions. ☐ Decreased parasympathetic innervation.
  - ☐ Decreased cognition awareness. ☐ Other _____
- ☐ Resident will be toileted q2h to minimize incontinence.
- ☐ Resident uses the following ☐ BR ☐ Urinal ☐ Bedpan ☐ Beside commode
- ☐ Bladder/Bowel training program ⊕
  - Date started _____ Date finished _____
  - Schedule _____

8. (ENEMAS, DOUCHES, etc.)

SERVICE	FREQ.
Manual removal	
Enema	
Douche	

9./10. RESPIRATORY THERAPY - use will be documented on Treatment Sheet

All care will be given per nurse.

TYPE	FREQ.	DUE TO
☐ TRACH CARE		REASON FOR TREATMENT
☐ SUCTIONING		
☐ OXYGEN		
☐ IPPB		

11. OSTOMY CARE:

- ☐ Ostomy Care will be done by nurse. Describe _____
  - Freq. _____ Type ☐ Colostomy ☐ Ileostomy ☐ Ureterostomy
- Describe stoma: _____
- ☐ Ostomy irrigation Type: _____ Freq. _____

12. INTRAVENOUS/SUBCUTANEOUS FLUIDS/HYPERALIMENTATION - will be recorded on the Parental Flowsheet.

SHORT TERM PROBLEMS AND GOALS
OVERALL PLAN OF CARE

Patient's Name

DATE IDENTIFIED	DEPT.	PROBLEM/NEED	GOAL/EXPECTED OUTCOME	INTERVENTION/APPROACH	TIME	SIGNATURE	RESOLVED	DATE SIGNATURE

FIGURE 6–9

Care plan for a patient in a nursing home. (Courtesy of Greenwood Pharmacy, Sharon, PA.)

and the entries are recorded in sequence. Your signature and title are placed at the end of the recording.

The health care institution in which you are employed will tell you what kind of charting is required during orientation. If you are not familiar with the kind of charting required, you should ask for help so that you can chart correctly.

Both subjective and objective terms are required in recording. Medical terminology and abbreviations should be used to save time reading and writing. Over time, care givers learn what is important information to include on the change of shift report.

The change of shift report is written as well as verbal. Important observations you write on this form might include

- present vital signs
- ability to perform ADLs

Pt. Name: *Art Holland*	**Pt. Name:** *Joe Harte*
Room #: *240*	Room #: *246*
Age: *81*	Age: *65*
Allergies: *NKA*	Allergies: *Aspirin*
Diagnosis: *Fx Hip (L)*	Diagnosis: *Fx Hip (R)*
Physician: *Cotton*	Physician: *Cotton*
Treatments: *Help c̄ bath / No walking*	Treatments: *Self care / U disq*
Tests: *↑ GI*	Tests: *—*
Diet: *Cl liq*	Diet: *Reg. -ate all*
I & O: *750 cc in / 675 cc out*	I & O: *—*
Vitals: *99⁸ 92 16 160/86*	Vitals: *98⁸ 88 20 148/90*
Observations: *Oriented "Pain in (L) hip" / Lying flat. Side rails ↑*	Observations: *Ambulated 50 ft. c̄ assist of 1*
Pt. Name: *Harriet Walk*	**Pt. Name:** *Margery Masher*
Room #: *247*	Room #: *248*
Age: *48*	Age: *72*
Allergies: *Mold*	Allergies: *Penecillin*
Diagnosis: *Dizziness*	Diagnosis: *Abd. pain*
Physician: *Lee*	Physician: *Carver*
Treatments: *Safety prec.*	Treatments: *Self-care*
Tests: *X-ray chest — done am.*	Tests: *BaE*
Diet: *NPO*	Diet: *NPO*
I & O: *90 cc in p̄ XR./400 cc out*	I & O: *400 cc out*
Vitals: *97⁶ 86 18 140/92*	Vitals: *100⁴ 102 20 150/85*
Observations: *"Not dizzy today" Slept all am. CXR done*	Observations: *Grasping abd., knees bent. / Vomited 50 cc cl. yellow XT.*

FIGURE 6–10

A sample preprinted form on which to write down information received during an oral report on your patients.

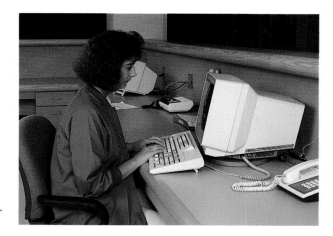

FIGURE 6-11
Using a computer to record patient information.

- dietary status
- scheduled treatments (for example, dressing change) or procedures (such as going for x-rays)

Often a preprinted form is provided for you to use (Figure 6-10).

As discussed earlier, graphic recording is generally reserved for recording the patient's vital signs, appetite, bowel movements, and intake and output. Graphic recording provides a quick visual reference about the patient's range of vital sign measurements over a period of 5 or more days.

FUNCTIONAL RECORDING

Functional recording is a method of recording patients' activities during each shift. This type of recording is usually done in a special tablet or binder. For example, nursing homes may keep a daily record of each patient's bowel movements in a separate place.

COMPUTER RECORDING

Computer recording is another method sometimes used to keep patient records. In some institutions, you may have access to a computer to record information about your patients (Figure 6-11).

COMPUTER
a device that electronically stores, retrieves, and processes information

ACCIDENT OR INCIDENT REPORT

Recording unusual events may require that you fill out a special form called an **accident or incident report** (Figure 6-12). If you are uncertain about completing an accident/incident report, make sure you ask the nurse in charge for directions. Examples of **accident** and **incident** events include

- any injury (for example, a fall) to the patient, a visitor, or yourself
- loss of a patient's personal belongings
- spilling of hot liquids (such as coffee or soup) on a patient
- not following physician's orders (such as allowing the patient to ambulate when the physician has ordered bed rest)
- performing skills incorrectly (for example, measuring vital signs without using the skills you were taught)
- allowing the patient to "wander" (this can occur when a patient is disoriented [confused]) or to "elope" (leave the nursing unit). A hospitalized

ACCIDENT/INCIDENT REPORT
facts written on a report to describe the event that caused an accident or injury

ACCIDENT
unforeseen or unplanned event
INCIDENT
an event, an unusual event when the result is likely to cause an accident

ACCIDENT/INCIDENT REPORT

Name _____ Sex _____ Age _____ Patient _____

_____ Visitor _____

_____ Employee _____

Date _____ Time _____ Other _____

Location of Incident _____

Name(s) of Person(s) Present _____

_____

_____

Brief Description of the Accident/Incident _____

_____

_____

_____

_____

_____

Signature of Person Making Report

_____.

Report by Examining Physician _____

_____

_____

_____

_____

Diagnosis and Treatment _____

_____

_____

_____

Referred For Further Treatment _____

_____

Signature of Supervisor

_____

If employee, to Health Service at _____

Disposition _____

_____

_____

Signature of Risk Mgr.

_____

Patient Stamp   Date _____

FIGURE 6–12
Accident/incident report form.

patient generally stays on the unit unless the physician writes an order to allow the patient to leave the unit for another part of the institution.

You must fill out an incident report for an accident or incident, regardless of whether you caused it. Any situation that violates a patient's rights should also be recorded on an incident report. The following behaviors will help you maintain patients' rights:

- Keep all information confidential.
- Identify the patient properly before you give care.

- Perform all procedures as you were taught.
- Remove safety hazards whenever you identify them.
- Keep patients safe when they cannot do so for themselves.
- Report all malfunctioning equipment to the appropriate department of the institution.
- Always use the safety practices you were taught.
- Report all errors you make to the nurse or supervisor.

Fill out the incident report as soon as possible after the unsafe situation occurs. Give facts only. You are asked for:

- the names of the people involved in the occurrence
- the date, time, and place of the occurrence
- a description of the event
- the steps taken to correct the situation

Report each situation to the nurse, who will direct you in filling out the incident report. Complete the incident report as thoroughly and factually as possible and give it to the nurse or supervisor.

RISK MANAGER

The person assigned to keep track of accident/incident reports is often called the *risk manager*. The risk manager uses the information from these reports to help pinpoint problem areas in the institution. The institution uses this information to take steps to prevent another accident or incident. The institution may do so by teaching special courses. For example, if the risk manager notices a number of back injuries among care givers, a course to teach the basics about body mechanics might be offered, or if a number of patient injuries occur from falls, a course in safety might be considered.

CARING COMMENT

A accident/incident report is not used to punish care givers. It is a report that is used to help all health team members and patients stay healthy and injury free.

DATE AND TIME OF THE RECORDING

An important part of recording is specifying the date and time of the recording. Each time you make a note or record on an official document or form, you should place the correct data in the appropriate column.

Some institutions use military time to record and report information instead of clock time. The abbreviations a.m. and p.m. are not used with military time. The following chart shows the conversion of military time to clock time.

THE CONVERSION OF MILITARY TIME TO CLOCK TIME	
Military Time (Hour)	**Clock Time (O'clock)**
0100	1:00 a.m.
0200	2:00 a.m.
0300	3:00 a.m.

Box continued on following page

THE CONVERSION OF MILITARY TIME TO CLOCK TIME *Continued*

Military Time (Hour)	Clock Time (O'clock)
0400	4:00 a.m.
0500	5:00 a.m.
0600	6:00 a.m.
0700	7:00 a.m.
0800	8:00 a.m.
0900	9:00 a.m.
1000	10:00 a.m.
1100	11:00 a.m.
1200	12:00 noon
1300	1:00 p.m.
1400	2:00 p.m.
1500	3:00 p.m.
1600	4:00 p.m.
1700	5:00 p.m.
1800	6:00 p.m.
1900	7:00 p.m.
2000	8:00 p.m.
2100	9:00 p.m.
2200	10:00 p.m.
2300	11:00 p.m.
2400	12:00 Midnight

For time not on the hour, use the number of actual minutes in place of the two 00's:

0115	1:15 a.m.
1030	10:30 a.m.
1545	3:45 p.m.
2155	9:55 p.m.

CHAPTER WRAP-UP

- The observations you make each day contribute to better nursing care of patients. You should become a keen observer and learn to report and record useful information about your patients.
  Observations can be subjective or objective.
  Subjective observations reflect what the patient says, while objective observations are what you actually see, hear, touch, taste, or smell.
- Examples of reporting include
  giving and receiving reports about patients
  change of shift reports
- Examples of recording include
  change of shift reports
  graphic charting
  functional charting
  computer recording

REVIEW QUESTIONS

1. Patients' feelings are subjective observations. Give three examples of subjective observations.

2. Objective observations involve use of the five senses. Give an example of an observation for each of the senses.

3. What is the difference between reporting and recording your observations?

4. How would you report and record changes in your patients' behavior using subjective terms? Objective terms?

5. What information is included in a written change of shift report?

ACTIVITY CORNER

Set aside about 10 minutes to sit and talk with another person. While you are talking, use your senses to gather important information. Write down all of your observations in the first column. Put a check in the second column if the observation is subjective; put a check in the third column if the observation is objective.

	Person's Statement (Subjective)	Observed Using My Senses (Objective)
_____	_____	_____
_____	_____	_____
_____	_____	_____
_____	_____	_____
_____	_____	_____
_____	_____	_____

Add more lines if you need them. Ask a classmate to check your work. Do you both agree that you checked the correct column? Review pages 115–117 if you have difficulty identifying observations.

Many agencies use military time. This activity will help you learn military quickly.

Write down your activities for a busy morning or afternoon or use the suggested activities below. List the times using the normal clock time in the first column. Convert to military time in the second column.

Hint: Use four digits for military time. For example, 1200 military time is 12:00 noon in clock time.

Activity	Clock Time	Military Time
Wake up	_____	_____
Leaving home	_____	_____
Eating lunch	_____	_____
Taking a break	_____	_____
Catching the bus	_____	_____
Cooking dinner	_____	_____
Taking a shower	_____	_____
Going to bed	_____	_____

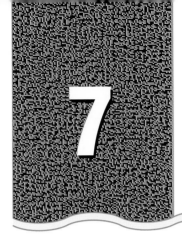

7 Understanding Medical Words

Objectives

AFTER YOU COMPLETE THIS CHAPTER, YOU WILL BE ABLE TO:

Identify common medical terminology and abbreviations.

Define the terms *prefix, root word,* and *suffix.*

State the meanings of the prefixes, suffixes, and roots commonly used in medical terminology.

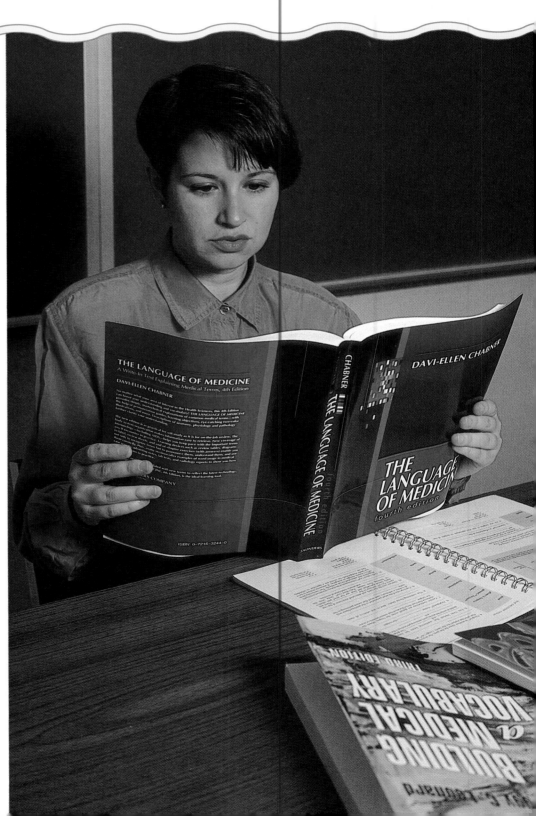

Overview By learning and using the medical terminology and abbreviations presented in this chapter, you will make the task of communicating with other health care team members easier for yourself. When you understand what the different parts of words mean, you can figure out the meanings of new words you see or hear.

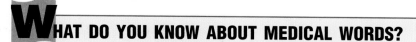

WHAT DO YOU KNOW ABOUT MEDICAL WORDS?

Here are four statements about medical words. Consider them to test your current ideas about medical terminology. If you think the statement is true, circle the T; if you think the statement is false, circle the F. Change the false statements to make them true.

1. T   F   A suffix is used at the beginning of a word.
2. T   F   The word ending *-itis* means "inflammation."
3. T   F   An abbreviation is a shortened word or group of words.
4. T   F   The abbreviation for complete blood count is CBC.

ANSWERS

1. **False.** A suffix is used at the end of a word; a prefix is used at the beginning of the word. To remember this, remember that *p* comes before *s* in the alphabet.
2. **True.** Any medical term with the ending *itis* means that inflammation is present in that place. For example, *appendicitis* means that inflammation is present in the appendix.
3. **True.** The definition of *abbreviate* is to make short.
4. **True.** CBC is the abbreviation for *complete blood count.*

MEDICAL TERMINOLOGY

MEDICAL TERMINOLOGY
the group of special terms used in the medical field

Health care workers communicate in a special language known as **medical terminology.** Medical terminology includes words or terms that describe the structure (anatomy) and function (physiology) of the human body, diseases, and treatments for diseases. You are probably already familiar with many common medical terms.

You must use proper medical terminology when you report and record information about your patients. With practice and experience, you will use medical terminology with greater understanding and confidence.

CARING COMMENT

Keep in mind that not all patients are familiar with medical terminology. Use simple terms when you interact with patients and their families.

WORD ELEMENTS

WORD ELEMENTS
parts of words

Medical terms are made up of **word elements.** When word elements are combined, words are formed. To learn about medical terminology, you need to understand and recognize the word elements. Each medical term is made up of one or more of the following word elements:

Prefix
Root word
Suffix

Prefixes

PREFIX
a word element placed before a root word that helps to describe the root word

A **prefix** is a word element placed before a root word that helps to describe the root word. The following diagram shows how a prefix is combined with a root word to form a new word.

Prefix	+	Root Word	=	New Word
tachy (fast)	+	*cardia* (heart)	=	*tachycardia* (a fast heart rate)
tachy (fast)	+	*pnea* (breathing)	=	*tachypnea* (fast breathing or respirations)

The more knowledge you have of prefixes, the more medical terminology you will be able to learn and understand. The chart of common prefixes gives examples of how to use these prefixes to make new words.

COMMON PREFIXES AND THEIR MEANINGS		
Prefix	**Meaning**	**New Word and Its Meaning**
a, an-	absence of, without	**a**symptomatic—without symptoms
ab-	away from	**ab**duct—take away from the middle part of something

COMMON PREFIXES AND THEIR MEANINGS *Continued*

Prefix	Meaning	New Word and Its Meaning
ad-	toward	**ad**duct—bring toward the middle part of something
ano-	pertains to anus and rectum	**ano**scope—instrument used to examine the anal canal
ante-	before	**ante**febrile—before a fever starts
anti-	effective against	**anti**anxiety—effective against anxiety
arterio-	pertains to arteries	**arterio**pathy—disease of an artery
auto-	self	**auto**clave—self-locking device that sterilizes something
bi-	two	**bi**lateral—having two sides
bio-	life	**bio**logy—study of living organisms
brady-	slow	**brady**cardia—slow heartbeat
cardio-	pertains to heart	**cardio**therapy—treatment of heart disease
circum-	around	**circum**duction—moving the arm or leg around in a circular motion
contra-	against, opposed	**contra**ception—prevention of conception
derma-	pertains to skin	**derma**titis—inflammation of the skin
dis-	away from	**dis**sect—cut away from
dys-	difficult, impaired	**dys**pnea—difficult breathing
en-	in, into	**en**ema—introducing fluid into the rectum
endo-	inside	**endo**cardial—inside the heart
eryth-	red	**eryth**rocyte—red blood cell
ex-	out, away from	**ex**cise—take away by cutting
gastro-	pertains to stomach	**gastro**enteritis—inflammation of the lining of the stomach and intestine
hemi-	half	**hemi**plegia—paralysis of one side of the body
hyper-	high, too much	**hyper**tension—high blood pressure
hypo-	low, less than	**hypo**tension—low blood pressure
inter-	between	**inter**vascular—between blood vessels
intra-	within	**intra**venous—within a vein
macro-	large	**macro**mastia—large breasts
mal-	bad, illness	**mal**ady—disease or illness
mega-	large	**mega**colon—enlarged colon
micro-	small	**micro**embolus—very small embolus (blood clot)
muco-	pertains to mucous membrane	**muco**lytic—something that destroys mucus
neo-	new	**neo**nate—newborn

Box continued on following page

COMMON PREFIXES AND THEIR MEANINGS *Continued*		
Prefix	**Meaning**	**New Word and Its Meaning**
neuro-	pertains to nerves	**neur**itis—inflammation of a nerve
olig-	scant	**olig**uria—scant amount of urine
patho-	pertains to disease	**patho**logist—specialist who studies diseases
peri-	around	**peri**oral—around the mouth
poly-	many, much	**poly**dipsia—excessive (much) thirst
post-	after	**post**natal—happening after birth
pre-	before	**pre**natal—happening before birth
retro-	backward, behind	**retro**lental—behind the lens of the eye
semi-	half	**semi**lunar—shaped like a half-moon
sub-	under, less than	**sub**normal—less than normal
super-	above, in addition to	**super**infection—infection in addition to an existing infection
supra-	above, over	**supra**spinal—above the spine
tachy-	fast, rapid	**tachy**pnea—rapid breathing
trans-	across, through	**trans**dermal—through the skin
ven-	pertains to veins	**ven**ipuncture—puncture of a vein

ROOT WORDS

ROOT WORD

the part of a word that indicates the disease or condition

The meaning of a medical term is found in the **root word.** The root word usually indicates the name of a disease or condition, as shown in the chart on the next page. You can combine a root word with a prefix, a suffix, or another root word to make new word combinations.

A vowel is the connector used to link two root words or a root word and a suffix. The vowel, called a combining vowel, helps make the newly combined words easier to pronounce. The most common combining vowel is *o.* For example, ger*o*ntology is the study of the elderly. Occasionally, *i* is used to link words, as in the following word diagram.

Root Word	+	Combining Vowel	+	Root Word	=	New Word
cyst	+	*i*	+	*form*	=	*cystiform* (resembling a cyst)
dent	+	*i*	+	*meter*	=	*dentimeter* (instrument for measuring teeth)
ven	+	*i*	+	*puncture*	=	*venipuncture* (puncture of the vein)

COMMON ROOT WORDS WITH THEIR COMBINING VOWELS

Root Word and Combining Vowel	Meaning
abdomin(o)	abdomen
aden(o)	gland
adren(o)	adrenal gland
arteri(o)	artery
arthr(o)	joint
bronch(o)	bronchus, bronchi
cardi(o)	heart
cerebr(o)	brain
cephal(o)	head
chol(e), chol(o)	bile
chondr(o)	cartilage
col(o)	colon, large intestine
cost(o)	rib
crani(o)	skull
cyan(o)	blue
cyst(o)	bladder, cyst
cyt(o)	cell
dent(o)	tooth
derm(a)	skin
duoden(o)	duodenum
encephal(o)	brain
enter(o)	intestine
fibr(o)	fiber, fibrous
gastr(o)	stomach
geront(o)	old age
gloss(o)	tongue
gyn(e), gynec(o)	woman
hem(a), hem(o), hemat(o)	blood
hepat(o)	liver
hyster(o)	uterus
ile(o)	ileum
lapar(o)	abdomen, flank, loin
laryng(o)	larynx
mamm(o)	breast
mast(o)	breast
men(o)	menstruation
my(o)	muscle
myel(o)	muscle
necr(o)	death
nephr(o)	kidney
neur(o)	nerve
ocul(o)	eye
oophor(o)	ovary
ophthalm(o)	eye
orth(o)	straight
oste(o)	bone
ot(o)	ear
path(o)	disease
ped(o)	child, foot
pharyng(o)	pharynx

Box continued on following page

COMMON ROOT WORDS WITH THEIR COMBINING VOWELS *Continued*

Root Word and Combining Vowel	Meaning
phleb(o)	vein
pneum(o)	lung, air, gas
proct(o)	rectum
psych(o)	mind
pulm(o)	lung
py(o)	pus
rect(o)	rectum
rhin(o)	nose
salping(o)	uterine or eustachian tube
splen(o)	spleen
sten(o)	narrow, constricted
stern(o)	sternum
stomat(o)	mouth
therm(o)	heat
thorac(o)	chest
thromb(o)	clot, thrombus
thyr(o)	thyroid
trache(o)	trachea
urethr(o)	urethra
urin(o)	urine
ur(o)	urine, urinary tract, urination
uter(o)	uterus
vas(o)	blood vessel
ven(o)	vein
vertebr(o)	spine, vertebrae

SUFFIXES

SUFFIX

a word element that, when placed after a root word, creates a new word

A **suffix** is placed at the end of a root word to form a new word. Suffixes usually indicate some action on or condition of the root word.

COMMON SUFFIXES

Suffix	Meaning
-algia	pain
-asis	condition, usually abnormal
-centesis	puncture and aspiration (sucking out) of
-ectasis	dilation, stretching
-ectomy	excision, removal of
-emia	presence of blood
-genic	producing, causing
-gram	record
-graph	diagram
-ism	condition
-itis	inflammation
-logy	study of
-lysis	destruction of
-megaly	enlargement

COMMON SUFFIXES *Continued*

Suffix	Meaning
-meter	measuring instrument
-ology	study of
-oma	tumor
-orrhaphy	surgical repair
-osis	disease
-ostomy	creation of an opening
-otomy	incision, cutting into
-pathy	disease
-penia	lack, deficiency of
-phobia	exaggerated fear
-plast	surgical repair
-plegia	paralysis
-pnea	breathing
-ptosis	falling, sagging, dropping down
-rrhage, rrhagia	excessive flow
-rrhaphy	stitching
-rrhea	profuse flow, discharge
-scope	examination instrument
-scopy	examination using a scope
-stasis	maintaining a constant level
-uria	condition of the urine

After you break apart the medical term, translate the suffix first. If the root word ends with a consonant, use a vowel to combine the word. The root *hem* uses an *a* or an *e* to link up with a suffix. H*ematest* is a common test for blood in the stool.

If the root word ends in a vowel and the suffix begins with a vowel, drop the vowel at the end of the root word to link the two, as in the word diagram that follows:

Root Word	+	Suffix	=	New Word
arthr(o) (joint)	+	*ectomy* (surgical removal of)	=	*arthrectomy* (surgical removal of a joint)
enter(o) (intestine)	+	*itis* (inflammation)	=	*enteritis* (inflammation of the intestines)

The following chart shows examples of how to use a suffix to form a new word.

USING COMMON SUFFIXES TO FORM NEW WORDS

Suffix	Example	Meaning
-ectomy	*appendectomy*	surgical removal of the appendix
	gastrectomy	surgical removal of the stomach or part of it
	vasectomy	removal of the vas deferens
-itis	*phlebitis*	inflammation of a vein

Box continued on following page

USING COMMON SUFFIXES TO FORM NEW WORDS *Continued*		
Suffix	**Example**	**Meaning**
-plegia	*rhinitis*	inflammation of the nose
	tracheitis	inflammation of the trachea
	hemiplegia	paralysis of one side of the body
	paraplegia	paralysis of the legs or lower part of the body
	quadriplegia	paralysis of all four limbs

COMBINING WORD ELEMENTS

Word elements are combined to form medical terms. The following general rules will help you interpret and understand medical terminology.

- A root word can be combined with another root word and with a prefix or a suffix.
- A prefix always combines with a root word and is never used alone.
- A suffix always combines with a root word or words and is never used alone.

USING ROOTS TO MAKE NEW WORDS		
Combination	**Example**	**Meaning**
Two Roots		
cardio + pulmonary	*cardiopulmonary*	pertaining to the heart and lungs
cardio + vascular	*cardiovascular*	pertaining to the heart and blood vessels
Prefix and Root		
pre + natal	*prenatal*	preceding birth
pre + operative	*preoperative*	preceding an operation
Root and Suffix		
cardio + logy	*cardiology*	study of heart disease
cardio + megaly	*cardiomegaly*	enlargement of the heart
cardi + itis	*carditis*	inflammation of the heart

When you hear a new word, write it down and try to break it into parts. First, identify the root word and try to recall what it means. Then, look at the prefix and/or suffix and try to figure out what each means. Put the meanings of all the parts together for the meaning of the new word.

ABBREVIATIONS

ABBREVIATION

a shortened form of a word or phrase used in place of the word or phrase

To "abbreviate" means to "make short." Thus, **abbreviation** is the making a word or a group of words shorter. The use of abbreviations aids in quick communication among health care team members. It is much easier and quicker to say or write "BM" than to say or write "bowel movement." Each health care institution has a list of accepted abbreviations. Always make sure the abbreviations you use are on the accepted list at your place of employment.

COMMONLY USED MEDICAL ABBREVIATIONS

Abbreviation	Meaning
$\bar{a}$	Before
abd	Abdomen
ac, a.c.	Before meals
ADL	Activities of daily living
ad lib	As desired
adm	Admission or administer
AM, a.m.	Morning
AMA	Against medical advice
amb	Ambulate
amt	Amount
AP, ap	Apical pulse
approx	Approximately
ASAP	As soon as possible
B&B	Bowel and bladder retraining
BaE, BE	Barium enema
b.i.d.	Twice a day
bld	Blood
BM, bm	Bowel movement
BP	Blood pressure
BR	Bed rest
BRP	Bathroom privileges
BS	Bowel sounds
BSC	Bedside commode
Bx, bx	Biopsy
$\bar{c}$	With
C	Centigrade, Celsius
Ca	Cancer
Cath	Catheter, catheterize
CBC	Complete blood count
CBR	Complete bed rest
cc	Cubic centimeter
CCU	Coronary care unit
CHF	Congestive heart failure
ck	Check
cl liq	Clear liquid
CO_2	Carbon dioxide
COPD, COLD	Chronic obstructive pulmonary disease, chronic obstructive lung disease
CPR	Cardiopulmonary resuscitation
CS	Central supply
CVA	Cerebrovascular accident, stroke
CXR	Chest x-ray
DAT	Diet as tolerated
dc, d/c	Discontinue
disch	Discharge
DM	Diabetes mellitus
DNR	Do not resuscitate
DOA	Dead on arrival
DOB	Date of birth
DR	Delivery room
drsg, dsg	Dressing

Box continued on following page

COMMONLY USED MEDICAL ABBREVIATIONS *Continued*

Abbreviation	Meaning
Dx	Diagnosis
ECG, EKG	Electrocardiogram
EEG	Electroencephalogram
EENT	Eye, ear, nose, throat
ER	Emergency room
F	Fahrenheit
F, FE	Female
fb	Foreign body
FBS	Fasting blood sugar
FF	Force fluids
fld	Fluid
FOB	Foot of bed
ft	Foot, feet
FUO	Fever of undetermined origin
Fx	Fracture
gal	Gallon
GI	Gastrointestinal
gtt	Drop
GU	Genitourinary
GYN	Gynecology
H_2O	Water
h/o	History of
HOB	Head of bed
hr	Hour
H.S., hs	Hour of sleep, bedtime
ht	Height
HTN	Hypertension
ICU	Intensive care unit
in	Inch
I&O	Intake and output
irr	Irregular
isol	Isolation
IV	Intravenous
K^+	Potassium
L	Liter or left
Lab	Laboratory
lb	Pound
L&D	Labor and delivery
liq	Liquid
LLQ	Left lower quadrant (abd)
LPN	Licensed practical nurse
lt	Left
LUQ	Left upper quadrant (abd)
LVN	Licensed vocational nurse
M	Male
MD	Medical doctor
Meds, meds	Medications
MI	Myocardial infarction, heart attack
mid, noc, noct	Midnight
min	Minute
ml	Milliliter

COMMONLY USED MEDICAL ABBREVIATIONS *Continued*

Abbreviation	Meaning
NA	Nursing assistant
Na⁻	Sodium
neg	Negative
n/g tube	Nasogastric tube
nil	Nothing, none
N	Noon
no, #	Number
noc, noct	Night
NPO	Nothing by mouth
O_2	Oxygen
OB	Obstetrics
OJ, oj	Orange juice
OOB	Out of bed
OR	Operating room
Ord	Orderly
os	Mouth
OT	Occupational therapy
oz	Ounce
$\bar{p}$	After
PAR	Postanesthesia room
pc, p.c.	After meals
PEDS	Pediatrics
per	By, through
PM, p.m.	Afternoon or evening
PMC	Postmortem care
p.o., per os	By mouth
postop, post op	Postoperative, after surgery
preop, pre op	Preoperative, before surgery
prep	Preparation
prn, p.r.n.	When necessary or needed
PT, pt	Patient
pt	Pint
PT	Physical therapy
q	Every
qam	Every morning
qd, q.d.	Every day
qh, q.h.	Every hour
q2h, q.2h.	Every 2 hours
q3h, q.3h.	Every 3 hours
q12h, q.12h.	Every 12 hours
qhs, q.h.s.	Every hour of sleep, every bedtime
qid, q.i.d.	Four times a day
qod, q.o.d.	Every other day
qs	Quantity sufficient
qt	Quart
R	Rectally or right
RLQ	Right lower quadrant (abd)
Rm	Room
RN	Registered nurse
r/o	Rule out

Box continued on following page

COMMONLY USED MEDICAL ABBREVIATIONS *Continued*

Abbreviation	Meaning
ROM	Range of motion
RR	Recovery room
RT	Respiratory therapy
RUQ	Right upper quadrant (abd)
R*x*	Prescription, treatment
$\bar{s}$	Without
S&A	Sugar and acetone
SOB	Short of breath
SOS	Sacrament of the sick
spec	Specimen
SSE	Soap suds enema
stat	Immediately
STD	Sexually transmitted disease
Surg	Surgery
S*x*	Symptoms
T&A	Time and amount
T, *temp*	Temperature
tbsp	Tablespoon
tid, t.i.d.	Three times a day
TLC	Tender loving care
TPR	Temperature, pulse, and respiration
tsp	Teaspoon
TWE	Tap water enema
T*x*	Treatment, traction
U/A, *u/a*	Urinalysis
UGI	Upper gastrointestinal series
VS, *vs*	Vital signs
WA	While awake
WBC	White blood cells
w/c	Wheelchair
WNL	Within normal limits
wt	Weight
×	Times
−	Negative
+	Positive

ung = ointment = in the eye.

CARING COMMENT

You should learn the abbreviations of words you use everyday, such as *with, without, before,* and *after,* as soon as you can. Use these abbreviations everyday when you write a note to yourself. Try to learn another new abbreviation each day. When you begin working, you will take notes and read important information in which abbreviations are used.

CHAPTER WRAP-UP

- Use appropriate terminology and abbreviations when reporting and recording information about your patients.
- Medical terminology includes the study of prefixes, roots, and suffixes.
- An abbreviation is a shortened form of a word or phrase.

REVIEW QUESTIONS

1. Define medical terminology. Give an example of when you would use medical terminology.

2. Break the following words into parts (root word/prefix/suffix) and figure out what the word means.

   pathology: _____

   urinalysis: _____

   hysterectomy: _____

   gastroenteritis: _____

   ophthalmologist: _____

3. What are the abbreviations for the following terms?

   with _____

   without _____

   before _____

   after _____

   head of bed _____

   nothing by mouth _____

   hour of sleep _____

ACTIVITY CORNER

Look in the glossary of this book. Write down five medical words in the spaces provided below. Circle the common root of each word.

   Check the list of common roots on pages 133 and 134 to see if you are correct.

   1. _____

   2. _____

   3. _____

   4. _____

   5. _____

Measuring
Vital Signs

8 Understanding Vital Signs

Objectives

AFTER YOU COMPLETE THIS CHAPTER, YOU WILL BE ABLE 1

List the vital signs.
Explain the importance of measuring vital signs.
Identify the factors that affect vital signs.
Tell when vital signs should b measured.

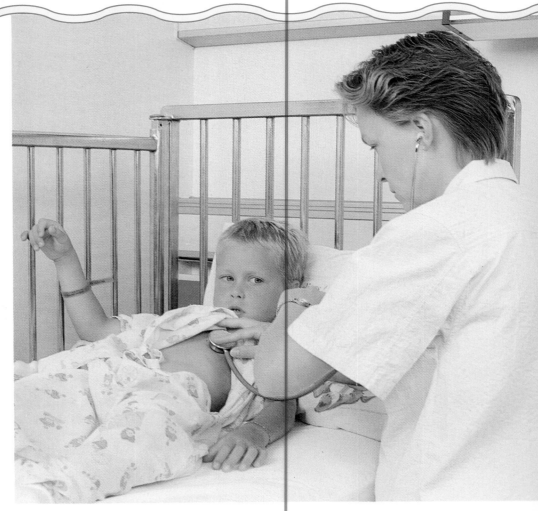

Overview Vital signs are also called the signs of life or cardinal signs. You will learn how to measure the vital signs: body temperature, pulse, respirations, and blood pressure. You will be expected to measure your patients' vital signs. The vital sign measurements you report to the nurse are important because they provide the entire health care team with information about how major systems in the body are functioning.

WHAT DO YOU KNOW ABOUT VITAL SIGNS?

Here are four statements about vital signs. Consider them to test your current knowledge about the vital signs of the body. If you think the statement is true, circle the T; if you think the statement is false, circle the F. Change the false statements to make them true.

1. T F Hand washing is part of the routine when vital signs are measured.

2. T F Vital signs include measurements of the temperature, pulse, and respiration only.

3. T F Exercise can cause changes in vital signs.

4. T F An infant's pulse is very low.

ANSWERS

1. **True.** Hands are always washed before and after a procedure. Vital sign measurement is a procedure.

2. **False.** Blood pressure measurement is also included in vital sign measurements.

3. **True.** Exercise makes the heart work harder. Count your pulse after you run up two flights of stairs.

4. **False.** The pulse is higher at birth. It goes down as the person grows and evens out to a normal adult range during the teen years.

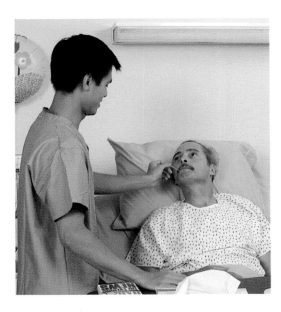

FIGURE 8–1
Vital signs are measured as often as needed for the individual patient.

VITAL SIGNS

the signs of life: temperature, pulse, respiration, and blood pressure

Vital signs, also called cardinal signs, are the measurements of the signs of life. The vital signs are important indicators of how well the major tissues of the body (the heart and lungs) are functioning. The vital signs are complex and closely related to each other. Most people's vital signs remain within a range that is normal for them during a 24-hour period.

Changes in one vital sign may indicate changes in other vital signs. The presence of a disease in the body can affect the vital signs (Figure 8–1).

Vital signs of major body functions include measurements of the body's

Temperature
Pulse
Respirations
Blood pressure

Measuring vital signs is an important responsibility of the nursing assistant. It is a function that you will perform often and the health care team will rely on to treat the patient. Vital signs are usually written as TPR (temperature, pulse, and respirations) followed by BP (blood pressure). The results of vital sign **measurement** are monitored closely to follow the patient's progress toward health. When the measurements are interpreted, they tell the health care team members how the patient's body systems are functioning.

MEASUREMENT

an extent or amount obtained by measuring

FACTORS THAT AFFECT VITAL SIGNS

Various factors inside and outside the body can affect the body's temperature, pulse, respiration, and blood pressure functions. These factors include

Age
Sex
Environment
Food and fluid intake
Exercise
Life-style
Fear and anxiety
Disease
Medication

TABLE 8–1   VITAL SIGNS ACROSS THE LIFE SPAN

Age	Temperature	Pulse	Respirations	Blood Pressure
Newborn	99.4	140	35	70/40
1 month–1 year	99.6	120	30	90/60
1 year–6 years	98.8	115	23	100/66
6 years–12 years	98.6	95	20	116/76
Adolescence	98.6	80	18	120/80
Adult range	98.6	60–100	14–20	120/80*
Adults over 70	96.8	60–100	14–20	120/80*

    * Diastolic pressure may increase.

AGE

The age of a person can give you a clue to the person's expected range of vital signs. (Table 8–1).

At birth, the pulse and respirations are very rapid, whereas the blood pressure is low. A baby's temperature is unstable because the body is not mature enough to keep a constant body temperature in hot or cold weather. As the baby grows into a child, the pulse and respirations slow down and the blood pressure rises. During adolescence, the vital signs approach the more familiar ranges of the adult.

With **aging,** vital signs may change in some persons. The blood pressure may be elevated because of changes that occur in the blood vessels. The elderly may also experience problems with temperature regulation; therefore you may observe a lower body temperature in some elderly persons.

AGING
the physical and psychological changes that occur as life continues

SEX

The sex of the person can affect certain vital signs. The body temperature of the female who is **ovulating** rises one-half to one degree. The average male adult has a slightly lower pulse than the average female adult.

OVULATING
the releasing of an ovum at intervals of about 28 days

ENVIRONMENT

A healthy body works to keep a constant temperature in hot or cold weather. The body's temperature can be higher simply because of hot weather. In addition, in warmer climates, the heart works harder to circulate the blood; therefore the blood pressure and pulse may also be higher. In high elevations, such as in the mountains, the rate of respirations (breathing) increases because less **oxygen** is available in the air.

ENVIRONMENT
the conditions, circumstances, or objects that surround a person

OXYGEN
a colorless, tasteless, odorless gas; the air we breathe is about 20% oxygen

FOODS AND FLUIDS

Eating and drinking very hot or very cold food or fluids can affect the body's temperature. The heat or cold can be retained in the oral cavity (mouth) for 15–20 minutes after food or fluids are taken in. For this reason, never measure the body temperature by mouth immediately after the patient has eaten or has had anything to drink.

EXERCISE

The rate of respirations increases in response to the demand for more oxygen. People who exercise regularly have a higher pulse rate than those who don't because the body works harder to deliver the extra oxygen that is demanded (Figure 8–2). Exercise can also increase the body temperature temporarily. After exercise, the body returns to its normal rate of functioning. You will observe a slower heart rate in people who follow an active exercise schedule because their hearts work more efficiently.

LIFE-STYLE

BEING OVERWEIGHT   Overweight individuals may find they have difficulty breathing when they exert themselves. The heart works harder to circulate blood in the overweight person.

CARBON DIOXIDE
an odorless, colorless gas that is expelled from the lungs

SMOKING   Smoking affects the exchange of oxygen and **carbon dioxide** in the lungs. There is an increase in the number of respirations and in the pulse rate of the person who smokes.

SEDENTARY LIFE-STYLE   A sedentary life-style is one in which a person is not active physically and does not plan for active exercise on a regular basis. The heart and lungs do not function efficiently in persons with a sedentary life-style.

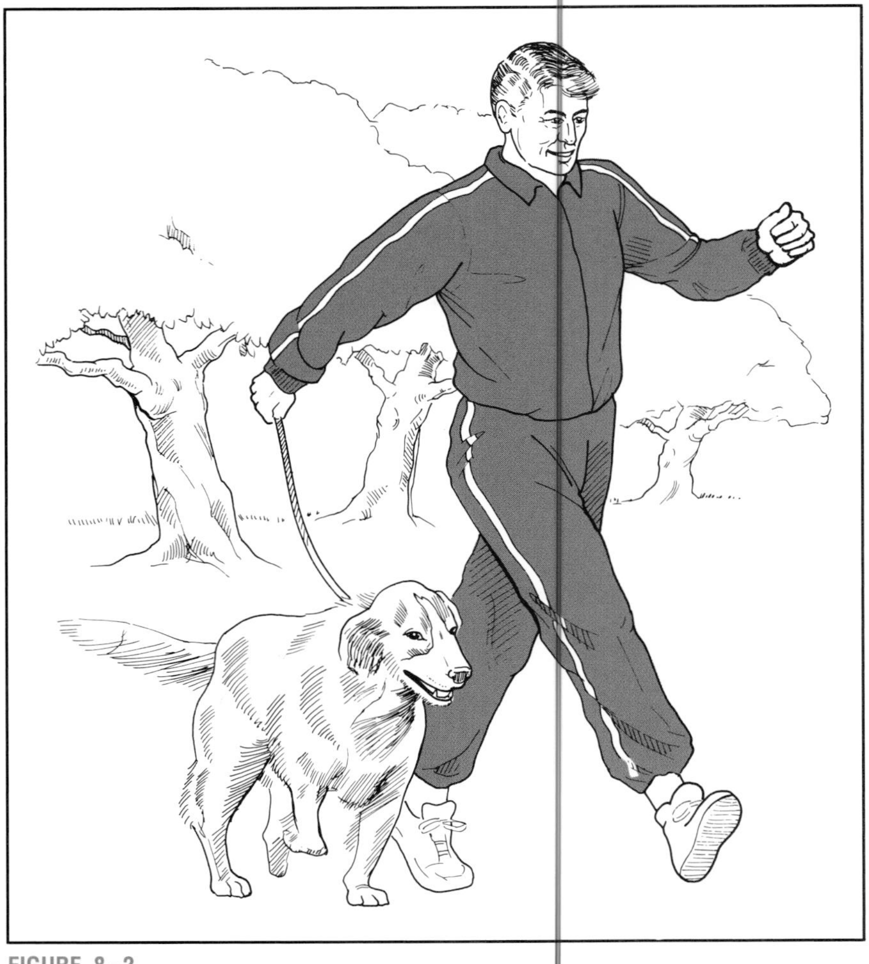

FIGURE 8–2
A brisk walk increases the heart rate.

In fact, the heart and lungs work harder to deliver the oxygen required by the body's tissues.

FEAR AND ANXIETY

Fear and **anxiety** are emotions that put stress on the body. Patients may feel their heart pounding because the heart responds to stress by increasing its overall activity. The force of the heartbeat and the pulse increases. The blood pressure also increases in response to stress. You may observe an increase in respirations in patients who are fearful or anxious. When the fear and anxiety are relieved, the pulse, respirations, and blood pressure return to the measurements that are normal for that patient.

ANXIETY
an uneasy feeling that comes from something that is going to happen or an individual believes might happen

DISEASE

Changes in a person's usual vital sign measurements can indicate that a **disease** process is at work in the body. During an infection, the body's temperature rises as the body attempts to fight off invading **microorganisms.** When the body temperature is elevated, the body needs more oxygen, and the pulse rate rises in response. When the lungs are not functioning properly, the body meets its need for more oxygen by increasing the rate of respirations. The heart is affected when it works against extra pressure caused by narrowed or non-elastic blood vessels. The result is hypertension.

DISEASE
sickness; a condition of the body or one of its parts that changes the way the body functions
MICROORGANISM
an organism so tiny it can only be seen under a microscope; capable of helping the body as well as causing disease

MEDICATIONS

Certain medications can affect the vital signs. You may be asked to measure body temperature after the nurse administers an aspirin or acetaminophen for your patient's fever. You would expect a lower temperature as a result of these medications. Other medications might be given to lower a patient's heart rate or blood pressure. It is very important that you measure the patient's vital signs accurately and report current measurements to the supervisor or nurse.

WHEN TO TAKE VITAL SIGNS

Vital signs are measured on a routine basis for all patients in a health care institution. Measurements are scheduled according to the hospital's routine, or they may be ordered at specific intervals by the physician.

Vital signs are commonly measured before and after any diagnostic test or procedure that invades the body. In addition, when you observe changes in a patient's physical or mental condition, you should remember to measure and record vital signs. Patients may tell you they have noticed a change in their body function, such as

- Shortness of breath
- Pounding of the heart
- Feeling warm
- Any other unusual or different feelings

Be sure to measure vital signs and record the results in the appropriate document and then notify the nurse in charge.

RECORDING VITAL SIGNS

The results of vital sign measurements may be recorded in several different places on the unit. When you take the measurements, you should immediately record them on your notepad. Include the patient's name and the time the vital signs were measured.

SAMPLE: Mrs. Greene, T 98.6, P 72, R 16, BP 120/84, 0600.

After you report the results of the vital signs to the nurse or supervisor, you should document them on the forms indicated by the health care institution. Such forms might include the graphic sheet and change of shift report (see Chapter 6), special forms like a postoperative flow sheet (See Chapter 26), and a unit worksheet. You may also be required to include the vital signs in the nurses' notes. Be sure you know the rules of the health care institution regarding charting vital signs.

CHAPTER WRAP-UP

- The vital signs are important indicators of how well the body's major tissues are functioning. Vital signs consist of measurements of
    Body temperature
    Pulse
    Respirations
    Blood pressure
- Vital signs can be affected by various factors, including
    Environment
    Ingestion of hot or cold food or fluids
    Exercise
    Disease
- It is important to read and report all vital sign measurements accurately.

REVIEW QUESTIONS

1. List the vital signs and their abbreviations.
2. List the factors that affect vital sign measurements.
3. Explain when vital signs should be measured.

ACTIVITY CORNER

Count your own and a friend's pulses and respirations at two times during the day. Write down the results.

	Time	Self	Friend
Pulse	_____	_____	_____
	_____	_____	_____

Respirations ____   ____   ____

          ____   ____   ____

Were pulse and respirations the same each time they were taken? Are the results for you and your friend the same? What factors might account for any differences?

9 Measuring Body Temperature

Objectives

AFTER YOU COMPLETE THIS CHAPTER, YOU WILL BE ABLE TO:

Identify the normal ranges of body temperature.

Use a variety of thermometers to measure body temperature.

Measure body temperature accurately and record results correctly.

Discuss the care of the patient who has a fever.

Explain how to give a cooling bath.

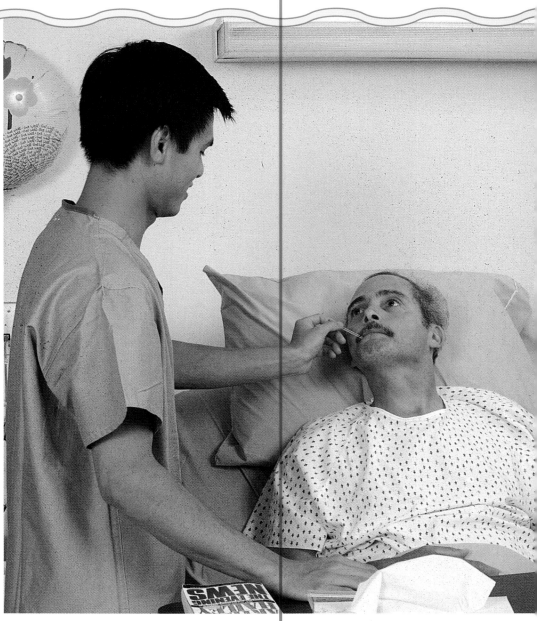

Overview Body temperature is an important indicator of health. Many things inside the body, such as an infection, can affect body temperature. Things outside the body, such as cold weather, can also affect the body's temperature. As a nursing assistant, you measure the body's temperature using a variety of thermometers. Many times you are the first person to observe that a patient's body temperature has changed. Other health care team members rely on you to report your observations about patients.

WHAT DO YOU KNOW ABOUT BODY TEMPERATURE?

Here are five statements about body temperature. Consider them to test your current knowledge of body temperature. If you think the statement is true, circle the T; if you think the statement is false, circle the F. Change the false statements to make them true.

1. T F A glass thermometer should be used to measure a 3-year-old's temperature by mouth.

2. T F Body temperature is highest in the early morning hours.

3. T F A temperature measured by mouth is the most accurate representation of the body's temperature.

4. T F If a patient drinks hot coffee, you should wait 15 minutes to measure the oral (in the mouth) temperature.

5. T F The person with a fever needs to drinks fluids.

ANSWERS

1. **False.** A 3-year-old is likely to bite down on the glass thermometer and be injured. Most health care institutions require that a rectal temperature be measured in children under 6 years of age.

2. **False.** The body's temperature is the lowest in the early morning hours; it is higher in the late afternoon and early evening hours.

3. **False.** The rectal temperature is the most accurate representation of the body's temperature.

4. **True.** When a person drinks hot or cold liquids, the temperature of the mucous membranes of the mouth are affected. The correct action is to wait 15 minutes and return to measure the temperature.

5. **True.** Fluids are lost when the body temperature is high and must be replaced by giving the patient fluids by mouth or through the veins.

WHAT IS BODY TEMPERATURE?

BODY TEMPERATURE
the degree of body heat or cold measured by a clinical thermometer
THERMOMETER
the instrument used to measure temperature
HYPOTHALAMUS
an area of the brain that controls body temperature
CIRCADIAN
occurring about every 24 hours

Body temperature is the degree of body heat or cold measured by a clinical **thermometer.** The measurement reflects the balance between the heat produced by the body and the heat it loses.

The **hypothalamus** in the central nervous system regulates the body's heat production. Located at the base of the brain, the hypothalamus functions as the body's thermostat (Figure 9–1). The hypothalamus controls the body's temperature so closely that it may vary only about 1° in a 24-hour cycle.

Individuals' body temperatures go up and down according to their **circadian** rhythm. You will notice that patients' body temperature measurements are the lowest during the early morning hours. Many health care institutions require that temperature measurements be taken at 6:00 a.m. to take advantage of this natural body cycle. On the other hand, the highest readings of body temperature occur between 4:00 and 7:00 p.m.

HEAT PRODUCTION

Heat is produced in the body's cells by the following activities:

* the breakdown of food
* the contraction of muscles during exercise
* the actions of certain hormones
* external factors, such as the sun beating down on a hot summer day

HEAT LOSS

When you care for very young or elderly patients, you may need to protect them against heat loss. The young person's system for regulating body temperature is immature; the elderly person's may be inefficient. Certain factors cause the body's cells to lose heat:

* Wind and snow are external factors that contribute to the loss of body heat.

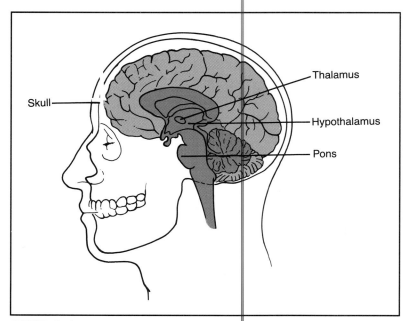

FIGURE 9–1
The hypothalamus regulates the body's temperature.

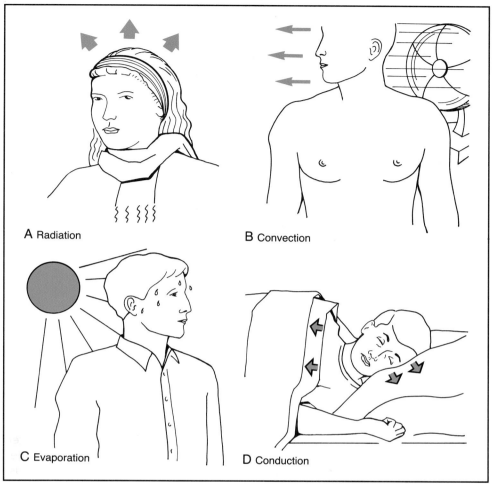

FIGURE 9–2

Heat loss. A, On a cold day, the body gives off heat (radiation). If not covered, the head acts as a chimney and allows heat to escape. B, Air from a fan or the wind blowing across the body takes heat away (convection). Never point a fan directly at a patient; aim the flow of air at the floor or ceiling. C, Heat is also lost when a person perspires (sweats). Small drops of body fluid appear on the skin and evaporate into the air (evaporation) and carry body heat away. D, The body can use its own heat to warm other objects (conduction). Climbing into bed and settling between the sheets cause the body to warm the surrounding sheets.

- Heat is lost through the skin and through breathing. In colder climates a person can see a puff of white steam whenever a breath is exhaled.
- Urine and feces, warm when exiting the body, add to heat loss.

Heat loss occurs because the body can transfer heat away from itself by using one of the following methods:

- **Radiation**—Heat is given off in rays by the body. The action is similar to heat coming out of an old-fashioned radiator during the winter (Figure 9–2A).
- **Convection**—Heat is moved away from the body on currents of air (Figure 9–2B).
- **Evaporation**—Body heat is converted (changed) into a vapor (beads of sweat). A hot day or active exercise creates extra body heat. The body loses the heat by perspiring (sweating) (Figure 9–2C).
- **Conduction**—Body heat is carried away through contact with an object. The body warms any object that it touches if the object's temperature is cooler than that of the body (Figure 9–2D).

RADIATION
a mechanism of heat loss in which heat is given off or thrown off by the body
CONVECTION
a mechanism of heat loss in which heat is moved away from the body on currents of air
EVAPORATION
a mechanism of heat loss in which body heat is converted into a vapor (beads of sweat)
CONDUCTION
a mechanism of heat loss in which body heat is carried away through contact with an object

CARING COMMENT

The very young and the elderly cool off much faster than persons in other age groups. Be certain to provide comfort and warmth for patients who are not comfortable in their environment.

MEASURING BODY TEMPERATURE

SCALES

FAHRENHEIT SCALE
a temperature scale with the freezing point at 32° and the boiling point of water at 212°; abbreviated F

CELSIUS SCALE
a temperature scale with the freezing point at 0° and the boiling point of water at 100°; abbreviated C

There are two scales of measurement you need to know. They are the **Fahrenheit (F)** and the **Celsius** or centigrade (C) scales. Your health care facility will use one of these scales. A special formula is available if you are asked to convert your reading from one scale to another.

FAHRENHEIT AND CELSIUS SCALE EQUIVALENTS

Fahrenheit		Celsius
95.9°		35.5°
96.8°		36.0°
97.7°		36.5°
98.6°	**Normal**	**37.0°**
99.0°		37.2°
99.5°		37.5°
100.4°		38.0°
101.3°		38.5°
102.2°		39.0°
103.1°		39.5°
104.0°		40.0°
104.9°		40.5°

FORMULA TO CONVERT TEMPERATURE MEASUREMENTS FROM ONE SCALE TO THE OTHER

To convert a Fahrenheit reading to a Celsius or centigrade reading, subtract 32 from the Fahrenheit reading and multiply by 5/9.

Example: 97.6° F = ?° C

$$97.6 - 32.0 = 65.6 \qquad 65.6 \times \frac{5}{9} = \frac{3280}{9} = 36.6° \text{ C}$$

To convert a Celsius or centigrade reading to a Fahrenheit reading, multiply the Celsius reading by 9/5 and add 32.

Example 39.0° C = ?° F

$$39.0 \times \frac{9}{5} = \frac{351.0}{5} = 70.2 + 32.0 = 102.2° \text{ F}$$

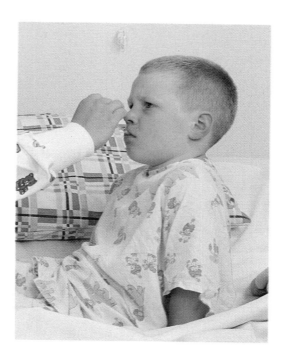

FIGURE 9–3
Measuring the temperature orally.

SITES FOR TAKING BODY TEMPERATURE

Body temperature is measured at four sites:

THE MOUTH (ORALLY) The mouth is the most frequently used site because it is convenient (Figure 9–3) and is comfortable for and accepted by the patient.

THE RECTUM (RECTALLY) The rectal temperature is the most accurate representation of the body's temperature (Figure 9–4). You should measure a rectal temperature in children under the age of 6 or according to the policy of your health care institution. A rectal temperature is measured whenever the patient situation demands it.

RECTUM
the last part of the large intestine that ends at the anal canal

UNDER THE AXILLA (AXILLARY) An axillary temperature is measured in the axilla (Figure 9–5). This method provides the least accurate measurement.

AXILLA
the armpit

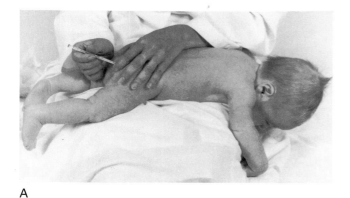

A

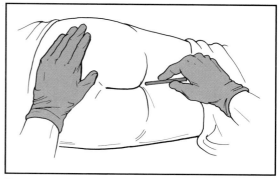

B

FIGURE 9–4
Measuring the temperature rectally. A, Infant (From Jarvis C: Physical Examination and Health Assessment. Philadelphia, W.B. Saunders Company, 1992.) B, Adult.

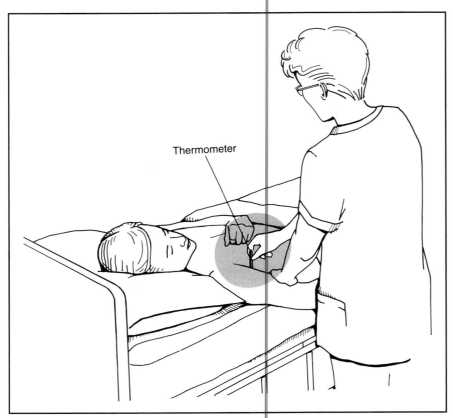

Thermometer

FIGURE 9–5
Measuring a temperature under the axilla.

TYMPANIC

pertaining to the eardrum

THE EAR (TYMPANIC) A tympanic temperature is measured by a special device that senses the body's temperature at the tympanic membrane (eardrum) (Figure 9–6).

Whenever the patient has difficulty breathing through the nose, always ask the nurse or supervisor if a rectal body temperature measurement should be taken.

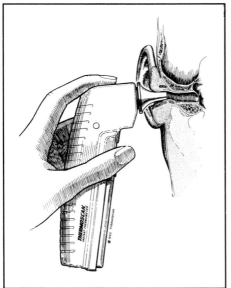
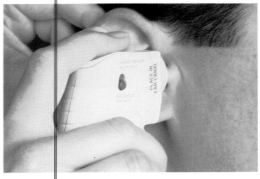

FIGURE 9–6
Measuring the temperature at the tympanic membrane. (Photo by Thermoscan.)

Do not take an oral temperature in the following situations:

- Nasal packing is present.
- The patient is under the age of 6.
- The patient is unconscious.
- Oxygen is being administered.
- The patient has a nasogastric tube.
- The patient is confused or disoriented.
- The patient breathes through the mouth.
- The patient is paralyzed as a result of a stroke.
- The patient has had surgery or injury of the face, mouth, nose, or neck.

AVERAGE BODY TEMPERATURE BY SITE

When measured by mouth, the average body temperature is 98.6° F or 37.0° C. When measured rectally, the average temperature is higher:

- 99.6° F (higher by 1° on the Fahrenheit scale)
- 37.5° C (higher by about .50° on the Celsius scale)

When an axillary (under the arm) measurement is done, the average temperature is lower than the average temperature by mouth.

- 97.6° F (lower by 1° on the Fahrenheit scale)
- 36.5° C (lower by about .50° on the Celsius scale)

The temperatures given above are only averages. Each site—mouth, rectum, and axillary—has a range of several degrees that are considered to be normal. The ranges are presented in the chart.

RANGES OF NORMAL BODY TEMPERATURES BY SITE		
Site	Fahrenheit Scale	Celsius or Centigrade Scale
Oral	97.6°–99.6°	36.5°–37.5°
Rectal	98.6°–100.6°	37.0°–38.1°
Axillary	96.6°–98.6°	36.0°–37.0°

TYPES OF THERMOMETERS

A thermometer is used to measure body temperature. You need to be familiar with and know how to care for, several different kinds of thermometers.

GLASS THERMOMETERS

The glass thermometer is a thin, hollow tube made of glass. One end contains a bulb filled with mercury. The outside of the glass tube is marked with a scale for measurement. When the heat in the body site (mouth, rectum, or under the arm) contacts the mercury in the bulb, it causes the mercury to expand and rise in the hollow tube. When the mercury stops rising, the measurement of body temperature is read on the thermometer.

There are three different kinds of bulbs (ends) on glass thermometers:

- One thermometer that is used to measure temperature in the mouth or under the arm has a thin, slender bulb (Figure 9–7).
- A red-topped thermometer that is used to measure the temperature rectally has a rounded stubby bulb (Figure 9–8).
- Another thermometer used in the mouth or under the arm has a pear-

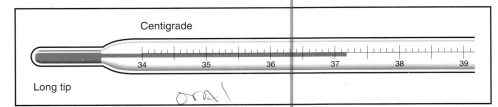

oral

FIGURE 9–7
Thermometer with a long tip.

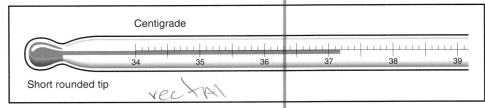

rectal

FIGURE 9–8
Thermometer with a short rounded tip.

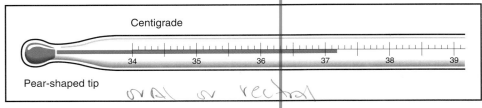

oral or rectal

FIGURE 9–9
Thermometer with a pear-shaped tip.

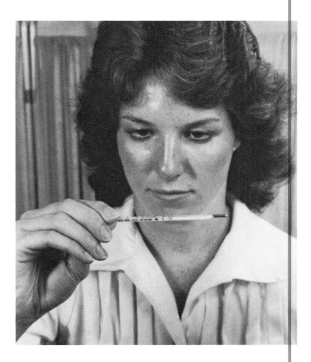

FIGURE 9–10
Read the glass thermometer at eye level for accurate results. (From Bonewit K: Clinical Procedures for Medical Assistants, 3rd ed. Philadelphia, W.B. Saunders Company, 1990.)

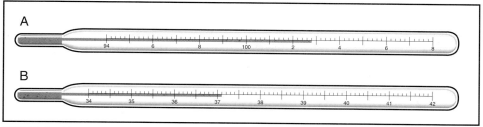

FIGURE 9-11

Thermometers with Fahrenheit (A) and Celsius (B) scales. The temperature on the Fahrenheit thermometer is 102.8°; the temperature on the Celsius thermometer is 37.1°.

shaped, stubby bulb. These thermometers often have a blue top (the end opposite the bulb) (Figure 9–9).

Reading a Glass Thermometer

A glass thermometer is best read by holding it at eye level (Figure 9–10). To read a glass thermometer, first look at the number scale (Figure 9–11). If the scale numbers start at about 94° and continue to 108°, it is a Fahrenheit scale. It is marked with long and short lines. The long lines mark the even degrees, and the short lines indicate two-tenths of a degree.

The Celsius or centigrade scale is numbered from 34° to 42°. It also is marked with long and short lines. The long lines mark the degree, and the short lines indicate one-tenth of a degree. Read the temperature at the top of the column of **mercury** and write it down on a piece of paper for accuracy.

MERCURY

a chemical agent that expands with heat

CARING COMMENT

When reading a glass thermometer, hold the shaded side of the thermometer away from you. This makes it easier to locate the mercury to read the results.

Care of Glass Thermometers

If your health care institution uses glass thermometers, one is kept in each patient's room and used for that patient only. This practice prevents the spread of infection. **Microorganisms** from the mouth, rectum, or axilla can **contaminate** the thermometer.

The glass thermometer must be cleaned before and after each use. A special solution is used to disinfect a thermometer. A thermometer used in the rectum can be cleaned in cool water after it is wiped with a tissue. Hot water can damage a thermometer because heat may cause the mercury to expand and break the thin glass. A **disinfectant** is applied to the thermometer before it is used again.

Examine the thermometer for cracks or chipped surfaces before each use.

In many health care institutions, a supply of thin plastic covers (also called **sheaths**) is provided for use with each glass thermometer (Figure 9–12). The covering protects the thermometer from contamination from body secretions and serves to keep the thermometer clean. The plastic covering is applied before the body temperature is measured. It is discarded after the temperature is read, and the thermometer is stored until needed again. Your health care institution may require that you disinfect the thermometer between use to control the spread of microorganisms.

MICROORGANISM

an organism so tiny it can only be seen under a microscope; capable of helping the body as well as causing disease

CONTAMINATE

to soil or infect by contact

DISINFECTANT

a chemical that destroys or disables microorganisms

SHEATH

a case or cover

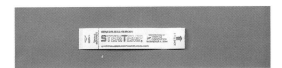

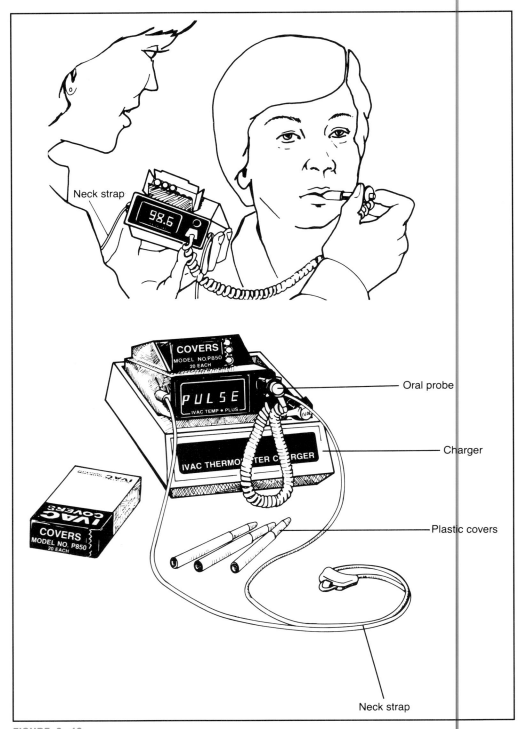

FIGURE 9–13

An electronic thermometer. (From DuGas BW: Introduction to Patient Care: A Comprehensive Approach to Nursing, 4th ed. Philadelphia, W.B. Saunders Company, 1983.)

ELECTRONIC THERMOMETERS

The electronic thermometer provides a quick, easy method for measuring body temperature. The **digital** display area lights up with the correct temperature reading when the probe senses the body's temperature. The electronic thermometer is a portable unit that stores in a battery charger or holding area when not in use. It can be carried in your hand and may have a cord that allows you to hang it around your neck if you are measuring a series of body temperatures (Figure 9–13).

DIGITAL
an electronic number display

Two detachable **probes** are supplied with the electronic thermometer: an oral (blue-tipped) and a rectal (red-tipped) probe. A rigid plastic sheath protector covers the probe when the patient's temperature is taken. The sheath protector is disposable and is used only once. A supply of sheath protectors is carried on the electronic unit.

PROBE
a slender instrument used to explore inside the body and send back information

The electronic thermometer registers the temperature quickly and beeps when the temperature is ready to be read. The digital display is accurate and easy to read. The greatest benefit of the electronic thermometer, though, is the reduction of the spread of microorganisms. The drawback is that this type of thermometer is expensive. Follow specific directions for cleaning and care of the electronic thermometer.

CARING COMMENT

Hold the electronic thermometer in the patient's mouth, because it is heavy and can be uncomfortable. If patients are able, they may hold it in their mouth themselves.

DISPOSABLE ORAL THERMOMETERS

A disposable oral thermometer is used only once. It contains a series of dots that react to the body's heat. When a certain temperature is reached, the reaction stops and the dots change colors. Unwrap the thermometer and place the end with the dots under the patient's tongue. Ask patients to close their mouth. An oral temperature can be measured in about 1 minute. Discard the thermometer after you read and write down the results.

TEMPERATURE-SENSITIVE TAPES

A temperature-sensitive tape also reacts to body heat. It is not read for an exact temperature measurement like the other thermometers. The color change indicates only whether the temperature is normal or above normal. The body temperature is registered about 15 seconds after you place the tape on the patient's forehead or abdomen.

TAKING AN ORAL TEMPERATURE

An oral temperature is the easiest, most convenient way to measure body temperature. Use a glass or an electronic thermometer to take an oral temperature in older children and adults.

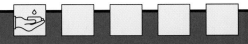

PROCEDURE

Taking an Oral Temperature with a Glass Thermometer

Explain to patients that you are going to measure their body temperature with a glass thermometer. You should wait 15 minutes to take an oral temperature if patients have just eaten, drunk, smoked, or chewed gum.

GATHER EQUIPMENT

Glass thermometer (usually blue-tipped or clear) and storage container
Tissues
Thin plastic thermometer sheaths (when available)

Paper
Pen

ACTION	RATIONALE
Preparation	
1. Wash hands.	Prevents spread of microorganisms.
2. Identify yourself and the patient.	Maintains patients' rights.
3. Provide privacy.	Maintains patients' rights.
4. Explain the procedure.	Informs patients what is happening.
Procedural Steps	
5. Use cold water to rinse the thermometer if it is soaked in disinfectant solution.	Hot water may cause mercury to expand and result in an incorrect measurement.
6. Use a tissue to dry the thermometer, moving from the flat top to the slender end (Figure 9–14).	Prepares the thermometer for placement in the patient's mouth.

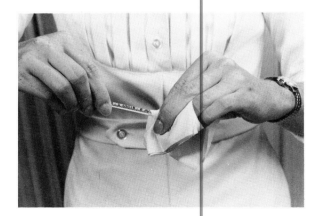

FIGURE 9–14

(From Bonewit K: Clinical Procedures for Medical Assistants, 3rd ed. Philadelphia, W.B. Saunders Company, 1990.)

7. Check the thermometer for damage to the glass.	Breaks or chips can cause injury to the mucous membranes of the mouth.
8. Shake down the thermometer. Hold thermometer firmly at the top (flat) end and shake it with a quick snap of your wrist.	The mercury should be at the bottom of the thermometer to ensure accurate results.

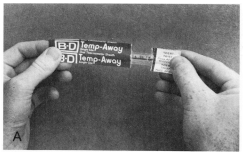

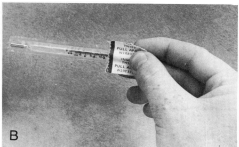

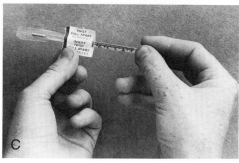

FIGURE 9–15

(From Bonewit K: Clinical Procedures for Medical Assistants, 3rd ed. Philadelphia, W.B. Saunders, 1990.)

9. Cover the thermometer with a thin plastic sheath, if available (Figure 9–15).

Helps prevent the spread of microorganisms.

10. Ask patients to wet their lips.

11. Place the bulb with the mercury end under the patient's tongue near the frenulum (the fold of tissue under the tongue) (Figure 9–16).

The area under the tongue contains a heat pocket that heats the mercury so that it expands up the glass column.

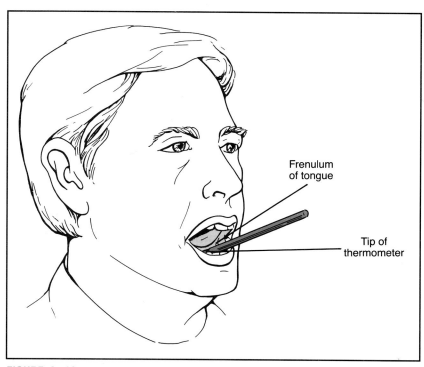

Frenulum of tongue

Tip of thermometer

FIGURE 9–16

Continued on following page

Taking an Oral Temperature with a Glass Thermometer *Continued*

12. Ask patients to close their lips gently around the thermometer.	Helps hold the thermometer in the mouth and trap the warmth in the mouth.
13. Let the thermometer remain under the tongue for 10 minutes.	Provides the most accurate measurement.
14. Remove the thermometer from the patient's mouth.	
15. Wipe the thermometer from the flat end down toward the bulb. If you used a plastic sheath, remove and discard it.	Wiping from the cleanest end to the dirtiest prevents the spread of microorganisms.
16. Read the thermometer at eye level.	Ensures accuracy.
17. Record the results and the patient's name and room number on the piece of paper.	Helps you recall the specific temperature for each patient.
18. Shake down the thermometer.	Prepares the thermometer for the next use.
19. Rinse and dry the thermometer.	
20. Replace the thermometer in the original storage container.	Reduces breakage.
21. Place the patient in a comfortable position with the call signal within reach.	Leaves the patient with a means to communicate.
22. Open the privacy curtains.	

Follow-Through

23. Wash hands.	Prevents the spread of microorganisms to you or other patients.
24. Report the results to the nurse.	The nurse is responsible for a decision based on the results of your measurement.
25. Record the temperature in the appropriate place.	Provides an official record of the results of a procedure.

PROCEDURE

Taking an Oral Temperature with an Electronic Thermometer

Explain to patients that you are going to measure their body temperature with an electronic thermometer. You should wait 15 minutes to take an oral temperature if patients have just eaten, drunk, smoked, or chewed gum.

GATHER EQUIPMENT

Charged electronic thermometer or self-contained unit
Blue-tipped oral probe

Supply of disposable probe covers
Paper
Pencil

ACTION	RATIONALE

Preparation

1. Wash hands.

    Prevents the spread of microorganisms.

2. Identify yourself and the patient.

    Maintains patients' rights.

3. Provide privacy.

    Maintains patients' rights.

4. Explain the procedure.

    Informs patients about what is happening.

Procedural Steps

5. Check that the oral probe is connected securely to the charged unit.

    The thermometer registers only if the probe connection is secure.

6. Remove the metal probe from the charged unit and insert it into a probe cover.

    The cover is discarded after one use to prevent the spread of harmful microorganisms.

7. Ask patients to open their mouth and raise their tongue slightly.

    Permits easy access to the heat pocket located at the base of the tongue.

8. Place the covered probe on either side of the tongue (Figure 9–17).

    Correct placement is necessary for the digital display to register an accurate measurement.

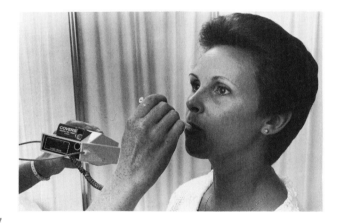

FIGURE 9–17

(From Bonewit K: Clinical Procedures for Medical Nursing Assistants, 3rd ed. Philadelphia, W.B. Saunders Company, 1990.)

9. Ask patients to close their mouth. Hold the probe in place for patients.

    Most probes are heavy and cause discomfort if left in the mouth with no support.

10. Listen for a tone or look for a flashing light that indicates the measurement is complete.

    Equipment varies from one health care institution to another.

11. Remove the probe from patients' mouth.

    The electronic thermometer does not continue to measure after the signal is activated.

12. Read the results on the digital display.

13. Eject the probe cover into the waste container and return the probe to the holder (Figure 9–18).

    Your hands should not touch a probe cover after it has been used.

14. Record the results and patients' name and room number on the piece of paper as soon as possible.

    Even a slight distraction may make you forget what the reading was.

Continued on following page

Taking an Oral Temperature with an Electronic Thermometer *Continued*

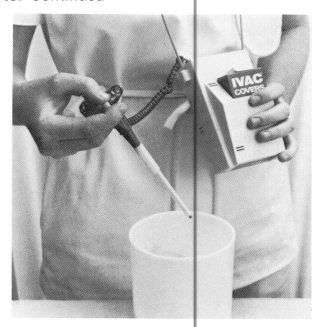

FIGURE 9–18

(From Bonewit K: Clinical Procedures for Medical Assistants, 3rd ed. Philadelphia, W.B. Saunders Company, 1990.)

15. Place patients in a comfortable position with the call signal within reach.	Leaves patients with the means to communicate.
16. Open the privacy curtains.	

Follow-Through

17. Wash hands.	Prevents the spread of microorganisms to you or other patients.
18. Replace the unit in the battery charger or holding area.	The unit charges until needed again. The holding area is a safe place for storage.
19. Report the results to the nurse.	The nurse is responsible for a decision based on the results of your measurement.
20. Record the temperature in appropriate place.	Provides an official record of the results of a procedure.

TAKING A RECTAL TEMPERATURE

A rectal temperature is the most accurate representation of the body's temperature. You use a glass or an electronic thermometer to take a rectal temperature in children under the age of 6 as well as in older children and adults in whom an oral measurement of body temperature is not indicated.

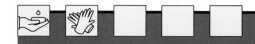

Taking a Rectal Temperature with a Glass Thermometer

Explain to patients that you are going to measure their body temperature by inserting the thermometer into the rectum.

GATHER EQUIPMENT

Glass thermometer (usually red-tipped) and storage container
Toilet paper
Tissues
Thin plastic thermometer covers (when available)

Water-soluble lubricant
Disposable gloves
Paper
Pen
Watch

ACTION	RATIONALE
Preparation	
1. Wash hands.	Prevents the spread of microorganisms.
2. Identify yourself and the patient.	Maintains patients' rights.
3. Provide privacy.	Maintains patients' rights.
4. Explain the procedure.	Informs patients about what is happening.
Procedural Steps	
5. Use cold water to rinse the thermometer if it is soaked in disinfectant solution.	Hot water may cause mercury to expand and result in an incorrect measurement.
6. Use a tissue to dry the thermometer from the flat top to the bulb-shaped end.	Prepares the thermometer for placement in patients' rectum.
7. Check the thermometer for damage to the glass.	Breaks or chips can cause injury to the mucous membranes of the rectum.
8. Shake down the thermometer.	The mercury should be at the bottom of the thermometer to ensure accurate results.
9. Cover the thermometer with a thin plastic sheath, if available.	Helps prevent the spread of microorganisms.
10. Lower the head of the bed and position patients on their left side.	A flat position for rectal measurement is comfortable for patients.
11. Put on disposable, clean gloves.	Protects hands from direct contact with fecal material.
12. Apply the water-soluble lubricant to the mercury (bulb) end of the thermometer.	Permits ease when inserting the thermometer and provides patient comfort.
13. Move linens to expose patients' buttocks.	
14. Raise the buttock to expose the **anus** (Figure 9–19).	Helps you visualize the anus before insertion.
15. Insert the lubricated bulb end 1 inch into the rectum. Remove hand from the buttock.	Creates a closed space and traps heat.
16. Hold the thermometer in place for 3–5 minutes.	Body heat in the rectum heats the mercury and causes it to expand up the glass column.

WATER-SOLUBLE LUBRICANT
a substance that reduces friction and dissolves in water

ANUS
the posterior opening of the body through which waste materials are expelled

Taking a Rectal Temperature with a Glass Thermometer *Continued*

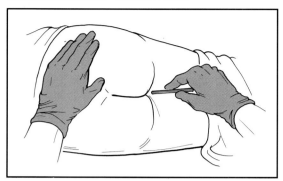

FIGURE 9–19

17. Remove the thermometer from the rectum.

18. Wipe the thermometer with the toilet tissue from the flat end toward the bulb end. If you used a plastic sheath, remove and discard it.

Wiping from the cleanest end to the dirtiest prevents the spread of microorganisms.

19. Place the used tissue on a paper towel and place the thermometer on another clean paper towel.

Keeps work surface clean while wiping patients' buttocks.

20. Wipe the anal area with tissue and discard used tissue into the toilet.

Removes lubricant and feces from the area.

21. Cover patients and reposition them if necessary.

Provides comfort and privacy.

22. Remove disposable gloves and discard them in an appropriate container. Soiled gloves in many institutions are being placed in a hazardous waste container.

Prevents the spread of microorganisms.

23. Read the thermometer at eye level.

Ensures an accurate reading of the results.

24. Record the results and patients' name and room number on the piece of paper.

Helps you recall the specific temperature for each patient.

25. Shake down the thermometer.

Prepares the thermometer for the next use.

26. Rinse and dry the thermometer.

27. Replace in the original storage container.

Reduces breakage.

28. Place patients in a comfortable position with the call signal within reach.

Leaves patients with a means to communicate.

29. Open the privacy curtains.

Follow-Through

30. Wash hands.

Prevents the spread of microorganisms to you or other patients.

31. Report results to the nurse.

The nurse is responsible for a decision based on the results of your measurement.

32. Record the temperature in the appropriate place. Write an *R* to signify the temperature was taken rectally (for example, 38° C—R).

Provides an official record of the results of the procedure.

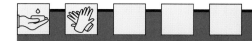

Taking a Rectal Temperature with an Electronic Thermometer

Explain to patients that you are going to measure their body temperature with an electronic thermometer. Explain that the thermometer will be inserted into the rectum for less than a minute.

GATHER EQUIPMENT

A charged electronic thermometer
Red-tipped rectal probe
Supply of disposable probe covers
Toilet tissue

Water-soluble lubricant
Disposable gloves
Paper
Pencil

ACTION	RATIONALE

Preparation

1. Wash hands.	Prevents the spread of microorganisms.
2. Identify yourself and the patient.	Maintains patients' rights.
3. Provide privacy.	Maintains patients' rights.
4. Explain the procedure.	Informs patients about what is happening.

Procedural Steps

5. Check that the rectal probe is connected securely to the charged unit.	The thermometer registers only if the probe connection is secure.
6. Remove the metal probe from the charged unit and insert it into a probe cover.	The cover prevents the spread of harmful microorganisms. It is discarded after use.
7. Lower the head of the bed and position patients on their left side.	A flat position for rectal measurement is comfortable for patients.
8. Apply the water-soluble lubricant to the tip of the probe cover.	Lubricant permits ease when inserting the thermometer and provides patients comfort.
9. Put on the disposable gloves.	Protects your hands from direct contact with fecal material.
10. Remove the linens to expose patients' buttocks.	
11. Raise the buttock to expose the anus.	Helps you visualize the anus before insertion.
12. Insert the lubricated end 1 inch into the rectum. Remove your hand from the buttock.	Creates a closed space and traps heat.
13. Hold the probe in place until a tone or flashing light indicates the measurement is complete.	Equipment varies from one health care institution to another.
14. Remove the probe from patients' rectum.	The electronic thermometer does not continue to measure after the signal is activated.
15. Read the results on the digital display.	
16. Eject the probe cover into the waste container and return the probe to the holder.	Prevents the spread of microorganisms.
17. Record the results and patients' name and room number on the piece of paper.	Helps you recall the specific temperature for each patient.

Continued on following page

Taking a Rectal Temperature with an Electronic Thermometer *Continued*

18. Wipe the anal area with tissue and discard used tissue into the toilet.	Removes lubricant and feces from the area.
19. Cover patients and reposition them if necessary.	Provides comfort and privacy.
20. Remove disposable gloves and discard in an appropriate container.	Prevents the spread of microorganisms.
21. Place patients in a comfortable position with the call signal within reach.	Leaves patients with the means to communicate.
22. Open the privacy curtains.	

Follow-Through

23. Wash hands.	Prevents the spread of microorganisms.
24. Replace the unit in the battery charger or holding area.	The unit charges until it is needed again. The holding area is a safe place for storage.
25. Report results to the nurse.	The nurse is responsible for a decision based on the results of your measurement.
26. Record the temperature in the appropriate place. Write an *R* to signify that the temperature was taken rectally (for example, 38° C—R).	Provides an official record of the results of a procedure.

TAKING AN AXILLARY TEMPERATURE

The axillary temperature measurement is the least accurate way to measure body temperature. It is used when the oral and rectal routes are not recommended. The axilla (armpit) must be dry, and the thermometer (glass or electronic) must be held in place until the temperature registers. In some patients, the arm must be held close to the body to create a warm air pocket. Because less heat is available in this area, you need to hold the glass thermometer in place for 10–11 minutes.

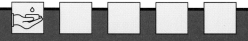

PROCEDURE

Taking an Axillary Temperature with a Glass Thermometer

Explain to patients that you are going to measure their body temperature by placing the thermometer in the axilla. You also need to tell patients that the thermometer must be placed next to the skin.

GATHER EQUIPMENT

Glass thermometer (usually clear or blue-tipped) and storage container	Tissues
	Paper
Thin plastic thermometer cover (when available)	Pen

ACTION	RATIONALE

Preparation

1. Wash hands.

Prevents the spread of microorganisms.

2. Identify yourself and the patient.

Maintains patients' rights.

3. Provide privacy.

Maintains patients' rights.

4. Explain the procedure.

Informs patients about what is happening.

Procedural Steps

5. Use cold water to rinse the thermometer if it is soaked in disinfectant solution.

Hot water may cause mercury to expand and result in an incorrect measurement.

6. Use a tissue to dry the thermometer from the flat top to the slender, thin end.

Prepares the thermometer for placement.

7. Check the thermometer for damage to the glass.

Breaks or chips can cause injury to the delicate skin under the arms.

8. Shake down the thermometer.

The mercury should be at the bottom of the thermometer to ensure accurate results.

9. Cover the thermometer with a thin plastic sheath, if available.

Helps prevent the spread of microorganisms.

10. Remove clothing on the side you select to measure the temperature.

Permits access to the axillary area.

11. Place the bulb end containing the mercury under the arm.

12. Place the arm close to the body and hold the thermometer under the axilla for 10–11 minutes.

The area under the arm forms a heat pocket. Providing adequate time ensures an accurate reading.

13. Remove the thermometer from under the arm.

14. Replace clothing.

15. Wipe the thermometer from flat end down toward the bulb end with tissue. Discard used tissue. If you used a plastic sheath, discard it.

Wiping from the cleanest end to the dirtiest prevents the spread of microorganisms.

16. Read the thermometer.

17. Record the results and patients' name and room number on the piece of paper.

Helps you recall the specific temperature for each patient.

18. Shake down the thermometer.

Prepares the thermometer for the next use.

19. Rinse and dry the thermometer.

20. Replace thermometer in the original storage container.

Reduces breakage.

21. Place patients in a comfortable position with the call signal within reach.

Leaves patients with a means of communication.

22. Open the privacy curtains.

Follow-Through

23. Wash hands.

Prevents the spread of microorganisms.

24. Report results to the nurse.

The nurse is responsible for a decision based on the results of your measurement.

25. Record the temperature in the appropriate place. Write an *A* to signify the temperature was taken by the axillary method (for example, 98.6° F—A).

Provides an official record of the results of a procedure.

PROCEDURE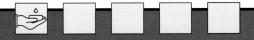

Taking an Axillary Temperature with an Electronic Thermometer

Explain to patients that you are going to measure their body temperature by placing the thermometer under the armpit. You also need to tell patients that the thermometer must be placed next to the skin.

GATHER EQUIPMENT

Charged electronic thermometer   Paper
Supply of probe covers   Pencil

ACTION	RATIONALE
Preparation	
1. Wash hands.	Prevents the spread of microorganisms.
2. Identify yourself and the patient.	Maintains patients' rights.
3. Provide privacy.	Maintains patients' rights.
4. Explain the procedure.	Informs patients about what is happening.
Procedural Steps	
5. Check that the oral probe is connected securely to the charged unit.	The thermometer registers only when the unit is connected securely.
6. Remove the metal probe from the charged unit and insert it into a probe cover.	The cover is discarded after one use to prevent the spread of harmful microorganisms
7. Remove clothing on the side you select to measure the temperature.	Permits access to the heat pocket under the axilla.
8. Place the arm close to the body and hold the thermometer under the axilla.	Ensures accurate results.
9. Listen for a tone or look for a flashing light that indicates the measurement is complete.	Equipment varies from one health care institution to another.
10. Remove the probe from under patients' arm.	The electronic thermometer does not continue to measure after the signal is activated.
11. Read the results on the digital display.	
12. Eject the probe cover into the waste container and return the probe to the holder.	Your hands should not touch a probe cover after it has been used.
13. Record the results and patients' name and room number on the piece of paper.	Helps you recall the specific temperature for each patient.
14. Replace clothing.	
15. Place patients in a comfortable position with the call signal within reach.	Leaves patients with the means to communicate.
16. Open the privacy curtains.	
Follow-Through	
17. Wash hands.	Prevents the spread of microorganisms.
18. Replace the unit in the battery charger or holding area.	The unit charges until it is needed again. The holding area is a safe place for storage.

19. Report results to the nurse.

The nurse is responsible for a decision based on the results of your measurement.

20. Record the temperature in the appropriate place. Write an *A* to signify the temperature was taken by the axillary method (for example, 98.6° F—A).

Provides an official record of the results of a procedure.

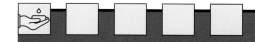

Taking a Tympanic Temperature with a Tympanic Thermometer

Explain to patients that you are going to measure their body temperature with a thermometer that is placed in the ear canal.

GATHER EQUIPMENT

Charged, electronic tympanic thermometer
Disposable probe covers

Paper
Pencil

ACTION	RATIONALE

Preparation

1. Wash hands.

Prevents the spread of microorganisms.

2. Identify yourself and the patient.

Maintains patients' rights.

3. Provide privacy.

Maintains patients' rights.

4. Explain the procedure.

Informs patients about what is happening.

Procedural Steps

5. Check that the tympanic probe is connected to the charged unit.

The thermometer registers only if the probe connection is secure.

6. Insert the cone-shaped end of the tympanic thermometer into a probe cover.

Probe covers are designed for single use to prevent the spread of microorganisms.

7. Ask patients to turn their head so that their ear is directly in front of you. If patients are unable to move their head, you should position their head so that it is directly in front of you.

Permits easy access for placement of the probe into the ear canal.

8. For adults, grasp the **pinna** and pull up and back. For infants, pull the pinna straight back (Figure 9–20).

Straightens the ear canal to allow the probe to seal the ear canal.

PINNA

the part of the ear that projects outside the head; also known as the auricle

9. Place the covered probe into the ear canal.

Correct placement ensures accurate results.

10. Listen for a tone or look for a flashing light that indicates the measurement is complete. If a tone or flashing light is not provided, the digital display itself may signify the measurement is complete by stopping or flashing.

Equipment varies from one institution to another.

11. Remove the probe from patients' ear.

The electronic thermometer does not continue to register after the signal is activated.

Continued on following page

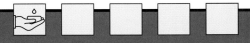

PROCEDURE

Taking a Tympanic Temperature with a Tympanic Thermometer *Continued*

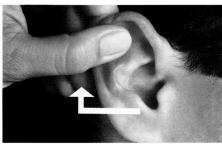

A

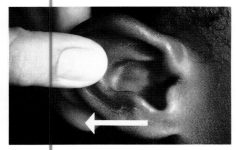

B

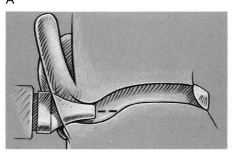

C

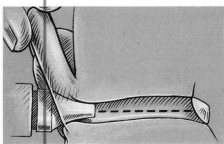

D

FIGURE 9–20

Tympanic temperature measurement. A, For an adult, grasp the pinna and pull up and back. B, For an infant, grasp the pinna and pull straight back. C, Ear canal alignment (horizontal view) before the ear is pulled back. D, Ear canal (horizontal view) after the ear is pulled back. (Photos courtesy of Thermoscan).

12. Read the results on the digital display.	
13. Eject the probe cover into the waste container.	Your hands should not touch a probe cover after it has been used.
14. Record the results and patients' name and room number on the piece of paper.	Record the results as soon as possible. Even a slight distraction may make you forget what the reading was.
15. Place patients in a comfortable position with the call signal within reach.	Leaves patients with the means to communicate.
16. Open the privacy curtain.	

Follow-Through

17. Wash hands.	Prevents the spread of microorganisms.
18. Replace the tympanic thermometer in the battery charger or the holding area.	The unit charges until it is needed again. The holding area is a safe place for storage.
19. Report results to the nurse.	The nurse is responsible for a decision based on the results of your measurement.
20. Record the temperature in the appropriate place. Write a *TY* or the specific abbreviation used in your agency to show a tympanic temperature was taken.	Provides an official record of the procedure.

CARE OF THE PATIENT WITH A CHANGE IN BODY TEMPERATURE

WHAT IS A FEVER?

A **fever** (also called pyrexia) is an elevation of the body's temperature. An elevation in temperature is the body's response to some diseases. When body temperature is elevated, you may observe the following in your patient (Figure 9–21):

- Hot, dry skin
- Flushed face
- Loss of appetite
- Thirst

FEVER

above-normal body temperature; also known as pyrexia

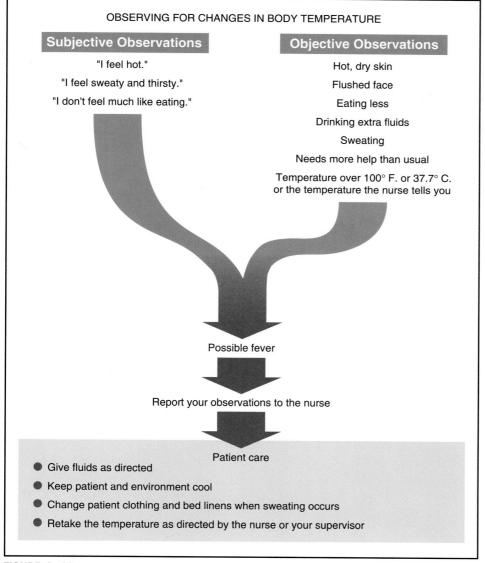

OBSERVING FOR CHANGES IN BODY TEMPERATURE

Subjective Observations

"I feel hot."

"I feel sweaty and thirsty."

"I don't feel much like eating."

Objective Observations

Hot, dry skin

Flushed face

Eating less

Drinking extra fluids

Sweating

Needs more help than usual

Temperature over 100° F. or 37.7° C. or the temperature the nurse tells you

Possible fever

Report your observations to the nurse

Patient care

- Give fluids as directed
- Keep patient and environment cool
- Change patient clothing and bed linens when sweating occurs
- Retake the temperature as directed by the nurse or your supervisor

FIGURE 9–21

Flow chart for fever.

- Sweating
- General weakness (malaise)

You should report such observations to the nurse or supervisor.

CARE OF THE PATIENT WITH A FEVER

When you care for a patient with a temperature elevation, you should follow the guidelines given by your supervisor or nurse. Some activities you might be asked to do are to keep the patient hydrated (give fluids as permitted) and cool (Figure 9–22). Remove or loosen the clothing or blankets. The physician may order a cooling bath with ice at the axilla and groin. Medications to reduce fever (such as aspirin or acetaminophen) are administered by the nurse if ordered by the physician.

Fluids

FLUIDS
liquids

DEHYDRATE
to remove or lose water

Fluids are an important part of the body. The heat produced by a temperature elevation can cause the body to lose fluids. Fluids are lost with each breath. They are also lost through the skin (sweating) during a fever. It is important that fluids lost during this time are replaced. If fluids are not taken in by mouth (or through the veins), the body becomes **dehydrated.** The loss of body fluids causes the cells to function incorrectly and die.

Water given by mouth is the best way to replace body fluids. You can offer your patient other fluids if there are no restrictions on the type or amount of fluid the patient can take in. Offer patients the fluids of their choice as frequently as possible. If patients can take in only small amounts, give the fluids as frequently as every 10 or 15 minutes. This action is especially important in children and in the elderly because they can become dehydrated very quickly.

External Temperature Controls

The body must be able to get rid of the extra heat it produces. Having too much clothing on or too many covers on the bed traps the body's heat, causing discomfort to patients. Therefore your nurse or supervisor may ask you to take the following measures:

- Avoid the use of blankets; keep a light linen cover on patients.

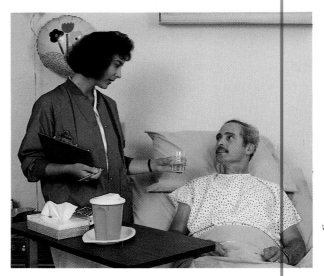

FIGURE 9–22
Offer the patient fluids at least every 2 hours.

- Remove or loosen heavy or extra clothing.
- Adjust the air temperature to a cool level of comfort for patients. Air conditioning and open windows can provide coolness to a room. During the winter, the temperature controls can be turned down because the body is producing extra heat. This allows the extra body heat to enter the cooler air of the surroundings and leave the body.

The physician may order other ways to help the body lower the temperature. You may be asked to give your patient a cooling bath to help bring the body temperature down to a more normal range.

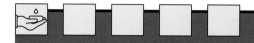

PROCEDURE

Giving a Cooling Sponge Bath

Explain to patients that you are giving them a cooling bath to help bring their body temperature down. Explain that the ice bags under the arms, on the **groin,** and on top of the head also help cool their body (Figure 9–23). A hot water bag is placed under the feet to prevent chilling.

GROIN

the area from the lower abdomen to the inner part of the thighs

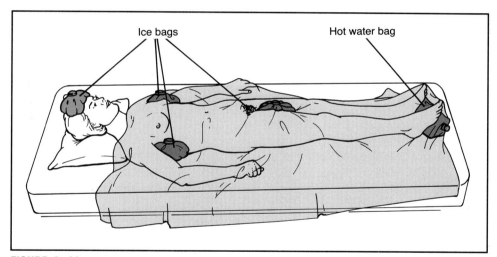

Ice bags   Hot water bag

FIGURE 9–23
Placement of ice packs to help lower body temperature.

GATHER EQUIPMENT

Bath basin
Bath thermometer
Two bath towels
Two washcloths
One hand towel
Clean patient gown
Bath blanket

Six cloth-covered or disposable ice packs
One hot water bottle
Thermometer to measure body temperature
Paper
Pen

ACTION   **RATIONALE**

Preparation

1. Wash hands.

   Prevents the spread of microorganisms.

2. Identify yourself and the patient.

   Maintains patients' rights.

Continued on following page

Giving a Cooling Sponge Bath *Continued*

3. Provide privacy.	Maintains patients' rights.
4. Explain the procedure.	Informs patients about what is happening.

Procedural Steps

5. Prepare a basin of water. Use a bath thermometer to measure the water temperature of 70–86° F.	The water temperature should be cooler than the body temperature of 98.6° F or higher.
6. Add alcohol, if ordered. The solution is one part alcohol and one part water.	Alcohol is rarely added to the bath water for this procedure. Alcohol evaporates at lower (than body) temperature, allowing rapid removal of body heat.
7. Fill the ice packs and the hot water bottles and place them in cloth-covered bags.	Preparation permits more efficient use of time and effort.
8. Bring the equipment to the over-bed table.	Provides easy access to supplies.
9. Lower the side rail on the side from which you are working.	
10. Measure patients' temperature, pulse, and respirations. Write the results and time on the paper.	Gives a baseline measurement for later comparisons.
11. Cover patients with the bath blanket and fold the bed linens to the bottom of the bed.	Provides patient privacy.
12. Remove patients' gown.	Helps the cooling procedure by releasing trapped body heat.
13. Place a bath towel under patients.	Protects bed linens.
14. Place a folded hand towel across patients' genitalia.	
15. Place the cloth-covered hot water bottle against patients' feet.	Helps prevent chilling.
16. Place the cloth-covered ice packs in the following positions: • one on the top of the head • one in each axilla • one over the groin • if ordered, one on each side of the neck	Promotes the loss of body heat.
17. Place the washcloth in the water or water-and-alcohol solution. Change to a cooled washcloth when the one in use becomes warm.	Promotes the loss of body heat. A cooled washcloth is always available.
18. Expose the arm farthest from you. Place a bath towel under the arm.	Bath towel absorbs drips.
19. Use long, smooth strokes to bathe the arm for 5 minutes. Alternate the cooled washcloths during the procedure.	
20. Do not dry off the skin.	Allows evaporation of body heat to occur naturally.
21. Replace the bath blanket over the newly bathed area.	Provides patient privacy.

22. Repeat the same procedure on the arm nearest you.

23. Cover patients' chest and abdomen with a bath towel. Fanfold the bath blanket down to expose the chest and upper abdominal area.

Provides patient privacy.

24. Bathe neck, shoulders, chest, and upper abdomen for 5 minutes.

25. Replace the bath blanket over newly bathed area.

Provides patient privacy.

26. Fanfold the bath blanket down over the groin.

27. Bathe the abdominal area for 5 minutes.

28. Replace the bath blanket over newly bathed area.

Provides patient privacy.

29. Expose the leg farthest from you. Place a bath towel under the leg. Bathe the leg for 5 minutes. Do not dry the skin.

Bath towel absorbs drips.

30. Replace the bath blanket over the newly bathed area.

Provides patient privacy.

31. Repeat the cooling procedure on the leg nearest you.

32. Replace the bath blanket over the newly bathed area.

Provides patient privacy.

33. Assist patients onto their side. Place the bath towel lengthwise next to patients' back.

Bath towel absorbs drips.

34. Bathe the back for 5 minutes.

35. Replace the bath blanket over the newly bathed area.

Provides patient privacy.

36. Assist patients to a comfortable position.

37. Remove the following:
    * hot water bottle
    * all ice packs
    * bottom bath blanket.

Allows patients to rest at the end of the procedure.

38. Replace bed linens if damp.

Ensures patient comfort.

39. Dress patient in a clean gown. Reposition the top linens and remove the bath blanket from the top of patients' body.

Ensures patient comfort.

40. Measure patients' temperature, pulse, and respirations. Write the results and time on the piece of paper.

Helps you recall the specific measurement for each patient.

41. Place patients in a comfortable position with the call signal within reach.

Leaves patients with the means to communicate.

42. Open the privacy curtains.

Follow-Through

43. Carry the soiled linens to the laundry area.

Prevents spread of microorganisms.

Continued on following page

Giving a Cooling Sponge Bath *Continued*

44. Clean and store equipment as directed in your health care institution's policy manual.

    Equipment is prepared for reuse if it is not disposable.

45. Wash hands. Report results and patients' reaction to the cooling bath to the nurse.

    The nurse is responsible for a decision based on the results of your measurement.

46. Return to patients in 30 minutes to measure their temperature, pulse, and respirations again. Write down and report the results to the nurse. Wash hands before and after this procedure.

    The nurse is responsible for a decision based on the results of your measurement.

47. Record the temperature, pulse, and respiration measurements in the appropriate place.

    Provides an official record of the results of the procedure.

48. Record and report any unusual observations you made during the cooling bath procedure.

    The nurse is responsible for a decision based on the observations.

Application of ice packs to the axilla and groin areas during the cooling bath also helps reduce the temperature of a fever. The nurse will advise you if the physician has ordered alcohol to be added to the bath water. The cooling bath is generally not given to very young or elderly patients because the regulation of body temperature is less stable at these ages.

CHAPTER WRAP-UP

- Fever is an elevation in body temperature.
- The balance between the heat the body produces and the heat it loses produces a body temperature reading within the normal range. A body temperature above or below the normal range may signal that a disease process is at work in the body.
- The average oral body temperature is 98.6° F or 37° C.
- An important part of the care of the patient with a fever is hydration (giving fluids).

REVIEW QUESTIONS

1. Identify the sites at which you can measure body temperature.
2. What two main types of equipment are used to measure body temperature?
3. What would you observe if your patient has a fever?

ACTIVITY CORNER

Measure and write down your temperature before and after the following activities.

	Before	**After**
Drinking a hot cup of coffee	_____	_____
Missing the bus or any activity that makes you very angry	_____	_____
Sleeping at night (take your temperature before going to bed and as soon as you wake up in the morning)	_____	_____

What caused the differences? _____

_____

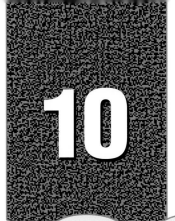

10

Measuring Pulse, Respirations, and Blood Pressure

Objectives

AFTER YOU COMPLETE THIS CHAPTER, YOU WILL BE ABLE TO:

Identify normal pulse ranges.
Count a pulse rate accurately and record it correctly.
Identify normal respiration ranges.
Count respiration rate accurately and record it correctly.
Define asthma, emphysema, and pneumonia.
Discuss the care of patients with common disruptions in respirations: asthma, emphysema, and pneumonia.
Explain the nursing assistant's responsibilities when giving a patient oxygen.
Explain how to set up and use a humidifier.
Identify normal blood pressure ranges.
Measure the blood pressure accurately and record it correctly.
Define myocardial infarction and cerebral vascular accident.
Discuss the care of patients with common disruptions in blood supply: myocardial infarction and cerebral vascular accident.

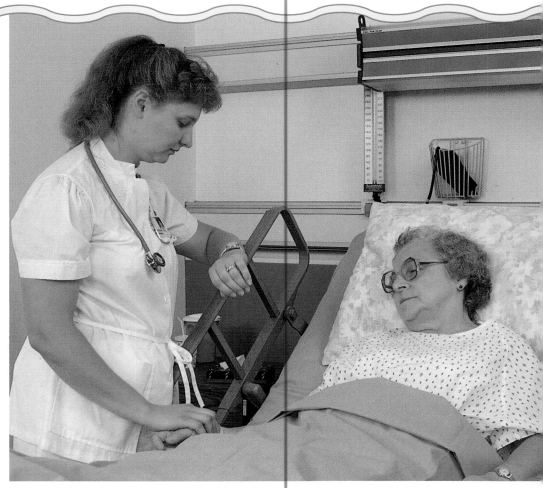

Overview The pulse, respiration, and blood pressure measurements tell how well the two major body organs, the heart and lungs, are functioning. These vital signs change when the heart and lungs are affected by disease or illness. When the heart and lungs do not function properly, the person may not be able to do such ordinary things as walking, sitting, or lying down.

Measuring these vital signs is an important responsibility of the nursing assistant and is performed often in the care of patients. Your observations of patients while you take vital signs are also important to patients' plan of care.

WHAT DO YOU KNOW ABOUT PULSE, RESPIRATIONS, AND BLOOD PRESSURE?

Here are seven statements about pulse, respirations, and blood pressure. Consider them to test your current knowledge about these vital signs. If you think the statement is true, circle the T; if you think the statement is false, circle the F. Change the false statements to make them true.

1. T F The pulse rate (number of heartbeats per minute) rises in response to exercise.

2. T F An infant's pulse rate is the same as an adult's.

3. T F The pulse rate counted when a stethoscope is placed over the tip of the heart is called the apical pulse.

4. T F People cannot control their rate of breathing.

5. T F The trachea, bronchi, and lungs are organs of respiration (breathing).

6. T F When the heart muscle contracts, the heart is at rest.

7. T F *Hypertension* is another name for high blood pressure.

ANSWERS

1. **True.** Exercise puts extra demands on the heart (and lungs) and thus the heart beats faster to meet the body's demand for more oxygen.

2. **False.** An infant's heart rate is over 100 beats per minute because the growing body cells of an infant create a great demand for oxygen. As a person matures, the heart rate slows down to somewhere between 60 and 100 beats per minute.

3. **True.** The pulse counted when a stethoscope is placed over the apex (tip) of the heart is called the apical pulse rate.

4. **False.** Although breathing is an involuntary function, people can control their rate of breathing, for example, when singing or crying.

5. **True.** The trachea, bronchi, and lungs are organs of breathing. They are assisted by other organs known as secondary organs of breathing.

6. **False.** *Contraction* is the term used for the heart at work; *relaxation* is the term for the heart at rest.

7. **True.** H*yper* means fast or high; thus *hypertension* is another name for high blood pressure.

Measurements of the pulse, respirations, and blood pressure tell how the heart and lungs are functioning. Changes in these vital signs can signify a change in body function. Your measurements as well as observations of the patient are an important part of patient care.

THE STRUCTURES OF CIRCULATION

The structures of circulation include the red blood cells, the blood vessels, and the heart (Figure 10–1).

RED BLOOD CELLS

OXYGEN
a colorless, tasteless, odorless gas; the air we breathe is about 20% oxygen

CARBON DIOXIDE
an odorless, colorless gas that is expelled from the lungs

Red blood cells are needed to carry **oxygen** to the body's cells and carry **carbon dioxide** away from the cells. The red blood cells and other cells are

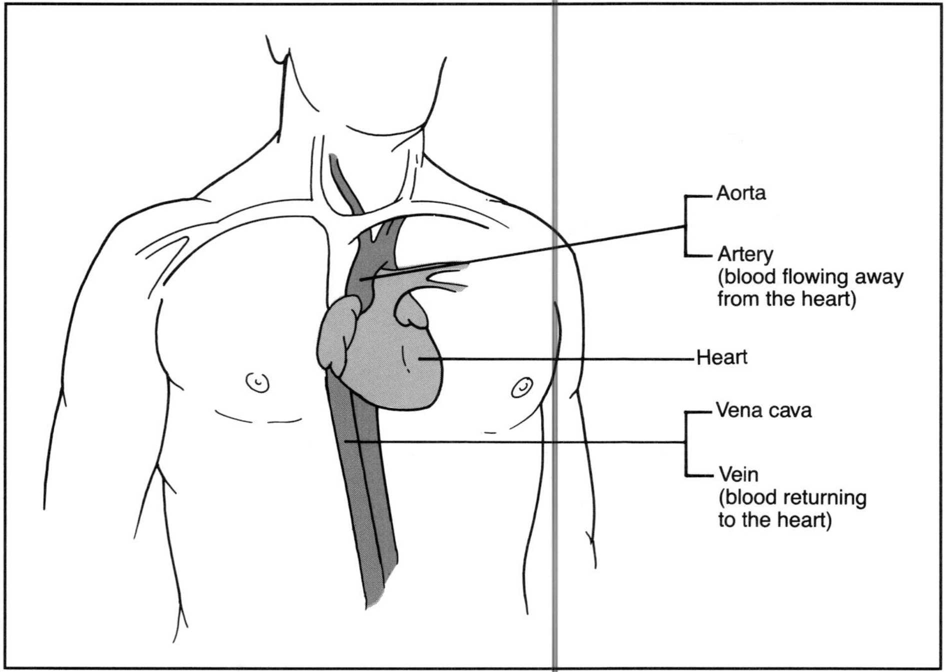

FIGURE 10–1
The heart and blood vessels.

suspended in a special fluid called *plasma*. Together, the cells and plasma form the blood. The term *bloodstream* refers to the flow of blood throughout the body. Blood is delivered to the body's cells through the blood vessels.

BLOOD VESSELS

The blood vessels are made up of the arteries and veins. An **artery**'s job is to carry blood from the heart so that oxygen is delivered to the cells. The blood in the arteries is carried through the body by the pumping action of the heart. The oxygen and carbon dioxide are exchanged at the smallest parts of the arteries **(arterioles)** and the **vein (venules).** The blood journeys back to the heart through the veins. The veins have small valves that stop the back-flow of blood. Blood is returned to the heart and sent to the lungs for fresh oxygen.

HEART

The **heart** is an electrical pump, especially designed to move blood in and out of itself and through the blood vessels of the body. The heart is located in the left side of the chest and is protected by the ribs. The wave of blood that creates the pulse is created by the alternate **contraction** and **relaxation** of the heart muscle.

The heart is a muscle that is divided into four chambers. Special valves are located at the entrance and exit of the heart and between the chambers. The valves snap shut with every beat of the heart to prevent any flow of blood back in the direction from which it came.

Each side of the heart has an upper chamber, called an **atrium,** and a lower chamber, called a **ventricle** (Figure 10–2). Thus there are two atria and

ARTERY
a blood vessel that carries blood away from the heart to the body's organs

ARTERIOLE
smallest part of the artery

VEIN
a blood vessel that carries blood from the body's organs to the heart

VENULE
smallest part of a vein

HEART
the hollow muscular organ located in the left side of the chest that is an electrical pump that controls the flow of blood

CONTRACTION
shortening or tightening of muscle fiber

RELAXATION
easing of tension; resting

ATRIUM
an upper chamber of the heart; there are two upper chambers of the heart (together called the atria)

VENTRICLE
a small chamber or cavity located in the heart or brain; the heart has two lower chambers (together called the ventricles)

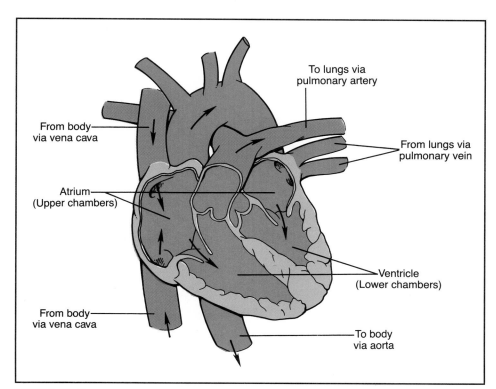

FIGURE 10–2
The chambers of the heart. Note the flow of blood through the chambers of the heart.

LUNGS

the two main organs of respiration

PULMONARY ARTERY

large artery that carries blood from the right ventricle to the lungs

PULMONARY VEIN

the large vein that carries oxygenated blood from the lungs to the left atrium of the heart

AORTA

the largest artery in the body; it rises from the left ventricle

VENA CAVA

the large vein that returns blood to the right atrium of the heart

two ventricles in the heart. The blood comes into the atrium on the right side of the heart from the veins in the body. It is then pumped into the right ventricle.

Because the red blood cells need oxygen, the heart pumps the blood to the **lungs** by way of a special blood vessel called the **pulmonary artery.** Oxygen reaches the lungs through the air we breathe in. The red blood cells give up the carbon dioxide they are carrying and receive the oxygen in the lungs. The carbon dioxide is breathed out into the air from the lungs. Another special blood vessel (called the **pulmonary vein**) delivers the blood that is carrying the fresh oxygen to the atrium on the left side of the heart.

The blood then enters the left ventricle ready to be pumped into the arteries. From here the blood enters the aorta. The **aorta** is the main artery that branches off into the other arteries of the body. The arteries are able to reach all body cells so that oxygen can be delivered. The red blood cells then return to small veins; in turn, certain veins enter into the **vena cava,** which delivers the blood directly into the right atrium. This is the cycle that is repeated with every heartbeat.

PULSE

PULSE

the beat of the heart as felt through the walls of the arteries

The **pulse** is a wave of blood rushing through the arteries. It is created by pumping action of the heart muscle as it contracts and relaxes. The wave that is created can be felt when slight pressure is applied at certain points of the body.

These points, known as pulse sites, are located wherever the artery lies

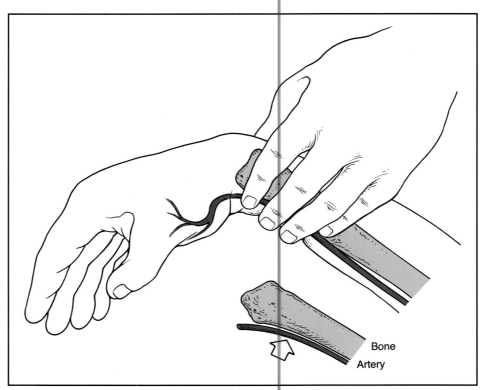

FIGURE 10–3

The radial artery lies close to the surface of the skin. (It is located over the radial bone.)

TABLE 10-1 PULSE RATES ACROSS THE LIFE SPAN

Age	Range	Average
Newborn	120–160	140
1 month–1 year	80–140	120
1–6 years	80–120	115
6–12 years	75–110	95
Adolescence–adult	60–100	80

close to a bone (Figure 10–3). When you apply slight pressure with your fingers on these areas, you can count the number of heartbeats in a minute.

The number of beats per minute is normally the same at any pulse site in the body. If the pulse can be measured at the feet (the site farthest away from the heart), you know that the blood is circulating and reaching the body's tissue with oxygen for the cells. The pulse is measured for the rate as well as the regularity or irregularity of the beat.

PULSE RATE AND REGULARITY

The **pulse rate** is the number of heartbeats per minute felt at a pulse site. It is the same as the heart rate. The heart rate can vary according to factors such as age, sex, and activity (discussed in Chapter 8). It is highest at birth and keeps decreasing until a person is fully grown (Table 10–1). For an adult, the normal heart rate ranges between 60 and 90 beats per minute.

When the heart's pumping action is inefficient, the result may be an abnormal heart rate or an irregular beat.

- The term **bradycardia** is used for any heart rate below 60 beats per minute.
- The term **tachycardia** is used for any heart rate over 100 beats per minute.

The amount of time between beats of the heart should be equal between each beat. When it is equal, the heart rate is called a "regular" pulse. A pulse that does not produce a regular pattern when you count the beats is called an "irregular" pulse.

You may also be asked to describe the "fullness" (thready or bounding) of the pulse. Use the following guidelines to determine pulse fullness.

HOW TO DETERMINE PULSE FULLNESS	
Term Used	**What You Feel at the Site**
Full and bounding	Gentle pressure of the fingers does not blot out the puise.
Weak and thready	Gentle pressure of the fingers eliminates the pulse easily.

You should report any pulse that is

- below 60 beats per minute
- over 100 beats per minute
- not regular when the beats are counted
- weak and thready

PULSE RATE

the number of heartbeats per minute felt at a pulse site; the same as the heart rate

BRADYCARDIA

a heart rate less than 60 beats per minute

TACHYCARDIA

a heart rate over 100 beats per minute

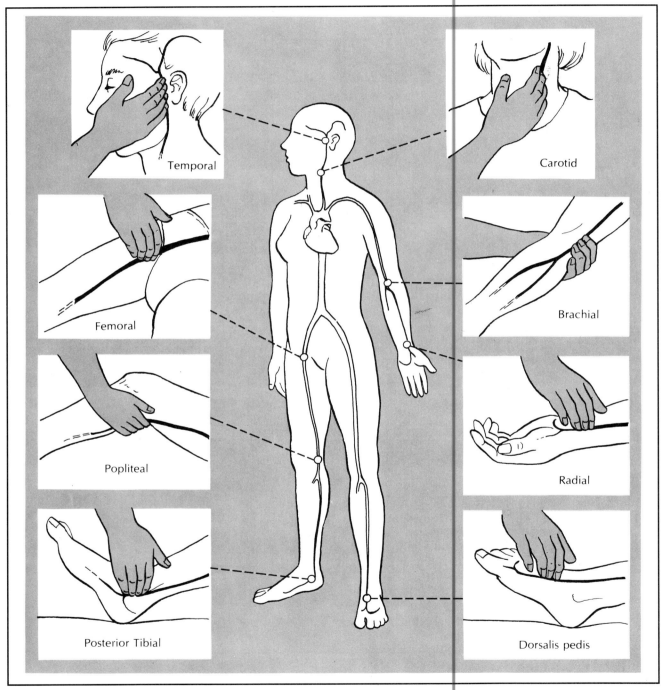

FIGURE 10–4

Peripheral pulse sites. (From Sorensen KC, Luckmann, J: Basic Nursing: A Psychological Approach, 2nd ed. Philadelphia, W.B. Saunders Company, 1986.)

PULSE SITES

Peripheral

The pulse can be counted at sites near the surface of the body. They are called **peripheral** sites; that is, they are located away from the heart. Peripheral pulses are found wherever an artery passes closely over a bone that is near the skin.

Peripheral sites you may use include the following (Figure 10–4):

Radial (wrist)
Brachial (antecubital)
Carotid (throat)
Temporal (temple)
Femoral (thigh)
Popliteal (knee)
Posterior tibial (back of the ankle)
Dorsalis pedis (foot)

The peripheral pulse site used most often is the radial site. The brachial pulse **(antecubital)** is used when you measure the blood pressure.

PERIPHERAL
outer edge

ANTECUBITAL
the inner part of the elbow

Apical

Another site you use is the apical site, that is, over the apex (tip) of the heart (Figure 10–5). You must use a **stethoscope** to listen to the apical heartbeat. The **apical pulse** is always counted

- for 1 full minute
- whenever the heart rate is irregular
- in infants and children up to age 1 (or as recommended in your institution's policy manual)
- if the patient is on cardiac (heart) medications
- whenever the heart rate is too fast to count at a peripheral site
- anytime you cannot count a radial pulse accurately

Note: The apical pulse rate is never lower than the radial pulse rate.

STETHOSCOPE
an instrument used to hear and amplify the sounds of an internal organ (heart, lungs, or bowels)

APICAL PULSE
pulse counted by listening through a stethoscope over the apex (tip) of the heart

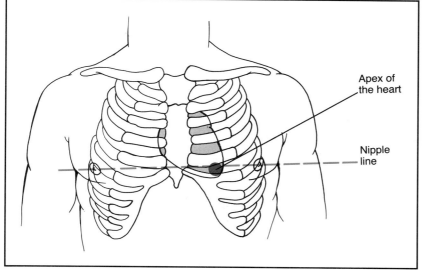

Apex of
the heart

Nipple
line

FIGURE 10–5
Location of the apical pulse. Place the stethoscope over the apex (tip) of the heart.

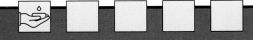

Counting the Radial Pulse

The radial pulse site is the most commonly used site because it is comfortable for the patient and easily reached by the care giver.

GATHER EQUIPMENT

Watch with a second hand   Pencil
Paper

ACTION	RATIONALE

Preparation

1. Wash hands.
2. Identify yourself and the patient.
3. Provide privacy.
4. Explain the procedure.

Prevents the spread of microorganisms.
Maintains patients' rights.
Maintains patients' rights.
Informs patients about what is happening.

Procedural Steps

5. Place patients in a comfortable position. (The arm can be placed across the chest.)

6. Locate the radial pulse by placing your first three fingers gently on the thumb side of the patient's wrist (Figure 10–6).

Use your fingers because the thumb has a pulse of its own.

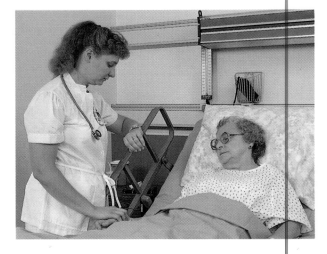

FIGURE 10–6
You should concentrate on counting and watching the second hand of your watch when you are taking the patient's pulse and respirations.

7. When you feel the pulse, place gentle pressure against the artery.

The radial artery lies close to the bone, allowing a pulse to be counted at the site. Gentle pressure ensures that you won't **obliterate** the pulse.

OBLITERATE
erase

8. Watch the second hand of your watch and count the number of beats you feel for 1 full minute. (In some health care institutions, you may be taught to count for 30 seconds and multiply by two for the result.)

Be sure to follow your institution's policy in regard to counting a peripheral pulse.

9. Remove your fingers when the pulse is counted and record the results and patients' name and room number on the piece of paper.

    Record the results as soon as possible. Even slight distraction may make you forget the results.

10. Place patients in a comfortable position with the call signal within reach.

    Leaves patients with the means to communicate.

11. Open the privacy curtains.

Follow-Through

12. Wash hands.

    Prevents the spread of microorganisms.

13. Report results to the nurse.

    The nurse is responsible for any decision that is based on the results of the measurement.

14. Record the pulse rate in the appropriate place. Include the rate, regularity, and fullness of the pulse in your recording.

    Provides an official record of the results of the procedure.

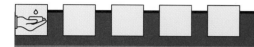

PROCEDURE

Counting the Apical Pulse

The apical pulse site, located at the apex (tip) of the heart, is used in specific situations. The nurse tells you when you should take an apical heart rate.

GATHER EQUIPMENT

Stethoscope   Paper
Alcohol swab   Pencil
Watch with a second hand

ACTION   RATIONALE

Preparation

1. Wash hands.

    Prevents the spread of microorganisms.

2. Identify yourself and the patient.

    Maintains patients' rights.

3. Provide privacy.

    Maintains patients' rights.

4. Explain the procedure.

    Informs patients what is happening.

Procedural Steps

5. Clean the ear pieces, bell, and diaphragm of the stethoscope with the alcohol swab (Figure 10–7).

    Helps disinfect the parts and prevents the spread of microorganisms.

6. Place the clean ear pieces in your ears. Hold the diaphragm in your hands for a few minutes to warm it.

    A warm stethoscope on the chest is more comfortable for patients.

7. Place the stethoscope (bell or diaphragm) on patients' bare chest to the left at the nipple line (Figure 10–8).

    Never listen and count through patients' clothing because other sounds might interfere with an accurate count.

8. Listen for the heartbeat.

    Locates the correct sound (lub-dub) before the count begins.

9. Watch the second hand of your watch and count for 1 full minute.

    An apical pulse rate is always counted for 1 full minute.

Continued on following page

Counting the Apical Pulse *Continued*

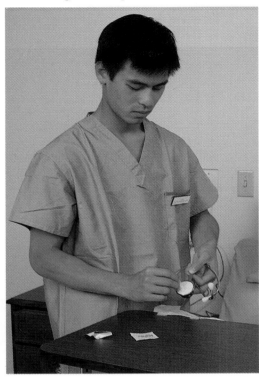

FIGURE 10-7
Clean the ear pieces, the bell, and the diaphragm of the stethoscope with an alcohol swab.

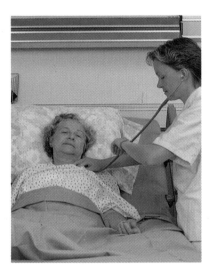

FIGURE 10-8
After you count the apical pulse for 1 minute, continue to listen through the stethoscope and count the patient's respirations while you watch the chest rise and fall.

10. Remove the stethoscope from patients' chest and the ear pieces from your ears.

11. Record the results and patients' name and room number on the piece of paper.

Record the results as soon as possible. Even slight distraction may make you forget the results.

12. Place patients in a comfortable position with the call signal within reach.

Leaves patients with the means to communicate.

13. Open the privacy curtains.

14. Clean the ear pieces and the bell or diaphragm of the stethoscope with an alcohol swab. Return the stethoscope to storage.

    Keeps equipment as free of microorganisms as possible.

Follow-Through

15. Wash hands.

    Prevents the spread of microorganisms.

16. Report results to the nurse.

    The nurse is responsible for any decision that is based on the results of the measurement.

17. Record the pulse rate in the appropriate place. Include the rate, regularity, and fullness of the pulse in the recording.

    Provides an official record of the results of the procedure.

USING A STETHOSCOPE

The stethoscope is especially made to magnify (make louder) sounds. It consists of three main parts, as shown in Figure 10–9.

HOW A STETHOSCOPE WORKS

Part	Use
Diaphragm or bell	Picks up sounds when placed over certain body parts
Tubing	Carries the magnified sound of the body part to the listener
Ear pieces	Deliver the sound to the listener's ears

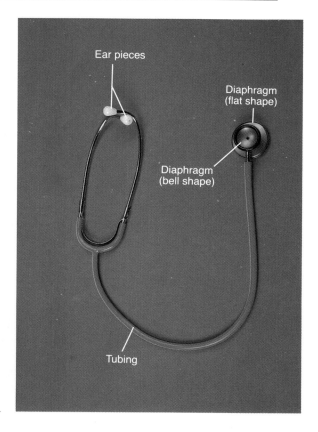

FIGURE 10–9

Parts of the stethoscope.

CARING COMMENTS

Any time you use a stethoscope to listen to a body sound, remember to clean the diaphragm or bell and both ear pieces before and after use.

Point the ear pieces of the stethoscope forward before you place them in your ears. This enables you to hear sounds through the stethoscope.

Taking a Pulse

When you listen to the heartbeat with a stethoscope, you hear two sounds.

"LUB"   The first heart sound heard is the "lub" of the "lub-dub." At the same time the ventricles of the heart contract to push the blood out of the heart into the circulation, the valves (**mitral** and **tricuspid**) between the atria and the ventricles snap shut to prevent the back-flow of blood into the atria. The "lub" is the sound the valves make when they close.

"DUB"   A soft sound occurs next. It is caused when the **semilunar valves** close to prevent the blood from flowing back into the ventricles. It is the "dub" of the "lub-dub."

When the heart becomes weakened by disease, it fails to send the usual wave of blood through the arteries. You may not be able to count the radial pulse and must listen with a stethoscope to count the heart rate. The apical site is located

- on the left side in front of the chest
- between the fifth and sixth ribs
- about the nipple line in men
- under the left breast below the nipple in women (see Figure 10–5)

Apical–Radial Pulse

You may be asked to assist with counting an apical–radial pulse. An **apical–radial pulse** is counted by two persons: one counts the radial pulse, and the other counts the apical pulse at the same time (Figure 10–10). The difference between the two pulses is the pulse deficit. A **pulse deficit** occurs when the heart beats so weakly that the pulse cannot be counted accurately at the radial (wrist) site. The box gives an example of how a pulse deficit is determined.

MITRAL VALVE
the valve between the left atrium and the left ventricle of the heart

TRICUSPID VALVE
the valve that is located between the right atrium and the right ventricle

SEMILUNAR VALVES
one valve that is located in the right ventricle and guards the entrance into the pulmonary trunk; one valve that is located in the left ventricle and guards the entrance into the aorta

APICAL–RADIAL PULSE
pulse counted by two persons (one person counts the apical pulse, and the second person counts the radial [wrist] pulse at the same time) to determine whether a pulse deficit is present

PULSE DEFICIT
the numerical difference between the radial pulse and the apical pulse

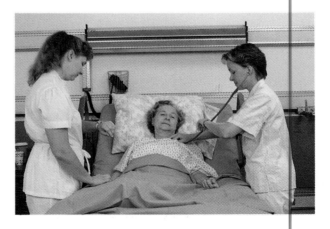

FIGURE 10–10
Two care givers count the apical-radial pulse.

> ### DETERMINING A PULSE DEFICIT
> 1. Care giver A counts an apical pulse of 100 beats per minute.
> 2. Care giver B counts a radial pulse of 96 beats per minute.
> 3. The pulse deficit is 4 (100 − 96 = 4).

Special equipment is available to count a pulse rate when it cannot be palpated (felt with the fingers). A Doppler is an instrument that works like sonar on a submarine. A water-soluble lubricant is placed on the skin over a pulse site. A wand is held on the skin over the area where a pulse needs to be counted. Sound caused by the wave action of the blood in the arteries bounces back and registers as a bleep that can be counted.

A cardiac monitor, used in special intensive care units, can also be used to record the pulse rate continuously on a screen.

THE STRUCTURES OF RESPIRATION (BREATHING)

The **nares, trachea, bronchi,** and the lungs are the organs of respiration (Figure 10–11). The purpose of respiration is to enable the exchange of oxygen and carbon dioxide in the lungs. The air that contains oxygen reaches the lungs by way of the nares, trachea, and bronchi. When air enters the nares, small particles are filtered out before it reaches the lungs. As air travels to the lungs, it is warmed by small blood vessels that line the mucous membranes of the passageways. The passageways become more narrow as the air enters the lungs.

The red blood cells must continually provide oxygen to the body's cells. Oxygen is needed by all body cells to live. When the oxygen is used by a cell, it is changed chemically into carbon dioxide, which is a waste product of the body. After the exchange in the cells of the lungs, the carbon dioxide leaves the body through the same structures by which it enters.

NARES
the nostrils; the external (outside) opening of the nasal cavity
TRACHEA
the air passage from the mouth to the lungs; the windpipe
BRONCHI
the air passageways in the lungs

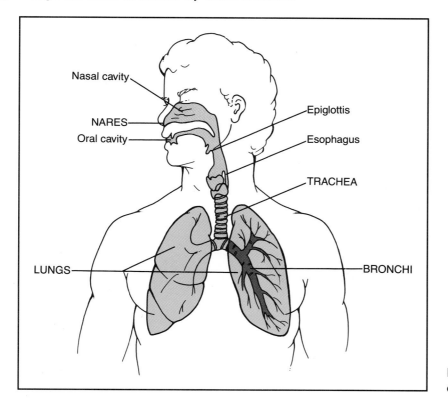

FIGURE 10–11
Organs of the respiratory tract.

RESPIRATION

RESPIRATION
the exchange of oxygen and carbon dioxide between the air and the body's cells
INSPIRATION
breathing in
EXPIRATION
breathing out
MEDULLA OBLONGATA
the respiratory control center in the brain

Respiration is the act of breathing. **Inspiration** is the act of breathing in oxygen that is distributed to the cells of the body. **Expiration** is the act of breathing out carbon dioxide. The exchange of oxygen for carbon dioxide occurs in the lungs. The **medulla oblongata** in the brain regulates the number of respirations. Respiration is automatic; yet we can adjust our breathing voluntarily when we sing or cry.

PATTERNS OF RESPIRATION

The normal pattern of breathing is quiet and regular. The normal range for breathing is 14–20 breaths per minute. The following terms are used to describe patterns of respirations:

- *bradypnea*—fewer than 14 breaths per minute
- *tachypnea*—more than 20 breaths per minute
- *dyspnea*—difficult breathing
- *apnea*—no respirations present
- *Cheyne-Stokes*—periods of deep breaths, followed by very short or no breaths, repeated in a cycle
- *stertorous*—noisy breaths that sound like snoring
- *shallow*—breaths that fill the lungs only partially with air

When you observe any of these patterns of breathing, you should report the breathing pattern to the supervisor or nurse.

When you count the patient's respirations, you should also observe for the following.

DEPTH OF BREATHING   Watch the rise and fall of the chest and note whether the

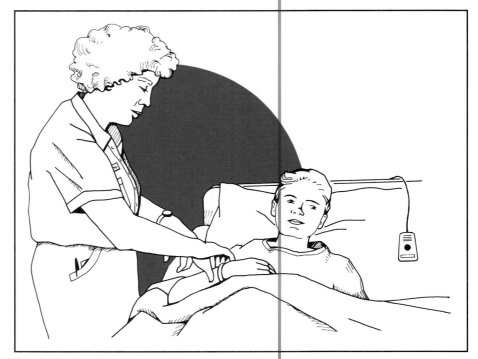

FIGURE 10–12

Counting respirations. By placing patients' arm across their chest, you can observe and count how many times the chest rises and falls.

breaths are deep (large amounts of air exchanged) or shallow (small amounts of air exchanged with minimal air movement).

SYMMETRY   Check to see that both sides of the chest rise and fall equally.

RHYTHM   Respirations should be evenly spaced and effortless.

ABNORMAL SOUNDS   You can hear two sounds without a stethoscope:
- wheezing—a whistling sound associated with breathing
- stridor—a shrill, harsh breath sound

You should count respirations before or after you measure the pulse rate (Figure 10–12).

SYMMETRY
balance

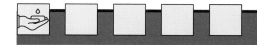

PROCEDURE

Counting Respirations

Count the number of respirations by watching the rise and fall of the chest. Use a watch with a second hand for this procedure.

GATHER EQUIPMENT

Watch with a second hand   Pencil
Paper

ACTION	**RATIONALE**

Procedural Steps

1. Count the respirations before or after you measure the pulse.

If patients know when respirations are being counted, they can choose to slow down or speed up respirations voluntarily.

2. Keep a steady, even pressure of your fingers on patients' wrist while you are counting the respiratory rate.

So patients do not know when you are counting respirations. You can therefore observe normal, involuntary breathing.

3. Observe respirations for the following:
- rate
- pattern
- depth
- symmetry of the chest
- rhythm or regularity
- unusual sounds

Always report any respirations that are not ordinary and effortless.

4. Record the results and patients' name and room number on the piece of paper as soon as possible.

Even a slight distraction may make you forget the results.

5. Place patients in a comfortable position with the call signal within reach.

Leaves patients with the means to communicate.

6. Open the privacy curtains.

Follow-Through

7. Wash hands.

Prevents the spread of microorganisms.

8. Report results to the nurse.

The nurse is responsible for any decision that is based on the results of the measurement.

9. Record the pulse rate in the appropriate place. Include the rate, regularity, and fullness of the pulse in your recording.

Provides an official record of the results of the procedure.

CARE OF THE PATIENT WITH COMMON DISRUPTIONS IN RESPIRATION

Common diseases that affect the organs of respiration are

Pneumonia
Asthma
Emphysema

Each disease can affect the oxygen–carbon dioxide exchange in the lungs. Patients whose bodies lack oxygen are tired and have little energy. They breathe faster (more respirations per minute) to keep up with their body's demand for oxygen.

PNEUMONIA

PNEUMONIA
an acute inflammation or infection of lung tissue

Pneumonia is an acute inflammation of lung tissue. It affects the tissues of the lower respiratory tract. The inflammation interferes with the exchange of oxygen and carbon dioxide in the lungs.

Pneumonia can be caused by viruses and other harmful microorganisms. These microorganisms may be present in the form of small droplets in the air and can be breathed into the lungs. The droplets can be breathed in from spray that comes out when people talk, cough, or sneeze. An inflammation response can occur if particles of food or fluid in the stomach or esophagus are **aspirated** into the lungs; this is called aspiration pneumonia. Unusual observations you will note in a patient with pneumonia are

ASPIRATION
a foreign body being drawn into the lungs; may occur in persons who are unconscious, under the effects of anesthesia, or having difficulty swallowing

PURULENT
containing pus

- fever that starts quickly
- shaking chills
- cough that may produce **purulent** sputum
- chest pain

Some patients may also become lethargic (sleepy) or weak and confused, and some may experience a loss of appetite and a loss of body fluid (dehydration).

The physician or the nurse can listen to the lungs; certain sounds indicate that oxygen and carbon dioxide are not being exchanged efficiently. The approximate location of the pneumonia can be determined from the sounds. Disease of the lungs can also be viewed and pinpointed on an x-ray if the physician orders it. The physician may order bed rest, fluids, and medications to treat the pneumonia and the fever.

ASTHMA

ASTHMA
a disease of the bronchi characterized by difficult, wheezing respiration

POLLEN
the substance that fertilizes flowering plants

DANDER
small particles from the hair or feathers of animals that may cause an allergy

Asthma is a disease of the bronchi (air passages) in the lungs. The cause of asthma is not clearly understood. It is known that the lungs respond to certain stimuli (irritants). Stimuli may be

- certain foods or dust
- **pollen**
- animal **dander**
- small scales from the hair or feathers of animals
- smoke
- any number of other irritants or pollutants in the environment
- stress

Not all persons respond with asthma to these stimuli. In people who do respond, the response causes

SPASM
a sudden contraction (tightening) of a muscle or group of muscles

- **spasm** of the bronchi
- swelling of the air passageways
- production of thick secretions

These responses make the air passageways more narrow, so it is difficult for enough oxygen to reach the lungs.

The major observation of a patient with asthma is dyspnea (difficulty breathing). Wheezing occurs often in asthmatic persons. Dyspnea or wheezing should be reported to the supervisor or nurse. During an asthma attack, the patient may experience the following:

- a feeling of fullness or tightness in the chest
- shortness of breath
- coughing
- fear and irritability
- profuse sweating
- extreme anxiousness
- an inability to talk because of lack of oxygen

The physician treats asthma in a patient by ordering certain medications that dilate (open) the air passageways so that oxygen can be delivered to the lungs.

EMPHYSEMA

Emphysema results from the destruction of the alveoli and enlargement of air spaces in the lung tissue. The oxygen and the carbon dioxide cannot move in and out of the lungs as usual.

Emphysema is classified as a chronic obstructive pulmonary disease. Because an obstruction (blockage) of the air passageways causes air to become trapped in the lungs, the patient cannot empty the lungs of air. It is a chronic disease (an illness that continues over a long period of time); the patient experiences periods of remission in which the disease is quiet and does not interfere with activities of daily living. These can be followed by an **exacerbation** of the emphysema.

In the early stages of emphysema, patients may arise in the morning, cough, and produce **sputum.** As the disease progresses, the cough and amount of sputum increase. Patients also become short of breath upon exertion.

In the late stage of emphysema, patients develop a persistent cough and produce large amounts of sputum. They are too tired to perform the activities of daily living because even a small amount of movement causes them to use their oxygen reserves quickly. Observations include

- a cough that may persist
- increased amounts of sputum
- increased shortness of breath upon exertion
- decreased ability to perform activities of daily living
- fatigue

Each of these becomes more severe as the disease progresses.

The main form of treatment of emphysema is a medication to dilate the air passageways. Depending on symptoms, other medications can be ordered to make patients comfortable and help them function. Oxygen may also be ordered (Figure 10–13).

EMPHYSEMA
destruction of the alveoli (tiny air sacs in the lungs) and enlargement of air spaces so oxygen and carbon dioxide cannot move in and out of the lungs

EXACERBATION
making more severe; a flare-up

SPUTUM
a mucous secretion from the lungs, bronchi, and trachea that is ejected (brought up) through the mouth

MONITORING RESPIRATORY RATE

Registered Nurse's Responsibilities

The registered nurse
- knows how to administer oxygen
- knows the amount of oxygen the physician has ordered

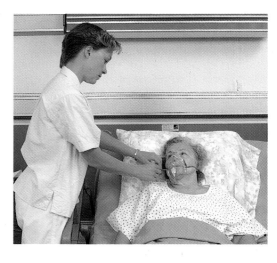

FIGURE 10–13
Adjust the elastic so that the oxygen delivery system (mask or nasal cannula) is comfortable for the patient.

- sets up and cares for the oxygen equipment
- monitors the oxygen administration

Nursing Assistant's Responsibilities

The nursing assistant

- checks to see that the oxygen is set at the ordered amount (Figure 10–14A)
- checks that the humidifier container is bubbling and the proper amount of distilled water is in the container
- keeps the tubing free so that it is not pinched off (Figure 10–14B)

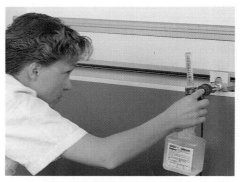

A

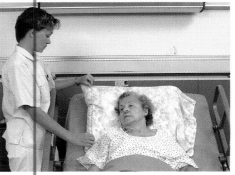

B

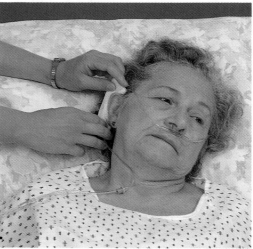

C

FIGURE 10–14
A, Read the oxygen setting at eye level. *Never adjust the flow meter*. B, Check the tubing frequently; the patient should not lie on the tubing. C, If the skin breaks down, the nurse may ask you to place a piece of gauze under the tubing to protect the patient's skin.

- gives the patient frequent oral care
- observes areas of the cheeks and ears where the plastic tubing touches the skin for redness and swelling (Figure 10–14C)
- reports any different oxygen setting to the nurse or supervisor
- reports any respiratory distress to the nurse or supervisor
- when using portable oxygen, checks the gauge to make sure adequate oxygen is in the tank

Note: The device (a nasal cannula or mask) that delivers the oxygen to the patient should never be removed.

GENERAL CARE OF THE PATIENT WITH BREATHING DISRUPTIONS

You can take certain actions to help the patient who is experiencing breathing problems (Figure 10–15).

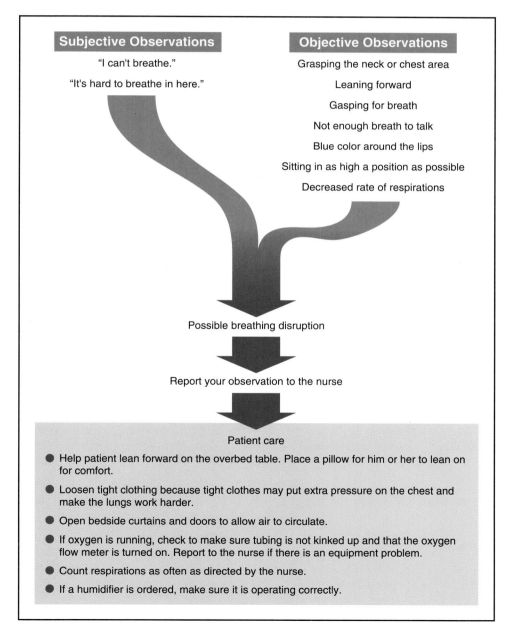

Subjective Observations

"I can't breathe."

"It's hard to breathe in here."

Objective Observations

Grasping the neck or chest area

Leaning forward

Gasping for breath

Not enough breath to talk

Blue color around the lips

Sitting in as high a position as possible

Decreased rate of respirations

Possible breathing disruption

Report your observation to the nurse

Patient care

- Help patient lean forward on the overbed table. Place a pillow for him or her to lean on for comfort.
- Loosen tight clothing because tight clothes may put extra pressure on the chest and make the lungs work harder.
- Open bedside curtains and doors to allow air to circulate.
- If oxygen is running, check to make sure tubing is not kinked up and that the oxygen flow meter is turned on. Report to the nurse if there is an equipment problem.
- Count respirations as often as directed by the nurse.
- If a humidifier is ordered, make sure it is operating correctly.

FIGURE 10–15

Flow chart for a patient with breathing problems.

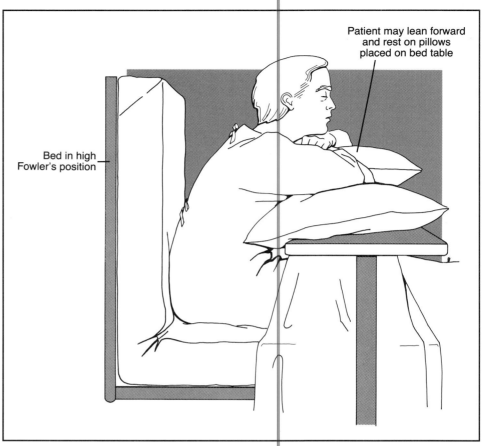

Patient may lean forward
and rest on pillows
placed on bed table

Bed in high
Fowler's position

FIGURE 10–16
Orthopneic position.

Position

Help the patient sit up in Fowler's position (sitting with head of the bed raised) or the **orthopneic position** (Figure 10–16). In the orthopneic position, the over-bed table is placed in front of the patient. A pillow can be placed on the table, and the patient can lean over the table. Both positions help the lungs expand more efficiently so there is better oxygen–carbon dioxide exchange.

Fluids

Extra fluids are helpful to the patient because they keep the body's tissues bathed in fluid. If there are thick secretions, the fluids help break them up, which allows them to be removed from the body more easily. Oral fluids are encouraged, and the patient may also receive fluids through a vein.

Air

Be sure air is moving in the patient's room. If curtains and doors are kept shut, the air becomes stale and stuffy. The patient will find it difficult to breathe.

Clothing

Loosen any tight clothing that can interfere with the patient's breathing. Bras and tight collars or ties can cause discomfort or difficulty breathing.

ORTHOPNEIC POSITION

an upright position supported by pillows; relieves difficulty in breathing

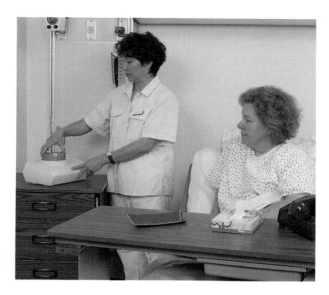

FIGURE 10-17
A humidifier adds moisture to the room air, which helps the patient breathe easier.

Oxygen

Oxygen is ordered by the physician to help the patient receive more oxygen than is present in the air. It is a *drug*. Check the setting on the **oxygen flow-meter**; it should be set at the amount the nurse tells you. Report any change in flow rate to nurse. D*o not* adjust the flow of oxygen.

OXYGEN FLOW-METER
a meter that regulates the amount of oxygen prescribed for delivery to a patient

Humidity

Air that contains moisture helps break up the mucous secretions that might be interfering with respirations. The physician may order a **humidifier** to be placed in the room (Figure 10-17). A humidifier is a special container that produces a fine mist of water particles. The mist enters the air that surrounds the patient. The **humidity**, in the form of mist, is breathed in by the patient. This added moisture helps to break up thick secretions and allows the patient to breathe more easily.

HUMIDIFIER
a device (run by electricity) that produces a fine mist of water particles
HUMIDITY
moisture

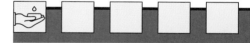

PROCEDURE

Monitoring a Humidifier

Place the water-filled humidifier on a stable surface out of the patient's reach. Check the cord and plug; they should be intact. Plug into the electrical outlet. Direct the spout toward the patient.

GATHER EQUIPMENT

Humidifier   Water

ACTION   **RATIONALE**

Procedural Steps

1. Make sure the humidifier is running.	The humidifier runs on electricity. Be certain the cord is plugged into the wall outlet.
2. Check the fluid indicator.	Fluid is needed in the container to produce the mist.

Continued on following page

Monitoring a Humidifier *Continued*

3. Check the position of the humidifier spout.

The mist should be available for the patient to breathe in.

4. Check the placement of the humidifier. It should be about 5–6 feet away from the patient.

The humidifier should be placed where it cannot be accidentally spilled.

5. Report any of the following to the nurse:
   - a humidifier that is not operating correctly
   - a level of fluid that indicates the need to add more fluid
   - any observations you make about the patient's breathing

The humidifier must operate correctly if it is to help the patient's respirations.

6. Record information about the humidifier in the appropriate place.

Provides an official record that the ordered equipment is operating.

BLOOD PRESSURE

BLOOD PRESSURE

pressure caused by the blood circulating against the arteries

Remember that oxygen-carrying blood must reach every cell of the body. The heart is a pump that must use a tremendous amount of pressure to force the blood to circulate through the arteries and veins.

The pressure the heart uses to pump against the resistance of the body can be measured. The result is a number called **blood pressure.** The physician and nurse can determine the heart's efficiency by interpreting the blood pressure numbers. The nursing assistant helps with this by measuring patients' blood pressure.

Blood pressure is caused by the blood pushing against the walls of the arteries as it travels through the body. Blood pressure is regulated by

- the amount of blood ejected from the heart with each beat
- the amount of blood available in the heart and blood vessels
- the elasticity (flexibility) of the arterial walls
- the size of the smallest parts of the arteries (arterioles and capillaries)

Factors that can result in a higher than normal blood pressure measurement are

- age
- sex
- heredity
- exercise
- physical and emotional stress
- pain
- conditions that interfere with the movement of blood in the body

Blood pressure can be lowered by:

HEMORRHAGE

the escape of blood from a ruptured blood vessel; uncontrolled bleeding

- rest
- not eating
- weight loss
- certain medications
- conditions that result in **hemorrhage**

SYSTOLIC AND DIASTOLIC PRESSURES

Blood pressure consists of two number measurements: systolic pressure and diastolic pressure.

Systolic Pressure

The first measurement is the **systolic pressure.** It is caused by blood circulating through the body when the heart contracts and ejects (pushes) the blood out of the left ventricle. The systolic pressure measures the heart at work—the working phase. The normal range for the systolic measurement is 100–150 mm Hg.

Diastolic Pressure

The second measurement is the **diastolic pressure.** It is caused when the heart relaxes between beats—the resting phase. There is always pressure in the blood vessels because the blood is kept moving by the heart's pumping action. The normal range for the diastolic measurement is 60–90 mm Hg.

SYSTOLIC PRESSURE
pressure caused by the blood circulating through the body when the heart contracts and ejects (pushes) the blood from the left ventricle

DIASTOLIC PRESSURE
pressure resulting when the heart rests between beats

CARING COMMENT

To help yourself and your patients understand systolic and diastolic pressure, think of the heart's action as like the ordinary garden hose you use to water a garden. If you bend it (like the heart contracts), you close off the flow of water between the bend and the faucet. The pressure builds up and is like the systolic pressure of the blood in the heart.

When you unbend the hose, the pressure of the bend is released, yet some pressure remains that forces water to flow through the hose. Diastolic pressure is like this—the heart is at rest, but some pressure is still moving the blood through the body.

EQUIPMENT THAT MEASURES BLOOD PRESSURE

Sphygmomanometer

Blood pressure is registered on a **sphygmomanometer** (Figure 10–18), also known as a blood pressure cuff. The cuff contains two pieces of tubing. One tube is connected to the measuring gauge, which contains a series of numbers you can read. The measuring gauge may be either a column of mercury or a round dial. The other tube is connected to a bulb that fits in the palm of your hand. The bulb contains a pressure control button that helps you regulate the release of air from the inflated bladder. The inflatable bladder is located inside the cuff.

The bladder is inflatable so that air can be pumped into it when the cuff is wrapped around the patient's arm. Cuffs are available in a variety of sizes (Figures 10–19), including cuffs for infants, children, adults, and adults who are built larger. *The size of the cuff used is very important, because the wrong fit can result in an inaccurate blood pressure measurement.* The cuff should not be too wide or too narrow. The width of the cuff should measure about two-thirds the diameter of the patient's upper arm.

There are two types of sphygmomanometer available (Figure 10–20):

- An aneroid sphygmomanometer has a round dial gauge.
- A mercury gravity sphygmomanometer has a mercury column gauge.

A sphygmomanometer may be installed in the patient's room, or a portable one may be available (Figure 10–21). Electronic sphygmomanometers are used in special care areas of the acute care health care institution (for example, the intensive care unit). These areas may also use special electronic equipment that measures all vital signs when attached to a patient.

SPHYGMOMANOMETER
instrument used to measure the arterial blood pressure

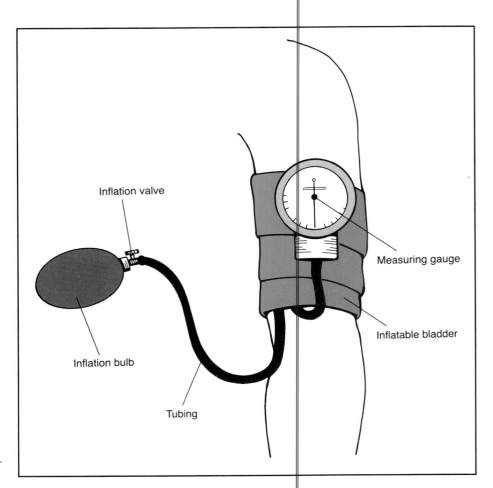

Inflation valve

Measuring gauge

Inflation bulb

Inflatable bladder

Tubing

FIGURE 10–18
The parts of the sphygmoma-nometer (blood pressure cuff).

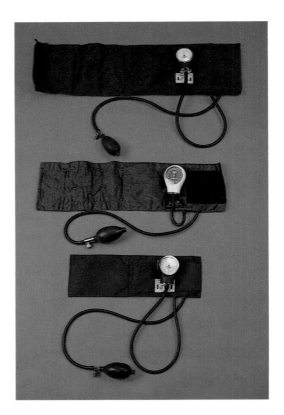

FIGURE 10–19
From top to bottom, an extra large cuff, an adult cuff, and a pediatric cuff.

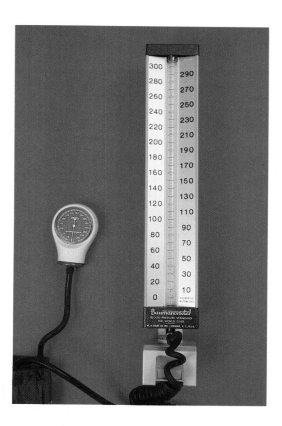

FIGURE 10-20

Sphygmomanometer gauges: aneroid (*left*) and mercury gravity (*right*).

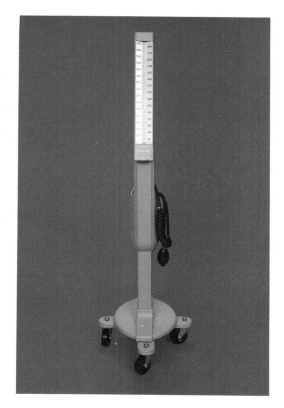

FIGURE 10-21

A portable sphygmomanometer with a mercury column gauge.

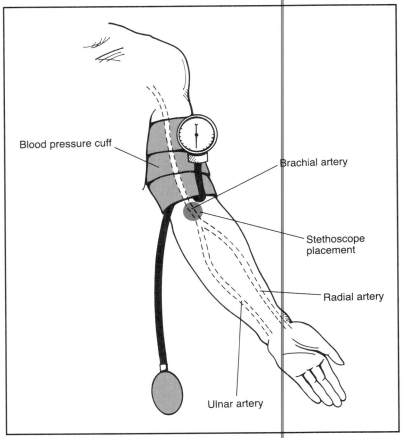

FIGURE 10–22

When you release the air while listening over the brachial artery with a stethoscope, you can hear the sound of the blood as it rushes to fill the artery. Note stethoscope placement.

Stethoscope

A *stethoscope* is another piece of equipment needed to measure the blood pressure. The pressure caused by the inflated cuff pushes against the brachial artery and stops the flow of blood. You listen by placing the stethoscope over the artery, and when you release the air you can hear the sound of the blood as it rushes to fill the artery (Figure 10–22). This rush creates the first clear sound, which is called the systolic pressure. The last sound you hear signifies that the artery is filled and blood is flowing evenly again. The point at which you hear the blood flowing evenly again is the diastolic pressure. While you are listening, you observe the numbers on the dial at which you hear the first clear sound and the last sound (Figure 10–23).

Ask for instructions to measure blood pressure in:

- patients whose arm is injured or paralyzed or who are receiving an intravenous infusion
- patients who have had a mastectomy (breast surgery) on that side (for example, if a patient has had the right breast removed, you should take the blood pressure on the patient's left arm)
- patients who are on **dialysis**

DIALYSIS

an artificial method of removing liquid waste products from the body when the kidneys produce little or no urine

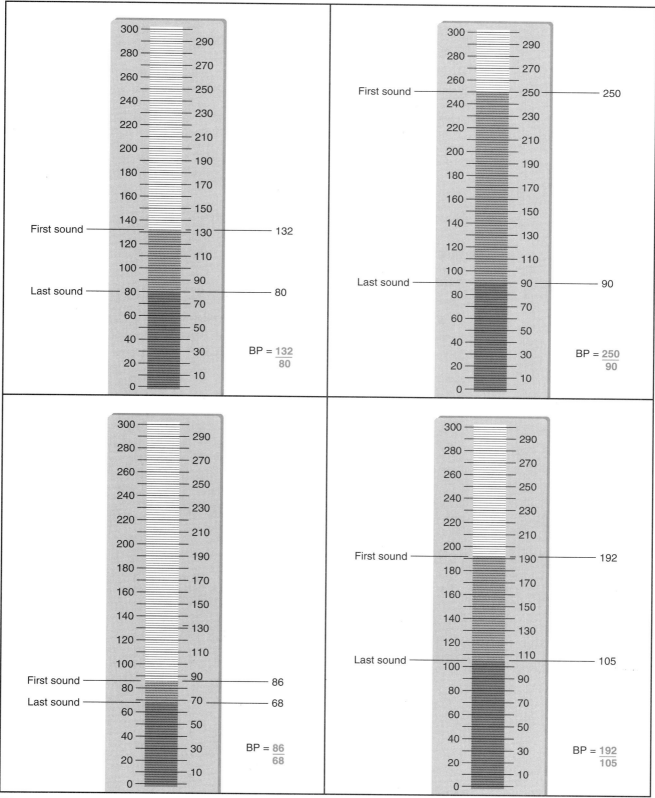

FIGURE 10–23

Reading the blood pressure gauge. While listening, note at which number on the gauge you hear the first clear sound and the last sound.

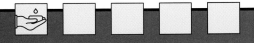

PROCEDURE

Measuring Blood Pressure

Explain to patients that you are going to measure their blood pressure. Remove any long-sleeved clothing from the arm or roll up the sleeve of the patients' gown about 5 or 6 inches above the elbow before the blood pressure is measured. A quiet environment is necessary for this procedure so that the measurement is accurate. Lower the volume on the television or radio and remove noisy distractions before measuring blood pressure. Make sure the patient has been resting at least 15 minutes.

GATHER EQUIPMENT

Sphygmomanometer   Paper
Stethoscope   Pencil
Two alcohol swabs

ACTION	RATIONALE
Preparation	
1. Wash hands.	Prevents the spread of microorganisms.
2. Identify yourself and the patient.	Maintains patients' rights.
3. Provide privacy.	Maintains patients' rights.
4. Explain the procedure.	Informs patients about what is happening.
Procedural Steps	
5. Place the patient in a comfortable position.	
6. Remove any clothing that may interfere with an accurate measurement. Roll the sleeve of the patients' gown up about 5 or 6 inches.	Clothing can constrict (flatten) the artery and result in an inaccurate measurement.
7. Position the blood pressure cuff on patients' upper arm about 1–1½ inches above the elbow. Fasten the Velcro closure or tie the cloth ties snugly. The tubing that leaves the cuff is positioned over the inner part of the arm.	This position places the cuff over the brachial artery.

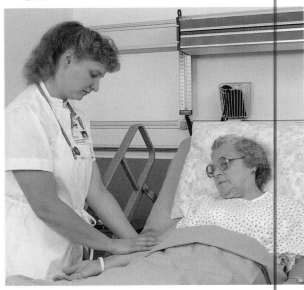

FIGURE 10–24
Palpating for the brachial pulse.

8. Clean the ear pieces and the diaphragm of the stethoscope with an alcohol swab. Place the ear pieces in the ears.

Prevents the spread of microorganisms.

9. Support patients' arm at the elbow while you palpate (feel) the pulse on the inner part of the elbow below the cuff (Figure 10–24). Place the arm on the bed or over the bed table for support (Figure 10–25). Place the diaphragm of the stethoscope over the pulse you feel in this spot.

The brachial artery is located in this area.

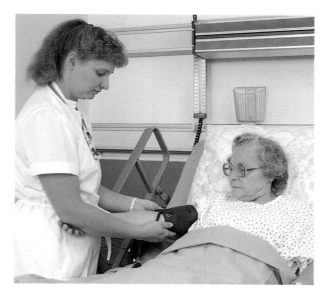

FIGURE 10–25

Patients who are able may feel more comfortable by placing their hand under your elbow to help keep their arm straight.

10. Grasp the bulb end of the sphygmomanometer, tighten the pressure control by turning it to the right (clockwise), and begin to pump air into the cuff. Watch the mercury rise in the column or the needle move on the dial of an aneroid gauge (Figure 10–26).

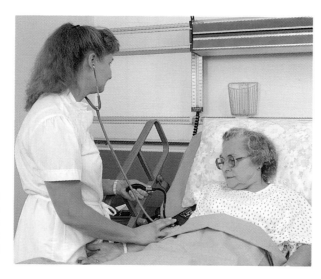

FIGURE 10–26

Grasp the bulb end of the sphygmomanometer and begin to pump air into the cuff. Watch the mercury rise in the column (or the needle move on the dial of an aneroid gauge).

Continued on following page

Measuring Blood Pressure *Continued*

11. When you know patients' usual blood pressure measurement, pump the air into the cuff. When the mercury or the needle on the dial registers 20 points above the usual measurement, stop pumping air. If the patient's blood pressure is not known, pump air into the cuff until the gauge registers at 200 mm Hg. Keep your fingers on the control located on the bulb. Begin to release air from the cuff by turning the control to the left. (Following these rules prevents patients' discomfort because too much air in the cuff can cut off circulation and cause pain or tingling and numbness.)

12. Slowly and evenly turn the pressure control screw to keep releasing air pressure while watching the sphygmomanometer. Listen for the sound caused by the first wave of blood.

Release of air allows the blood to flow again.

13. Note the line on the mercury or aneroid gauge where the first sound is heard. Be sure to read the gauge at eye level.

Accuracy is promoted by reading gauges at eye level.

14. Continue to release air from the cuff at a steady rate until no sound is heard. Note where on the gauge the last sound is heard.

15. Continue to turn the pressure control screw on the bulb until all the air is released.

Readies the cuff for the next use.

16. Remove the blood pressure cuff from patients' arm and replace or reposition clothing as needed (Figure 10–27).

Provides patient comfort.

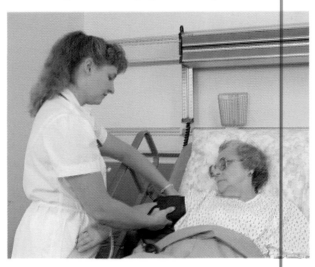

FIGURE 10–27
Always remove the cuff when you are finished. It should not be left on the patient's arm even if you need to retake the blood pressure in a few minutes.

17. Write the results of the blood pressure measurement and patients' name and room number on the piece of paper

Even a slight distraction may make you forget the measurement.

as soon as possible. The results are written like a fraction, with the higher number (systolic pressure) always written as the top number of the fraction. The lower number (diastolic pressure) is always written as the bottom of the fraction. For an example, $\dfrac{120}{80}$

18. Place patients in a comfortable position with the call signal within reach.	Leaves patients with the means to communicate.
19. Open the privacy curtains.	
20. Clean the ear pieces and the diaphragm with the other alcohol swab; then store the equipment appropriately.	Prevents the spread of microorganisms.

Follow-Through

21. Wash hands.	Prevents the spread of microorganisms.
22. Report results to the nurse.	The nurse is responsible for any decision that is based on the results of the measurement.
23. Report any problems with measuring a blood pressure to the nurse.	The nurse is responsible for any decision that is based on problems with measurement.

Note: If you are unsure of or missed the reading, wait 1–2 minutes before you retake the blood pressure.

24. Record the blood pressure measurement in the appropriate place on the chart.	Provides an official record of the results of the procedure.

BLOOD PRESSURE READINGS

The average adult blood pressure measurement is 120/80. However, the normal range of blood pressures is 110/60–140/90.

A blood pressure lower than 90/60 indicates that the person may have **hypotension.** Treatment is ordered only when the signs and symptoms interfere with the person's activities of daily living.

The condition known as **hypertension** occurs when the adult blood pressure consistently measures 140/90 or over. Hypertension is treated in ways that maintain the blood pressure within normal ranges.

Whenever you are unsure of a blood pressure measurement, report the results to the nurse and ask that the patient's blood pressure be measured again by another care giver. Blood pressure measurements can be in error for many reasons (see Problems with Blood Pressure Measurement and Ways to Avoid Them chart).

HYPOTENSION
low blood pressure
HYPERTENSION
persistent high blood pressure

PROBLEMS WITH BLOOD PRESSURE MEASUREMENT AND WAYS TO AVOID THEM

Problem	Solution
Improper cuff size	Choose the correct cuff size. It should be two-thirds the diameter of the patient's arm.
Incorrect placement of the cuff	The tubing that leads out of the

Continued on following page

PROBLEMS WITH BLOOD PRESSURE MEASUREMENT AND WAYS TO AVOID THEM *Continued*

Problem	Solution
	cuff should be placed over the brachial artery.
Improper wrapping of the cuff	Wrap the cuff for a snug fit. It should not be loose (you should be able to fit one finger under the edge of the cuff).
Air leakage	Check cuff bladder, tubing, and bulb for a hissing sound that may indicate air is leaking. Send the equipment to the appropriate place for repair.
Improper positioning of the arm	Support the patient's forearm at the level of the heart. Place the patient's hand palm up.
Not reading the gauge at eye level	Position yourself to make it easy for you to read the gauge at eye level.
Using the arm for more than one blood pressure reading within a short period of time	Wait 1–2 minutes before taking another blood pressure measurement.
Reading the diastolic pressure at the wrong time	The sound might fade for 10 or 15 mm Hg after the first sound is heard. It starts again. This is known as the auscultatory gap. Continue listening for the last sound.
Unsure of your accuracy in the blood pressure reading	Ask the nurse to measure the blood pressure to verify accuracy.

PATIENTS WITH COMMON DISRUPTIONS IN BLOOD SUPPLY

The heart muscle and blood vessels can be affected by disease. You will care for patients with such common disruptions as

- orthostatic hypotension
- hypertension (high blood pressure)
- myocardial infarction (heart attack)
- cerebral vascular accident (stroke)

ORTHOSTATIC HYPOTENSION

ORTHOSTATIC HYPOTENSION
a dizzy feeling caused by a fall in blood pressure; occurs when a person sits or stands too quickly

Orthostatic hypotension is a fall in blood pressure that causes dizziness, syncope (fainting), and blurred vision when a person stands or sits down quickly (Figure 10–28). It can also occur when a person stands still for long periods of time. Observations may include

- statements such as "I feel dizzy" or I'm light-headed"
- sudden loss of muscle tone in patients while you are assisting them
- falling from a position of sitting or standing

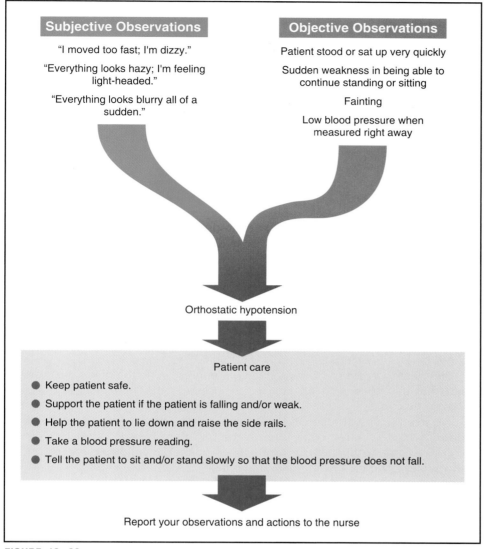

Subjective Observations

"I moved too fast; I'm dizzy."

"Everything looks hazy; I'm feeling light-headed."

"Everything looks blurry all of a sudden."

Objective Observations

Patient stood or sat up very quickly

Sudden weakness in being able to continue standing or sitting

Fainting

Low blood pressure when measured right away

Orthostatic hypotension

Patient care

● Keep patient safe.

● Support the patient if the patient is falling and/or weak.

● Help the patient to lie down and raise the side rails.

● Take a blood pressure reading.

● Tell the patient to sit and/or stand slowly so that the blood pressure does not fall.

Report your observations and actions to the nurse

FIGURE 10-28

Flow chart for the patient who has orthostatic hypotension.

You might notice the preceding behaviors in the following situations:

- when patients sit up or stand too quickly
- the first time patients get out of bed after surgery
- the first time patients get out of bed after bed rest is discontinued
- in patients who have problems with circulation
- in patients who are receiving certain medications

The nurse may tell you these patients have a history of orthostatic hypotension. You should observe patients closely and keep them from harm. If you see that the patients move quickly when changing positions, remind them to sit or stand more slowly. Even if the patients do not have a history of orthostatic hypotension, you should be alert to the possibility of orthostatic hypotension.

HYPERTENSION

A persistent blood pressure measurement higher than 140/90 is called *hypertension*. When the blood puts too much pressure against the walls of the artery, hypertension or high blood pressure results.

Hypertension is called the silent killer because the person may not feel symptoms or changes in the body early in the disease. It can affect people of any age but occurs often in people as they age.

The cause of most cases of hypertension is not known. In some cases, disease is a contributing factor or a definite cause. Treatment of the disease may help lower the blood pressure. It can help prevent future complications, such as myocardial infarction and cerebral vascular attack. The physician may order

- rest
- weight loss
- decreased stress
- decreased fat in the diet
- decreased salt in the diet
- medications to lower the blood pressure
- medications to rid the body of extra fluid
- medications to lower the level of cholesterol in the blood

MYOCARDIAL INFARCTION

INFARCTION

an area of dead or dying tissue due to a lack of blood supply

An **infarction** occurs when there is a lack of blood supply to the body's tissues. Lack of blood supply caused by blockage in the heart's arteries (called coronary arteries) results in the death of tissue. When tissue dies, it can no longer perform its usual function.

MYOCARDIAL INFARCTION

death of cells of the heart due to obstruction of the blood supply to the heart

The death of tissue that occurs in the muscle of the heart is called a **myocardial infarction** or heart attack. The tissue in the heart muscle dies and no longer functions.

The heart's normal function is to pump blood with a regular beat. During a myocardial infarction, the heart pumps with an irregular beat. Because death of tissue is occurring, the patient experiences pain. The following are important observations to report to the nurse immediately:

- chest pain the patient describes as crushing, stabbing, squeezing, or piercing
- pain that radiates to the left arm, hand, and shoulder and neck and jaw
- nausea and vomiting
- profuse sweating
- anxiety and a feeling of impending doom

ELECTROCARDIOGRAM

a recording of the heart's electrical activity

The physician begins to diagnose a myocardial infarction on the basis of the patient's sign and symptoms, the results of an **electrocardiogram,** and certain blood studies. The physician uses other tests to pinpoint the area of infarction.

The patient is placed on bed rest and given oxygen. Medications are ordered to decrease pain and to prevent further damage to the heart muscle. After the acute stage, the patient may be encouraged to

- lose weight
- decrease stress
- decrease fat in the diet
- decrease salt in the diet
- exercise daily by walking

CEREBROVASCULAR ACCIDENT

CEREBROVASCULAR ACCIDENT

when the blood stops going to the brain, causing brain tissue to die; a stroke

A **cerebrovascular accident** is the stoppage of the blood supply to the brain that results in the death of brain tissue. The brain needs a rich supply of blood to function at its best. The interrupted flow of blood can be caused by a

Cerebrovascular hemorrhage
Blood clot
Tumor

TUMOR
growth of tissue

The brain needs the oxygen that blood brings in order to function normally. Because the brain is the command center of the body, areas of the brain that are not getting oxygen cannot perform their usual sending of commands to the body's tissues. Each side of the brain controls certain body functions. The patient's signs and symptoms tell the physician which side of the brain was affected by the lack of blood.

The following are important patient observations to report to the nurse immediately:

* loss of consciousness
* loss of function, weakness, and paralysis on either side of the body
* inability to communicate or understand the spoken word; changes in the ability to see
* any other changes, however small, that you notice when you care for the patient, such as slurring of words that had previously been spoken clearly
* slight weakness in one side of the body when you help the patient move

The physician diagnoses a cerebrovascular accident through the use of sophisticated tests. Such tests can determine how large the area of infarction is and its location. The physician orders measures designed to keep the patient alive during the actual stroke.

Following the acute stage (immediately after the stroke), the patient may face a long period (6 or more weeks) of rehabilitation. **Rehabilitation** is a health care service that helps the patient return to as normal a life as possible. During rehabilitation, the patient may need to relearn how to do such basic things as

REHABILITATION
a program that helps a patient
return to as normal a life as possible

Eat
Dress
Move
Walk

GENERAL CARE OF PATIENTS WITH DISRUPTIONS IN BLOOD SUPPLY

Patients who have a disruption in blood supply need anywhere from very little assistance to total assistance with daily needs. The following are actions you can take to help patients experiencing problems with blood supply:

* Provide personal care when patients are unable to satisfy their own needs.
* Help patients remain safe in their environment.
* Provide adequate amounts of rest.
* Help patients reduce stress.
* Assist patients with an exercise program (ambulation) if ordered.
* Observe for possible side effects of medications as instructed by the nurse.
* Teach patients to sit up slowly and rest before rising if they have orthostatic hypotension.
* Follow instructions from the physical or occupational therapist.

You may care for patients in the acute care setting, when all personal care and assistance with moving must be provided. As soon as possible, patients are referred to a rehabilitation center where they learn or relearn how to

* use their arms and legs to be able to care for themselves
* control the bladder and bowel

- walk
- talk, if speech is affected

Patients with a disruption in blood supply are encouraged by all care givers to do as much for themselves as possible. When patients have been discharged to a nursing home or to their own home, you need to find out how much they have learned and how much they are able to do on their own. Give praise and encouragement when patients are successful, and be ready to help when they need you.

CHAPTER WRAP-UP

- The pulse is produced by the wave action of the blood as it passes through the arteries. It can be palpated (felt) and counted in places where the arteries lay close to a bone. A pulse above or below the normal range signals a breakdown in the heart as a pump or in the blood vessels as the delivery system. The exchange of oxygen and carbon dioxide is also affected by the pulse rate.
- Respiration is the process of breathing air in to provide oxygen to the lungs and breathing air out to remove carbon dioxide from the body. Respirations can be counted by watching the rise and fall of the chest or through the use of a special monitoring device. When the number of respirations in 1 minute is above or below the normal range, the body is performing its oxygen–carbon dioxide exchange in a less efficient way.
- The force of the circulating blood against the arterial walls is called the blood pressure. The highest pressure (systolic) is produced when the blood is pumped into the aorta and the rest of the body's arteries. The lowest blood pressure (diastolic) occurs when the heart rests between beats and the pressure drops.
- A blood pressure measurement above or below the normal range indicates a problem in the heart or the blood vessels or both. A consistently high blood pressure indicates that the heart and blood vessels do not function effectively. They are unable to deliver enough blood to accomplish adequate oxygen–carbon dioxide exchange.
- The patient with asthma, emphysema, or pneumonia may prefer to sit in Fowler's position or the orthopneic position.
- Extra fluids are important for patients who have disruptions in breathing.
- Hypertension is also known as high blood pressure.

REVIEW QUESTIONS

1. Name the peripheral sites available for counting a pulse.
2. Where is the stethoscope placed when you count an apical pulse rate?
3. What actions can you take to help a patient breathe more comfortably?
4. Describe how the sphygmomanometer works.
5. When patients wish to know their blood pressure, how do you give them this information?
6. Name four problems that can occur when you perform a blood pressure measurement. What are the solutions to these problems?
7. Describe the actions you can take to help a patient who has had a disruption in blood supply.

ACTIVITY CORNER

Count and write down your pulse and respirations when you wake up and after you eat dinner

Wake up _____

After dinner _____

Are the rates the same? If they are different, what might be the cause? Are the rates within the normal range for an adult?

Watch three people when you are waiting for the bus or eating out. Can you count their respirations without their knowing it?
Write down the number of respirations and the approximate age of each person. Are there differences? If so, why?

	Approximate Age	Respirations
Person 1	_____	_____
Person 2	_____	_____
Person 3	_____	_____

UNIT FOUR

Giving Basic Care

11

Preventing the Spread of Infection

Objectives

AFTER YOU COMPLETE THIS CHAPTER, YOU WILL BE ABLE TO:

Define the term *microorganism.*

Identify the links in the infection chain.

Describe how the body protects itself from infection.

Define medical asepsis.

Use medical aseptic techniques when caring for all patients.

List and explain the category-specific isolation procedures that prevent the spread of infection.

Describe the universal precautions used by all health care workers.

Use category-specific isolation procedures and universal precautions to prevent the spread of infection.

Provide care for a patient with an infectious disease.

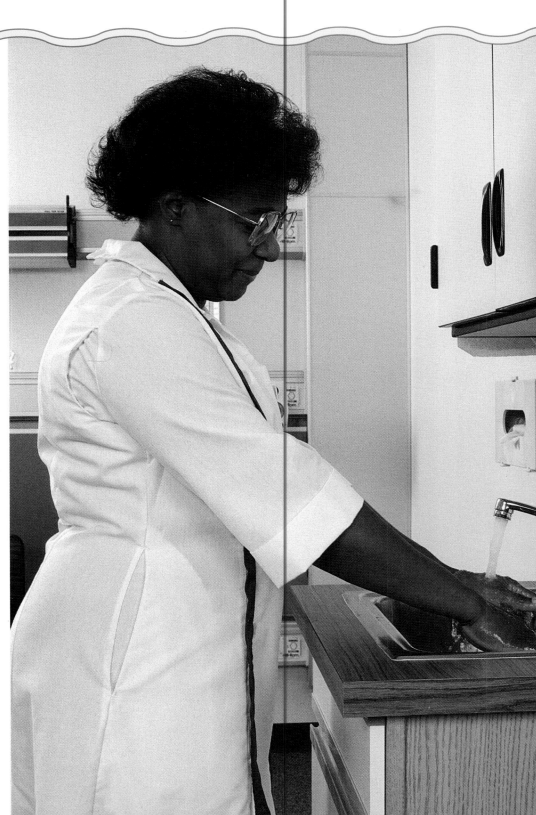

Overview As a nursing assistant, you care for many patients who have infectious diseases. They require special procedures to stop the infection and to prevent its spread to you, to other patients, and to other health care workers.

WHAT DO YOU KNOW ABOUT THE SPREAD OF INFECTION?

Here are eight statements about infection control. Consider them to test your current ideas about infection and infection control. If you think the statement is true, circle the T; if you think the statement is false, circle the F. Change the false statements to make them true.

1. T F Microorganisms are spread only by direct contact with the infected patient or contaminated objects.

2. T F A pathogen is a microorganism that is helpful to the body.

3. T F The body has its own defense system against harmful microorganisms.

4. T F A nosocomial infection is an infection that is acquired in a health care institution.

5. T F Hand washing before and after each patient contact is an effective way to prevent the spread of infection.

6. T F Only running water and a cleansing agent are necessary for thorough hand washing.

7. T F Hand washing is not necessary if you wear clean gloves for protection.

8. T F Spills of blood and body fluids are cleaned with hot water and soap.

ANSWERS

1. **False.** Microorganisms are also spread by droplets put into the air when a person sneezes.

2. **False.** A pathogen is a disease-producing microorganism.

3. **True.** The immune system is the body's defense system.

4. **True.** Nosocomial means "originating in the hospital." Ill persons' immune systems are weakened, so they are more easily infected by harmful microorganisms that thrive in the hospital setting.

5. **True.** Hand washing is the first line of defense against the spread of infection.

6. **False.** Vigorous rubbing of the hands (friction) is also needed for success in hand washing.

7. **False.** You should wash your hands each time you remove gloves.

8. **False.** Effective cleaning of blood and body spills requires a solution that contains household bleach.

MICROORGANISMS

MICROORGANISM

an organism so tiny it can be seen only under a microscope; capable of helping the body as well as causing disease

PATHOGEN

any agent or microorganism that causes disease

SALIVA

watery substance secreted from the salivary glands; moistens food and makes it easier to swallow

Microorganisms are living organisms that cannot be seen with the naked eye. Microorganisms may also be called *microbes*. They are seen and identified under a microscope. Some microorganisms have a beneficial effect on the body, some have a harmful effect, and some have no effect whatsoever on the body. Bacteria, fungi, yeast, and viruses are examples of microorganisms that have a harmful effect—infectious disease. A harmful microorganism is called a **pathogen**, or germ. Pathogens live and multiply in warm, dark, moist places.

Microorganisms grow in many places. Some places are familiar, for example, the bodies of humans and animals. On the bodies of humans and animals they often grow in drainage from body openings, such as (Figure 11–1)

- Nasal drainage
- **Saliva**

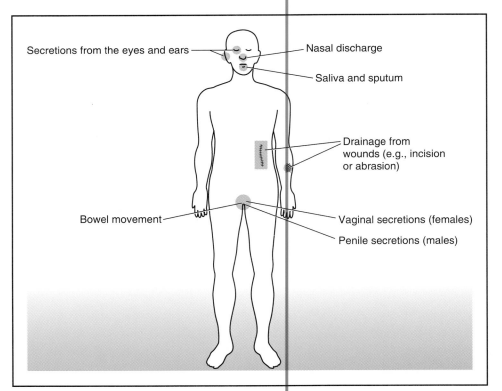

FIGURE 11–1

Drainage from body openings is a possible source of infection.

- **Sputum**
- Urine
- Vaginal drainage
- Penile drainage
- Fecal material
- Drainage from any opening in the skin

Other familiar places in which microorganisms thrive are foods and fluids and **feces**. Even clothing and other objects, such as a baby's bottle and children's toys, can provide shelter to microorganisms.

NORMAL FLORA

It is normal for certain types of microorganisms to live in certain places in the body. Each **body system** is a host to a variety of microorganisms because it provides them with a place to live and enough nutrition and oxygen to thrive. These microorganisms are called the **normal flora** of a body system. If the normal flora of one body system move to another system, however, they may be harmful to the body tissues in that system. For example, the **gastrointestinal** system provides the ideal environment for bacteria called *Escherichia coli* (E. *coli*). E. *coli* are considered normal flora when they remain within the gastrointestinal system. However, if the bacteria are transferred to the urinary system, a urinary tract infection occurs because this microorganism is very harmful to the tissues in the urinary system.

TYPES OF MICROORGANISMS

There are a great variety of microorganisms living in the human body and the environment. When examined under the microscope, a microorganism is identified by its shape and size and how it reproduces (Figure 11–2). It is important for physicians to know the name of the microorganism found in a specimen. This is how they know which medication to order to treat an illness. Common types of microorganisms are

Bacteria
Virus
Fungus
Protozoa

SPUTUM

a mucous secretion from the lungs, bronchi, and trachea that is ejected (brought up) through the mouth

FECES

waste eliminated from the body through the anus

BODY SYSTEM

a group of organs that work together to complete a certain function (for example, in the urinary system the kidneys produce urine and the bladder stores urine)

NORMAL FLORA

microorganisms that belong in a specific body site

GASTROINTESTINAL

pertaining to the stomach and intestines

ESCHERICHIA COLI

a bacteria found in the large intestine of humans

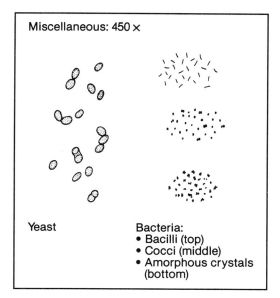

FIGURE 11–2

Microorganisms come in different shapes and sizes. (From Kinn ME, Derge EF: The Medical Assistant: Administrative and Clinical, 6th ed. Philadelphia, W. B. Saunders, 1988.)

BACTERIA

microorganisms that reproduce by cell division; also called germs

IMMUNE SYSTEM

the body's defense system against harmful microorganisms

NUTRITION

the study of food's relationship to health; the act of providing food to nourish the body

OXYGEN

a colorless, tasteless, odorless gas; the air we breathe is about 20% oxygen

AEROBIC

needing oxygen to live and grow

ANAEROBIC

able to live and grow without oxygen

VIRUS

a microorganism that needs living tissue in order to reproduce

ANTIBIOTIC

a substance that kills or stops the growth of certain microorganisms

INFLUENZA

a communicable disease caused by a virus; the flu

ANTIBODY

a substance that the body produces as a weapon against a specific microorganism; part of the body's immune system

FUNGUS

a microorganism that uses spores to reproduce

PROTOZOA

microscopic single-celled organisms

TRICHOMONIASIS

a sexually transmitted disease caused by a protozoa

INFECTION

the body's response to invasion by microorganisms and their multiplication in the body

Bacteria

Bacteria are a class of microorganisms that reproduce by cell division. The skin, respiratory tract, and gastrointestinal system are hosts to a variety of bacteria that are considered normal flora in those body systems. In these areas, either the bacteria are harmless or they can protect the body system by interfering with the growth of harmful bacteria. When the bacteria travel to another system, the body's **immune system** goes to work. The immune system attempts to destroy the harmful bacteria because they cause inflammation (warmth, redness, an increase in body temperature, swelling, and pain) and disease.

Bacteria seek a favorable environment in which to grow and thrive. To grow, bacteria prefer

Warmth
Darkness
Moisture

The body provides just the right environment. At 98.6° F, it is warm, and it contains many dark, moist places that encourage bacterial growth. Bacteria seek dark places for growth because exposure to light destroys them. They also prefer moist places, and the body has many such areas. Other moist places in which bacteria thrive are in drains, on sinks, and in soap dishes. Foods and fluids also provide the kind of environment that bacteria like. Foods and fluids and the warm bodies of humans and animals provide bacteria with nourishment (**nutrition**). Most bacteria also need **oxygen** for growth (**aerobic**), but certain ones can survive without oxygen (they are **anaerobic**).

Virus

A **virus** is an infectious agent that is distinguished by its extreme smallness. It is smaller than bacteria and cannot reproduce itself outside living tissue. Viruses are identified by their shape and size. Unlike bacteria, a virus is not killed by **antibiotic** treatment. The flu (**influenza**) is caused by a virus; penicillin (an antibiotic) cannot destroy a virus. A person can be immunized against some viruses. Immunization makes a person's body develop a special type of cell called an **antibody** that protects the body from infection by a particular virus.

Fungus

A **fungus** is a microorganism that uses spores (bacteria protected by a hard outer casing) to reproduce. Fungi are present in air, soil, and water. Very few kinds of fungi cause infection. A common fungus infection in humans is athlete's foot. Another fungus that grows on a certain kind of mushroom produces an infection that may be life-threatening if the mushrooms are eaten.

Protozoa

Protozoa are microscopic single-celled organisms. They are parasites that thrive in areas with poor sanitation of water and sewage. Protozoa cause the sexually transmitted disease known as **trichomoniasis.** Malaria and African sleeping sickness are also caused by protozoa.

INFECTION

Infection occurs as a result of the invasion and growth of a pathogenic (harmful) microorganism. An infection can affect a specific body part or the entire body. Certain signs and symptoms can be observed when a person develops an infection:

- **pain** over the affected area
- warmth over the affected area
- redness over the affected area
- swelling over the affected area
- tenderness over the affected area
- drainage from the affected area
- elevated **body temperature** and chills
- Gastrointestinal disturbances:
    Nausea
    Vomiting
    Diarrhea

PAIN
a feeling of discomfort, suffering, or agony

BODY TEMPERATURE
the degree of body heat or coldness measured by a clinical thermometer

THE INFECTION PROCESS

An infection is a disease that results from the presence of pathogens in or on the body. Certain conditions must be present for pathogens to survive and grow. A pathogen can be transmitted from one person to another. A disease that is transmitted from one person to another is called a **communicable disease.** Examples of common communicable diseases are measles and hepatitis. Actions can and should be taken to prevent the transmission of communicable diseases. When actions fail to prevent the transmission of an infectious disease to a patient in a health care institution, the infection the patient acquires (gets) is called a nosocomial infection.

COMMUNICABLE DISEASE
an illness that can be transmitted to another person

NOSOCOMIAL INFECTION

A **nosocomial infection** is an infection that a person acquires while in a health care institution. Nosocomial infections can range from simple, uncomplicated infections to major, life-threatening infections. Patients are at risk for developing a nosocomial infection because of the following reasons:

- their immune system may be too weak to fight off the infection
- medication or bed rest may weaken patients' response to infection
- the health care institution contains people and objects that may carry and transmit microorganisms that cause infection (Figure 11–3)

NOSOCOMIAL INFECTION
any infection acquired in a health care institution

THE INFECTION CHAIN

Consider the infection process as a chain of events that occur to help harmful microorganisms produce an infection in the body (Figure 11–4). The infection chain consists of

1. An infectious agent
2. A reservoir (source)
3. A portal of exit from the reservoir
4. A method of transmission
5. A portal of entry to the host
6. A susceptible host

When the chain is broken, the infection process is disrupted and the microorganism cannot continue to grow. By washing your hands after you touch an infected person or soiled object, you break the chain of infection. When you use a special cleansing agent (an antiseptic or antimicrobial), you also break

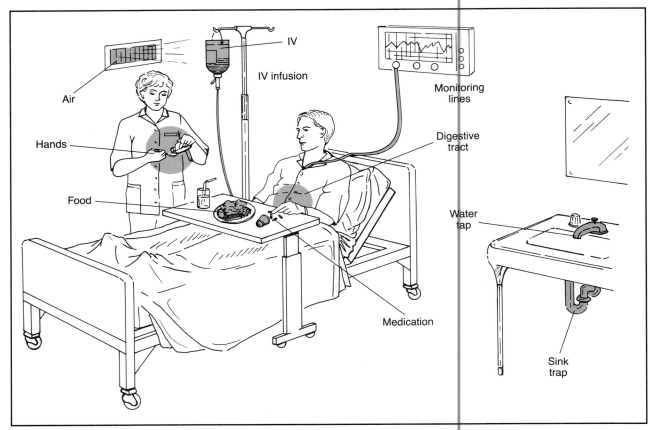

FIGURE 11–3

Sources of contamination are present in the hospital environment. The hands of care givers are the chief source of contamination. (Redrawn from Craven RF, Hirnle CJ: Fundamentals of Nursing: Human Health and Function. Philadelphia, J. B. Lippincott, 1992.)

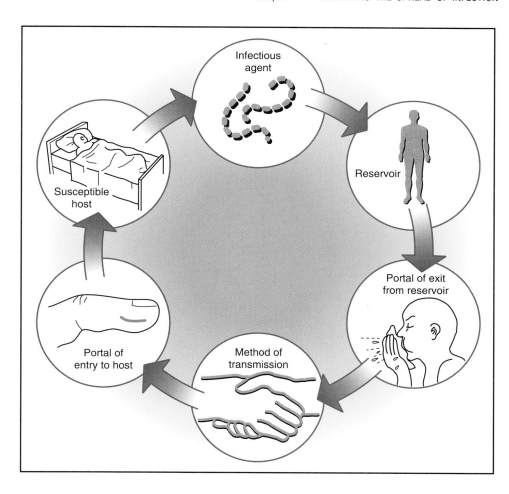

FIGURE 11–4
The infection chain.

the chain of infection (Figure 11–5). Cleansing agents work in the following ways:

- **Antiseptics** prevent (stop) the growth of bacteria.
- **Antimicrobials** kill or slow down the growth of microorganisms.

Infectious Agent

An **infectious agent** is a harmful microorganism that takes its nourishment from healthy tissues. Factors that affect the growth of microorganisms are:

- their number (how many there are)
- their strength
- their ability to enter the body and live there
- the body's inability to resist the microorganisms

Reservoir

A **reservoir** is a place where microorganisms thrive. Reservoirs are present in many areas that are dark, warm, and moist, such as your own body, other humans, animals, plants, and the environment. The most common source of harmful microorganisms is humans. Insects, birds, and animals are also common sources. Food and fluids, such as milk and water, and feces also are reservoirs. The reservoir must have a suitable environment for growth:

- food and water
- correct temperature

ANTISEPTIC
a substance that prevents the growth of bacteria
ANTIMICROBIAL
a substance that kills or slows down the multiplication of a microorganism
INFECTIOUS AGENT
a harmful microorganism that takes its nourishment from healthy tissue

RESERVOIR
a holding place

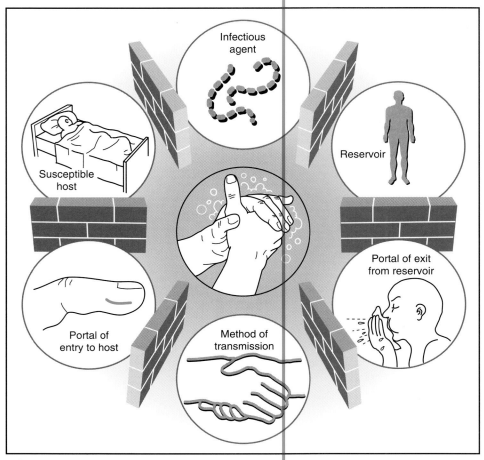

FIGURE 11-5
Hand washing breaks the chain of infection.

• oxygen (although some microorganisms can survive without oxygen)

PORTAL
an opening

Portal of Exit

To find another place in which it can live and grow, a microorganism must first find an exit from the reservoir. A number of portals of exit are available in humans, depending on the location of the reservoir. Examples of portals of exit include

• drainage from a wound
• droplets from sneezing or coughing

Method of Transmission

There are four main routes of transmission (movement from one place to another) for microorganisms (Figure 11-6):

Direct contact
Carrier (indirect contact)
Airborne
Vector

DIRECT CONTACT Transmission occurs when a weakened person (a person whose

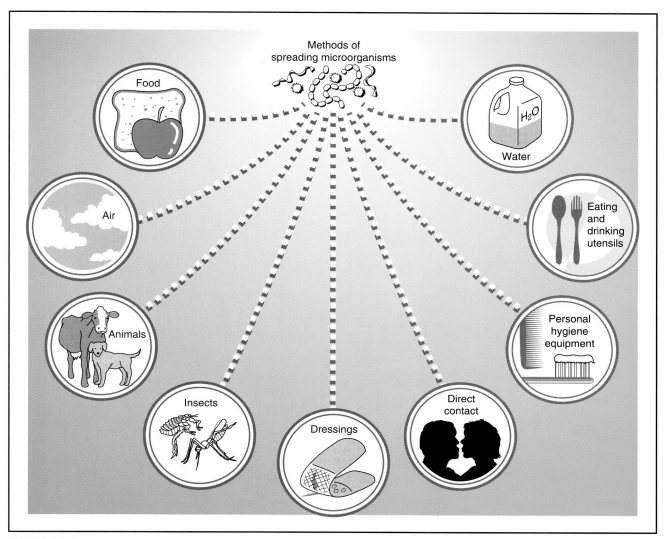

FIGURE 11–6
Methods of transmission of microorganisms.

immune system is unable to fight off the microorganism) touches an infected person.

CARRIER Transmission occurs when a weakened person touches a soiled (contaminated) object.

CARING COMMENT

Food, water, and blood are carriers by which microorganisms can invade a weakened person's body. It is essential to do everything possible to prevent coming in contact with carriers. Prevention methods are discussed throughout this chapter.

AIRBORNE **Airborne transmission** occurs when a weakened person comes in close contact with droplets put into the air by infected persons. When contaminated droplets or dust are present in the air within about 3 feet of a person, the person can inhale (breathe in) the harmful microorganisms.

AIRBORNE TRANSMISSION
sending or transferring something through the air

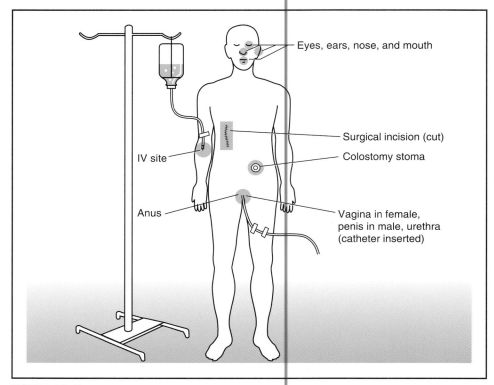

Eyes, ears, nose, and mouth

Surgical incision (cut)

Colostomy stoma

IV site

Anus

Vagina in female,
penis in male, urethra
(catheter inserted)

FIGURE 11–7
Body orifices (openings) are portals of entry for harmful microorganisms.

VECTOR
a carrying agent

VECTOR   Transmission occurs by way of a carrying agent. Animals and insects are **vectors** in the transmission of harmful microorganisms.

Portal of Entry

Microorganisms often enter one body by the same route they used to exit another body. Any break in the skin or opening in the body can provide a portal of entry (Figure 11–7). Remember that intact (no breaks) skin provides a barrier to the entry of microorganisms. When a harmful microorganism enters the body and thrives, a person becomes infected.

Susceptible Host

SUSCEPTIBLE
unable to resist

Any person who is at risk for infection is a **susceptible** host. A host provides the proper conditions for growth of microorganisms. Factors that increase the risk of being a susceptible host include the following:

- age (the very young and the elderly)
- high level of stress (for example, from work or school)
- poor nutrition (either malnutrition or chronic obesity; both place a person at risk because good nutrition helps the body resist disease)
- preexisting diseases (cancer or chronic lung disease)
- impaired immune system (the impairment may be present at birth or may be acquired)
- surgical treatment (for example, after a heart transplant)
- radiation (too much exposure to x-rays or certain cancer treatments)
- certain medications and medical treatments (such as **chemotherapy** for cancer)

CHEMOTHERAPY
the use of chemical agents to treat
disease and illness

Any disease that has depleted the body's ability to fight infection places the person at risk. As already discussed, anyone who is hospitalized is at risk for contracting a nosocomial infection. One of the most common kinds of nosocomial infection is the **urinary tract infection** that results from the use of **catheters** (a tube into the bladder), urine collection bags, and connections. Any patient with a urinary catheter is at risk for a urinary tract infection.

URINARY TRACT INFECTION
infection of the urinary tract, especially the bladder and urethra

CATHETER
a flexible tube passed into body openings to allow fluids to enter or exit the body

CARING COMMENT

You can prevent nosocomial infections by washing your hands before and after every patient contact.

PROTECTION FROM INFECTION

The body is equipped with special defenses against infection. For example, tears provide a cleansing and flushing action as protection for the eye against infection. **Cerumen** in the ears traps tiny particles that invade the ear canal. A sneeze or cough expels microorganisms forcefully into the air. The **cilia** that line the respiratory organs produce a wavy upward movement that brings mucus up and out of the body. Thus the mucus is a form of protection. Stomach acid is so strong that it destroys most microorganisms.

CERUMEN
ear wax

CILIA
tiny hairs that protect the respiratory tract by making a wavelike upward motion to carry mucus up and out of the body

In addition, all humans depend on their immune system to protect them from infection. The immune system responds to foreign material in the body. Special cells that are part of the immune system work to eliminate the foreign material from the body. In some cases, this may not be desirable. For example, when a person receives a transplanted organ (for example, a heart or kidney), special cells recognize that something is different and work to eliminate the transplanted body organ. Patients must take special medication the rest of their life to prevent rejection of a transplanted body organ.

Ways to help the immune system function effectively include eating a balanced diet and getting proper rest and sleep. **Immunizations** such as those against measles also help the body's immune system.

IMMUNIZATION
a procedure that helps the body develop an antibody against a specific harmful microorganism

PREVENTING THE SPREAD OF INFECTION

There are a variety of ways to prevent the spread of infection. As a care giver, it is *extremely* important for you to know and practice ways to prevent infection. Common methods to prevent infections are

Medical asepsis (hand washing)
Universal precautions recommended by the Centers for Disease Control (CDC)
Isolation
Barrier practices

MEDICAL ASEPSIS

Asepsis is the absence of harmful microorganisms. **Medical asepsis** comprises the techniques health care workers use to limit the number, growth, and spread of harmful microorganisms. "Clean technique" is another name for medical asepsis. By practicing medical asepsis, health care workers reduce the presence of harmful microorganisms on their body. Hand washing is the most common form of medical asepsis.

ASEPSIS
the absence of harmful microorganisms

MEDICAL ASEPSIS
clean technique; the techniques health care workers use to destroy or limit the spread of harmful microorganisms

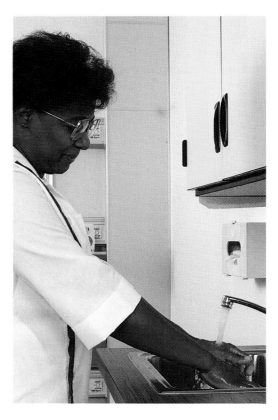

FIGURE 11–8

When washing hands, it is important *not* to touch the sink or cabinet with your body. Learn to hold your body away from the sink to prevent contact with contaminated surfaces during hand washing. Note the wall-mounted container of clean disposable gloves.

Hand Washing

Hand washing is the most important way to break the chain of infection. It is an effective, easy, and inexpensive way to control the spread of infection in the home and the institution (Figure 11–8). Remember that your hands contact many people and objects in the course of a day (Figure 11–9). They can easily carry harmful microorganisms to persons who are in a weakened state and at risk of developing an infection.

The three main ingredients for effective hand washing are (Figure 11–10)

- running water
- cleaning agent
- friction (rubbing the hands and fingers together)

The most important part of washing your hands is thorough, vigorous rubbing. Your hands are moist and warm, and the areas between your fingers are dark (Figure 11–11). As already mentioned, microorganisms grow and thrive in dark, warm, moist places. Because hand washing is so important, many local hospitals sponsor programs that teach children how to wash their hands correctly. Many children know "Scrubby Bear," who teaches them how, why, and when to wash their hands.

CARING COMMENT

You are at risk and put others at risk when you do not practice effective hand washing. The CDC recommends vigorous rubbing of the hands under a running stream of water with a cleansing agent. Your institution provides a supply of the cleansing agent it uses in each patient area. The CDC recommends that you wash your hands for at least 10 seconds. The best way to protect your patients and yourself is to wash your hands before and after every patient contact.

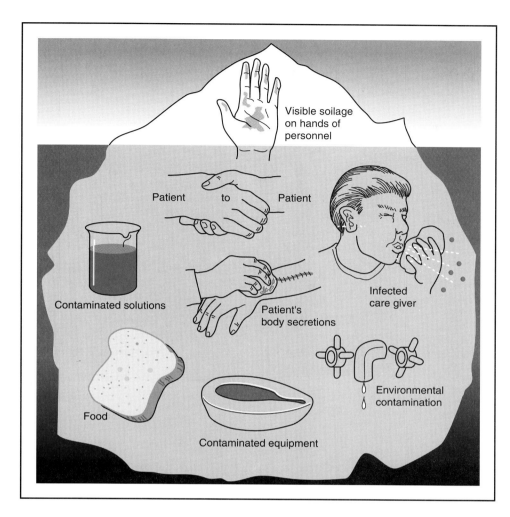

FIGURE 11–9

Contamination iceberg. The soilage (dirt) you see on the hands of care givers is only the tip of the iceberg. Many times the risk for carrying infection is hidden. (Redrawn from Craven RF, Hirnle CJ: Fundamentals of Nursing: Human Health and Function. Philadelphia, J. B. Lippincott, 1992.)

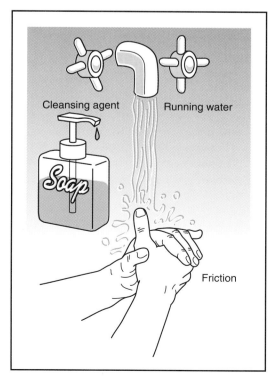

FIGURE 11–10

Items needed for effective hand washing.

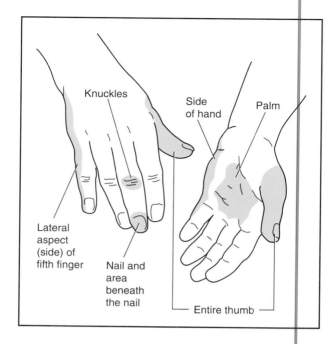

Knuckles

Side
of hand

Palm

Lateral
aspect
(side) of
fifth finger

Nail and
area
beneath
the nail

Entire thumb

FIGURE 11–11
Concentrate on the areas that
are the hardest to clean during
hand washing.

PROCEDURE

Hand Washing

Hand washing is performed to prevent the spread of harmful microorganisms. It is performed before and after every patient contact.

GATHER EQUIPMENT

Cleansing agent (liquid soap or other cleansing agents are supplied in dispensers located near each sink)

Warm running water
Paper towels
Waste container

ACTION	RATIONALE
Preparation	
1. Keep fingernails short.	Long fingernails harbor microorganisms. In addition, they can scratch the patient and cause discomfort. Trim your nails straight across and use an emery board to file off rough edges.
2. Remove jewelry. A plain wedding band is usually permitted by the health care institution. You can slide your watch above your elbow while you are washing.	Jewelry provides a place for microorganisms to grow.
3. Check your hands. Look for breaks in the skin, such as hangnails or cuts. Report to your supervisor if there are breaks in your skin. You may wear gloves if you have breaks in your skin, or your supervisor may change your assignment. Review your health care institution's policy about breaks in the skin.	Skin breaks provide a portal of entry for microorganisms. Gloves are a barrier to microorganisms.

4. Use lotion to keep your skin soft.

Procedural Steps

5. Turn on the water. Adjust for an adequate flow and a comfortable warm temperature (Figure 11–12).

Hot water is harsher on the skin because it removes the protective coating of oil on the skin.

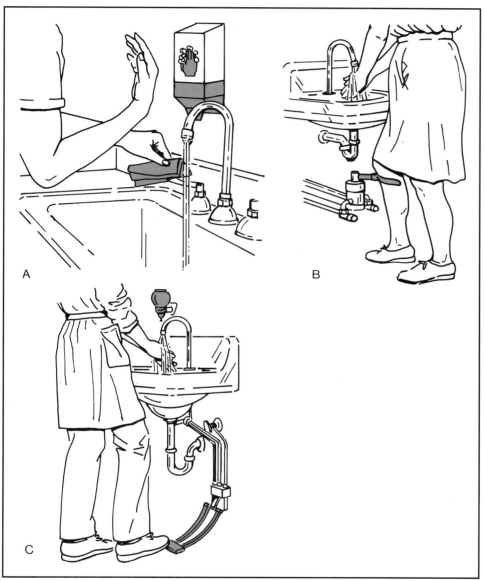

FIGURE 11–12

You may find different kinds of water faucet controls in the facility in which you work: A, Hand-operated control. Use a paper towel to touch the faucet to adjust the flow and temperature. The following two types of faucet control save steps in hand washing. There is less chance of contamination of clean hands with these kinds of controls. B, Knee control. Movement of the knee is used to control the flow and temperature. C, Foot-pedal control. Pressure on the pedals regulates flow and temperature.

6. Wet your hands and wrists. Use running water to get your hands thoroughly wet (Figure 11–13).

Water should flow from the least soiled to the most soiled area. The hands are considered the most soiled.

Continued on following page

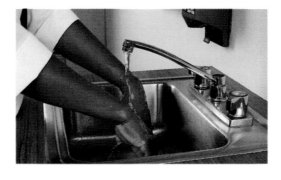

FIGURE 11–13
Hold your arms lower than your elbows so that water runs from arms (considered clean) toward fingertips (soiled).

7. Apply cleansing agent. Use about one teaspoon of cleansing agent to work up a lather. If you use bar soap, work up a lather and then rinse the bar of soap before you return it to the soap dish.

Microorganisms are removed from the bar of soap when you rinse it.

8. Wash all surfaces. Include the palms, back of the hands, and the wrist area of both hands. Use vigorous rubbing (Figure 11–14). Interlace your fingers and thumbs to clean the areas between your fingers and thumbs.

The friction and circular motion are necessary to remove microorganisms.

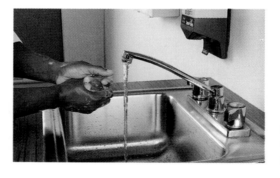

FIGURE 11–14
Vigorous rubbing produces the friction needed to release debris.

9. Wash hands vigorously for a minimum of 10 seconds. Rub all surface areas of the hands and 2 inches above the wrist.

The CDC recommends this amount of time to ensure the removal of microorganisms.

10. Clean under your fingernails. Use an orange stick to remove debris.

The area under fingernails is ideal for the growth of microorganisms.

11. Rinse your hands. Do not raise your hands so that they are even with or above the elbows.

Allow water to run off your fingertips so that you do not soil the clean areas above them.

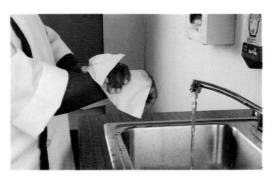

FIGURE 11–15
Start drying hands at the fingertips and work toward the wrist.

12. Dry your hands with paper towels. Pat dry; do not rub. Use a minimum of two paper towels for each hand (Figure 11–15). Discard soiled paper towels into the waste container. *Note:* The sides of the waste container are soiled, and clean hands must not touch that area.

Rubbing hands with paper towels leads to chapped hands and potential breaks in the skin.

13. Turn off the water. Use a clean, dry paper towel in each hand to do so (Figure 11–16).

Using paper towels prevents your hands from touching harmful microorganisms that may be present on the faucet handles.

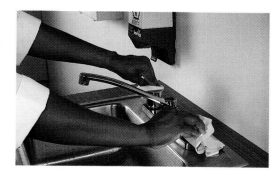

FIGURE 11–16
Use a paper towel barrier whenever you open or close a faucet.

14. If you accidentally touch the sink or faucets, start the hand-washing procedure over.

CARING COMMENT

When you use a soap dispenser, place a clean paper towel in your hand to push the bar that releases the liquid soap into your other hand (Figure 11–17), because there may be microorganisms growing on the bar.

UNIVERSAL PRECAUTIONS

The CDC-recommended **universal precautions** are measures taken in advance by all health care workers to prevent the spread of infection (Figure 11–18). The CDC recommends the consistent practice of the universal blood and body fluid precautions listed in the following chart. You must use these universal precautions for every contact with patients' blood and body fluids.

UNIVERSAL PRECAUTIONS
measures taken in advance by all health care workers to prevent the spread of infection

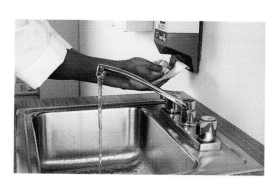

FIGURE 11–17
A paper towel barrier helps prevent contamination when you press the soap bar before you wash your hands.

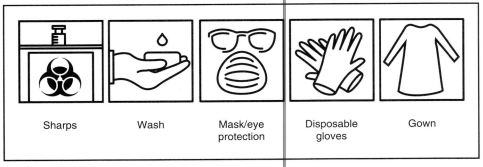

FIGURE 11-18

Centers for Disease Control Blood and Body Fluid Universal Precautions. (Adapted from Lane K: Saunders Manual of Medical Assisting Practice. Philadelphia, W. B. Saunders Company, 1993; and courtesy of Brevis Corporation, Salt Lake City, UT.)

UNIVERSAL BLOOD AND BODY FLUID PRECAUTIONS

Wear gloves before touching blood, body fluids, mucous membranes, and broken skin.

Wash hands immediately after removing gloves.

Always wash hands and other skin surfaces immediately if contaminated with blood or other body fluids.

Wear a gown when you are likely to come in contact with blood or body fluids and when working with patients in isolation.

Wear masks and protective eyewear if you expect to be around splashing blood or other body fluids and when working with patients in isolation.

Discard needles with syringes and other sharp objects in a puncture-resistant container.

All contaminated objects should be double-bagged and disposed of according to your institution's policy.

CARING COMMENTS

Use universal precautions to prevent the spread of infection from the very first contact with your patients. This is an excellent habit to develop.

Treat all blood and body fluids—saliva, sputum, urine, feces, wound drainage, etc.—as if they are infectious.

Gloves

A box of disposable plastic gloves is kept at the entrance of each patient's room for you to use. Clean, disposable gloves *must* be worn in the following situations:

- when touching blood and body fluids
- when touching patients' **mucous membranes** (for example, in the mouth or anus)
- if patients' skin is broken
- when cleansing a patient's **genital** or **rectal** area
- when discarding any material (linens, paper, gowns) soiled by blood and body fluids

MUCOUS MEMBRANES
the covering of skin that lines the organs of the gastrointestinal organs (from lips to anus)

GENITAL
pertaining to the genitalia

RECTAL
pertaining to the rectum

CARING COMMENTS

If you **contaminate** your bare hands with blood or body fluids, wash your hands immediately and thoroughly!

Always wash your hands when you remove your gloves.

CONTAMINATE
to soil or infect by contact

Dispose of soiled gloves before you leave the room. Use the appropriate waste container, not the patient's waste can, for disposal. Always wash your hands before putting on and after taking off disposable gloves.

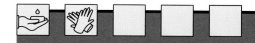

PROCEDURE

Putting On and Removing Gloves

Gloving is done to provide a barrier between clean hands and potentially harmful body fluids and blood.

GATHER EQUIPMENT

A pair of clean, disposable gloves

ACTION	RATIONALE

Procedural Steps

Putting on gloves

1. Wash your hands.

   Prevents the spread of microorganisms.

2. Remove a clean pair of gloves from the supply box (Figure 11–19).

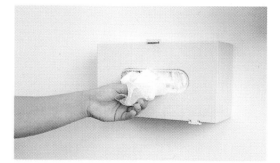

FIGURE 11–19

Health care institutions provide a supply of clean disposable gloves in patients' rooms.

3. Put one on each hand.

   You use both of your hands in most procedures. Since the hands are considered clean after washing, and gloves are considered clean inside, the result is putting a clean surface to a clean surface.

Removing gloves

4. With one gloved hand, grasp the glove on the other hand at the palm (Figure 11–20).

   Prevents you from touching the soiled outside surface of the glove with a clean hand.
   Prevents the spread of microorganisms.

Continued on following page

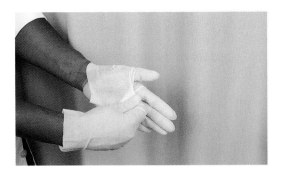

5. Remove glove while maintaining a firm grip on it with the gloved hand (Figure 11–21).

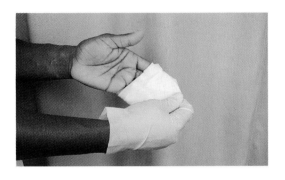

6. Continue holding the removed glove with the gloved hand (Figure 11–22).

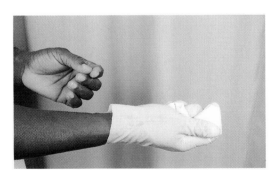

7. Use two fingers of the de-gloved hand to reach under the glove at the wrist. Pull off the glove while holding the first

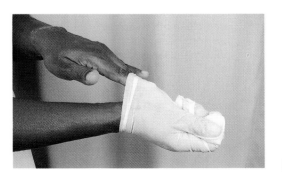

glove. (The second glove will be inside out with the first glove wrapped in it; Figure 11–23.)

8. Dispose of the soiled gloves in the appropriate waste container (Figure 11–24).

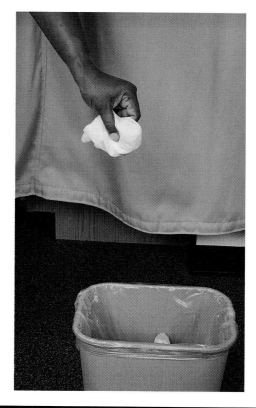

FIGURE 11–24

Gown

A gown protects your clothing from becoming soiled while you are caring for the isolation patient. Special gowns are provided by your facility for this purpose. They are usually yellow, made with knit cuffs, and large enough to cover all of your clothing. To prevent the spread of infection, *never* wear soiled gowns outside the room. The isolation gowns are worn only one time and then placed in a specially marked linen hamper before you leave the room.

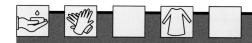

PROCEDURE

Putting On and Removing a Gown

The special isolation gown is worn to prevent your uniform from becoming soiled with harmful microorganisms.

GATHER EQUIPMENT

Isolation gown (washable or disposable)   Disposable gloves

ACTION	RATIONALE
Preparation	
1. Wash your hands.	Prevents the spread of microorganisms.
Procedural Steps	
2. Unfold the gown (Figure 11–25).	All ties are needed to secure the gown over your uniform.

Continued on following page

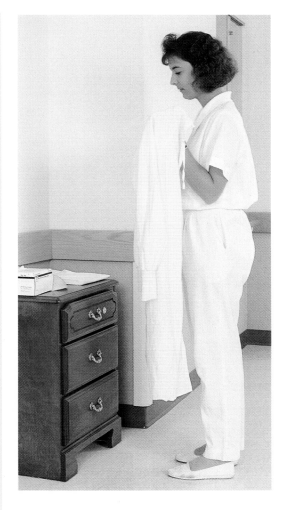

FIGURE 11–25

3. Put on the gown (Figure 11–26). Reach back and tie the ties at the neck (Figure 11–27). Tuck in the back edge (with no ties) and overlap. Reach back and tie the ties at the waist.

Protects your uniform from getting soiled during care of the patient.

4. Put on gloves, making sure they go over the cuff of the gown (Figure 11–28).
Note: *Never* leave a patient's room with an isolation gown on.

Prevents entry of microorganisms under the cuff of the sleeve.
Prevents spread of microorganisms outside the patient's room.

5. To remove a gown, take off gloves and discard. Then untie the back ties and loosen the gown.

Makes proper removal easier.

6. Withdraw one hand slightly into the cuff and grasp the other sleeve with the hand that is slightly inside the cuff. Pull the sleeve, freeing that arm. Hold the gown away from your body and ease the other arm out of the sleeve. Do not turn the sleeve inside out.

Prevents the soiled area from touching clean areas while removing the gown.

7. Loosen the gown away from your body. Hold it away from yourself.

8. Fold the gown with the soiled sides together.

Keeps the microorganisms inside the isolation gown.

FIGURE 11–26

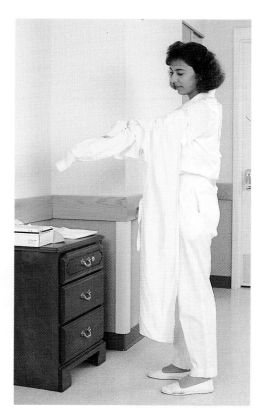

FIGURE 11–27

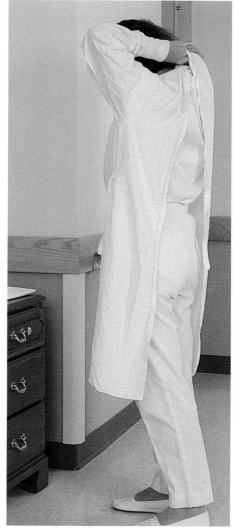

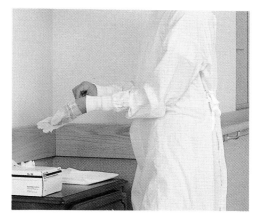

FIGURE 11–28

Continued on following page

9. Roll the gown into a loose ball while holding it away from your body. Dispose of the gown in the appropriate linen hamper.   Prevents soiling of clean objects.

10. Wash your hands.   Prevents the spread of microorganisms.

Mask

A mask prevents contact with airborne particles that may be infected. When masking is required, a box of disposable masks is kept at the entrance to the room. Remember that masks are never worn outside the room and never worn hanging around the neck after use. Dispose of the mask in the waste container before you leave the room.

PROCEDURE
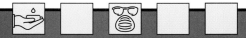

Putting On and Removing a Mask

A mask is worn to prevent the inhalation (breathing in) of harmful airborne microorganisms. A mask also helps prevent the spread of microorganisms if the health care worker is feeling ill.

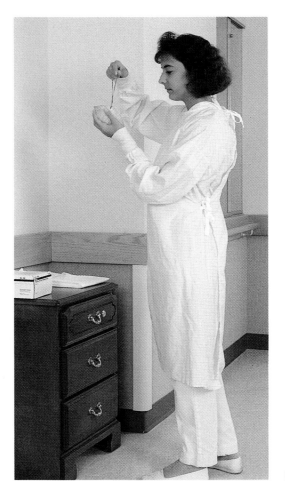

FIGURE 11–29

GATHER EQUIPMENT

Disposable face mask (most have a thin
metal strip at the top)

ACTION	RATIONALE
Preparation	
1. Wash your hands.	Prevents the spread of microorganisms.
Procedural Steps	
2. Open the mask if it is the folded type. Locate the metal strip at the top edge and bend it slightly (Figure 11–29).	
3. Place the mask over your nose and mouth with the metal edge over the nose. Adjust the mask over your nose for security and comfort.	Prevents transmission of airborne droplets.
4. Place the elastic band securely across the back of your head. (Figure 11–30). For a mask with ties, tie in two places—at the top of the head and the back of the head.	

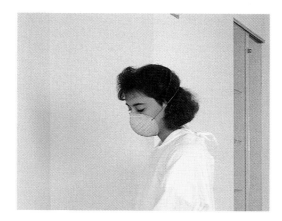

FIGURE 11–30

5. To remove the mask, untie it at both places if it has ties. Remove the mask by slipping two fingers under it and grasping the inside (clean) part of the mask.	Keeping the clean hand on the inside of the mask prevents soiling your hand with microorganisms.
6. Dispose of the mask by dropping it into the appropriate waste container.	Prevents the spread of microorganisms from a soiled area.
7. Wash your hands.	Prevents the spread of microorganisms.

Eye Protection

Because the eye is a portal of entry, for any care you give that could result in
splashing of fluids, protective eye wear should be used. Goggles are provided
by your health care institution for this purpose. The goggles should be large
enough to cover your eyes and form a seal around them for protection. A
see-through plastic shield similar to a welder's mask may also be provided.

Cleaning Blood Spills

DISINFECTANT
a chemical agent that destroys or disables microorganisms

Always wear clean disposable gloves to clean blood spills, and wash your hands after removing the gloves. Blood spills must be cleaned immediately with a **disinfectant** such as a household bleach and water (1 part bleach to 10 parts water) solution or the solution your institution's policy requires.

Double-Bagging

DOUBLE-BAGGING
placing a bag of contaminated waste inside a clean bag to prevent the escape of microorganisms

Any item that leaves the isolation room must be double-bagged and handled as your institution requires. Items that are sent to other areas of the institution are double-bagged to prevent indirect contact with harmful microorganisms by others who are not aware of the potential danger. Specially marked containers alert other health care workers to take special precautions when they see such a container. The proper containers for **double-bagging** are provided in the isolation set-up.

PROCEDURE

Double-Bagging

Linens and other objects used in the isolation room are double-bagged at the doorway of the room. The double-bagged items are kept away from other soiled items. They are treated in a special way by the workers in the laundry and janitorial service departments.

GATHER EQUIPMENT

Linen bag
A helper

Another linen bag (usually marked with a red stripe or ties)

ACTION	RATIONALE
Procedural Steps	
1. Enter the room wearing an isolation gown and gloves.	Prevents transmission of microorganisms from soiled linen to your uniform.
2. Place the soiled linen in the linen bag in the room and tie the top securely.	Keeps the soiled linens in a secure place away from other soiled linens.
3. The helper stands outside the room's entrance with a clean bag that may be marked with red stripes or ties and is soluble.	The marked bag alerts the laundry staff that the linens have been soiled by harmful microorganisms.
4. The helper holds the bag with the edges folded back to form a cuff over his or her own hands.	Prevents the spread of microorganisms to the helper's hands.
5. The helper holds the bag open while the gowned person places the soiled linen bag in the soluble (melts in water) laundry bag (Figure 11–31).	The gowned person remains inside the room's entrance to prevent the spread of microorganisms.
6. The helper secures the marked bag.	Keeps soiled linens secure during transfer of laundry.
7. The helper hands the gowned person a clean linen bag for replacement.	Provides a container for newly soiled linens.
8. The helper sends the marked bag to the laundry and washes his or her hands.	

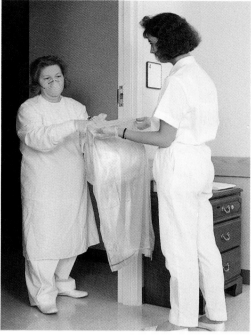

FIGURE 11-31

Note: Double-bagging is also used for other objects that may be contaminated. The procedure is the same as used for soiled linens. Use a plastic bag (or another special bag as designated by your institution) for the disposal of objects that are contaminated. You should check your institution's policy on how to handle disposable objects (dishes, wash cloths, etc.) and reusable objects (stethoscope, blood pressure cuff, etc.)

ISOLATION

When a patient is diagnosed as having or is strongly suspected of having an infectious disease, some form of **isolation** is ordered. The patient who is in isolation is in a room (or a part of a room) that is separated from other patients. This is intended to prevent the spread of infection to care givers, family members, visitors, and other patients. Isolation applies to not only the patient but also the items the patient touches or uses. A patient might touch or use linens, meal supplies, hygiene supplies, and personal items. It is extremely important to take special precautions when caring for patients in isolation to keep from spreading infectious diseases.

ISOLATION
being separated

CARING COMMENT

All of the universal precautions must be followed when you are doing procedures in isolation.

- hand washing
- gloving
- gowning
- masking
- eye protection
- double-bagging

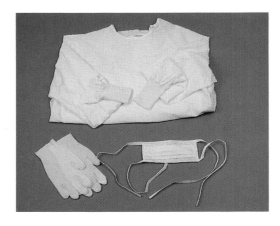

FIGURE 11–32
Gown, gloves, and masks are the commonly used isolation supplies. Note the mask with ties.

Isolation Set-Up

CATEGORY-SPECIFIC ISOLATION
the infection control measures practiced for a group of infectious diseases that have similar characteristics

When isolation precautions are required, the nurse orders isolation supplies from the supply area of the institution (Figure 11–32). A small portable cabinet, kept at the entrance to the room, contains the items needed to follow the guidelines posted at the entrance to the room (Figure 11–33). Depending on the kind of **category-specific isolation** ordered, the following supplies may be kept in or on the cabinet:

- isolation gowns
- masks (disposable)
- clean gloves (disposable)
- goggles or eye shield
- linen hamper
- waste can for trash disposal
- supply of specially marked laundry bags (meltable)
- supply of specially marked disposable trash bags

SPHYGMOMANOMETER
the instrument used to measure the arterial blood pressure
STETHOSCOPE
an instrument used to hear and amplify the sounds of an internal organ (heart, lungs, or bowels)

The following equipment is kept in the patient's room:

- glass thermometer
- **sphygmomanometer**
- **stethoscope**
- dressing supplies, if needed
- any other special supplies

Notify the nurse or supervisor when supplies are low.

CARING COMMENT

A person who is isolated is isolated for a reason. Most often, the reason is to prevent the spread of infection to others.

Category-Specific Isolation

INFECTION CONTROL
procedures enacted to control the spread of infection, particularly nosocomial (originating in the hospital) infections

Infectious diseases with common characteristics that require similar measures for **infection control** are grouped together. The diseases are assigned to a specific category of isolation procedures. Each category involves a particular combination of gloving, gowning, masking, eye protection, and double-bagging procedures to control the spread of infection. Hand washing is *always* done

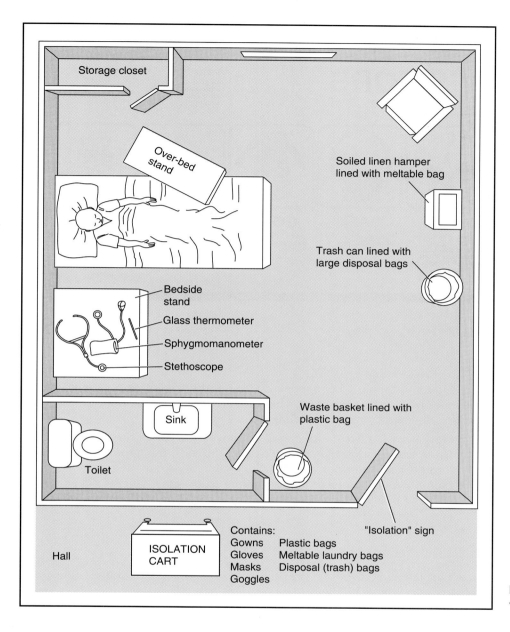

Storage closet

Over-bed stand

Bedside stand

Glass thermometer

Sphygmomanometer

Stethoscope

Sink

Toilet

Hall

ISOLATION CART

Contains:
Gowns   Plastic bags
Gloves   Meltable laundry bags
Masks   Disposal (trash) bags
Goggles

Soiled linen hamper lined with meltable bag

Trash can lined with large disposal bags

Waste basket lined with plastic bag

"Isolation" sign

FIGURE 11–33
The isolation room.

before and after each patient contact. A color-coded category-specific isolation sign is posted at the door to the patient's room and over the bed. The categories of isolation are:

- strict isolation
- contact isolation
- respiratory isolation
- AFB (tuberculosis) isolation
- drainage/secretion precautions
- **enteric** precautions
- reverse isolation

ENTERIC

pertaining to the small intestine

Strict Isolation

Strict isolation is used when the infection (such as chickenpox or shingles) is highly contagious (Figure 11–34). It is also ordered when a patient is at risk for

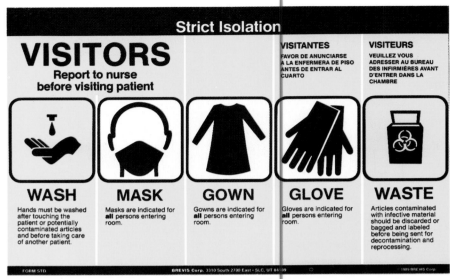

FIGURE 11–34

Strict isolation sign. (Courtesy of Brevis Corporation, Salt Lake City, UT.)

infection, for example, the patient on chemotherapy or the patient who receives a bone marrow transplant. The patient is in a private room with the door kept closed. Follow these procedures:

- Wear gowns, gloves, and masks whenever you are in the room.
- Discard all disposable contaminated articles in the appropriate container located near the door of the room.
- Perform good hand-washing technique to maintain strict isolation.
- Dispose of contaminated articles as indicated on the card identifying the category of isolation.

Contact Isolation

Contact isolation is used to prevent spread of infection that occurs mostly through direct contact (Figure 11–35). This patient is in a private room or shares a room with another patient who is infected with the same disease, such as an acute respiratory tract infection in infants. Follow these procedures:

- Wear masks when you are close to the patient (for example, when giving a bath) and a gown if soiling is likely.
- If you touch soiled objects, wear gloves.
- Dispose of contaminated articles as indicated on the card identifying the category of isolation.
- Use good hand-washing technique.

Respiratory Isolation

Respiratory isolation is used to prevent the transmission of airborne droplets by direct or indirect contact (Figure 11–36). A private room is needed. Sharing a room shared with another person who has the same infection, such as mumps or measles, is also permitted. Follow these procedures:

- Wear masks when you are close to the patient (for example, when giving a bath).

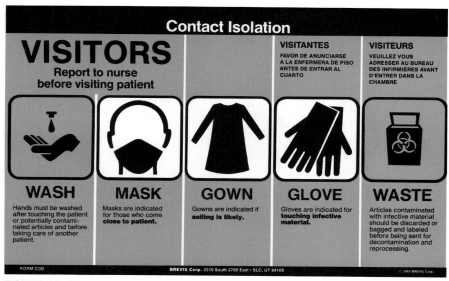

FIGURE 11–35

Contact isolation sign. (Courtesy of Brevis Corporation, Salt Lake City, UT.)

- Wear gloves when you dispose of soiled facial tissues.
- Use good hand-washing technique.
- Dispose of contaminated articles as indicated on the card identifying the category of isolation.

AFB (Tuberculosis) Isolation

Acid-fast bacilli (AFB) (tuberculosis) isolation prevents the transmission of **tuberculosis** in patients with active disease or who are strongly suspected of having it (Figure 11–37). Tuberculosis is on the rise among persons who have **acquired immune deficiency syndrome** (AIDS). A private room with special

TUBERCULOSIS
an infectious, inflammatory lung disease

ACQUIRED IMMUNE DEFICIENCY SYNDROME
the advanced stage of an infection by the human immunodeficiency virus, which destroys the cells of the immune system

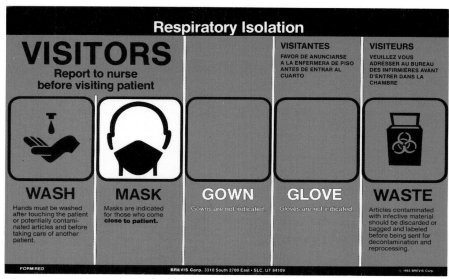

FIGURE 11–36

Respiratory isolation sign. (Courtesy of Brevis Corporation, Salt Lake City, UT.)

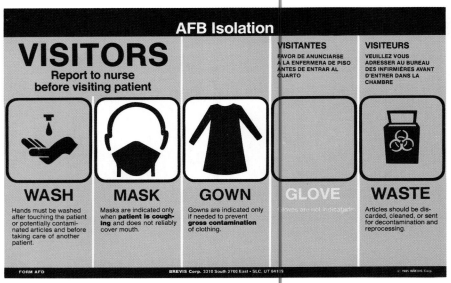

FIGURE 11–37

AFB (tuberculosis) isolation sign. (Courtesy of Brevis Corporation, Salt Lake City, UT.)

ventilation is needed, although two patients with active tuberculosis can share the same room. Follow these procedures:

- If the patient coughs without covering the mouth well, wear a mask.
- Gowns are necessary only if gross contamination is expected.
- Gloves are sometimes necessary. If you are unsure, ask the nurse or your supervisor for direction.
- Use proper measures to discard soiled objects as indicated on the card identifying the category of isolation.
- Perform good hand-washing technique.

Drainage/Secretion Precautions

Drainage/secretion precautions are used to prevent the spread of infection from infected blood or body fluids (Figure 11–38). An infected burn or surgical incision may require drainage/secretion precautions. A private room may be ordered if the patient's hygiene is poor. Follow these procedures:

- Wear masks and gowns if splashing or soiling is expected.
- Use the proper hand-washing technique before and after patient care and the handling of soiled objects.
- Dispose of contaminated articles as designated on the card identifying the category of isolation.

Enteric Precautions

Enteric precautions are used to prevent the spread of infection caused by contact (direct or indirect) with feces (Figure 11–39). Enteric precautions are usually ordered for the patient who has diarrhea. The microorganisms that cause disease can be spread quickly by contact with feces. Follow these procedures:

- Wear gloves when you care for the patient of any age who has diarrhea.
- Wear gloves any time you give care to the **perineal area** of the patient who has been **incontinent** of stool.
- Wear a gown if soilage (contact with stool) may occur.

PERINEAL AREA
the area between the legs, including the genitals and anus

INCONTINENT
unable to respond to the urge to eliminate the waste products of the body

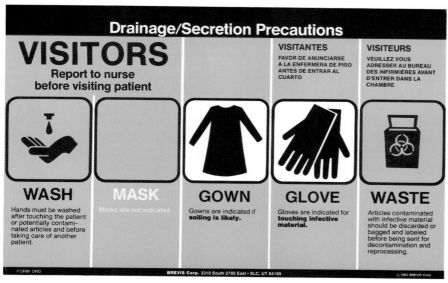

FIGURE 11-38

Drainage/secretions precautions sign. (Courtesy of Brevis Corporation, Salt Lake City, UT.)

- Wash hands thoroughly before and after contact with feces (even when gloves were worn).
- Dispose of articles (linens, disposables, etc.) as indicated on the card identifying the category of isolation.

Reverse Isolation

Reverse isolation is used to prevent infection in the patient with an impaired immune system. Because the patient's body cannot protect itself against infection, it is at high risk for infection. High-risk patients include

- patients receiving certain medications, such as those for cancer treatment

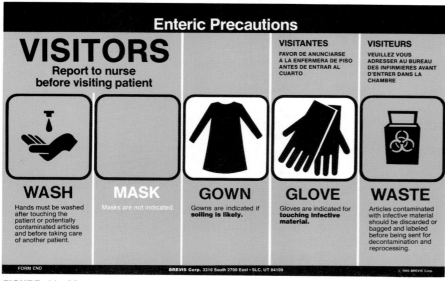

FIGURE 11-39

Enteric precautions sign. (Courtesy of Brevis Corporation, Salt Lake City, UT.)

- patients receiving radiation treatment
- burn patients

The patient is placed in a private room, and the environment is kept as free as possible from harmful microorganisms. Follow these procedures:

- Hand washing is required of all persons coming into the room.
- All persons who come in contact with the patient must wear gloves, masks, and gowns.
- Use proper measures to dispose of soiled articles as indicated on the card identifying the category of isolation.

Care of the Patient in Isolation

When you are assigned to care for a patient in an isolation room, it is important for you to follow the instructions on the card posted at the doorway of the room. The category-specific procedures tell you how to protect yourself from that infection.

If you are required to measure vital signs on an isolated patient, you need to see your watch. In this case, before going into the room, put your watch in a small, clear plastic bag and carry it into the room. You can read the second hand through the clear plastic without touching the watch. The watch can be dropped from the bag into the clean hands of another person at the doorway who can hold the watch for you until you leave the room.

In some instances, patients in isolation receive their meals on disposable trays. The dishes and silverware, if plastic, are also disposable. Before disposing of these articles in the waste container in the room, empty all the liquids from the containers into the toilet and flush. Then place the soiled articles and food in the waste container in the room. If the patient is on intake and output, record the amount of liquid the patient has taken on the intake and output record.

If you are asked to collect a urine or stool specimen from the patient in an isolation room, follow the usual routine you learned. In addition, follow these guidelines:

- Always wear gloves to collect a specimen.
- Double-bag a specimen at the doorway before it is taken to the laboratory.
- A specimen or any object from an isolation room is not permitted to leave that room without double-bagging when this is noted on the category-specific isolation card posted at the entrance to the patient's room.
- Follow the double-bagging procedure presented earlier for any item that leaves the patient's room.
- Label the specimen with the type of the category-specific isolation that has been ordered.

Transferring the Patient Who Is in Isolation

A patient who is in isolation may be taken to another part of the health care institution for diagnostic studies. The patient is not transferred to a cart. The usual procedure is to take the patient to the area of testing in the patient's own bed.

TRACHEOSTOMY
an artificial opening into the windpipe

If the patient is in respiratory isolation, a mask is placed over the patient's mouth and nose. If the patient has a **tracheostomy**, a mask is placed over it. You should wear a gown, gloves, and/or mask as required by the specific kind of isolation ordered by the physician. The nurse tells you what special care is needed for the patient who is being transferred and what precautions you should take during the transfer.

You accompany the patient to the testing area. You and the patient should be the only persons on an elevator. When others try to enter, ask them to take the next elevator. The care givers in other areas of the health care institution should also wear gloves, gowns, and/or masks as required.

Consider how the patient might feel about being in isolation. Keep in mind that the person in isolation may become very lonely and depressed because of the lack of outside contact. Some patients may feel as if they are being punished when they are in isolation. A book, radio, TV set, or a telephone may help the patient keep occupied. Use touch with isolation patients and talk to them. Even stopping in the doorway to say hello sends a message of value and worth to the patient.

BARRIER PRACTICES

Barrier practices are activities you do to help prevent the spread of infection. These activities include

- Using the clean and soiled utility rooms appropriately.
- Providing a receptacle (bag or other container) for used tissues and other small items used by the patient.
- Providing personal care items for individual patient use.
- Encouraging the patient to use hygiene practices.
- Practicing proper hand washing.
- Encouraging proper food preparation.
- Recognizing the importance of disinfection and sterilization.

BARRIER
a way of blocking something; an obstruction

Clean and Soiled Utility Rooms

In the health care institution, items that are clean—that is, never used before —are stored in the "clean" utility room (Figure 11–40). Objects that are soiled

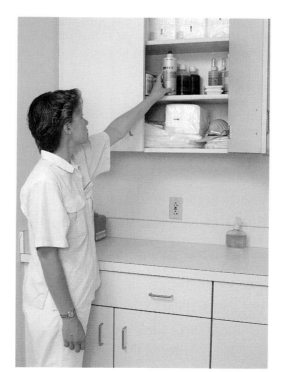

FIGURE 11–40
Any equipment or supplies that you may need are stored in the clean utility room.

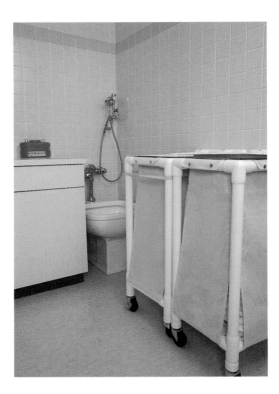

FIGURE 11–41

FIGURE 11–41
A soiled utility room. Note the large hampers for soiled linens and the hopper with a spray cleaner for rinsing large soiled items.

or used are returned to the "soiled" (also called "dirty") utility room. Never take soiled objects into the clean utility room, because you may bring harmful microorganisms to a clean area. Remember to place soiled linen and equipment in designated soiled containers in the soiled utility room (Figure 11–41).

Receptacles for Soiled Items

When you sneeze, cough, or blow your nose, always cover your mouth and nose with a clean facial tissue to prevent the spread of airborne droplets. Many hospitals provide each patient with a supply of facial tissues. Hang a paper bag within the patient's reach if the patient uses facial tissues (Figure 11–42). The patient can place other small soiled objects in the bag too.

Personal Care Items

Every person, whether at home or in an institution, needs an individual supply of personal care items. Such items are towels and washcloths, toothbrushes and toothpaste, and a drinking glass. This practice prevents the spread of infection through indirect contact with a soiled object.

Regular Hygiene Practices

Bathing, shampooing, and nail care contribute to a sense of well-being in addition to removing potentially harmful microorganisms from the body. It is important that patients as well as care givers wash hands after going to the toilet.

Food Preparation

The use of clean technique in the preparation of food helps prevent the spread of harmful microorganisms. In the hospital, wash your hands when you help

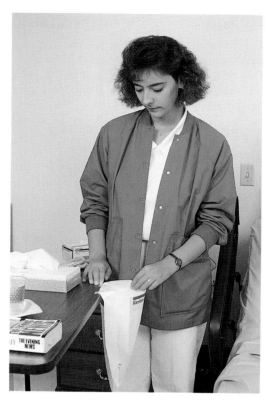

FIGURE 11-42
Use tape to secure the small bag for tissue disposal in a place convenient to the patient.

patients with food on their tray or when you prepare foods or feed them. In the home, always wash your hands before preparing food. Wash all fruits and vegetables before eating them. Cook meats thoroughly. Refrigerate foods that spoil easily, especially if they contain mayonnaise or eggs. Clean dishes and silverware are also important to good health and the prevention of infection.

Disinfection and Sterilization

Disinfection destroys *some* **pathogenic** microorganisms. When objects are boiled in water for 15 minutes, they are disinfected. Another way to destroy some harmful microorganisms is through the use of chemicals. Chemical disinfectants are used to clean equipment after a patient has been discharged.

Sterilization destroys *all* harmful microorganisms. Special sterilizing equipment, for example an **autoclave,** provides steam under pressure to ensure destruction of all harmful microorganisms. Items processed in an autoclave are considered sterile.

INFECTIOUS DISEASES

Infectious diseases are more commonly known as **communicable diseases.** These are disruptions in the body's immune system. Examples include **chickenpox,** tuberculosis, and **scabies.** These three cause many problems because they spread very quickly in health care institutions. When a person is ill, the body's immune system is affected and the body is at risk for infection. If you contact a person with a communicable disease, report this to your supervisor and follow instructions. Other common communicable diseases include the common cold, bacterial infections, hepatitis B, and AIDS.

DISINFECTION
the process of destroying or disabling harmful microorganisms
PATHOGENIC
relating to any disease-producing agent or microorganism
STERILIZATION
the process of killing all harmful microorganisms on an object by placing it in an autoclave
AUTOCLAVE
a device that sterilizes reusable objects through steam pressure

COMMUNICABLE DISEASE
an illness that can be transmitted to another person
CHICKENPOX
a highly contagious viral disease spread by contact with a blister or by droplet infection
SCABIES
a contagious disease that causes itching in folds of skin, such as the groin and under the breasts

COMMON COLD

The common cold is an acute (having a short and relatively severe course) and highly contagious infection of the upper respiratory tract. It is caused by a virus. There is no effective treatment to prevent or cure the common cold. The common cold lasts 7–10 days, and treatment is directed at the symptoms. Observations to note include

- runny nose
- sneezing
- watering of the eyes
- slight headache
- perhaps a slight fever
- tiredness and **lethargy**
- difficulty concentrating

Not all patients display the same symptoms because each person can react differently to the same virus. Rest, fluids, and medication are the accepted treatment for the common cold. Antibiotics are not effective against a virus.

BACTERIAL INFECTIONS

Staphylococcus and **Streptococcus** (also known as staph and strep) infections are the most common bacterial infections in humans. Observations to note include

- rise in body temperature
- warmth, redness, and swelling over the infected part
- possible pain
- reluctance to use or move the part
- **purulent** drainage if, for example, the infection is in an **incision** (wound)

Bacterial infections are treated with antibiotics, according to the kind of bacteria the laboratory identifies from the specimen it has examined. Other treatment is given according to the patient's symptoms. You need to provide plenty of fluids (if the patient's condition permits fluids), comfort, and rest for the patient with a bacterial infection.

HEPATITIS B

Hepatitis is an inflammation of the liver. **Hepatitis B** is an inflammation of the liver caused by the hepatitis B virus found in contaminated blood products or objects contaminated by blood (such as needles and surgical instruments). The virus enters the body after contact with contaminated objects through several routes:

- mouth
- feces
- direct contact
- sexual contact
- breast milk
- needle puncture

In the first stage of hepatitis B, flu-like symptoms are observed. These include

- lethargy
- mild fever

LETHARGY
abnormal drowsiness and indifference

STAPHYLOCOCCUS
a harmful microorganism that looks like grape clusters when seen through a microscope

STREPTOCOCCUS
a harmful microorganism that looks like pairs or chains when seen through a microscope

PURULENT
containing pus

INCISION
a cut or wound made by a sharp instrument

HEPATITIS
inflammation of the liver

HEPATITIS B
an inflammation of the liver caused by the type of virus that is transmitted only through blood and blood products

- chills
- cough
- possible loss of appetite
- some nausea and vomiting
- diarrhea or constipation

During the next stage of the disease, **jaundice** appears, as a result of damage to the liver. The urine becomes dark colored and the stools are clay colored because of the liver damage. During the later stages of hepatitis B, the jaundice clears up but the patient remains tired.

Treatment of hepatitis B depends on the symptoms present. If the patient is extremely fatigued, bed rest is ordered and activity is slowly increased as tolerated. You should provide fluids, comfort, and rest time. Other symptoms are usually cared for through treatment ordered by the physician, so be certain to report your observations to the registered nurse accurately.

Prevention

A preventative measure for hepatitis B, called hepatitis B immune **globulin,** is available and given to any person exposed to hepatitis B through a needle puncture, direct contact with feces or oral secretions, or sexual contact. Also a vaccine against hepatitis B is available; persons who give direct patient care can receive the vaccine. If you are exposed to hepatitis B, you must report the exposure to the appropriate person (usually the infection control nurse) in your institution. Your best protection is to practice good hand-washing technique and universal precautions at all times.

ACQUIRED IMMUNE DEFICIENCY SYNDROME

When a person has AIDS, the person's body can no longer defend itself against invasion by harmful microorganisms. The virus that causes AIDS attacks the immune system. About 3–6 months after exposure to the virus, the patient experiences flu-like symptoms:

- fever
- sore throat
- swollen lymph nodes
- pain in the joints
- skin rashes
- diarrhea

Before AIDS actually develops, a period of up to 10 years may pass. No cure for AIDS has been discovered. Researchers hope to learn more about AIDS and find better treatment and a cure. AIDS-related complex (ARC) is another syndrome that has been identified recently. It is similar to AIDS, but the person with ARC is not as sick as the person with AIDS. Most researchers believe the person with ARC will eventually develop a full-blown case of AIDS. One drug has been discovered that reduces repeat episodes of common ARC infections.

Because the weakened immune system cannot fight off other diseases, some AIDS patients develop **Kaposi's sarcoma** and **pneumocystic pneumonia.** There is also an increased incidence of tuberculosis among persons with AIDS.

Patients with AIDS are treated according to their symptoms and are made comfortable. You must wear clean gloves when you give oral care to patients with AIDS and assist them with toileting. In addition, if the patient has open lesions, be sure to wear clean gloves when you bathe the patient. AIDS is spread through direct contact with body fluids, such as blood, and through sexual contact.

JAUNDICE
yellowness of the skin, sclerae (whites of the eyes), mucous membranes, and body excretions caused by an accumulation of bile pigment in the blood

GLOBULIN
a protein

KAPOSI'S SARCOMA
a rare form of skin cancer, associated with acquired immune deficiency syndrome

PNEUMOCYSTIC PNEUMONIA
a lung infection, associated with acquired immune deficiency syndrome

CARE OF PATIENTS WITH A DISRUPTION IN THEIR IMMUNE SYSTEM

For most patients with a disruption in their immune system, care is directed to the relief of symptoms. For example, if the patient has a fever, the physician may order fluids and a medication to reduce the body temperature. Such care helps make the patient comfortable and gives the body time to heal. It is critical that you prevent the spread of microorganisms to other patients, visitors, staff, and yourself. The following guidelines will help you give physical as well as psychologic care:

- Practice effective hand washing.
- Practice the universal blood and body fluid precautions at the very first contact with all patients and consistently thereafter.
- Follow the directions on the sign for each type of category-specific isolation.
- Keep the patient comfortable and offer support.
- Provide appropriate stimulation (music, reading, talking, and touch).
- Observe vital sign measurements, skin condition, appetite, elimination patterns, and emotional state.
- Report your observations to the nurse or supervisor.

CHAPTER WRAP-UP

- Microorganisms are present in the environment and in and on the body.
- Some microorganisms are harmful and produce disease in the body.
- The body protects itself from infection by using its own defense system: the immune system.
- Most of the infections in hospitalized patients are caused by a virus or bacteria.
- Common observations of infection are
  elevated body temperature
  warmth
  redness
  swelling
  pain or tenderness at the site of the infection
- Practice universal precautions from the very first contact with all patients.
- Category-specific isolation is ordered for persons with a specific infectious disease. Each category of isolation requires a particular combination of gloving, gowning, masking, and eye protection.
- Follow the instructions on the card indicating the category of isolation posted in the patient's room and at the doorway.
- The most effective way to prevent the spread of infection is hand washing.
- One of your major responsibilities as a nursing assistant is to practice precautions that prevent the spread of infection to yourself and others.

REVIEW QUESTIONS

1. How are microorganisms recognized?
2. List the six links of the infection chain. At which point in the process can infection occur? How?

3. Name four methods of transmission of microorganisms.

4. What is a nosocomial infection?

5. Name the most commonly used clean technique to prevent the spread of infection in the home and health care institution.

6. List the universal precautions. When are they used?

7. What is the correct way to clean blood spills?

8. Why are the category-specific isolation procedures important?

ACTIVITY CORNER

1. Count how many times you touch your mouth, eyes, and nose during the day. Write down the number. _____

2. Count how many times you touch objects in the environment, such as pencils, faucets, door knobs, etc. Write down the number. _____

3. Count how many times you wash your hands in one day. Write down the number. _____

4. How many times during the day did you touch something and pick up microorganisms on your hands? To determine this, add the numbers from questions 1 and 2. _____

5. How many times did you prevent the spread of infection by washing your hands? Write down the number from question 3. _____

6. Subtract the number in question 5 from the number in question 4 to find out how many times you were exposed to the spread of microorganisms.
What should you do to prevent the spread of microorganisms?

12

Giving Safe Care

Objectives

AFTER YOU COMPLETE THIS
CHAPTER, YOU WILL BE ABLE TO:

Identify safety needs across the
   life span.
Describe activities that help keep
   patients safe.
Explain how protective devices
   are used.
Describe environmental safety.
Give examples of an unsafe
   work environment.
Explain the need for fire safety.
Describe the care of patients
   during a fire.
Describe the care of patients
   during a disaster.
Give safe patient care.

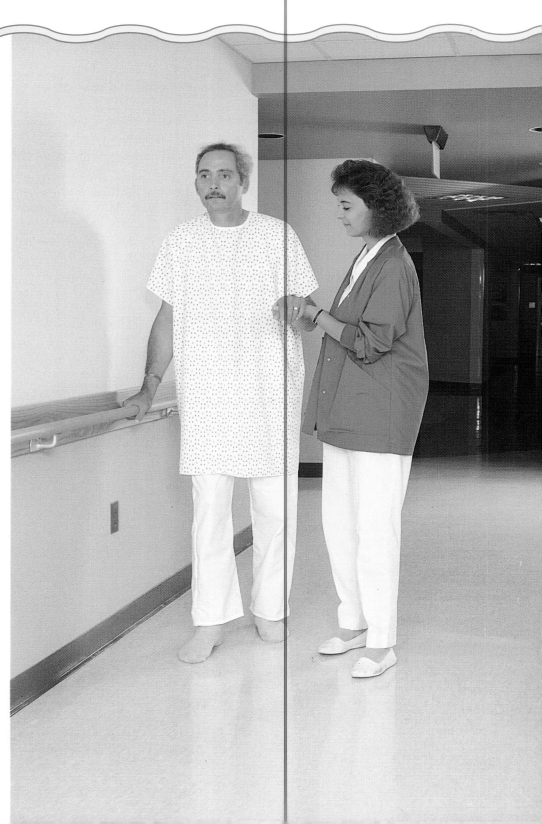

Overview Safety is an important concern in health care institutions. Young and elderly patients have the greatest need for protection from accidents. Part of your job as a nursing assistant is to help keep patients safe from injury. You need to watch for and report any broken equipment and/or electrical and fire hazards that pose a threat to safety.

You will participate in programs about safety. During fire and disaster drills, you will have the opportunity to practice helping evacuate patients to safety should the need arise.

WHAT DO YOU KNOW ABOUT SAFETY?

Here are nine statements about safety. Consider them to test your current knowledge of safety. If you think the statement is true, circle the T; if you think the statement is false, circle the F. Change the false statements to make them true.

1. T F The nursing assistant is concerned with the safety needs of all patients.
2. T F A patient in a bed in a high position with the side rails raised is safe from harm and injury.
3. T F A nursing assistant can apply a protective device.
4. T F A square knot is the best way to secure a protective device.
5. T F Protective devices are released every 2 hours to check the patient's circulation.
6. T F A nursing assistant is responsible for checking and reporting electrical hazards.
7. T F Fire drills are performed for the benefit of the fire department.
8. T F Health care workers should know the disaster plan of their health care institution.
9. T F Shelter and warmth are the critical needs during a disaster.

ANSWERS

1. **True.** The nursing assistant is responsible for patients' safety needs. Safety practices protect patients from injury or harm.
2. **False.** Any patient who is left alone while the bed remains in a high position is at great risk for injury even though the side rails are raised. Always lower the bed to the lowest horizontal position whenever you must leave the patient for any reason.
3. **True.** A nursing assistant can apply a protective device under the direction of the nurse, who in most cases gets the order to apply protective devices from the physician. Never decide on your own to place a protective device on a patient.

4. **False.** The recommended knot for securing a protective device is a slip knot. If the patient needed to be released in an emergency, the square knot would need to be untied, using precious time. A slip knot can be released in seconds if necessary.

5. **True.** Protective devices must be released at least every 2 hours so that the skin and circulation at the site of the device can be monitored.

6. **True.** Each health care worker is responsible for taking actions that prevent the potential for a fire hazard.

7. **False.** Fire drills allow health care workers to practice the actions that must be undertaken in the case of a fire in the health care institution. Persons who do not know what to do in the event of a fire may cause harm or injury to others.

8. **True.** The disaster plan clearly outlines the actions required to safeguard patients and workers during a disaster.

9. **False.** Air, water, and food are the critical needs of people during a disaster. Once these basic needs are satisfied, shelter and warmth should be provided.

SAFETY

SAFETY
the status of being safe from experiencing or causing hurt, injury, or loss

Safety is the condition of being free from experiencing or causing hurt, injury, or loss. Everyone has a need for safety. Your patients stay safe because of measures you take to limit or prevent hurt, injury, or loss. Safety practices are important for your safety as well. Common activities that keep a person safe are

MICROORGANISM
an organism so tiny it can be seen only under a microscope; capable of helping the body as well as causing disease

- not walking across wet floors because a fall could result in injury
- keeping foods refrigerated to prevent the growth of harmful **microorganisms** in certain foods. When the contaminated (spoiled) food is eaten, illness may occur (see Chapter 11)
- checking electrical cords for frayed cords or exposed wires
- helping small children or weak elderly persons down steps because you know they cannot manage walking down stairs alone

ENVIRONMENT
the conditions, circumstances, or objects that surround a person

Many daily safety activities are performed automatically. Part of the comfort of your own home is created by the safety practices you perform for yourself and those you love, for example, keeping sharp knives in a safe place. In the health care institution, you use many of these safety activities and learn others to create a safe **environment** for yourself and your patients. You need to learn about the safety needs of people of all ages. You are responsible for keeping patients and their environment safe so that no one is hurt or injured.

SAFETY NEEDS ACROSS THE LIFE SPAN

SAFETY FOR INFANTS AND TODDLERS

INFANT
the person at the beginning of life (from birth to 1½ years), for whom all needs are met by others
TODDLER
the child from 1½ to 3 years of age
PROBLEM-SOLVING PROCESS
the systematic method used to resolve problems

Infants and **toddlers** need a safe environment in which to thrive. Infants and toddlers are too young to use the **problem-solving process** to save themselves from harm. Therefore, adults (the parents or care giver) must create a safe environment for them. In this age group (from birth to about 3 years), children face many unsafe and potentially life-threatening situations. Accidents often occur because parents mistakenly think the infant can or cannot do something.

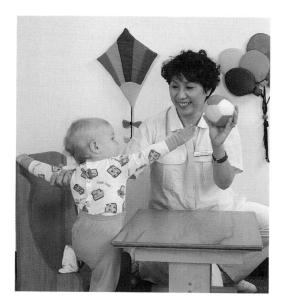

FIGURE 12-1

A young child tries to balance while climbing onto a small chair.

Typical Accidents

FALLS Infants who are learning to roll over are interested in the "how" of rolling. They are not aware that they are on a changing table, crib, bed, or couch and can roll off. Infants and toddlers do not like to be restricted in their movement and try to climb out of high chairs, walkers, and cribs without realizing the potential for a fall (Figure 12-1). Infants and toddlers can injure themselves if they are carrying a sharp object or a broken toy when they fall. Falls may result in broken bones or head injuries.

BURNS Infants do not fully understand the concepts of hot and cold. The handle of a pot on the stove looks inviting to them. They may pull it down and spill hot food or fluids on themselves, resulting in a serious burn. Infants and toddlers see extension cords, cigarettes, burning candles, and **humidifiers** (because they are noisy and steamy) as items worthy of investigation.

SUFFOCATION **Suffocation** occurs when an object does not allow air to enter the lungs. A common item like a plastic bag pulled down over the head can block the entry of air into the lungs and cause death. Infants and toddlers love to snuggle into soft things, such as pillows, which can block the entry of air. A small amount of water in a bathtub or a puddle can also block the entry of air and cause accidental death by drowning. The risk of suffocation is also high for the infant who is in a bed with a sleeping adult.

ASPIRATION Infants and toddlers love to explore by putting objects in their mouths. A small object like a peanut may be breathed into the air passages and block the entry of air into a part of the lungs. A whole hot dog given to an infant or toddler to munch on is dangerous because, if swallowed, it can block the air passages so completely that no air gets to the lungs. Infants and toddlers should have toys that are appropriate to their age. Any small objects, especially toys with small parts, should not be given to them.

POISONING Infants and toddlers are busy exploring their surroundings and often get into things that can cause them harm. Colorful pills may look like candy. Harmful fluids may look like soda pop or juice to these age groups, especially if packaged in a similar-shaped bottle. If these substances are swallowed, a child could become seriously ill or even die if not treated quickly and properly. Make sure harmful fluids are kept out of reach to prevent accidental poisoning.

HUMIDIFIER
a device (run by electricity) that produces a fine mist of water particles

SUFFOCATION
a stop in breathing due to a lack of oxygen

ASPIRATION
the act of inhaling vomitus, mucus, or a small object into the respiratory system; may occur in persons who are unconscious, are under the effects of general anesthesia, or have difficulty swallowing

POISONING
a condition produced by swallowing or breathing in a harmful substance; may also be produced by injection by a stinging insect

MOTOR VEHICLE ACCIDENTS The best safety practice, now required by law in many states, is the use of safety car seats for all infants, toddlers, and young children. Infants and toddlers like to move around. While exploring, they quickly learn how to unbuckle the belts. This creates an unsafe situation. Accidents can also occur when children crawl or walk unattended in areas (such as roads, driveways, and alleys) where moving vehicles can cause serious injury or loss of life.

Practices to Keep Infants and Toddlers Safe in the Home and Health Care Institution

Infants and toddlers are at high risk for accidents at home and in the health care institution. Table 12–1 lists safety measures that you should practice to provide a safe environment for infant and toddler patients.

TABLE 12–1 SAFETY MEASURES FOR INFANTS AND TODDLERS

Activity	Common Hazard	Safety Activity
Climbing	Crib	**To prevent falls:** Raise side rails before you leave the room (Figure 12–2).
	High chair	Use the safety belt to buckle the child in and do not leave the child unattended.
	Playpen	Do not leave a child unattended.
Rolling and reaching	High flat surfaces (such as the changing table, bed, or sofa)	**To prevent falls:** Do not leave child unattended. Never turn your back on a child.
	Crib	**To prevent suffocation:** Replace a crib if it has wide spaces between the rails because an infant may slip through the rails. Keep crib away from venetian blinds and/or curtain cords
Crawling and walking	Steps	**To prevent falls:** Carry a child up and down the steps until strength and coordination develop.

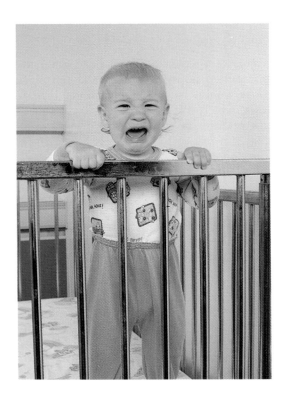

FIGURE 12–2
Raise the side rails before you leave an infant or young child in a crib.

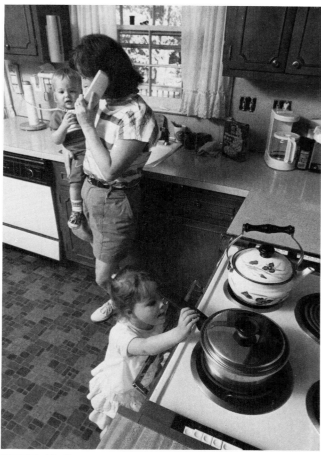

FIGURE 12-3

A curious child may want to examine an object that is out of reach. In the attempt to reach for it, an accident can happen. (From Foster RLR, Hunsberger MM, Anderson JJT: Family-Centered Nursing Care of Children. Philadelphia, W. B. Saunders Company, 1990.)

		Use gates at top and bottom of stairs.
Running	Floor clutter	**To prevent falls:**
		Remove sharp objects (furniture and toys) and loose carpets.
Eating	Propping a bottle of formula	**To prevent aspiration:**
		Hold the infant or toddler while feeding formula.
	Adult snacks (popcorn, peanuts, hard candy, and gum)	Offer snacks like applesauce or toast.
	Solid foods (such as hot dogs, bread, and fruit)	Cut foods into bite-size pieces.
	Hot foods and fluids	
		To prevent burns:
		Test for temperature before feeding infants or allowing toddlers to feed themselves.
Exploring and investigating	Any noisy, colorful, eye-catching objects and equipment	**To prevent burns:**
		Turn pot and pan handles out of sight (Figure 12-3).
		Keep hot items (coffee, cigarettes, matches, ash trays, etc.) out of reach.
		Cover electrical outlets.
		Keep electrical equipment unplugged when not in use.
		To prevent suffocation:
		Keep plastic bags out of reach and out of sight.
		Do not store toys in plastic bags.
		Do not leave child or toddler unattended near water (tub, sink, pool, toilet, or any container of fluid).
		Do not permit the use of pillows at this age.
		To prevent aspiration:
		Examine toys (or other objects the infant or toddler might handle) for loose, missing, or small parts and remove them from reach.

Continued on following page

TABLE 12–1   SAFETY MEASURES FOR INFANTS AND TODDLERS (Continued)

Activity	Common Hazard	Safety Activity
		Do not allow children of this age to play with objects like balloons or rubber bands.
	Pills and other medications	**To prevent poisoning:** Keep all medications locked and out of reach. Do not tell a toddler a medication is a candy.
	Household cleaning items	Keep cleaning items (solutions, crystals, etc.) locked or stored in a special place the child cannot get to.
	Poisonous objects/substances	Post the number of your local Poison Control Center in a convenient place by a telephone. Keep objects like rat pellets away from infants and toddlers. Keep the following plants out of reach: English ivy Rhododendron Philodendron Mistletoe Holly (berries) Poinsettia Hydrangea Rhubarb leaves Take any child who eats or drinks a poison or a suspected poison for professional medical treatment.

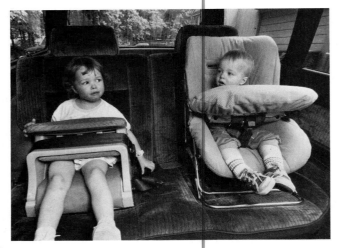

FIGURE 12–4

Serious injury can be prevented when infants and children are secured in car seats. (From Foster RLR, Hunsberger MM, Anderson, JJT: Family-Centered Nursing Care of Children. Philadelphia, W. B. Saunders Company, 1990.)

Activity	Common Hazard	Safety Activity
	Motor vehicles (car, motorcycle, etc.) and moving vehicles (gurney, hospital beds, and heavy equipment)	**To prevent injury:** Secure the infant and toddler in a safety approved car seat (according to the laws of your state) (Figure 12–4). Never leave a child alone in a vehicle.

SAFETY FOR PRESCHOOL-AGE CHILDREN

PRESCHOOL AGE
the child from 3 to 6 years of age

Children ages 3–6 face many of the same risks for injury as infants and toddlers do. Preschool-age children are at additional risk when they discover the outdoors and leave the safety of home.

Typical Accidents

FALLS Preschool-age children are stronger and more involved in the world of play than are infants and toddlers. In fact, they are so eager to move about they do not see where they are going. They run and try to jump while carrying toys or food, and this can result in a fall.

BURNS Preschoolers have a better understanding of the concepts of hot and cool than toddlers do. They can associate each word with its idea; for example, if you tell them something is "hot," they will hesitate and be more cautious. On their own, however, they may be so preoccupied with playing they might not realize that something really is hot. They are curious about how things work and try to master new concepts like turning lamps off and on, putting items in toasters and turning them on, and handling other electrical items that are left unattended. Matches and fire are especially attractive to children of this age. Preschool-age children do not understand about fire and how quickly it can spread.

ASPIRATION Preschool-age children chew and swallow much better than infants and toddlers, but because they are so active they are still at risk for aspiration. As children get closer to the age of 6, their improved hand–eye coordination allows them to cut their own food.

POISONING Preschool-age children may understand that the word *poison* means something bad, but they may not recognize a poison when they see one. They are curious and like to open and close boxes and bottles. They are quick to taste foods and fluids even when they do not know what they are. They may innocently taste something that is poisonous.

MOTOR VEHICLE ACCIDENTS Preschool-age children can explore their world on a tricycle or with a wagon. They are so intent on the activity that they do not see danger. They may fall off a tricycle or wagon or ride into the path of a motor vehicle. Children may be required to use car seats until they reach a certain weight as indicated by individual state law.

Practices to Keep Preschoolers Safe in the Home and Health Care Institution

You can protect preschoolers from harm by using many of the same safety activities you use for infants and toddlers (see Table 12–1). Table 12–2 lists additional practices to consider as the preschooler grows and develops.

TABLE 12–2 **SAFETY MEASURES FOR PRESCHOOLERS**

Activity	Common Hazard	Safety Activity

Running and jumping	Any object that interferes with freedom of movement	**To prevent falls:**
		Do not permit children to run and jump with food in their mouths or toys in their hands or underfoot.
		Offer quiet play activities such as:
		    Listening to stories
		    Coloring
		    Building with building blocks or an Erector Set
		    Playing with clay

Playing	Action without thought for safety	**To prevent burns:** Turn on and adjust the flow of hot water for bathing. Caution a child when near hot items. Take special precautions with lighters and matches.

Continued on following page

TABLE 12–2 **SAFETY MEASURES FOR PRESCHOOLERS** *Continued*

Activity	Common Hazard	Safety Activity
Eating	Putting large pieces of food in the mouth	**To prevent aspiration:** Teach the child to ask an adult to cut food into bite-size pieces. Allow children to cut food as they approach 6 years of age.
Exploring		**To prevent poisoning:** Introduce preschoolers to Mr. Yuk (Figure 12–5).

FIGURE 12–5

Children as young as preschool age can recognize the Mr. Yuk symbol. It means DO NOT TOUCH—DANGER IS PRESENT. (Permission to reproduce Mr. Yuk granted by Children's Hospital of Pittsburgh.)

Attach Mr. Yuk labels to dangerous bottles and boxes.
Keep hazardous substances out of reach.
If poisoning occurs, call your local poison control center for information (Figure 12–6).

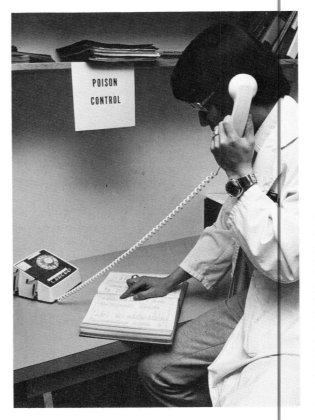

FIGURE 12–6

The poison control center gives information over the telephone about poisoning. The poison control nurse will urge anyone who is accidentally poisoned to seek professional help from a physician or the local emergency department. (From DuGas BW: Introduction to Patient Care: A Comprehensive Approach to Nursing, 4th ed. Philadelphia, W.B. Saunders Company, 1983.)

| | Never leave a child alone in a room where there are harmful substances. |
| Bathing/swimming | **To prevent drowning:** Do not leave a preschooler unattended in a tub or swimming pool. |

SAFETY FOR SCHOOL-AGE CHILDREN

From ages 6 to 12, children's motor coordination continues to develop. Problem-solving and decision-making skills continue to increase as school-age children learn to cope with the world at home and at school. Physical, active play is common for school-age boys and girls, including running, jumping, swimming, and other sports that sharpen the competitive spirit. Many of the safety concerns for school-age children are the same as for children in younger age groups, including falls, burns, drowning, and motor vehicle accidents. However, school-age children take more control of their behavior and might be tempted to do things or go places that their parents might disapprove of; this could increase the risk of harm.

Typical Accidents

FALLS Because school-age children are so quick and curious and like to test their strength, many falls result in what are known as sports injuries. Sports injuries affect the muscles and bones used in competitive and close-contact sports.

BURNS Children between the ages 6 and 12 are still attracted to fire. They are able to manipulate (handle) small objects quite well and may strike a match or light a lighter just to watch the flame. They want to be able to control the length of time the flame lasts.

DROWNING As with the younger age groups, drowning may occur in the school-age child. Children this age still need to be supervised when they are near water.

MOTOR VEHICLE ACCIDENTS Remember that children are competitive at this age. They may run out into traffic from between two cars. Children may also ride a bicycle or skateboard or glide on roller skates into traffic. Wheelchair races are a common attraction and a release from boredom in a health care institution.

PERSONAL SAFETY Children who are ill may not have control over their environment. There are many unfamiliar people in a health care institution. Many children are trusting, and because they are in a health care institution they may go with any person who comes into the room with a wheelchair or **gurney**. Children could be in danger if they leave their room with anyone who is not associated with the health care institution.

Practices to Keep School-Age Children Safe in the Home and Health Care Institution

Table 12–3 lists practices to keep school-age children safe from harm or injury.

SAFETY DURING ADOLESCENCE

Adolescents, or teenagers, are maturing physically and mentally (Figure 12–7). They like to copy each other in their activities. Smoking, drinking alcohol, and

SCHOOL AGE
the child from 6 to 12 years of age (the years before adolescence)

GURNEY
a cart used to transfer patients

ADOLESCENT
the child who is maturing; teenager

TABLE 12–3   SAFETY MEASURES FOR SCHOOL-AGE CHILDREN

Activity	Common Hazard	Safety Activity

Increasing responsibility for own activity	Temptation to do things over and above their ability	**To prevent falls:**
		For children confined to bed, provide activities that allow a lot of movement and large muscle use, such as:
		    Painting and drawing
		    Coloring
		    Building
		Do not allow roughhousing or racing in the halls.
		To prevent burns:
		Store any items that start fires in a secure, preferably locked, place.
		Do not allow school-age children to handle electrical equipment alone.
		To prevent drowning:
		Never leave children alone in a tub or shower when they are weak and need extra assistance with bathing.
		To prevent injury:
		Monitor the activities of school-age children in the health care setting.
		Provide activities that offer competition:
		    Spelling contests
		    Simple card games
		To improve personal safety:
		Place the call signal within reach and teach the child to call for the care giver for help with unfamiliar people and their requests.

ADOLESCENCE

a time of transition from childhood to adulthood

using drugs are great temptations during **adolescence** because "everyone else is doing it." Although they are still at risk for problems like younger children, adolescents accept more responsibility for their behavior. They may resort to smoking, drinking alcohol, or using drugs while they are a patient in the health care institution. Monitor visits from other adolescents and young adults. Observe for signs of such activities.

CARING COMMENT

Although school-age children and adolescents can take some responsibility for their own safety, you should remain alert to the possibility of unsafe situations.

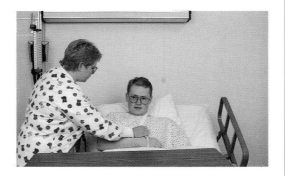

FIGURE 12–7

Teenagers have safety needs when they are ill. You should follow the nurse's instructions on keeping the side rails raised.

SAFETY IN YOUNG AND MIDDLE-AGED ADULTS

From the early 20s through the 60s (as well as older adults), the person who is a patient in the health care institution may be exposed to danger as a result of smoking, drinking alcohol, or abusing drugs. These are all considered substance abuse. Be alert to signs of undesirable behaviors such as the following:

- the smell of cigarette or cigar smoke in the room
- the presence of matches in the wastebasket
- lighters on the bedside stand
- the presence of medications from home
- unusual behavior
- inappropriate answers to simple questions

Ill persons may see themselves as stronger and more capable than they really are. Encourage patients to use the **call signal** to bring help for transfers and walking or any other assistance that might be needed.

CALL SIGNAL
a communication tool used by patients who must remain in bed or in a chair; also called a call light or call bell

CARING COMMENT

Everyone should strive to prevent injury to patients and others. Always report a potentially unsafe situation to the nurse or supervisor as soon as possible. Examples are a wet floor without a warning sign and a patient who wants to smoke while drowsy.

SAFETY IN THE ELDERLY

The number of **elderly** persons in the population is growing. People are living longer because they are taking better care of themselves and because of new medical technology. The combination of being ill and taking medication can cause an elderly person to become confused and disoriented. Confused elderly persons may not be able to provide a safe environment for themselves. Weakness and illness contribute to high risk for injury among the elderly in the home and in the health care facility (Figure 12–8) (see Chapter 31). Table 12–4 provides guidelines to help keep the elderly patient safe.

ELDERLY
a term frequently used to refer to older adults, usually individuals older than age 65

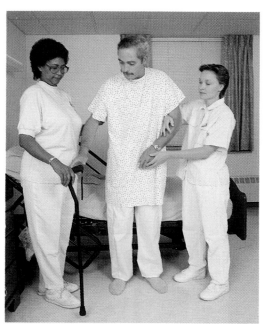

FIGURE 12–8
The use of hand rails and canes helps protect patients who may be weak or ill.

TABLE 12-4 KEEPING THE ELDERLY SAFE

Potential Safety Hazard	Safety Activity
Bed	**In the health care institution** • Place the call signal within patients' reach before you leave the room. • Instruct patients to call you for help in and out of bed. • Keep all side rails raised and the bed in low position. • Respond to the call signal as soon as possible so that patients' needs are met. **In the home** • Place a bell within patients' reach. • Instruct patients to call you for help in and out of bed. • Place the bed against one wall and use portable side rails that fit under the mattress on the other (unprotected) side. • Respond to the call bell as soon as possible.
Ambulating	**In the health care institution** • Place call signal within reach and tell patients to call you for assistance in walking. • Assist any patient who is weak or confused. • Place sturdy shoes on patients' feet. • Show patients how to use handrails. • Provide walkers, canes, crutches, and braces when ordered by the physician. **In the home** • Perform the same safety activities as in the health care facility. • If handrails are not installed in the home, sturdy furniture may be used.
Floor clutter	**In the health care institution** • Keep floors clear of equipment and personal belongings. • Place footwear in patients' closet or under the bed. • Use soft lighting to show a pathway whenever the room is darkened. • Keep floors clean and dry. Wipe all spills immediately. **In the home** • Perform the same safety activities as in the health care facility. • Remove all small rugs, runners, and carpets.
Mealtime	**In the health care institution** • Stir food to cool it before serving or feeding a meal to patients. • Cool fluids such as coffee, tea, and soup with an ice cube. • Be aware of patients who have difficulty swallowing. You may need to feed these patients a special diet (consisting of thickened liquids and strained or pureed foods) if ordered by the physician. **In the home** • Perform the same safety activities as in the health care facility. • Serve a cooked meal while you are on duty in the home and prepare and refrigerate the next meal (one that can be eaten without heating).
Tub bathing	**In the health care institution** • Test bath water with a bath thermometer before you assist patients into the tub. • Show and tell patients about the emergency call signal next to the tub. • Place a bath mat next to the tub for patients to step onto when exiting the tub. • Instruct patients not to adjust the water temperature. • Stay with patients who are weak, dizzy, or confused. **In the home** • Perform the same safety activities as in the health care facility. • With patients, establish a way they can call for assistance. A handheld bell, a verbal call, or a time limit may be chosen.

Toileting	**In the health care institution**

* Assist patients on and off the toilet or bedside commode as needed.
* Show and tell patients about the emergency call signal in the bathroom; place a call signal within reach of patients who are using a bedside commode.
* Remind patients to use any special equipment installed in the bathroom for safety purposes (for example, handrails, shower seat, and toilet extender).

In the home

* Perform the same safety activities as in the health care facility.
* With patients, establish a signal that they can use to call for help in getting off the toilet or bedside commode. A handheld bell, a verbal call, or a time limit may be chosen.
* Respond to patients' call for assistance at once.

Smoking   **In the health care institution**

* Assist patients (if they are permitted) to smoke in designated areas.
* Stay with patients whose smoking or use of matches has been restricted by the physician. (Patients who are weak, confused, or on certain medications may have restrictions on smoking.)

In the home

* Perform the same safety activities as in the health care facility.
* Decide with patients and their families how restrictions will be enforced by all care givers.

Response time   **In all situations:**

* Remember that elderly persons may need time to respond or make their needs known to you.
* Allow patients extra time to express themselves.
* Do not make any quick movements that could harm patients.
* Answer the call signal quickly.

PATIENTS AT RISK

Infants, toddlers, and preschool- and school-age children are at risk for injury while they are patients in a health care institution. At the other end of the life span, the elderly are also at great risk for injury when they are patients. Think about your patients on an individual basis in terms of their age and how they might react when ill. You may observe and care for patients who are confused, who wander, or who are weak. These patients are at risk whether they are young or old. Patients may be at risk because of their **disease** and its treatment. For example, a brain tumor might interfere with the nerves of the eyes, dimming or blurring a patient's sight. Such patients are at risk because they can no longer see normally. Other patients might be on a powerful medication that makes them feel drowsy and weak. They are also at risk for injury. As a nursing assistant, you are responsible for practicing safety activities that protect your patients.

DISEASE
sickness; a condition of the body or one of its parts that causes a change in the body's functioning

SAFETY CONCERNS IN THE ENVIRONMENT

Hazards in the environment can lead to unsafe care of or injury to patients. You may recognize some of the same hazards in your home. Common hazards in the environment include (Figure 12–9)

HAZARD
a source of danger

* damaged electrical equipment
* improper use of electrical equipment

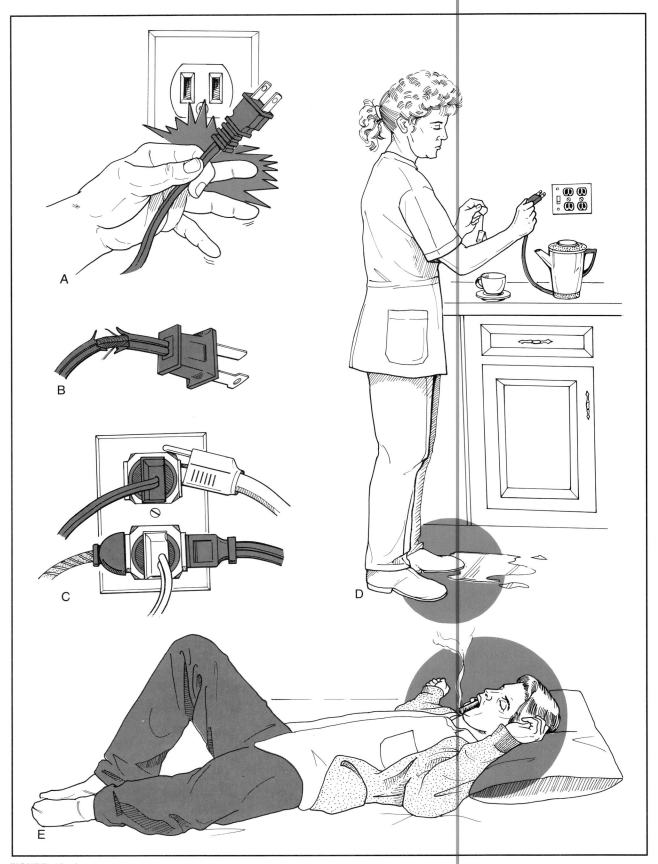

FIGURE 12–9

Common hazards. A, Feeling an electrical shock when you unplug an appliance. B, Bare wires or frayed electrical cords on appliances. C, Too many extension cords in use, or too many cords in one electrical outlet. D, Standing on a wet floor when plugging the cord into an outlet. E, Trying to smoke while in bed or while sleepy.

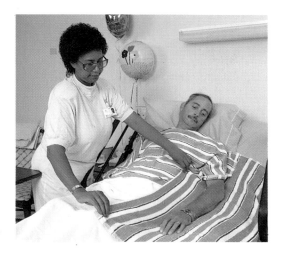

FIGURE 12-9 *Continued*

- smoking when sleepy or **confused**
- cluttered areas
- wet floors
- unplugged call signal
- serving very hot liquids such as soup, coffee, or tea
- poor lighting
- difficulty in regulating hot water flow

CONFUSED

not being oriented to time, place, or person; disoriented

CARING COMMENT

Prevent accidents by using common sense and following the safety policies of your health care institution.

PERSONAL SAFETY

Each person in the health care institution has the right to safety.

Smoking

The nurse will give you special instructions on how to handle patients who smoke cigarettes or cigars. The patients who are sedated are not permitted to smoke unless a care giver is present. If patients are confused or wandering, you may be asked to remain with them while they smoke. You should perform the following safety measures in this case:

- Provide a proper container for the disposal of ashes while patients smoke.
- Do not discard cigarette or cigar butts or ashes into plastic waste containers.
- Place the burning end into a container of sand to extinguish the fire.
- Store matches, lighters, cigarettes, and cigars in a safe place.

Some health care institutions desire a smoke-free environment and do not allow any smoking on the premises. Other institutions may permit smoking in designated areas of the building. Always follow the nurse's direction regarding patients or visitors who smoke.

CARING COMMENT

When persons are ill, they might not recognize an unsafe situation. You must strive to keep patients' environment as safe as possible.

Medical Equipment

All equipment that you or the patient use should be in good working order. Each patient unit contains equipment for that patient. You should never use one patient's equipment in the care of other patients. Check all equipment (glass, plastic, metal, and electrical) for damage that could injure someone. Chips and cracks in equipment provide a place for harmful microorganisms to thrive. A chip or crack in a glass may cut a person's lips. Each health care institution has a procedure to be followed for the repair or disposal of faulty equipment. You are responsible for knowing how to use equipment correctly and safely. Seek the nurse or your supervisor whenever you need to learn about a new piece of equipment.

ELECTRICAL SAFETY

Electrical safety is a concern for everyone in the health care institution. The institution has written rules on the care and safety of electrical equipment. Read and follow all safety rules of the institution. Appliances from home, such as radios and hair dryers, may not be permitted in the institution. In some institutions, the electrician can check patients' appliances to determine whether they may be used. Remember that electrical hazards can be the cause of a fire. Take the following steps to ensure electrical safety in your institution:

- Check all cords for breaks, metal wires, or loosening from plug before plugging them into an outlet.
- Do not attempt to use appliances or equipment with metal wires showing or frayed cords.
- Many electrical cords have plugs that have three prongs to fit into a grounded outlet. Do not use the cord if the extra prong has been removed from the plug. Never remove the third prong from an electrical plug.
- Report any time you felt an electrical charge when you plugged a piece of equipment into an outlet or when sparks flew out of the outlet when you unplugged the equipment. An electrical charge can interfere with the heartbeat and can thus harm you and/or patients. Do not attempt to use the equipment until the electrician has checked it for safety.
- Be on guard when your patient is receiving **oxygen** treatment. Because oxygen supports combustion (the act of burning), a spark from electrical equipment can be very dangerous.
- Plug all electrical equipment directly into an outlet. Do not use extension cords in the health care institution or home.

OXYGEN
a colorless, tasteless, odorless gas; the air we breathe is about 20% oxygen

THE ACCIDENT/INCIDENT REPORT

ACCIDENT/INCIDENT REPORT
a report in which the event that caused an accident or injury is described

An **accident/incident report** is a special document or form provided by the health care institution that must be completed for any situation that results in

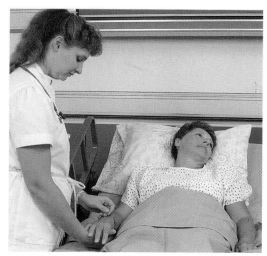

FIGURE 12–10
Patients receive an identification band when they are admitted to a health care institution.

injury. If anyone (patient, visitor, or staff) is injured or hurt in any way, the situation must be documented on the incident report (see Chapter 6). Nursing assistants are responsible for completing this form for any accidents involving themselves or their patients.

SAFETY PRACTICES FOR NURSING ASSISTANTS IN THE HOME OR HEALTH CARE SETTING

The practice of safety is important in the home as well as in the institution. The nursing assistant plays an important role in keeping patients safe from harm. Safety practices are a part of giving basic patient care. They include

- identifying the patient correctly (Figure 12–10)
- preventing the spread of harmful microorganisms
- preventing injury

IDENTIFYING THE PATIENT

When individuals are admitted to a health care institution, an identification bracelet is placed on their wrist. It is designed to provide the following basic information about each patient (Figure 12–11):

Name
Age
Sex
Room number
Allergies
Special hospital or institutional numbers

A long-term care institution, such as a nursing home, may identify the patient by using a current photograph. The photograph (with the patient's name and room number) may be placed in the patient's room. Another photograph is placed in the patient's record. The photograph should be updated on a schedule determined by the institution. When photographs are used for identification, bracelets are not necessary.

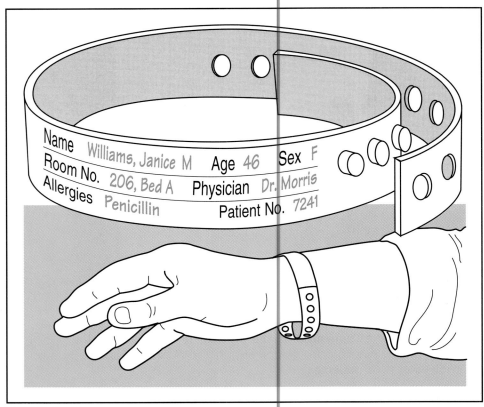

FIGURE 12-11

The identification band contains basic information about the patient who wears it. A red identification band should alert you to a patient allergy, which will be printed on the band.

CARING COMMENT

It is very important for all care givers to identify patients by checking their identification bracelet before giving a treatment (for example, a dressing change) or performing a procedure (for example, a bed bath). This is the best way to identify your patients correctly. It is also wise to call patients by name while checking their bracelet.

Remember that a confused patient may answer "yes" to any question or request. Your unit may have two patients with the same surname (last name). In such situations, you should be extra careful in identifying these patients. You must tell the nurse of any patients who do not have an identification bracelet on their wrist. The nurse takes steps to obtain an identification bracelet for these patients.

PREVENTING THE SPREAD OF HARMFUL MICROORGANISMS

INFECTION CONTROL
procedures used to control the spread of infection, particularly nosocomial (originating in the hospital) infections

When people are ill, their normal body defenses are weakened. They cannot easily fight off harmful microorganisms. The most important practice for you is to always wash your hands before and after every patient contact (Figure 12–12). The many ways you can prevent the spread of harmful microorganisms are a part of **infection control** (see Chapter 11).

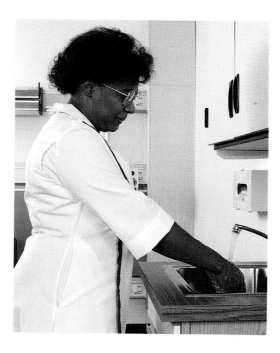

FIGURE 12-12
Washing hands before and after each patient contact helps prevent the spread of infection.

PREVENTING INJURY

Falls are a common cause of injury in patients in the health care institution. Be alert to the potential danger in the bathroom and other areas of the home or health care institution. You should practice the following safety measures to prevent injury and keep patients safe whether in the health care institution or in the home.

Bed

The hospital bed should never be left in a high position with a patient lying in the bed. Always lower the bed to its lowest **horizontal** position before you leave the patient. Even a fall from the lowest position can result in injury to the patient.

HORIZONTAL
a flat or even view one sees when looking at a bed or the horizon

Side Rails

Side rails are provided on all hospital beds to help prevent patients from falling out of bed (Figure 12-13). Patients who are weak and ill, confused or

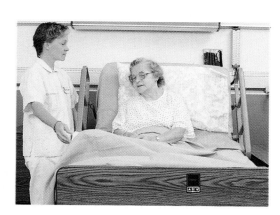

FIGURE 12-13
Raise side rails on beds to decrease the risk of the patient's falling out of bed.

DISORIENTED
unaware of self, time, or place; confused

SELF-IMAGE
your idea of who you are and what your role in life is

disoriented, or receiving certain medications are at risk of falling out of bed. You can lower one side when you are giving care, but make sure you raise it before you leave the patient. It is especially important for you to remember to raise the side rails when you finish caring for an infant or small child. Patients over or under a certain age are required to have raised side rails in some institutions. Be familiar with your institution's policy for the use of side rails. Nurses are permitted to make a decision regarding the use of raised side rails for patients who are alert and in stable condition. Patients who regard side rails as a threat to their **self-image** and self-esteem may be permitted to sign a release form, which releases the health care institution from legal responsibility in case of an accidental fall from bed.

CARING COMMENT

While changing a baby's diaper, always keep one hand on the child to prevent the child from rolling out of bed.

Handrails

Handrails line the corridors of many health care institutions. They are secured to the walls at about waist height. They give support to patients who begin to walk once their strength starts to return (Figure 12–14). When you walk with patients, ask them to place one arm on the handrail to support themselves. You can then provide support under the other arm as needed.

If patients have an intravenous fluids (IV) line attached to them and need to walk, you can show them how to push a portable IV pole with one hand and use the handrail for support with their other hand. Patients feel like they are more independent when they can walk this way. As their strength returns, patients can walk more often and for longer distances on their own.

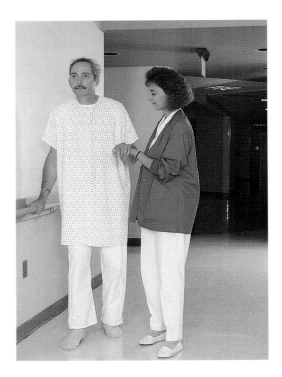

FIGURE 12–14
Encourage your patient to use hand rails for support.

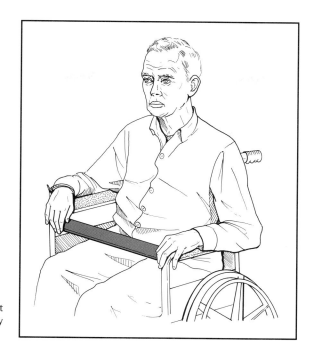

FIGURE 12–15

A safety belt or bar is used to prevent patients from injuring themselves by falling or sliding out of a wheelchair.

Chairs

Patients who are weak or confused may be encouraged to sit in a special chair known as a *geri-chair*. The geri-chair is a high-backed chair on wheels. A geri-chair can be a straight back or reclining type of chair. The back can be adjusted for patient comfort if it is a reclining chair. A tray is available to attach to the front of the chair.

When patients sit or are transported in a wheelchair, the safety belt should be secured to prevent them from slipping out of the chair. The safety belt is similar to a car seatbelt. A wheelchair safety bar may also be available to secure across the front of the wheelchair to remind a patient to stay seated (Figure 12–15).

Protective Devices

A **protective device** is designed to be placed on patients who need protection from harm they may possibly cause themselves or others. It may also be known as a safety device. It is not meant to be used as a restraining device to restrict patients' freedom of movement. The protective device also serves as a reminder to patients not to pull at any tubes or appliances attached to their body. If patients try to climb out of bed without help, the protective device reminds them to call for help.

There are legal considerations associated with the application of protective devices. You cannot decide to apply a protective device on your own. A physician's order is needed before any protective device can be applied. The patient or a family member may view the use of a protective device as unlawful restraint. The nurse tells you when a patient needs a protective device. In caring for patients for whom a protective device has been ordered, you are responsible for the following care actions:

- Check and remove the protective device at least every 2 hours.
- Exercise the **extremity** through range of motion exercises while the protective device is loosened, or allow patients to move the extremity on their own.
- Check the condition of the skin under the protective device.

PROTECTIVE DEVICE

a piece of equipment designed to prevent patients from harming themselves or others; formerly called a restraint

EXTREMITY

a limb of the body; an arm or leg

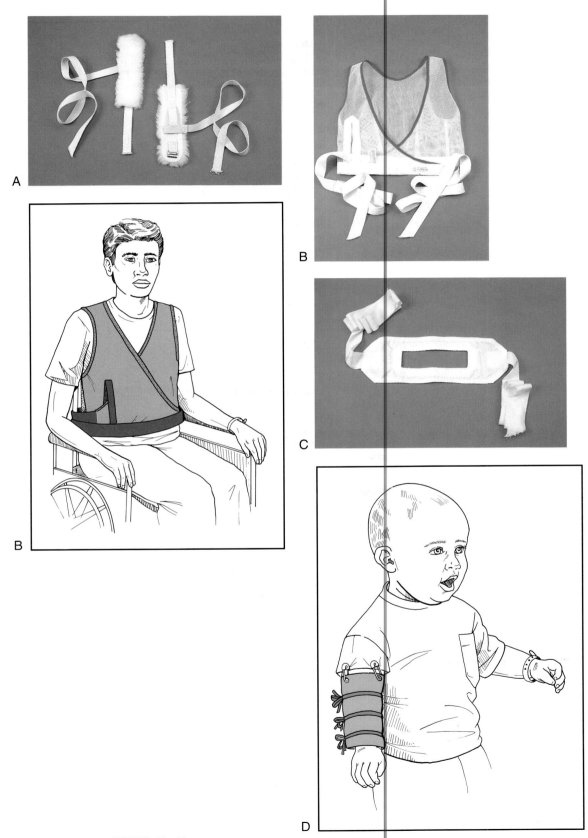

FIGURE 12–16

Common protective devices: A, Wrist. B, Vest. C, Belt. D, Elbow immobilizer (usually used with children).

- Make sure the protective device is not too tight.
- Document that you have taken the above actions.
- Document what protective device is in place and the extremity to which it is applied.
- Report patients' response and any problems to the nurse.

Protective devices are available in washable fabrics; soft, disposable material; and leather. They are made in several sizes and are applied for protective purposes only. The following are the most commonly used protective devices:

- **Wrist**—used to restrict the movement of one or more extremities (Figure 12–16A). Disposable or washable protective devices are available. Or you can make one out of soft padding and a strip of gauze.
- **Vest**—used to restrict total body movement. (Figure 12–16B). The extremities are free; patients can move their arms and legs. The protective vest is washable.
- **Belt**—used to restrict total body movement (Figure 12–16C). The extremities are free, and patients can move their body from side to side.
- **Elbow**—used to keep the arm(s) in a straightened position so that patients cannot pull equipment off their body (Figure 12–16D).

A *mummy wrap* is a protective device used for infants, toddlers, and preschool-age children (Figure 12–17). It holds a child's body in place when certain procedures are used. A *mitt* is used to cover a patient's hands (Figure

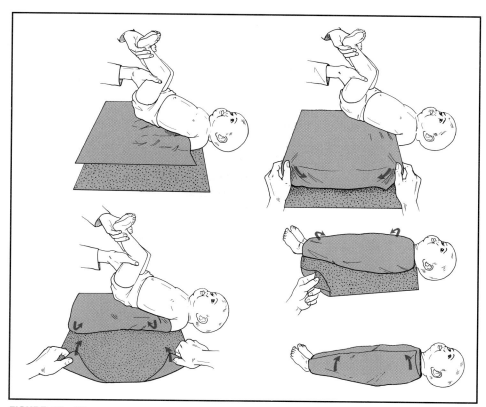

FIGURE 12–17

A child who is wrapped in a mummy wrap is ready for any procedure in which it is important that the child lie still. A, Use a small sheet (or a draw sheet folded in half) and place the infant on it as shown. Fold the sheet back, pinning the arms down. B, Tuck the sheet back under the child's left arm. C–E, Wrap the sheet around the child's body and secure the sheet with adhesive tape or pins. If there is an excess of material at the feet, secure with adhesive tape or pins. (Redrawn from Smith DW: Introduction to Clinical Pediatrics, 2nd ed. Philadelphia, W. B. Saunders Company, 1977.)

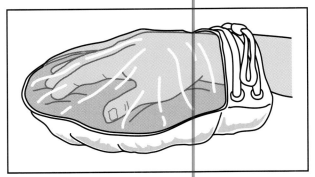

FIGURE 12–18

A mitt device restricts the use of fingers. The patient is able to move the arm easily

12–18). A net protector may be draped over a crib, or a bubble may be placed on top (Figure 12–19) to keep infants and toddlers safe.

Patients may have changes in their emotional status because of the protective device; they may feel helpless, sad, imprisoned, or angry. It is important that you explain to patients how the protective device is helping them.

CARING COMMENT

The term "restraint" does not tell patients and their family that the device is used for protection. Rather, it evokes visions of being tightly tied to a bed or chair. Use the term "protective device" to emphasize the purpose of protection.

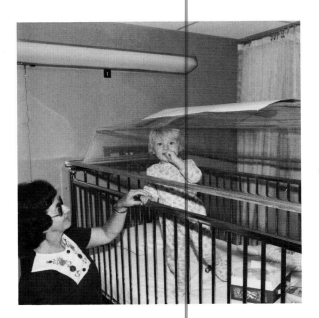

FIGURE 12–19

The net protector covers the entire crib and is secured at each corner just below the main frame of the crib. It is made of a fishnet type of material. The crib might also be covered with a special, clear plastic that helps keep a child safe. (From Foster RLR, Hunsberger MM, Anderson JJT: Family-Centered Nursing Care of Children. Philadelphia, W. B. Saunders Company, 1990.)

The following chart lists rules for applying protective devices safely.

RULES FOR APPLYING PROTECTIVE DEVICES

Rule	Reason
Apply protective devices only when the nurse directs you to do so. Never apply them on your own.	Use of a protective device without the physician's order is illegal.
Select the correct size for the patient.	If the protective device is too large, the patient may slip out of it. If it is too small, it can cut off the **circulation.**
Place the device on so that it is snug but not tight. Follow the test shown in Figure 12–20.	This simple test helps prevent damage to the patient's skin that can be caused by decreased circulation of blood in the area of the protective device.

CIRCULATION
the movement of blood through the body caused by the heart's pumping action

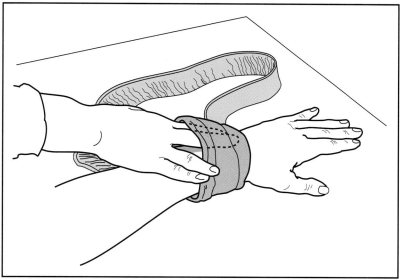

FIGURE 12–20
Place your fingers between the protective device and the patient's skin to make sure the device is not stopping circulation.

Use a slip knot to secure the protective device (Figure 12–21).	The slip knot can be untied quickly in an emergency.
Release the protective device every 2 hours or more often, as directed by the nurse.	This allows you to check the skin under the device and permits the patient to be unrestricted for up to 20 minutes.
While the device is released (loosened), change the patient's position.	Changing position helps improve blood circulation and loosen **secretions** that may be in the lungs.
Stay with the patient until the protective devices are reapplied.	Your presence helps keep the patient safe.

SECRETION
drainage material that leaves the body through an opening

Continued on following page

RULES FOR APPLYING PROTECTIVE DEVICES *Continued*

Rule	Reason

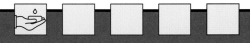

FIGURE 12-21

The slip knot is used because it can be released quickly in an emergency.

Secure the protective device to the main frame of the bed or chair.	The main frame is the most stable part of certain pieces of furniture. If you secured the protective device to a side rail, the patient's hand could be pinched in the space you create when you raise and lower the side rail.
Ask patients if they are comfortable.	This allows patients to tell you if there is any problem with the protective device.

PROCEDURE

Applying a Protective Wrist or Ankle Device

The physician orders a protective wrist or ankle device to restrict patients' movement of an extremity. It may be ordered to protect patients from pulling out tubes (such as a **catheter** or feeding tube) or from injuring themselves or others.

CATHETER
a flexible tube passed into body openings to allow fluids to enter or exit the body

GATHER EQUIPMENT

Protective device of the correct size and type (washable, disposable, or leather)

ACTION	RATIONALE
Preparation	
1. Wash hands.	Prevents the spread of microorganisms.
2. Identify yourself and the patient.	Maintains patients' rights.
3. Provide privacy.	Maintains patients' rights.
4. Explain the procedure.	Informs patients what is happening.

Procedural Steps

5. Apply the protective device to the correct extremity or extremities (Figure 12–22).

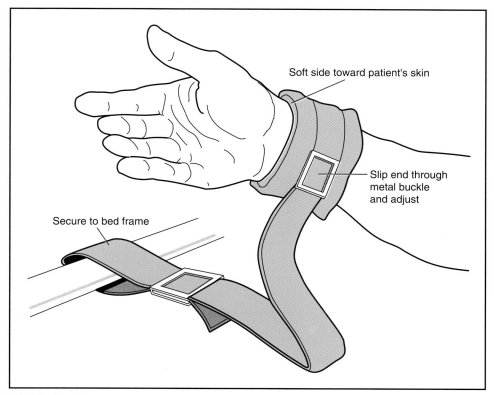

Soft side toward patient's skin

Slip end through metal buckle and adjust

Secure to bed frame

FIGURE 12–22
Applying a wrist protective device.

6. Place your fingers under the device.	Checks for tightness. You should be able to fit two fingers under the device.
7. Measure the long tie ends from the wrist or ankle to the frame of the bed or chair.	Allows for range of motion of the extremity.
8. Use a slip knot to secure the long ends of the device to the main frame of the bed or chair.	The slip knot allows quick removal of the device in case of emergency. The main frame is the strong, safe place to secure a slip knot out of patients' reach.
9. Place patient in a comfortable position with the call signal within reach.	Leaves patients with a means to communicate.
10. Open the privacy curtains.	

Follow-Through

11. Wash hands.	Prevents the spread of microorganisms.
12. Record the time you applied the protective device, the extremity on which you applied it, and the type of device.	Provides an official record of the completion of a procedure.
13. Report patient's response to the nurse.	

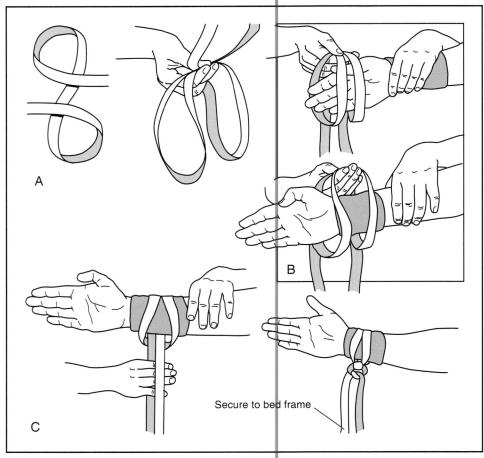

FIGURE 12-23

Making a clove hitch. A, Lay or hold gauze in a straight line. Make a loop by bringing one end across straight line. Bring other end across straight line, making a loop on opposite side of straight line. Pick up both loops at once. B, Bring loops together and let loops drop down. Place fingers through both loops and pull ends firmly. C, Slip clove hitch over padded extremity. Tighten gauze by pulling alternately on the ends of the gauze. The knot is firmly secured against the padded extremity but should not impair circulation. (Redrawn From Sorensen KC, Luckmann J: Basic Nursing: A Psycholophysiologic Approach, 2nd ed. Philadelphia, W. B. Saunders Company, 1986.)

You may be asked to apply limb protection using soft padding and a strip of gauze. The padding is held in place when you place gauze over it and make a clove hitch to secure it around the extremity (Figure 12-23).

CARING COMMENT

Always record the following in your nurses' notes when you release the protective device:

- how the skin looks when the protective device is removed
- the length of time you kept the protective device off
- that you encouraged movement of the extremity or performed range of motion exercise

Applying a Protective Mitt Device

The physician orders a protective mitt device to restrict patients' use of the fingers on one or both hands. Patients can move their arms but cannot use their fingers. The mitt may be secured the same as the protective wrist or ankle device (that is, to the bed frame) if movement of the arm must also be restricted.

GATHER EQUIPMENT

Protective device of the correct size (infant, child, or adult) and type (washable or disposable)

Device to support the hand in the correct anatomical position while it is in the mitt (for example, a cone-shaped object like a Styrofoam cup)

Note: In some institutions, you may be asked to make a device out of a rolled washcloth.

ACTION	RATIONALE
Preparation	
1. Wash hands.	Prevents the spread of microorganisms.
2. Identify yourself and the patient.	Maintains patients' rights.
3. Provide privacy.	Maintains patients' rights.
4. Explain the procedure.	Informs patients what is happening.
Procedural Steps	
5. Wash and dry patient's hand if needed.	If the hand is not clean and dry, microorganisms can grow. Remember, the area under a protective device is warm, moist, and dark.
6. Place the hand in the correct anatomical position.	Helps prevent **contracture** of the hand.
7. Slip the hand into the mitt.	
8. If hand motion is to be restricted, secure the long ties to the main frame of the bed or chair with a slip knot.	The slip knot allows quick removal of the device in case of emergency. The main frame is a strong, safe place to secure a slip knot out of patients' reach.
9. Place patient in a comfortable position with the call signal within reach.	Leaves patients with a means to communicate.
10. Open the privacy curtains.	
Follow-Through	
11. Wash hands.	Prevents the spread of microorganisms.
12. Record the time you applied the protective device, the extremity on which you applied it, and the type of device.	Provides an official record of the completion of a procedure.
13. Report patient's response to the nurse.	

CONTRACTURE
a shortening of muscle that causes a permanent disability of an extremity; the extremity loses flexibility and becomes frozen in position

PROCEDURE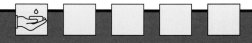

Applying a Protective Belt Device

The physician orders a protective belt device to restrict patients' movement of the trunk of the body. A protective belt device permits patients to roll from side to side but prevents them from leaving the bed without assistance. It prevents patients from falling out of the bed.

GATHER EQUIPMENT

Protective belt device of a soft washable fabric as directed by the nurse

ACTION	RATIONALE
Preparation	
1. Wash hands.	Prevents the spread of microorganisms.
2. Identify yourself and the patient.	Maintains patients' rights.
3. Provide privacy.	Maintains patients' rights.
4. Explain the procedure.	Informs patients what is happening.
Procedural Steps	
5. Place the loop (created by opening the belt near the center) over patient's head and around the trunk and position it at the waist (Figure 12–24).	

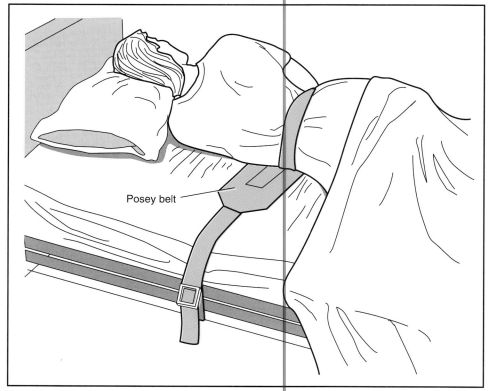

Posey belt

FIGURE 12–24

The patient in a belt device is able to turn freely from side to side. (Redrawn From DuGas BW: Introduction to Patient Care: A Comprehensive Approach to Nursing, 4th ed. Philadelphia, W. B. Saunders Company, 1983.)

6. Use a slip knot to secure the ties to the main frame of the bed. Secure one tie to each side of the bed.

7. Place patient in a comfortable position with the call signal within reach.

8. Open the privacy curtains.

Follow-Through

9. Wash hands.

10. Record the type of protective device you applied and the time you applied it.

11. Report patient's response to the nurse.

The slip knot allows quick removal of the device in case of emergency. The main frame is a strong, safe place to secure a slip knot out of patient's reach.

Leaves patients with a means to communicate.

Prevents the spread of microorganisms.

Provides an official record of the completion of a procedure.

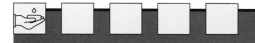

PROCEDURE

Applying a Protective Vest Device

The physician orders a protective vest device to restrict body movement to a certain area (a bed or chair). It allows adequate movement of the body for patients who should not get out of bed without assistance. It is used to prevent falls from a bed or chair.

GATHER EQUIPMENT

Protective device of a soft washable fabric in a size that fits the patient (medium or large adult size).

ACTION

RATIONALE

Preparation

1. Wash hands.
2. Identify yourself and the patient.
3. Provide privacy.
4. Explain the procedure.

Prevents the spread of microorganisms.
Maintains patients' rights.
Maintains patients' rights.
Informs patients what is happening.

Procedural Steps

5. Apply the protective vest device by putting patient's arms through the armholes. The opening of the vest should be in front of the patient.

6. Adjust the vest for fit and comfort.

7. Use a slip knot to secure the ties to the main frame of the bed or chair. Secure one tie to each side of the bed or chair.

8. Place patient in a comfortable position with the call signal within reach.

9. Open the privacy curtains.

Prevents accidental choking if patients slip forward in a wheelchair.

The slip knot allows quick removal of the device in case of emergency. The main frame is a strong, safe place to secure a slip knot out of patients' reach.

Leaves patients with a means to communicate.

Continued on following page

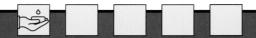

PROCEDURE	

Applying a Protective Vest Device *Continued*
Follow-Through

10. Wash hands.   Prevents the spread of microorganisms.

11. Record the type of device you applied   Provides an official record of the comple-
    and the time you applied it.   tion of a procedure.

12. Report patients' response to the
    nurse.

PROCEDURE	

Applying an Elbow Immobilizer

The physician orders an elbow immobilizer to prevent patients from bending their arm at the elbow. An elbow immobilizer may also be ordered to prevent patients from removing any tubes or bandages.

GATHER EQUIPMENT

IMMOBILIZER
a device that keeps someone or
something from moving

Elbow **immobilizer** in a size appropriate for the patient (a disposable elbow immobilizer or one made of a soft, washable fabric may be available; the washable elbow device is made with slots in which wooden tongue blades can be inserted to give the elbow area strength and stability).

ACTION	**RATIONALE**

Preparation

1. Wash hands.   Prevents the spread of microorganisms.

2. Identify yourself and the patient.   Maintains patients' rights.

3. Provide privacy.   Maintains patients' rights.

4. Explain the procedure.   Informs patients what is happening.

5. If a washable elbow device is being
   used, insert the wooden tongue
   blades into the slats to provide extra
   strength and stability to the elbow.

Procedural Steps

6. Place the immobilizer around patient's
   elbow (Figure 12–25). Allow enough
   room for slight flexion of the elbow.

7. Adjust the immobilizer around the
   elbow and secure the device in place
   by tying the ends in bows or connect-
   ing the Velcro edges together.

8. Place patient in a comfortable position   Leaves patients with a means to commu-
   with the call signal within reach.   nicate.

9. Open the privacy curtains.

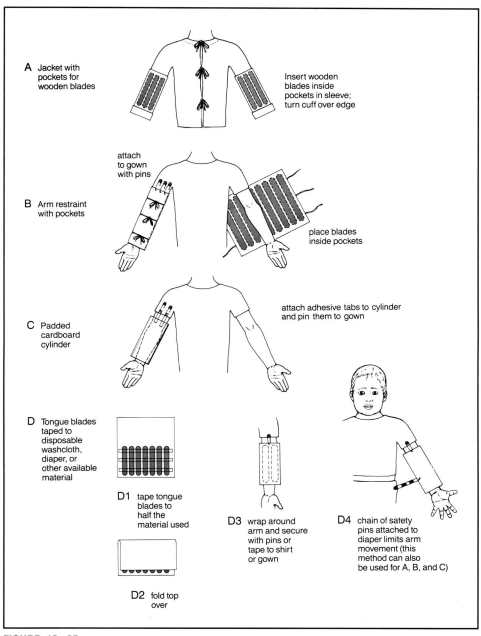

FIGURE 12-25

Various elbow-immobilizing devices. (From Foster RLR, Hunsberger MM, Anderson JJT: Family-Centered Nursing Care of Children. Philadelphia, W. B. Saunders Company, 1989.)

Follow-Through

10. Wash hands.	Prevents the spread of microorganisms.
11. Record the type of device you applied and the time you applied it.	Provides an official record of the completion of a procedure.
12. Report patients' response to the nurse.	

CARING COMMENT

Most institutions have a policy that guides the recording of the application of a protective device. Make sure you know the proper rules for your facility. You should record the kind of protective device you used, the time you released it, and for how long it was released. You should also record your observations of patients' skin.

OTHER SAFETY PRACTICES

There are hazards in all patient environments that can contribute to patient injuries. Poor lighting, wet floors, and damaged equipment are a few of the hazards that you should be particularly aware of. The following safety measures help prevent injury.

CALL SIGNAL (CALL BELL)

Call signals are installed next to each patient bed. The call signal should be within patients' reach at all times (Figure 12–26). It is patients' link to the world outside their room. When patients have a need, they use the call signal to seek help. You are responsible for answering the call signal and attending to patients' needs as soon as you possibly can.

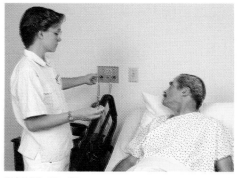
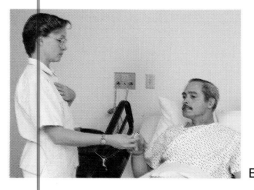

A   B

FIGURE 12–26
The call signal: A, Orient the patient to the call signal system as part of the admission process. B, Ask the patient to practice working the call signal before you leave the room.

NIGHT LIGHTING

Night lighting, an important safety feature in health care institutions, is generally placed about 12–18 inches from the floor. A dim light at night allows patients to see large objects and have a general recognition of their surroundings. Such a practice is useful not only for the patient, but also for the care giver who gives care through the night. A small night light in the home is also a good safety practice. The benefits of night lighting far outweigh the inexpensive cost of the electricity used to keep a night light on.

OBSTACLE-FREE TRAFFIC AREAS

Clear traffic areas, including hallways, corridors, and elevators, are another important aspect of safety. The areas of a patient unit and the corridors should be free of obstacles such as wastebaskets, hampers, supply carts, or any unnecessary equipment. Traffic areas should also be kept clean and dry (Figure 12–27). Spills must be cleaned up immediately so that no one slips and falls. Wet floors must be clearly identified with a "Wet Floor" or "Slippery Floor" sign (Figure 12–27).

STURDY FOOTWEAR

Patients need firm traction to prevent injury when they walk in their room or in the corridors (Figure 12–28). Nonskid shoes or slippers are preferred. Sneakers also provide good traction for walking on hard surfaces. Shiny-soled footwear should not be worn because it does not give the needed traction for safe walking.

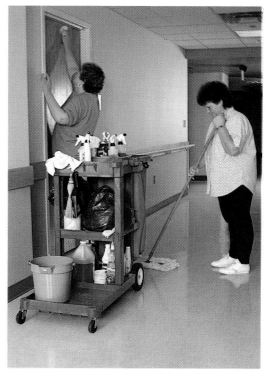

FIGURE 12–27
Traffic areas must be kept clear and dry.

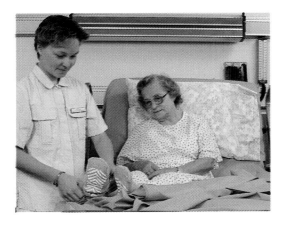

FIGURE 12–28
Apply protective footwear if the patient is unable to put on shoes or slippers.

MONITORING DEVICES

In some health care institutions (such as nursing homes and adult day care centers), patients are allowed to walk anywhere on the unit. Confused or wandering patients may not be able to recognize or react to danger without assistance. If a hazard exists in another area of the building or outdoors, an electronic monitoring device can be worn by these patients to prevent them from going there. The device triggers an alarm when the person attempts to pass through doorways in which a special beam or a mat on the floor has been installed (Figure 12–29). Care givers are alerted by the signal and can take action to bring the person back to the unit. These devices are similar to the device attached to clothing that sets off an alarm at the doors of a department store.

Bed alarms can also be used for confused or disoriented patients. A special pad is placed under the patient. If the patient attempts to get out of bed, an alarm rings at the nurses' station. The care givers are alerted and can check the patient's safety.

OXYGEN
a colorless, tasteless, odorless gas; the air we breathe is about 20% oxygen

OXYGEN SAFETY

The use of oxygen therapy in the home or health care institution presents the possibility of a fire hazard. **Oxygen** is combustible (able to burn). In the rooms

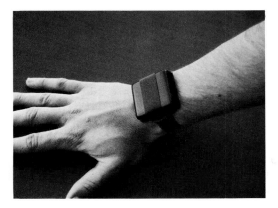

FIGURE 12–29
Electronic monitoring device that may be worn by patients who wander. (Photo courtesy of RF Technologies, Inc., Milwaukee, WI.)

of patients who are receiving oxygen, steps must be taken to reduce the possibility of fire. You may be asked to post "No Smoking" signs above the patient's bed and at the entrance to the room. You need to take measures to reduce the risk of sparks in the room; for example, offer male patients a rechargeable shaver rather than an electric razor. Patients and visitors are prohibited from smoking when oxygen therapy is in use in the room.

FIRE SAFETY IN THE HEALTH CARE INSTITUTION

Fire safety is a major concern in health care institutions. Most fires are caused by faulty electrical equipment or by accidents involving smoking. You are responsible for providing environmental safety for each of your patients. As part of your job, you receive fire safety instructions and take part in fire safety drills. Fire prevention is also an important part of your fire safety responsibilities.

- Remain with patients who smoke when they are confused, disoriented, drowsy, weak, or sedated.
- Keep matches away from children and patients who might use them unsafely.
- Provide ash trays when smoking is permitted. (Do not let patients use paper or foam dishes.)
- Place used cigarettes, cigars, and their ashes in containers of sand or water.
- Follow your institution's safety procedures regarding the use of oxygen therapy.
- Follow your institution's procedures for electrical safety.

CARING COMMENT

Take immediate action whenever you smell smoke or see fire.

WHAT TO DO IN CASE OF FIRE

In the event of a fire in the health care institution, you should follow the policies and procedures of the institution. You must be aware of the institution's procedures and how and when to carry them out. Wherever you are employed, you need to know the locations of the following (Figure 12–30):

- fire alarms (usually red)
- fire extinguishers
- fire hoses (usually in a red case)
- fire blankets (usually dark green)
- emergency exits (red lettering)

FIRE DRILLS

Every health care institution holds unannounced fire drills on all shifts so employees can practice the steps to take in case of fire. Team work is important. Each health care institution expects its staff to respond to a fire drill. You need to know what actions are expected of you during a drill. Until the all-clear

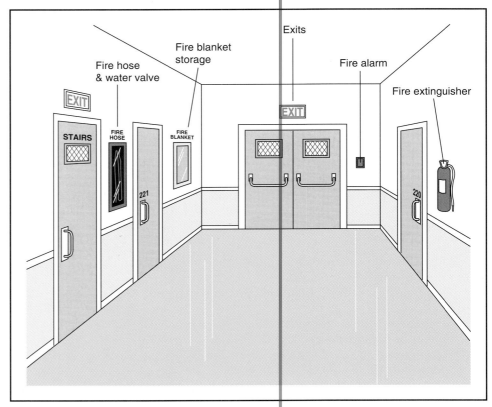

FIGURE 12–30

Always locate the fire safety equipment on your unit: fire alarm, fire extinguishers, fire blankets (usually wall mounted), and fire hoses (often located near a stairway exit and all exits from the unit).

signals sound after a fire drill, you should act as though a real fire is burning in the institution.

If you ever spot a fire, you should immediately do the following:

1. Sound the nearest fire alarm.
2. Notify the appropriate person of the fire's location.
3. Assist patients to a safe place away from the fire by using stairways. N*ever* use the elevator during a fire.
4. Use a fire extinguisher when the fire is small and nearby on the unit.
5. Turn off electrical equipment in the area of the fire (if it is safe to do so).
6. Turn off any oxygen in use (if it is safe to do so).
7. Close doors and windows.

USING A FIRE EXTINGUISHER

You will learn how to use a fire extinguisher when you are hired by the health care institution. Different types of fires require different types of fire extinguishers. A special fire extinguisher is needed for each of the following kinds of fires:

Wood or paper
Oil or grease
Faulty electrical equipment

Know the ABCs of fire extinguisher types:

A **extinguishes** wood or paper fires

B extinguishes oil or grease fires

C extinguishes electrical fires

EXTINGUISH
to put an end to

The directions for using a fire extinguisher are printed on the container. General directions for using a fire extinguisher follow.

PROCEDURE

Using a Fire Extinguisher

Use a fire extinguisher to put out a fire. Select the correct fire extinguisher to put out a fire caused by oil or grease, faulty electrical equipment, or wood or paper.

GATHER EQUIPMENT

Proper fire extinguisher for the type of fire

ACTION	RATIONALE
1. Remove the safety pin.	Allows extinguisher to be activated.
2. Push down the handle on the top of the extinguisher.	
3. Direct the open end of hose toward the *base* of the fire (Figure 12–31).	Helps extinguish the fire at its hottest part.

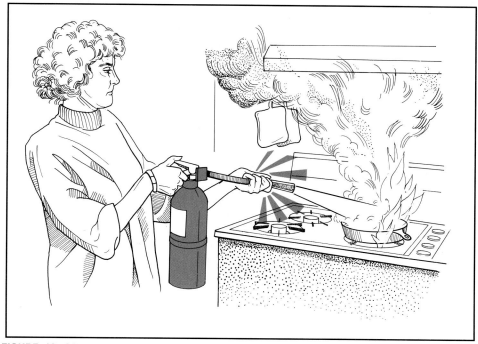

FIGURE 12–31

The proper way to use a fire extinguisher is to aim the hose toward the base of the fire while using a sweeping motion.

Continued on following page

PROCEDURE

Using a Fire Extinguisher *Continued*

4. Keeping the hose directed on the *base* of the fire, make a *sweeping motion* until the fire is out.

USING A FIRE HOSE

A fire hose is made to release water under pressure. It should be used only on a fire caused by wood, paper, or rags. The fire hose is usually used only by fire fighters because the water is under very high pressure. Without instructions, most people lose control of the nozzle and can cause injury. The fire hose is directed at the fire until the water reduces the heat of the fire by soaking. A blanket can be used to smother the flames of a fire. Cover the burning area with the blanket. Flames need oxygen to keep burning; the blanket helps stop the fire by cutting off the supply of oxygen.

CARING COMMENT

During a fire, the air near the floor is less smoky. You and your patients should crouch down so you can breathe easier.

USING A FIRE BLANKET TO EVACUATE PATIENTS

EVACUATE
to empty or remove something or someone

When you need to **evacuate** weak patients during a fire with a lot of smoke, you can use a fire blanket to take them to safety. Fire blankets are stored where they are easily accessible. They may be mounted on walls in hallways and are labeled "Fire Blanket."

PROCEDURE

Using a Fire Blanket to Evacuate Patients

Two care givers are more effective for this procedure. Take the fire blanket to patient's room and unwrap it.

GATHER EQUIPMENT
Fire blanket

ACTION	RATIONALE
1. Lower the side rail on the side nearest you.	To reach patients easily.
2. Roll patient on side away from you.	Fire blanket can be placed under patients.

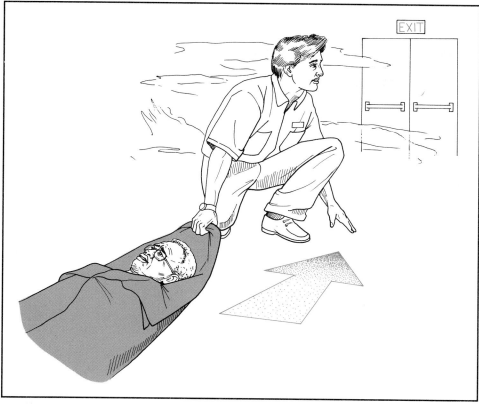

FIGURE 12–32

Patients can be taken to safety during a fire or a disaster when they are wrapped in a fire blanket and pulled along the floor.

3. Place fire blanket diagonally under patients.

4. Roll patients onto their backs.
5. Wrap patients in the fire blanket.

6. Loosen bottom bed linens and use them to lower patients to the floor if smoke is present.

7. Stay close to the floor while you are moving patients to safety. Pull patients along by using the edge of the fire blanket (Figure 12–32).

To wrap patients. (The same wrap method is used that is used for wrapping a baby in a blanket.)

Positions patients for wrapping.

Prepares patients for transport and offers protection against injury.

More oxygen is available near the floor.

CARING COMMENT

You can use a fire blanket to evacuate four or five babies at the same time during a fire in the nursery of the health care institution. Place the babies side-by-side on the fire blanket, cover them if protection is needed, and pull them to safety as you crawl along the floor.

CARRYING PATIENTS TO SAFETY

Another way to remove patients from the scene of a fire (or a disaster) is to carry them. The following are the most common methods of carrying patients to safety:

- **Cradle carry**—The cradle carry is used to carry a child or young person to safety. It may also be used to carry an adult who is light in weight (Figure 12–33A).
- **Piggyback carry**—Patients place their arms around the care giver's neck. They place their legs around the care giver's hips where the care giver can grasp and support them (Figure 12–33B).
- **Swing carry**—Two care givers make a seat by interlocking their hands in a certain position (Figure 12–33C).
- **Pack-strap carry**—Patients are carried on the care giver's back so the care giver must lean forward. Patients are held in place when the care giver grasps their wrists. Patients' feet dangle free (Figure 12–33D).

DISASTERS

DISASTER

a sudden extraordinary event that brings great damage, loss, or destruction

A **disaster** is a sudden extraordinary event that brings great damage, loss, destruction, and injury to people and their environment. Natural disasters include

Flood
Tornado or hurricane
Snow or ice storm
Earthquake

Natural events cannot be controlled. The most that can be done is for the authorities to be on guard and warn the population of the coming disaster. People can be taught how to protect themselves from certain disastrous events when they receive enough warning before the disaster strikes.

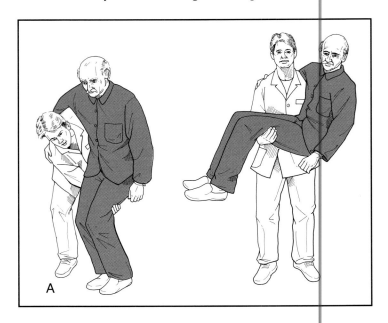
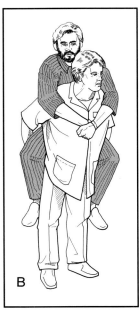

FIGURE 12–33

Common ways to carry a patient to safety: A, Cradle carry. B, Piggy back carry. C, Swing carry. D, Pack-strap carry. (Redrawn from DuGas BW: Introduction to Patient Care: A Comprehensive Approach to Nursing, 4th ed. Philadelphia, W. B. Saunders Company, 1983.)

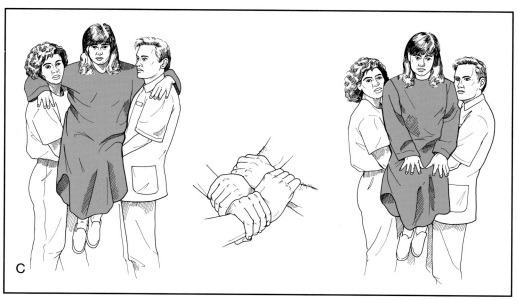

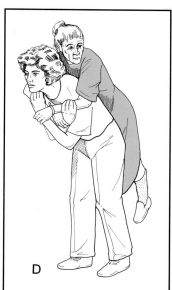

FIGURE 12–33 *Continued*

Disasters that are caused by people rather than nature include

- accidents involving transport vehicles
- accidents at nuclear power plants
- gas or chemical leaks
- fires and explosions
- riots and wars

Human-originating disasters can sometimes be controlled. The best action is for people to behave responsibly toward one another.

DISASTER PLAN

Each health care institution develops its own disaster plan. Your institution will teach you its disaster plan, and you will participate in disaster drills to prepare you in case a disaster should arise. You are responsible for knowing what action to take in case of a disaster. Disaster plans are developed for communities as well (local, state, and national). Disaster drills prepare you to

- take action in different types of disasters
- work with others as a team to provide a safe environment for everyone involved in a disaster
- learn how and whom to call for help
- act as befits your knowledge and experience

CARING COMMENT

You should become familiar with the disaster plan of your institution, because your role is important. In a disaster, teamwork, staying calm, and knowing what to do are vital responses that help prevent injuries and save lives.

A disaster plan includes a written plan of action that is available to all care givers in the health care institution. The plan includes procedures for

- evacuation or discharge of patients to a safer environment
- provision of air, water, food, and medication to people affected by the disaster
- notification of police, fire, and other local and national organizations that help during a disaster event

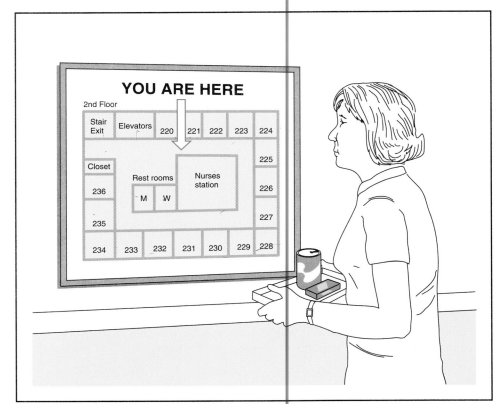

FIGURE 12-34

Drawings that show the way to the nearest exit are posted in strategic areas in all health care institutions.

- notification of the appropriate personnel of the institution
- safety and storage of records
- emergency care for people who are injured during the event
- the care giver's duties in the disaster

Evacuation or Discharge

All patients in the health care institution must be removed from the scene of the disaster and taken to a safe environment. Care givers and other staff are responsible for helping patients and visitors to safety. Look for the nearest exit:

- Red EXIT lights are above every door leading to the outside.
- Floor plans mounted on the walls throughout the building indicate the nearest exit (Figure 12–34).

In some communities, structures (for example, bomb shelters) have been built with specific disasters in mind. In other communities, buildings (such as schools) in the area may be temporarily converted to provide emergency shelter during a disaster. When possible, patients whose home is in a safe area may be discharged from the health care institution.

CARING COMMENT

Know the evacuation plan in each area of the health care institution where you work. Make a note of the EXIT signs on your unit.

Supplying Basic Needs

An emergency shelter provides people with basic needs during a disaster. The basic needs are air, water, and food. The disaster plan takes into account the possibility of certain disasters in various parts of the world. Planners make sure supplies are available on an ongoing basis. Water and food may be restricted until more supplies arrive.

The disaster shelter may provide additional items such as

- clothing and blankets for warmth
- facilities for hygiene
- toilet
- bedding
- a method to communicate with others
- medical supplies

In some institutions, the nursing assistant may be responsible for helping to collect needed supplies to take with the patient.

Support During a Disaster

When a disaster occurs, local police and fire departments are notified. If a disaster involves a great number of people and lasts a long time, other organizations (e.g., the Red Cross) are called in or volunteer to help. Various organizations accept a portion of the responsibility for providing care and supplies during a disaster.

Administrative Personnel

The administrative **personnel** of the health care institutions are notified that a disaster has occurred. These people contact emergency helpers and other

PERSONNEL
the people employed in an organization

agencies for assistance. Their contributions include the coordination and communication necessary to bring all people through the disaster safely.

CARING COMMENT

Each person in a health care institution is assigned a task during a fire or other disaster. You must have a clear understanding of your assignment in order to contribute to the team effort to help patients and visitors to safety.

Safety and Storage of Records

Records about patient care and services should be moved to a safe, dry place during a disaster. One or two persons may be assigned this responsibility once patients and visitors are safe. Important documents may be carried to safety by placing them on carts or wheelchairs and in linen bags or other easy-to-move containers. As more computers are placed in health care institutions, patient records are saved in the computer and can be retrieved when needed. Special procedures ensure that records are saved even if electrical power is lost, flooding occurs, or any other event interferes with computer operations.

Emergency Medical Care

TRAUMA
an injury

Injured persons must be treated according to the extent of their injuries. People with the most life-threatening problems are treated first. A doctor or nurse decides who needs immediate treatment and who can wait to be treated. A team is established to provide care on the basis of the doctor's or nurse's decisions. Seriously injured people are treated quickly at the scene of the disaster and are then taken to an area hospital or **trauma** center where they can get more complete treatment and care. Supplies for providing temporary, immediate help are included as part of the disaster plan.

CHAPTER WRAP-UP

- Safety is an important feature of caring for patients. You need to know what can cause patient injury and how to take action to keep patients safe.
- Infants and children are prone to injury from accidental poisoning or falls.
- Adolescents and young adults are usually injured as a result of automobile accidents.
- Elderly people are prone to falls caused by weakness and reduced vision and hearing.
- Patients who are weak and confused or who wander need greater protection from injury than others.
- Use common safety actions to prevent
  falls
  burns
  aspiration
  suffocation
  poisoning

- When a fire does erupt, fire safety procedures are critical.
- Participating in frequent drills is the best way to know the fire safety procedures. These procedures are
    Sound the alarm.
    Evacuate patients.
    Use a fire blanket when indicated.
    Use fire extinguishers.
    Save important papers.
- A disaster is an event that results in injury to or the loss of life and property for a great number of people.
- Disaster preparation includes a written plan and practice drills.

REVIEW QUESTIONS

1. What can you do to prevent injury to persons in each age group? Give two examples for each age group.
2. When are protective devices used? What patient care is needed for the patient who is wearing a protective device?
3. What are your responsibilities when you care for a patient for whom a protective device has been ordered?
4. Name the seven steps you must take when a fire starts.
5. Identify the special needs of patients who are involved in a disaster.

ACTIVITY CORNER

The next time you are assigned a patient's care in the health care institution, keep safety in mind. When your care of the patient has ended, review your safety practices. What activities kept your patient safe? How many times did you repeat each activity? The following is a list of common safety activities. In the space provided, write down the number of times you did each activity to keep your patient safe.

_____ Raised all side rails

_____ Placed the bed in low position

_____ Cooled hot foods and fluids

_____ Checked the temperature of the bath water

_____ Identified the patient before doing a procedure

_____ Placed the call signal within the patient's reach

_____ Answered the patient's call signal as soon as possible

Are there one or two safety activities you do most often?

_____ Yes _____ No

If yes, what are they? _____
Remember that your actions are very important in keeping patients safe from injury.

13

Giving Personal Care

Objectives

AFTER YOU COMPLETE THIS
CHAPTER, YOU WILL BE ABLE TO:

Explain the structure and
function of the skin.

Identify the normal observations
of the skin.

Identify unusual observations of
the skin.

Identify the common disruptions
in skin function.

Explain how common skin
disruptions are prevented.

Give care that prevents
decubitus ulcers.

Meet patients' hygiene and
personal care needs.

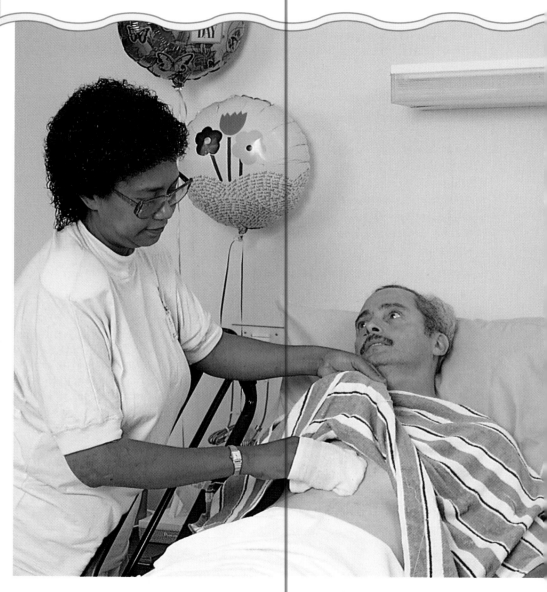

314

Overview Because many patients are too ill or too weak to meet their own hygiene needs, it is the nursing assistant's duty to help bathe and shave them; care for their hair, nails, and teeth; and dress them. When you do this in a careful and caring way, you help patients feel and look better and prevent painful and dangerous breaks in their skin.

WHAT DO YOU KNOW ABOUT PERSONAL CARE?

Here are eight statements about hygiene. Consider them to test your current ideas about giving personal care. If you think the statement is true, circle the T; if you think the statement is false, circle the F. Change the false statements to make them true.

1. (T) F   The skin is a protective organ of the body.
2. (T) F   The ultraviolet (UV) rays of the sun assist with the body's absorption of vitamin D.
3. T (F)   Observations of skin condition are not important.
4. (T) F   Dry skin is more easily injured than moist skin.
5. (T) F   The term "bed bath" means an actual bath is given while a person remains in bed.
6. (T) F   A back rub is usually part of the morning routine.
7. (T) F   The best treatment for decubitus ulcers (skin breakdowns) is prevention.
8. (T) F   Decubitus ulcers can form in a patient who stays in one position without moving or turning for long periods of time.

ANSWERS

1. **True.** The skin is the body's first line of defense against infection.
2. **True.** The body can only absorb vitamin D when it is exposed to the rays of the sun. Too much exposure to rays can damage the cells of the skin and increase a person's potential for skin cancer, however.
3. **False.** The nurse uses reports of skin condition in planning patient care.
4. **True.** Dry skin is more prone to injury than moist skin.
5. **True.** In a bed bath, a person is bathed from head to toe while in bed.
6. **True.** A back rub is a relaxing end to the morning's hygiene routine. Because relaxation is also desirable at the end of the day, a back rub is also given at the hour of sleep.

7. **True.** To prevent decubitus ulcers, care givers turn and position patients regularly and apply heel and elbow protectors when ordered.

8. **True.** The pressure created on an area by the force of the body when it stays in one position for a long period of time can interfere with the circulation of blood to the tissues. Adequate blood circulation is needed to keep the skin in good condition and ensure proper healing of damaged skin tissue.

GROOMING
making one's appearance neat and attractive

CIRCULATION
the movement of blood through the body caused by the heart's pumping action

HYGIENE
the practice of cleanliness to promote health

MUCOUS MEMBRANES
the covering of skin that lines the organs of the gastrointestinal organs (from lips to anus)

ILLNESS
sickness; a condition different from the normal health state; any change, temporary or long-lasting, in a person's physical, mental, emotional, or spiritual health and well-being

PERINEAL AREA
the area between the legs, including the genitals and anus

Think of all the things you do everyday for yourself. With scarcely any thought you bathe, brush your teeth, eat, dress and perform **grooming**, and go to the bathroom. Persons who are weak and ill cannot do such ordinary tasks without assistance. Some patients' conditions may even require that care givers do everything for them. As soon as patients are able, they are encouraged or taught how to take care of themselves. You may be required to help while allowing patients to do as much self-care as possible.

Individuals who can care for themselves benefit in two ways. First, the movement required by dressing and bathing helps the **circulation** of the blood and the flexibility of the joints. Encourage patients to do as much as possible for themselves because even a small amount of movement helps the circulation of blood to the body's tissues. Second, the pleasure they receive from dressing and bathing is a psychological benefit.

WHAT IS HYGIENE?

Hygiene is the practice of cleanliness to promote health. Cleanliness includes bathing and care of the skin and teeth and **mucous membranes** of the mouth and grooming of the hair and nails. Hygiene practices are learned during the growing-up years. They are based on the habits and practices of a person's family and social and cultural group. A good clean feeling can help a person look healthy and feel great.

The person who is ill may not have the energy needed for daily hygiene care. **Illness** changes how we feel about ourselves and how we react to others. The energy of an ill person is directed toward healing and becoming well, rather than on grooming. You may often be asked to help patients with their hygiene. You provide either complete or partial personal care, according to patients' needs. You may be asked to perform or help with any or all of the following personal care procedures:

- bathing
- care of the **perineal area**
- oral care
- combing and shampooing the hair
- dressing
- changing the bed linens

Performing personal care procedures gives you many opportunities to make observations about patients' condition. During this time, observe for the following:

What are the color, texture, degree of moisture, and temperature of the skin?

How much did patients participate in their hygiene care? What part of the care did patients do independently?

How well did patients tolerate the care?

How tired did they become during the bath?

Were patients reluctant to move?
How well were patients able to move their extremities (arms and legs) and
    move in bed without help?
Did patients say they felt refreshed after the bath?

When patients look good, they feel good. Feeling good helps give them a positive
self-image.

PERSONAL CARE ROUTINES

Before you give complete or partial personal care to patients, you need to
know what their usual routine is. The patient, a family member, or the nurse
directs you. A patient may require a special soap or special linens on the bed.
A patient may ask for the room to be warmed during the bath. During the day,
personal clothing may be worn instead of a patient gown. The usual routine in
acute care institutions (hospitals) is a morning bath. Hygiene needs are cared
for early so that when diagnostic testing or surgery occurs, patients' hygiene
needs have already been met. In addition, more care givers are available to
give hygiene care during the morning hours. In some facilities, patients can
choose the time for their bathing and grooming. In a long-term care setting such
as a nursing home, baths and showers may be in the morning or evening.

Bed baths are sometimes given at bedtime. This may be done for patients who are
restless and unable to sleep, because it may help them fall asleep more easily. Or it may
be done for patients whose at-home bedtime routine needs to be continued in the health
care setting.

Routines help patients meet certain personal care needs while they are in
the health care institution. Hygiene routines are classified in the following ways:

AM Care

1. Greet patients by name.
2. Position patients by moving them up in bed (Figure 13–1) and placing
   their body in proper alignment (see Chapter 16).
3. Offer a bedpan or urinal or assistance to the bathroom/commode.
4. When patients are finished, offer them a warm, wet washcloth and a
   towel so they can freshen up before breakfast.
5. Put glasses, dentures, or hearing aids in a reachable place.
6. Straighten the bed linens and clear the over-bed table.
7. Ask patients if they need something before breakfast.
8. If allowed, you may give patients coffee, tea, milk, or juice before
   breakfast.

Morning Care

Morning care consists of the routine of bathing and grooming procedures as
directed by the institution.

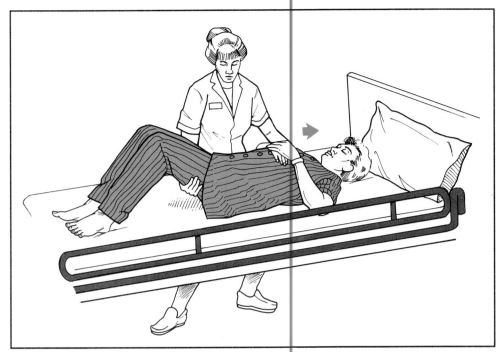

FIGURE 13-1

Moving a patient up in bed. The patient should cross arms over the chest. Notice the nursing assistant's good use of body mechanics.

PM Care

PM care may also be called hour of sleep (HS) care.

1. Provide patients with warm water, a washcloth, bath towel, articles for oral care, and a clean gown or personal sleep wear.
2. Give a relaxing back rub with lotion.
3. Place patients in a comfortable position.
4. Straighten the bed linens and provide patients with an extra blanket if desired.
5. Assist patients in following their usual home routine of preparing for sleep. (This may include watching television, listening to music, or reading a book.)

THE SKIN

SKIN
the body's protective outer covering
EPIDERMIS
the outer layer of the skin
DERMIS
the inner layer of the skin; the layer below the epidermis
INTACT
complete, whole, no breaks
MICROORGANISM
an organism so tiny it can be seen only under a microscope; capable of helping the body as well as causing disease

The **skin** is the body's protective outer covering. It is one of the most visible organs of the body. The skin is made up of two basic layers (Figure 13-2):

Epidermis
Dermis

EPIDERMIS

The epidermis, the outer layer or surface of the body, is the body's first line of defense. When the skin is **intact** (does not have cuts or breaks), it protects the body from invasion by harmful **microorganisms.** In places where the skin gets a

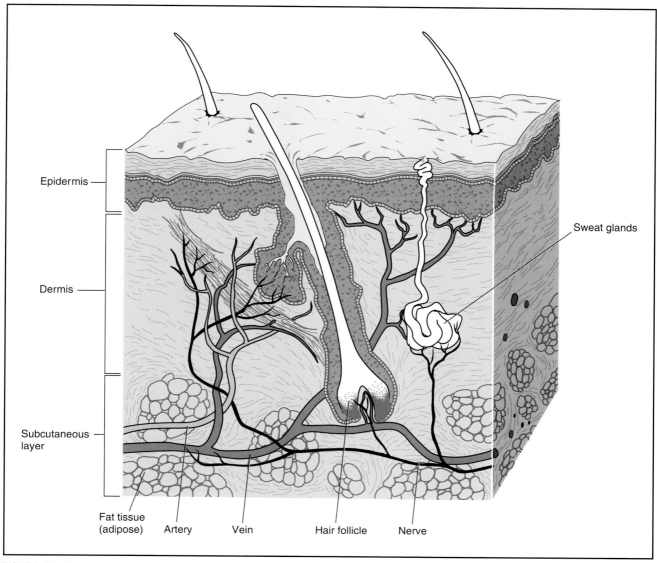

Epidermis

Dermis

Subcutaneous layer

Sweat glands

Fat tissue (adipose) Artery Vein Hair follicle Nerve

FIGURE 13–2
Structure of the skin.

lot of use, such as the palms of the hands and the soles of the feet, it is thicker to provide more protection.

The epidermis is made up of several layers of cells. One layer acts as a waterproof covering for the body. This layer of cells flakes off as a result of **friction** from washing the skin or wearing clothes. The discoloration of the fabric inside the neckline and cuffs of clothing is a collection of old cells that have rubbed off. As cells are lost, new cells push up from below to take their place.

Certain cells in this layer of skin contain a skin **pigment**. These cells determine our skin color. Human skin comes in many shades of black, brown, white, red, and yellow. Skin color is inherited from our parents. We can change our skin color when we expose it to sunlight. The sun's ultraviolet (UV) rays temporarily darken or tan the skin. When exposure is stopped, the skin returns to its normal color. Prolonged exposure to UV light is dangerous because it has been linked to the development of skin cancer. However, some sunlight is needed to help the body use **vitamin** D.

FRICTION
the rubbing of one object against another
PIGMENT
a substance that gives color to something
VITAMIN
an organic substance that is essential is small amounts to the body's health

If you look closely at your fingertips, you can see fine ridges or fingerprints. These ridges help you grasp and hold objects. They also serve to identify individuals. The ridges on the palms of the hands and bottom of the feet are permanent and never change unless an injury occurs.

DERMIS

The layer of skin below the epidermis is the dermis. This inner layer is thicker than the epidermis. The thickness of the dermis varies in different parts of the body. The dermis is the layer that contains the stronger tissues of the body, nerve endings, fat cells, muscles, hair follicles, and oil and sweat glands (see Figure 13–2). The subcutaneous layer lies below the dermis and contains the stronger tissues of the body, as listed above.

OTHER PARTS OF THE SKIN

INTEGUMENT

a covering, such as skin

The formal name for skin is the **integument.** Hair, nails, and sweat and oil glands are considered to be a part of the integument. In humans, hair is distributed over most of the body. Note that hair is not found in the palms of the hands and soles of the feet. Hair is found in a variety of textures (fine to coarse) and colors. People from Asia are yellow skinned and have straight black hair. African people have brown or black skin and brown or black hair that may be straight or curly. Caucasian (white) people's skin color ranges from very pale to deep olive; their hair color ranges from white to black and may be straight or curly.

PERSPIRATION

sweat; moisture excreted through the pores of the skin

The nails cover the ends of the fingers and toes. They continue to grow unless the cells of the dermis are damaged. Sweat glands exist to remove waste products from the body. Sweat is called **perspiration** and is the water lost through the skin. Pain or physical exercise can cause a person to lose water through sweating. When the body needs to throw off heat, it does so by sweating. Certain other glands in the skin secrete oil. The oil is needed to keep the skin soft.

Substances such as medications can enter the body through the skin. You may notice that some patients wear medication patches. This is similar to the patch commonly worn behind the ear by people traveling on boats to help prevent seasickness.

The nerve endings in the skin help the body monitor its surroundings for heat and cold, pain, and pressure. They alert the body to pleasure as well as danger. Skin acts as a screen to block some of the harmful UV rays of the sun from the internal organs of the body. It is also the body's blanket because it protects against heat loss.

OBSERVATIONS OF THE SKIN

TEMPERATURE

the degree of heat or cold, expressed in terms of a specific scale

Patients' skin should be observed for color, texture, moisture, and **temperature.**

Normal Observations

Observe for a pink color or a natural yellow tone to the skin. People with olive-colored skin and some people with black skin have a yellow tone to their skin. The skin should be soft and moist to the touch. Because the body continuously throws off its extra heat, the skin should be pleasantly warm (Figure 13–3).

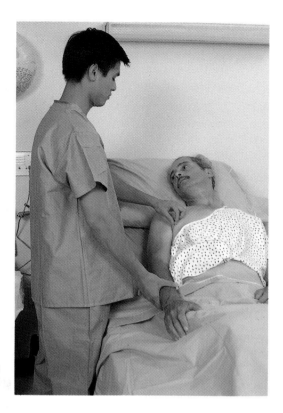

FIGURE 13-3

Each time you touch the patient during care, you make an observation about the skin.

Unusual Observations

Rashes; reddened areas; abrasions; open areas; dry, flaky areas; and color and temperature changes are unusual observations you might note in your patients' skin (Table 13–1). Ask yourself the following questions when you observe patients' skin:

* Is the skin red with small raised areas, or are large blotches and swelling visible?
* Is the skin ecchymotic (black and blue)?

TABLE 13–1 CHANGES IN SKIN

Characteristic	Healthy Skin	Change
Color	Pink White, olive, yellow, brown, black	Pale Ashen (gray) Jaundice (yellow) Cyanosis (blue) Flushed (pink, red)
Temperature	Warm to touch	Hot Cool or cold
Texture	Soft and moist	Dry Clammy, wet Scaly Wrinkled
Intactness	No visible breaks	Rash Bruising (black and blue) Reddened area Open area Abrasion Incision Drainage

- How large is the unusual area you observe?
- Is there an abrasion, with the top layer of skin scraped off?
- Are there any open areas of the skin? If so, how large are they? Where are they located?
- Is there any odor? If so, how would you describe it?

RASH A **rash** is a group of reddened spots close together on the skin. The spots may be flat or raised. A rash may be a response to a medication, food, or other substances with which the patient comes in contact. Report and record what you see.

REDDENED AREAS Reddened areas are usually noted where bones are close to the skin surface and the patient remains in one position for too long (more than 1 or 2 hours).

ABRASION An **abrasion** is a wound that results from rubbing or scraping the skin. In an abrasion, the top layer of the skin is accidently removed. The result may be bleeding, seeping body fluids, and, after a short while, discoloration in the area surrounding the injury.

DRY, FLAKY SKIN You should also report dry, flaky skin because it can crack and allow harmful microorganisms to enter the body.

COLOR When a person lacks enough red blood cells or iron in the blood, the skin may appear white or pale. You may observe an **ashen** color to the skin. Skin that is yellowed is called **jaundiced.** When a person has a disease that causes jaundice, a yellowness in the whites of the eyes is observed. **Ecchymosis** is skin that is black and blue or purplish in color.

TEMPERATURE Feel for the skin's temperature. When the body is throwing off excess heat, the skin can feel hot to the touch. A mother might say her child is "burning up." Feel the skin for perspiration. Sometimes perspiration or sweat can be felt as well as seen.

Older people's skin may feel cool or cold to the touch. This is because their blood does not circulate to the surface of the body as well as it used to. The body keeps the heat deeper inside, where it might be needed by the major body organs. In addition, as people age, their brain does not regulate body temperature as efficiently as it did in the past. More clothing may be needed to keep the older person sufficiently warm, even on a warm day.

PATIENTS' COMMENTS The comments patients make about their skin are important and should be reported to the nurse. Patients may show you a rash and tell you it "itches." You may observe patients scratching their skin. Patients may tell you that their skin feels hot, cold, or drier than usual. They may report the loss of feeling in their hand or fingers or may tell you that they cannot tell the difference between hot and cold or sharp and dull objects.

RASH
reddened spots close together on the skin; spots can be flat or raised

ABRASION
a wound that results from rubbing or scraping the skin

ASHEN
gray skin color
JAUNDICE
yellowness of the skin, sclerae (whites of the eyes), mucous membranes, and body excretions caused by an accumulation of bile pigments (substances that provide color) in the blood
ECCHYMOSIS
skin that is black and blue or purplish

CARING COMMENT

Always report what you see and hear regarding the condition and temperature of a patient's skin to the nurse. The nurse takes the responsibility for any decision about skin care.

BATHING

Your patients have developed routines that satisfy their particular needs for personal hygiene. When you help them to accomplish this routine, you help them feel better about themselves.

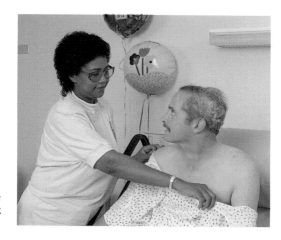

FIGURE 13-4
Helping the patient put on or remove clothes is included when you are giving complete patient care.

THE COMPLETE-CARE PATIENT

Patients who cannot perform or assist in their own care are called total-care or complete-care patients. These patients have all their personal care needs met by the care giver (Figure 13-4). All care is given while the patient is in bed; thus you may hear this procedure referred to as a "bed bath." When a bed bath is indicated for a patient, you should find out from the nurse or your supervisor whether the patient is allowed to do any personal care at all. It is important to encourage patients to do as much as possible for themselves.

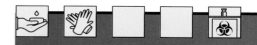

PROCEDURE

Giving the Complete-Care Patient a Bed Bath

Bathe patients from head to toe. Wash, rinse, and dry each body part before you proceed to the next. Take precautions to provide privacy for patients. Keep the room warm and draft free by closing windows and doors and shutting off any fans in the room. Change the water whenever it becomes dirty or soapy or cools off.

GATHER EQUIPMENT

Basin
Bath **thermometer**
Two washcloths
Two towels
Soap or another cleansing agent patients desire
Soap dish
Body lotion or powder
Clean gown and bottoms (if available) or personal sleep wear

Bath blanket
Clean linens
Two pairs of disposable gloves
Deodorant
Comb or brush
Nail clippers and file
Shaving cream
Razor

THERMOMETER
the instrument used to measure temperature

ACTION	RATIONALE

Preparation

1. Tell patients what you are going to do. Offer the bedpan or **urinal** before you begin the procedure.

An explanation helps gain patients' cooperation when a procedure is planned. Patients are more comfortable if their toileting needs are attended to before a procedure begins.

URINAL
a container into which a person urinates

Continued on following page

PROCEDURE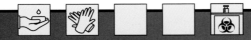

Giving the Complete-Care Patient a Bed Bath
Continued

2. Wash hands.

3. Identify yourself and the patient. Check patients' identification band.

4. Provide privacy when you bathe patients. You can ask visitors to leave for a short time and pull the curtains around the bed or close the door for privacy.

Prevents the spread of microorganisms.

Verifies that the correct patient is receiving the procedure. Maintains patients' rights.

Maintains patients' rights.

Procedural Steps

5. Position the over-bed table so that needed items are within your reach. Wipe and dry (damp dust) the over-bed table with dampened paper towels (Figure 13–5).

Helps with your **body mechanics.** Prevents spilling and dropping things on patients.

BODY MECHANICS

the use of the body to push, pull, or lift objects

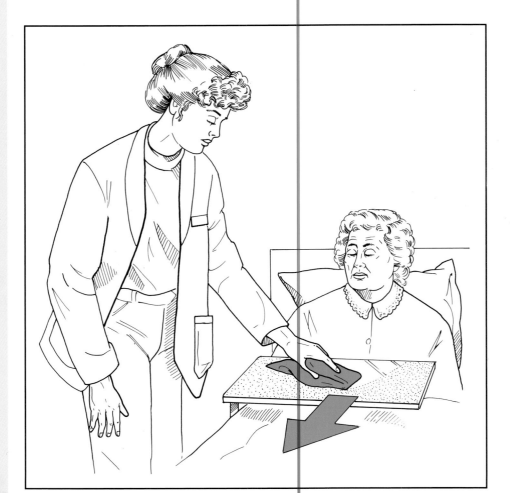

FIGURE 13–5

Damp dusting. Wipe and dry with a single stroke, using a motion directed away from yourself.

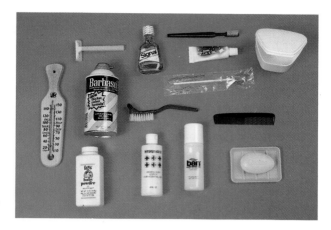

FIGURE 13–6

Common supplies to use for hygienic (bathing) care.

6. Arrange supplies on the over-bed table (Figure 13–6). Bring in linens and towels and place them on a clean chair near the bed (Figures 13–7 and 13–8). (Arrange them in the order of use.)

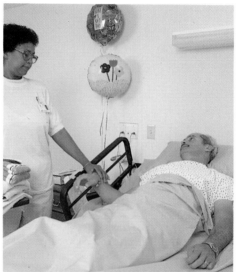

FIGURE 13–7

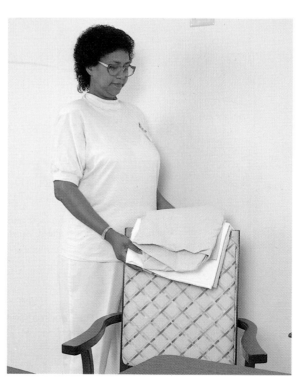

FIGURE 13–8

Continued on following page

SAFETY
the status of being safe from experiencing or causing hurt, injury, or loss

BODY ALIGNMENT
the body's correct, straight position

7. Raise the bed to a comfortable working height. Keep side rails raised until you are working.

Working at waist level prevents strain or pull on your back muscles. Side rails are kept raised for patient **safety.**

8. Place patients in a comfortable position that includes correct **body alignment.**

9. Loosen the top linens. Remove and fold the bedspread and blanket. Place them on the back of a chair.

The bedspread and blanket are reused if not soiled.

10. Unfold the bath blanket and place it over patients and top sheet (Figure 13–9).

Provides privacy and warmth.

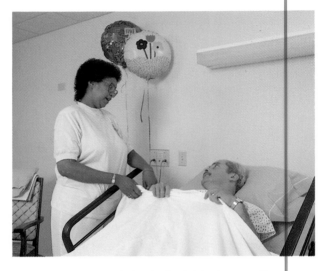

FIGURE 13–9
Ask the patient to grasp and hold the top edge of the bath blanket.

11. Ask patients to hold the bath blanket while you remove the top sheet from the bed (Figure 13–10). Roll the sheet, examining it for personal items while doing so. Place rolled sheet in a hamper.

The linens may be used again if not soiled. Items like pills, jewelry, or glasses as well as body discharges (such as blood) are often observed.

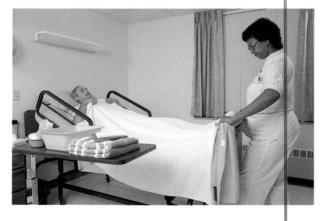

FIGURE 13–10
Stand at the foot of the bed and pull out the top sheet from under the blanket.

12. Oral or mouth care can be performed at this point (see Oral Hygiene).

13. Fill the basin with warm water and use a bath thermometer to check the water temperature (Figure 13–11). (The temperature should range from 105° to 110° F.)

Hot water may injure patients' skin. Cold water may be uncomfortable and cause a chill.

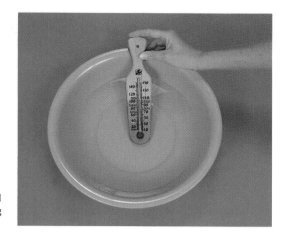

FIGURE 13–11
Check water temperature with a special bath thermometer each time you bring fresh water to the bedside.

14. Position patients toward the side of the bed where you are standing. Patients can move toward you themselves if able.

15. Place a clean towel across patients' chest.

16. Ask patients if they want soap used. Place the washcloth in the water. Squeeze excess water from the washcloth.

17. Fold washcloth into a mitt (Figure 13–12).

Allows you to bathe patients without extra bending over.

Patients' skin might be sensitive to certain soap.

Loose edges may allow water to drip on patients or bed linens.

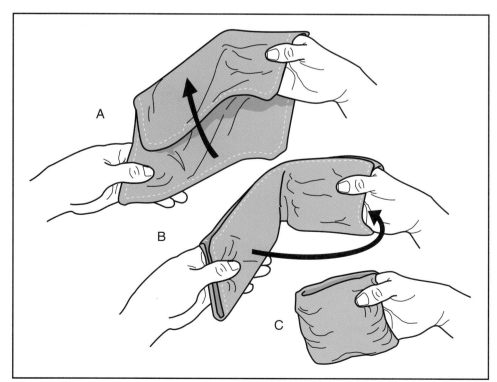

FIGURE 13–12
Folding a washcloth into a mitt: A, Secure one edge of the cloth with a thumb. B, Bring the other edge over the palm and secure it with your thumb. C, Bring the top folded edges down to the palm of your hand and tuck under to form a mitt. (From Sorensen KC, Luckmann J: Basic Nursing: A Psychophysiologic Approach, 2nd ed. Philadelphia, W. B. Saunders Company, 1986.)

Continued on following page

PROCEDURE

Giving the Complete-Care Patient a Bed Bath
Continued

18. Begin the bath by washing patients' eyes. Wash the eye farthest from you. Stroke from the inner part (bridge of the nose) to the outer part of the eye to prevent microorganisms from affecting the cleaner inner parts of the eyes (Figure 13–13). Then wash the eye nearest you, using another corner of the washcloth to avoid spreading microorganisms. Follow the same order to rinse. Pat dry with the towel. Place the washcloth in the basin of water.

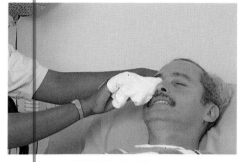

FIGURE 13–13

19. Squeeze the excess water out of the washcloth, fold the washcloth into a mitt, and wash patients' ears. Wash the ear farthest away from you, then the ear nearest to you (Figure 13–14). Wash the face and neck. Rinse and dry the face, neck, and ears.

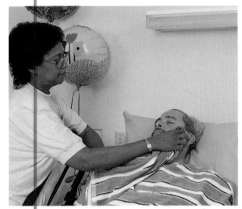

FIGURE 13–14

20. Loosen the ties of patients' gown and remove the gown or personal sleep wear (Figure 13–15).

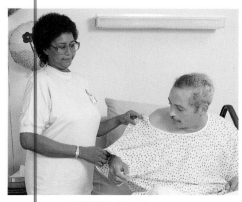

FIGURE 13–15

21. Fold back the bath blanket to expose the arm. Place the towel lengthwise under the arm farthest away from you. (Figure 13–16). Using long strokes from the shoulder down, wash the upper arm. Such strokes help increase the circulation. Wash the armpit.

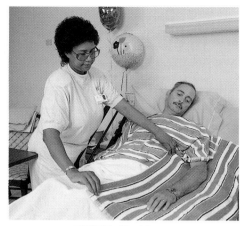

FIGURE 13–16

22. Rinse and dry by wrapping the towel around the arm and patting dry (Figure 13–17). Apply **deodorant/antiperspirant** if permitted by your institution. Cover the arm with the bath blanket.

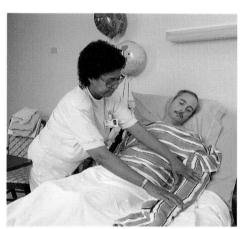

FIGURE 13–17

DEODORANT
a preparation that destroys unpleasant odors
ANTIPERSPIRANT
a preparation that reduces excessive perspiration

23. Wash from the elbow to the wrist. Rinse and pat dry (Figure 13–18).

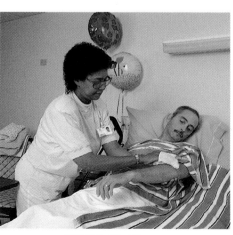

FIGURE 13–18

Continued on following page

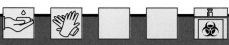

PROCEDURE

Giving the Complete-Care Patient a Bed Bath
Continued

24. Place the hand in the warm basin of water and wash and rinse. Remove from basin and pat dry. Push back the cuticle (excess skin at the base of the fingernails) with the towel. Cover the arm with the bath blanket.
25. Wash the other arm and hand the same way.
26. Place the towel across patients' chest. Fold the bath blanket to the waist. Lift the towel enough to wash, rinse, and dry patients' chest (Figure 13–19).

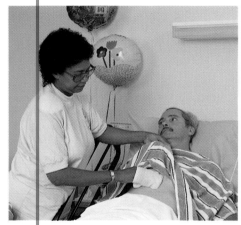

FIGURE 13–19

27. Check the area below the female patients' breasts for changes in the skin. Apply powder to your hands and pat the powder on the area under the breasts. Use only a small amount of powder, and be certain the area is completely dry before powder is applied.
28. Fold the bath blanket down to the pubic area and expose the abdomen. Wash, rinse, and dry the abdomen. Pull the bath blanket up to patients' chin and remove the towel from under the blanket.
29. Expose the leg farthest from you and place the bath towel under it. Wash, rinse, and dry the thigh. Work from the knee up to the thigh area. Place the basin of water on the second towel.
30. Place patients' foot in the basin (foot soak). Wash the leg from the knee down; then wash the foot (Figure 13–20). Perform nail care as allowed by your institution (see Nail Care). Rinse and dry. Be certain to dry the areas between the toes thoroughly. Cover leg with the bath blanket.

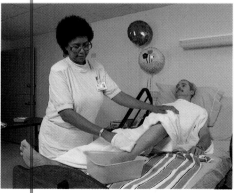

FIGURE 13–20

31. Apply lotion to the feet, especially if dry skin is present (Figure 13–21).

32. Repeat the same steps with the other leg and foot.

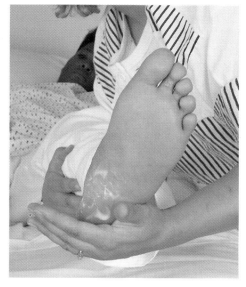

FIGURE 13–21

33. Position patients in the center of the bed and help them turn on their side. Expose the back and place the bath towel lengthwise next to patients' back. With clean warm water, use long strokes to wash, rinse, and dry patients' neck, back, and buttocks (Figure 13–22).

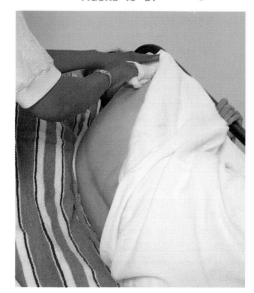

FIGURE 13–22

34. After washing patients' lower back, follow with a back rub (see Back Rub).

35. Place the bath towel under the buttocks and upper thighs. Position patients onto their back. If patients are able, ask them to complete the bath by washing the **genitalia.** When patients are unable to care for themselves, you are responsible for cleansing the **perineum** (see Perineal Care). Put on a pair of disposable gloves and use a clean washcloth. For female patients, wash with soap and water from front to back. Rinse and dry the perineal area thoroughly. For male patients, wash the penis, scrotum, and the **groin** area. Rinse and dry thoroughly.

GENITALIA
the external organs of the reproductive system
PERINEUM
the pelvic floor, extending from the pubic bones at the front of the body to the coccyx (tailbone) at the back
GROIN
the area from the lower abdomen to the inner part of the thighs

Continued on following page

PROCEDURE

Giving the Complete-Care Patient a Bed Bath
Continued

36. Discard the towel and washcloth in a laundry hamper. Discard the gloves in a waste container.

Note: Anytime patients tire or become short of breath during the bath you should stop and give them time to rest.

Follow-Through

37. Perform **range of motion** exercises as directed by the nurse (see Chapter 16).

38. Place a towel over patients' pillow. Groom hair by brushing or combing it (see Hair Care).

39. Help patients into clean clothing or night wear (see Dressing).

40. Place patients in a comfortable position that includes correct body alignment (see Chapter 16).

41. Clean all equipment. Replace equipment and supplies in the bedside stand or follow your institution's procedure so that everything is ready for next use.

42. Change the bed linens. (Follow the occupied-bed procedure; see Chapter 14.)

43. Place all soiled linen in a laundry hamper.

44. Lower the bed and place the call signal within patients' reach so that patients have a means to communicate needs.

45. Ask patients if anything else is needed. Follow through on their request if it is for something they are permitted.

46. Wash your hands to prevent spread of microorganisms.

47. Report and record the following (to provide a legal record that procedure was done).
    - patients' name
    - time of the bed bath
    - patients' response

Report any unusual observations to the nurse.

RANGE OF MOTION
the range, measured in degrees like a circle, through which a joint can be extended and flexed (bent)

Bathing and range of motion procedures are done on a daily basis for patients in the acute care facility. In the long-term care setting or in the home, the patient may receive a complete bed bath only once or twice a week, unless a bath is needed more often, for example, if the patient was sweating a lot.

CARING COMMENT

You should be aware of the difference between a deodorant and an antiperspirant. A deodorant is a preparation used to destroy unpleasant odors. An antiperspirant is a preparation used to reduce excessive perspiration (sweating). Some products are both a deodorant and an antiperspirant.

SPECIAL CONSIDERATIONS

ELDERLY PATIENTS Elderly patients in nursing homes or patients who need assisted personal care at home often receive a bath only once a week because receiving a complete bath daily would dry out the skin. Check nails for rough edges and trim them once a week.

PATIENTS WITH INTRAVENOUS TUBES If an intravenous (IV) line is set up when you go to bathe a patient, follow these steps:

1. Remove the free arm from the sleeve.
2. Slip the other sleeve down over the patient's arm or hand to which the IV is connected.
3. Remove the IV solution container (bottle or bag) from the pole or holder; then slip the gown over the length of tubing and the IV solution container.
4. Hang the container back on the pole until bathing is finished and it is time to put a clean gown on the patient.
5. Perform steps 1–4 in reverse. Then place a clean gown on the patient.

CARING COMMENT

When working with a patient who is connected to an IV line, be certain to handle all tubing gently. Pulling or tugging can cause injury to the IV site.

THE PARTIAL-CARE PATIENT

Patients who can attend to some of their hygiene needs themselves are called partial-care patients or patients who need assistance in hygiene needs. Patients may be able to wash, rinse, and dry parts of their body if you are present to assist them. Change the water as often as needed and be sure all supplies are within patients' reach. Placing necessary items within patients' reach reminds them to pay attention to certain needs. It is your responsibility to complete the washing, rinsing, and drying of any body part the patient cannot reach or is too tired to finish.

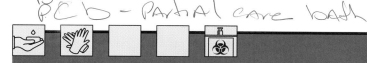

PROCEDURE

Assisting with a Partial-Care Patient's Bath

Encourage the patient to do as much self-care as possible or as permitted by the physician. If the patient becomes tired during the procedure, you might need to help finish the bathing procedure.

GATHER EQUIPMENT

Basin
Bath thermometer
Two washcloths
Two towels
Soap or another cleansing agent the patient desires
Soap dish
Body lotion or powder
Clean gown and bottoms (if available) or personal sleep wear

Bath blanket
Clean linens
Two pairs of disposable gloves
Deodorant
Comb or brush
Nail clippers and file
Shaving cream
Razor

Continued on following page

PROCEDURE

Giving the Complete-Care Patient a Bed Bath
Continued

ACTION	RATIONALE
Preparation	
1. Tell patients what you are going to do. Offer the bedpan or urinal before you begin the procedure.	An explanation helps gain patients' cooperation when a procedure is planned. Patients are more comfortable if toileting needs are attended to before a procedure begins.
2. Wash hands.	Prevents the spread of microorganisms.
3. Identify yourself and the patient. Check patients' identification band.	Verifies that the correct patient is receiving the procedure. Maintains patients' rights.
4. Provide privacy when you bathe patients. You can ask visitors to leave for a short time and pull the curtains around the bed or close the door for privacy.	Maintains patients' rights.
Procedural Steps	
5. Position the over-bed table so that needed items are within your reach. Wipe and dry (damp dust) the over-bed table with dampened paper towels.	Helps with your body mechanics. Prevents spilling and dropping things on patients.
6. Arrange supplies on the over-bed table. Bring in linens and towels and place them on a clean chair near the bed. (Arrange them in the order of use.)	
7. Raise the bed to a comfortable working height. Keep side rails raised until you are working.	Working at waist level prevents strain or pull on your back muscles. Side rails are kept raised for patient safety.
8. Place patients in a comfortable position that includes correct body alignment.	
9. Loosen the top linens. Remove and fold the bedspread and blanket. Place them on the back of a chair.	The bedspread and blanket are reused if not soiled.
10. Unfold the bath blanket and place it over patients and top sheet.	Provides privacy and warmth.
11. Ask patients to hold the bath blanket while you remove the top sheet from the bed. Roll the sheet, examining it for personal items while rolling. Place rolled sheet in a hamper.	The linens may be used again if not soiled. Items like pills, jewelry, or glasses as well as body discharges (such as blood) are often observed.
12. Assist with oral care as needed (see Oral Hygiene).	
13. Encourage patients to perform as much self-care as possible. Remain available to change water and help patients as needed.	
14. Always assist with bathing the back and legs and any other parts patients have difficulty reaching.	These areas are difficult for most patients to reach.

Follow-Through

15. Finish with the steps in the Follow-Through section of the procedure for giving a complete-care patient a bed bath.

16. Report to the nurse how much assistance patients required with the bath.

Keeps the nurse informed about patients' ability for self-care.

17. Report the condition of the skin.

THE SELF-CARE PATIENT

Patients who are able to perform their own personal hygiene are called self-care patients. Self-care patients may be able to bathe or shower themselves. If

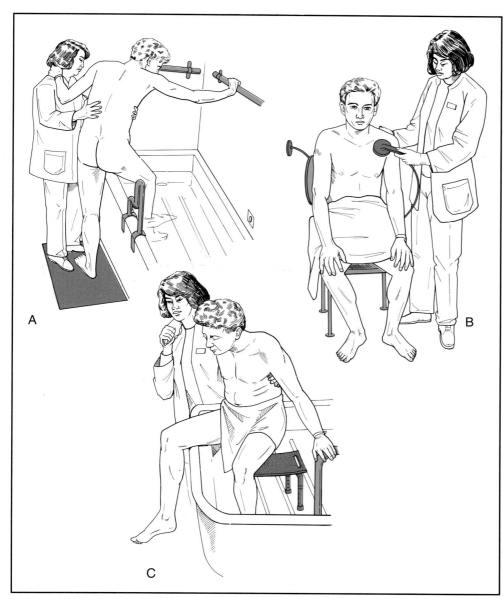

FIGURE 13–23

A, Safety hand rails help the patient get in and out of the tub. The patient can grasp a high hand rail while standing for a shower in the tub. B, The patient can sit on a stable chair during a shower. C, A small stool in the tub makes it easier for the patient to climb in and out of the tub. Nonslip strips at the bottom of the tub give a firmer surface when the patient stands up in the tub after bathing.

patients must stay in bed, you may need to provide them with the necessary items so that they can perform their self-care while in bed (or at the sink, if they are allowed to sit in a chair). You may be asked to assist self-care patients with a tub bath or a shower.

Special devices are designed to make bathing safe and more comfortable for patients. These include

- safety rails—These are placed within patients' reach on the walls around the tub and near the toilet. A special handrail can be mounted on the outside edge of the tub (Figure 13–23A).
- shower chair—This chair has rubber-tipped legs and is placed in the shower to allow patients to sit while showering (Figure 13–23B).
- small stool—This can be placed in the tub. The rubber-tipped legs keep the stool from sliding (Figure 13–23C).
- nonslip strips—These prevent slipping and are be applied to the bottom surface of the tub.
- nonslip shower/tub mats—These prevent slipping and absorb water.
- call signal—The call signal is placed within patients' reach in case they need to call for assistance.

PROCEDURE

Assisting a Self-Care Patient with a Tub Bath

If a tub is not available in patients' room, reserve a patient tub room by displaying the "Occupied" sign on the door. Check that the tub is clean; clean it if necessary. Arrange supplies on a shelf or other place provided in the room. Locate the emergency pull cord so that you can show patients how to use it. The nurse tells you about patients with whom you need to remain in the room during the bath.

GATHER EQUIPMENT

Bath towel
Washcloth
Soap or other cleansing agent
Deodorant and other toilet articles patients
  need

Clean gown or personal sleep wear
Nonslip slippers
Robe
Bath thermometer
Disposable or rubber bath mat

ACTION	RATIONALE
Preparation	
1. Place a rubber mat on the bottom of the tub if one has been provided by the agency.	Helps prevent accidental injury from a fall.
2. Place the disposable tub mat on the floor next to the tub.	Helps absorb water when patients are getting out of the tub.
3. Return to the patient's room.	
4. Wash hands.	Prevents the spread of microorganisms.
5. Identify yourself and the patient. Call patients by name and check their identification band.	Verifies that the correct patient is receiving the procedure. Maintains patients' rights.
Procedural Steps	
6. Provide privacy by closing the curtains or door of the room.	Maintains patients' rights.

7. Assist patients to a sitting position. Put their robe and nonslip slippers on them if they cannot do so themselves.

8. Assist patients to the room reserved for the tub bath. Seat them in a chair in the room.

9. Fill the tub ⅓–½ full with warm water. Use the bath thermometer (the water should measure 105–110°F).

   Hot water can injure patients' skin as well as cause fainting or dizziness.

10. Help patients undress if they cannot do it themselves.

11. Assist patients into the tub.

    Prevents injury from falls.

12. Place the bath supplies within patients' reach.

13. Show patients how to use the signal cord or button and tell them to signal if they need help or when they have finished bathing.

    The signal cord is a form of communication when help is needed.

14. Remind patients not to
    • add hot water
    • get out of the tub without help
    • stay in the tub longer than 20 minutes

    Protects patients from harm.

15. Keep door unlocked.

    Provides quick access to patients if necessary.

16. Leave the room and wash your hands. Check on patients every 5 minutes (For patients who are weak, remain at the tub until bathing is completed.)

    A safety precaution to prevent injury.

17. Return when patients signal that the bath is complete.

    Patients might be tempted to get out of the tub without help.

18. Assist patients out of the tub. Seat them in the chair next to the tub. Tuck a bath towel or bath blanket around them.

    Assistance helps steady patients while they are getting out of a slippery tub. The bath blanket prevents chilling and provides privacy.

19. If needed, help patients finish the bath by drying the skin and applying deodorant, lotion, or powder as desired. Assist patients into clean garments, slippers, and robe.

    Promoting independence is important for those who are able to complete the bath themselves.

20. Assist patients back to their room and provide a back rub (see Back Rub).

    A back rub is part of the bathing procedure and should be included to help patients relax. Also provides an opportunity for observation of the skin.

21. Place patients in a comfortable position, lower the bed, and raise the side rails. Place the call signal within patients' reach. Open privacy curtains.

    Prevents falls. Provides patients with a means to communicate.

22. Return to the tub room and clean the tub. Place soiled articles in the laundry hamper. Place disposable articles in the waste container.

    Prepares the room for use by the next patient.

23. Return personal care items to patients' room for storage. Ask patients if anything else is needed.

Continued on following page

PROCEDURE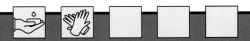

Assisting a Self-Care Patient with a Tub Bath
Continued

Follow-Through

24. Wash hands.	Prevents spread of microorganisms.
25. Report the following observations to the nurse: • the condition of the skin • how much assistance patients required • patients' response to the tub bath	Any change you notice is important for the day-to-day observations of each patient.

PROCEDURE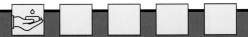

Assisting a Self-Care Patient with a Shower

If a shower is not available in patients' room, reserve a room with a shower by displaying the "Occupied" sign on the door. Check that the shower is clean; if soiled, clean it before bringing patients to the room. Arrange supplies on a shelf or other place provided in the room. Locate the emergency bell pull cord so that you can show patients how to use it. The nurse tells you which patients with whom you must remain in the room during the shower. *You must remain with any patient in a shower chair or on a shower cart.*

GATHER EQUIPMENT

Bath towel	Nonslip slippers
Washcloth	Robe
Soap or other cleansing agent	Bath thermometer
Deodorant and other personal care items patients desire	Disposable bath mat
	Shower chair or cart when preferred
Clean clothing or personal sleep wear	Waterproof footwear for yourself

ACTION	RATIONALE
Preparation	
1. Place a rubber mat on the floor of the shower if one has been provided by the agency.	Helps prevent accidental injury from a fall.
2. Place the disposable tub mat on the floor next to shower.	Helps absorb water when patients are getting out of the shower.
3. Return to patients' room.	
4. Wash hands.	Prevents the spread of microorganisms.
5. Identify yourself and the patient. Call patients by name and check their identification band.	Verifies that the correct patient is receiving the procedure. Maintains patients' rights.
Procedural Steps	
6. Provide privacy by pulling the curtains around the bed or closing the door.	Maintains patients' rights.
7. Help patients to a sitting position. Put their robe and nonslip slippers on them if they cannot do so themselves.	
8. Help patients to the room reserved for	

the shower. Seat them in a chair in the room. If patients are in a shower chair or on a shower cart, they can be washed without being transferred to another chair.

9. Turn on the shower and adjust the water until it is warm to the touch. Test with the bath thermometer (the water should measure 105–110° F).

Hot water can injure patients skin as well as cause fainting or dizziness.

10. Help patients undress if they cannot do it themselves.

11. Assist patients into the shower if necessary. Put on boots if you remain in the shower with patients. If patients sit in a shower chair or on a shower cart, assist them during the shower.

12. Place the shower supplies within patients' reach.

13. Show patients how to use the signal cord or button and tell them to signal when they need help or when the shower is finished.

14. Remind patients not to
    • add hot water
    • get out of the shower without help
    • stay in the shower longer than 20 minutes

Protects patients from harm.

15. Keep door unlocked.

Provides quick access to patients if necessary.

16. Leave the room and wash your hands. Check on patients every 5 minutes.

A safety precaution to prevent injury.

17. Return when patients signal that the shower is complete.

Patients might be tempted to get out of the shower without help.

18. Assist patients out of the shower. Seat them in a chair in the room.

Assistance helps steady patients while they are getting out of a slippery shower.

19. Help patients finish the shower by drying the skin and applying deodorant, lotion, or powder as desired. Assist patients into clean garments, slippers, and robe.

20. Assist patients back to their room and provide a back rub (see Back Rub).

A back rub is part of the bathing procedure and should be included to help patients relax. Also provides an opportunity for observation of the skin.

21. Place patients in a comfortable position, lower the bed, and raise the side rails. Place the call signal within patients' reach. Open the privacy curtains.

Prevents falls. Provides patients with a means to communicate.

22. Return to the shower room and clean the area. Place soiled articles in the laundry hamper. Place disposable articles in the waste container.

Prepares the room for use by the next patient.

23. Return personal care items to patients' room for storage.

Continued on following page

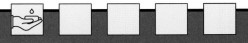

PROCEDURE

Assisting a Self-Care Patient with a Shower
Continued

24. Ask patients if anything else is needed. Follow through on their request if it is something you are permitted to do.

Gives patients the opportunity to express other needs they might have.

Follow-Through

25. Wash hands.

Prevents the spread of microorganisms.

26. Report the following observations to the nurse:
    • condition of the skin
    • how much assistance patients required
    • patients' response to the shower

Any change you notice is important for the day-to-day observation of each patient.

PERINEAL CARE — Peri - Care.

It is important to keep the perineal area clean and dry at all times to prevent breakdown and chafing of the skin. You should cleanse the perineum of any complete-care or partial-care patients or any patients who cannot do this for themselves.

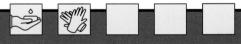

PROCEDURE

Cleansing the Perineal Area

This procedure is included in complete or partial bath care or whenever patients are unable to cleanse themselves. The perineal area should also be cleansed, rinsed, and dried thoroughly after each time the patient has been **incontinent** of bowel or bladder.

INCONTINENT
unable to respond to the urge to eliminate the waste products of the body

GATHER EQUIPMENT

Basin of water
Bath thermometer
Washcloth or disposable wipes
Soap or another cleansing agent

Bath towel
Bed protector
Disposable gloves

ACTION

RATIONALE

Preparation

1. Wash hands.

Prevents the spread of microorganisms.

2. Identify yourself and the patient.

Verifies that the correct patient is receiving the procedure. Maintains patients' rights.

3. Provide privacy.

Maintains patients' rights.

4. Explain the procedure.

Informs patients what is happening.

Procedural Steps

5. After you've completed giving or assisting with the bed bath, ask patients whether they are able to clean the perineal area.

For patients who are able to cleanse the perineum themselves:

6. Fill the basin with warm water (105–110° F). (Use a bath thermometer to measure the water temperature.)

7. Ask patients if soap can be used, or follow institution's policy.

Soap is used sparingly because it can irritate the skin in the perineal area.

8. Place the basin of water, soap or other cleansing agent, the washcloth or wipes, and towel on the over-bed table. Place the protective pad under patients. Pull the privacy curtains or close the door and leave the unit.

9. Return in 5 minutes to see whether patients have finished. If they have, remove, clean, and store the equipment.

10. Place the soiled linen in the laundry hamper. (Always wear disposable gloves when you handle soiled linen.)

For patients who cannot cleanse the perineal area themselves:

11. Fill the basin with warm water (105–110° F). (Use a bath thermometer to measure the water temperature.)

Keeping the perineal area clean and dry helps prevent skin **excoriation** and breakdown.

12. Place all equipment on the over-bed table within your reach.

Helps with your body mechanics.

13. Raise the bed to a comfortable working position for yourself and lower the side rail on the side nearest you.

Working at waist level prevents strain and pull on your back muscles.

14. Place the protective pad and the towel under patients' buttocks.

15. Put on the disposable gloves.

Prevents hands from coming in contact with body secretions.

16. Wet the washcloth or wipes and squeeze out excess water; then apply soap or cleansing agent.

For female patients:

17. Put on a pair of gloves.

18. Wash the pubic area from the front to the back using single strokes. The first stroke should wipe down the center (Figure 13–24A). The next strokes should wipe down each side. Turn the washcloth to another corner with each stroke. Spread the **labia majora** while you are cleansing the perineal area. Repeat enough times to rinse, using new wipes or a new part of the same washcloth for each stroke. Dry the area thoroughly.

Prevents microorganisms from the anal area from being carried forward to the urinary meatus (opening) and the **vagina,** where they could cause an **infection.**

19. Place the washcloth or wipes in the water.

20. Ask patients to turn over or assist them to turn.

21. Squeeze the excess water from the washcloth or wipes, apply soap or other cleansing agent to the wash

EXCORIATION

scratched or abraded (rubbed off) area of the skin

VAGINA

the canal in females that extends from the vaginal opening up to the cervix; stretches during intercourse and childbirth

INFECTION

the body's response to invasion by harmful microorganisms and their multiplication in the body

LABIA MAJORA

long outside folds of skin surrounding the urinary meatus and vagina in females

Continued on following page

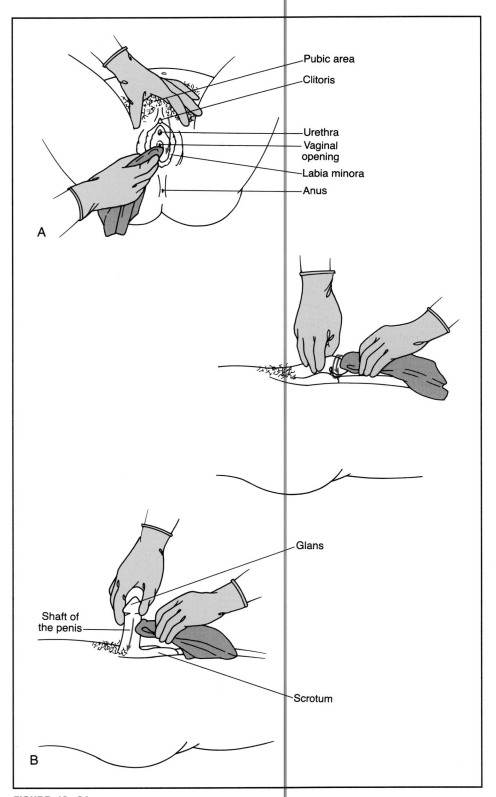

FIGURE 13–24

A, Performing perineal care on a female patient. Expose the urethral meatus (opening) and vaginal opening by spreading the labia with two fingers. Cleanse from pubic area to anal area in one stroke. Use a clean area of the washcloth each time you repeat the stroke. B, Perineal care of a male patient. Grasp the shaft of the penis and cleanse the tip from the urethral opening outward in a circular motion. Cleanse the shaft of the penis from the tip down.

cloth, and cleanse the anal area. Wipe from front to back. Repeat enough times, using a new wipe or new part of the same washcloth each time, to wipe clean. Dry the anal area.

For male patients:

22. Put on a pair of gloves. Grasp the shaft of the **penis** and wash in a circular motion from the top down (Figure 13–24B). Rinse the washcloth or wipes and cleanse the **scrotum.** Repeat enough times to wipe clean, and then dry thoroughly.

23. Place the washcloth or wipes in the basin of water.

24. Ask patients to turn over or assist them to turn.

25. Squeeze the excess water from the washcloth or wipes and cleanse the anal area. Repeat once to rinse, and then dry.

26. When cleansing the perineal area, observe for odor, redness, and swelling of the skin and any discharge.

Especially important for any patients who cannot complete their perineal care or who are incontinent.

27. Remove the protective pad and the towel from under patients.

28. Place patients in a comfortable position that includes correct body alignment. Raise the side rail and place the bed in the lowest position.

Prevents falls.

29. Place the call signal within patients' reach and open the privacy curtain.

Leaves patients with a means to communicate.

30. Discard dirty water into the toilet. (Never use the sink for disposal of water.) Cleanse and dry the equipment. Place the soiled linens in the laundry hamper.

Prevents spread of microorganisms.

31. Remove the disposable gloves and discard them in the waste container.

32. Ask patients if anything else is needed. Follow through on their request if it is something you are permitted to do.

Gives patients the opportunity to express other needs they might have.

Follow-Through

33. Wash hands.

Prevents the spread of microorganisms.

34. Record that perineal care has been completed and report your observations to the nurse.

The nurse is responsible for a decision in the case of unusual observations.

PENIS
external organ of urination and copulation in males

SCROTUM
the pouch (sac) that contains the testicles and their accessory organs in males

BACK RUB

You may give a massage (back rub) after you perform or assist with the bathing of any patient. It may also be given at the hour of sleep. A patient may request a back rub at other times as well.

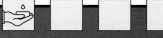

PROCEDURE

Giving a Back Rub

Use long strokes and apply firm pressure during a back rub. A back rub is comforting and relaxing for patients, decreases stress, and increases the blood supply to the tissues of the back. Be sure to warm your hands under warm water. You can warm the lotion by holding the container in the palms of your hands or floating the container in warm water for about 5 minutes.

GATHER EQUIPMENT

Body lotion   Bath blanket
Bath towel

ACTION	RATIONALE
Preparation	
1. Wash hands.	Prevents the spread of microorganisms.
2. Identify yourself and the patient.	Maintains patients' rights.
3. Provide privacy.	Maintains patients' rights.
4. Explain the procedure.	Informs patients what is happening.
Procedural Steps	
5. Warm your hands and the lotion.	A cold sensation on the patient's back can cause discomfort.
6. Raise the bed to a comfortable working position. Lower the rail on the side where you are standing.	Working at waist level prevents strain or pull on your back muscles.
7. Position patients on their abdomen. If patients cannot tolerate the prone position, assist them to their side, facing away from you.	Patients may not be able to breathe comfortably or may experience pain if placed in the prone position.
8. Untie the ties or snaps of the gown and expose the back. Drape back with the bath towel. (Place the bath towel near the back of patients who are positioned on their side.)	
9. Put lotion on the palms of your hands and rub together slightly to spread the lotion.	
10. Tell patients the lotion may feel cool.	Room temperature is cooler than body temperature.
11. Use long, firm strokes with both hands. Keep your hands in contact with patients' skin during the entire back rub (Figure 13–25).	
12. Begin at the buttocks midway between the spine and the hips. Stroke in an upward motion toward the shoulders. Complete a circle with your hands and at the shoulders and massage over the upper arms. Bring hands back over the shoulders and stroke down the back with a hand on each side (Figure 13–26). Complete a circle over the buttocks and repeat the above cycle for 3–5 mintues.	Long strokes help relax patients.

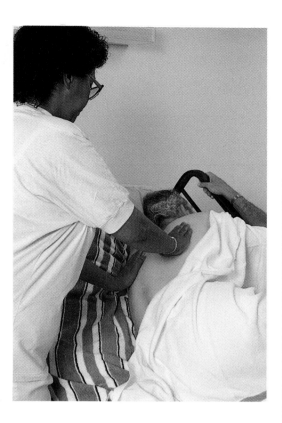

FIGURE 13-25

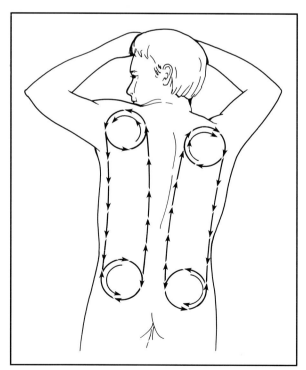

FIGURE 13-26
Use long, smooth strokes when you give a back rub.

13. Use your first two fingers and thumb to **knead** the skin on each side of the spine (Figure 13-27). Begin at the base of the spine and move upward with a smooth kneading motion. Com-

The faster kneading stroke is stimulating.

KNEAD
to press down with the hands

Continued on following page

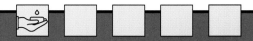

PROCEDURE

Giving a Back Rub *Continued*

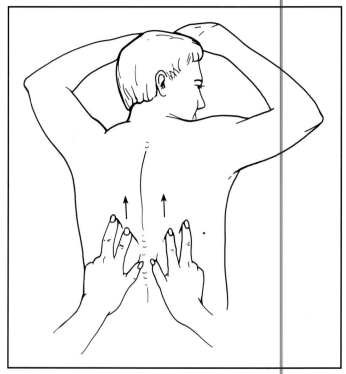

FIGURE 13–27
Use short strokes to knead the skin.

plete a circle at the shoulders and return to the buttocks as during step 12.
Repeat the kneading motion two more
times.

14. Massage bony areas by using a circular motion with the tips of your fingers.	Helps stimulate the blood supply to the areas of massage.
15. Tell patients when the back rub is near completion.	
16. Retie or snap the gown to cover patients' back.	
17. Remove the bath blanket and the bath towel.	
18. Place patients in a comfortable position that includes correct body alignment.	
19. Raise the side rails and lower the bed.	Prevents falls.
20. Store the lotion in patients' bedside stand.	Use the same supply of lotion for one patient.
21. Open the privacy curtains and place the call signal within patients' reach.	Leaves patients with a means to communicate.
22. Place used linen in a laundry hamper.	Provides for proper care of soiled supplies.

Follow-Through

23. Wash hands.	Prevents the spread of infection.
24. Report to the nurse that the back rub has been completed and report any unusual observations and patients' response to the back rub.	The nurse is responsible for a decision in the case of unusual observations.

ORAL HYGIENE

Oral hygiene, an important part of daily hygienic care, is a procedure in which the mouth is cleaned and all **debris** and **secretions** are removed. It is performed each morning, after each meal, and each evening at bedtime. It is refreshing for patients and keeps the mucous membranes of the mouth cleaned. If patients can perform their own oral hygiene, arrange the following articles for them in the bathroom or on the over-bed table at the bedside:

- toothbrush and toothpaste
- glass of water with a straw
- **dental floss**
- mouthwash
- small towel
- **emesis** basin (kidney-shaped basin needed when oral hygiene is completed while in bed)

Provide privacy for patients and check to see whether any help is needed. After oral hygiene is completed, return the equipment to patients' bedside stand or other designated storage area.

You may be required to perform some patients' oral hygiene care. Be sure to observe patients' **oral cavity** while you perform oral hygiene. Table 13–2 lists normal and abnormal observations of the oral cavity. If a patient requires total oral hygienic care, you are responsible for the following procedures:

- **Brushing the teeth**—Brushing cleans the teeth, helps prevent plaque build-up, and stimulates the gums (see Figure 13–29) The teeth are brushed after each meal or snack.
- **Flossing the teeth** (see Figure 13–32)—Flossing (using a special string to clean between the teeth) is done after each meal or snack.
- **Cleaning dentures** (see Figure 13–34)—Dentures are cleaned after each meal or snack. While you are cleaning the dentures, provide patients

ORAL
pertaining to the mouth

DEBRIS
dirt

SECRETION
discharge; drainage material that leaves the body through an opening

DENTAL FLOSS
a special string used to clean between the teeth

EMESIS
stomach contents brought up and expelled from the mouth; vomitus

ORAL CAVITY
the opening in the body that consists of the mouth, salivary glands, tongue, and teeth

TABLE 13–2 **OBSERVATIONS IN THE ORAL CAVITY**

Part of Oral Cavity	Normal	Abnormal
Lips	Pink, moist, and intact	Chapped, dry, cracked, swelled, or bleeding
Mucous membranes of the mouth	Pink and moist	Dry, cracked, or swelled
Tongue	Pink and moist	Coated, white, gray, or black
Teeth	Present and not loose	Dental caries (cavities) or loose or missing teeth
Gums	Firm and moist, pink to red in color	Spongy, pulling away from teeth, whitish color, swelled, or bleeding
Dentures	Snug fitting, with all teeth secure in the denture, not loose	Loose fit, dark red spots on gums when dentures removed, or chipped or broken dentures
Breath	No odor	Foul, or fruity (**acetone**)

ACETONE
a by-product of a certain acid; produced in abnormal amounts by persons with diabetes mellitus

- with water, a basin, and mouthwash. If patients cannot rinse their mouth, you should follow the procedure for cleansing the oral cavity of an unconscious patient.
- **Cleansing the inside of the mouth** (see Figure 13–31)—This procedure is done to remove any accumulation of debris. The mouth should be cleaned after any intake of food. For the patient who is unconscious, clean the mouth at least once a shift or as many times as needed to keep the mouth clean.

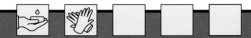

PROCEDURE

Brushing the Teeth of a Conscious Patient

The toothbrush cleans debris from the surfaces of the teeth. Toothpaste is used because it polishes the surfaces of the teeth and freshens the breath. Toothpaste with fluoride helps prevent cavities. Water swished in the mouth and then spit into the basin removes debris. The action of the bristles of the toothbrush stimulates the circulation of blood to the gums.

GATHER EQUIPMENT

Toothbrush
Toothpaste
Glass of water and a straw
Mouthwash if desired

Emesis basin
Lip moisturizer
Small towel
Disposable gloves

ACTION	RATIONALE
Preparation	
1. Tell patients what you are going to do. Offer the bedpan or urinal before you begin the procedure.	An explanation helps gain patients' cooperation when a procedure is planned. Patients are more comfortable when their toileting needs have been met before a procedure begins.
2. Wash hands.	Prevents the spread of microorganisms.
3. Identify yourself and the patient.	Verifies that the correct patient is receiving the procedure. Maintains patients' rights.
4. Provide privacy by pulling the curtains around the bed or closing the door.	Maintains patients' rights.
Procedural Steps	
5. Position the over-bed table so that needed items are within your reach.	Helps with your body mechanics.
6. Arrange supplies on the over-bed table in the order of use (Figure 13–28).	
7. Raise the bed to a comfortable working height. Keep all side rails raised until you begin the procedure.	Working at waist level prevents strain or pull on your back muscles.
8. Raise the head of the bed to a comfortable height for patients.	Permits the head movement needed to complete the procedure.
9. Apply a ribbon of toothpaste to the toothbrush. Put on the disposable gloves.	
10. Place the small towel across patients	

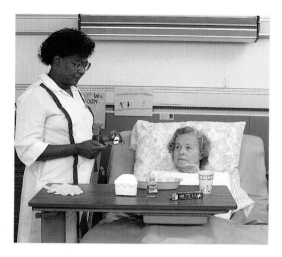

FIGURE 13-28

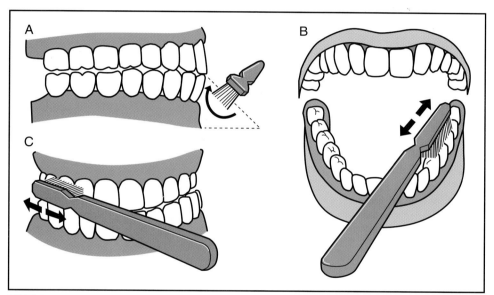

FIGURE 13-29

Toothbrush position. A, Hold the toothbrush at a 45° angle and brush from gum line to the top of each tooth. B, Hold the toothbrush even with the biting and chewing surface and brush in a back and forth motion. C, Hold the toothbrush against the outside surface of the teeth and brush back and forth.

chest. Brush all surfaces of patients' teeth (Figure 13-29).

11. Offer water for patients to rinse the oral cavity. Hold the basin under the chin to receive the water and debris (Figure 13-30).

12. If they desire, patients may use mouthwash at this time. Pour a small amount of mouthwash into a clean glass. Patients should swish the mouthwash around and spit it out into the basin. They may wish to repeat the procedure or may ask to have water added to the mouthwash.

Continued on following page

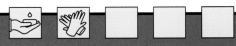

PROCEDURE

Brushing the Teeth of a Conscious Patient
Continued

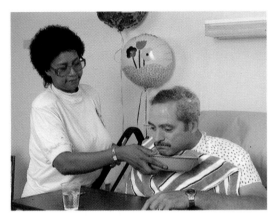

FIGURE 13–30

13. Lower the bed and place the call signal within reach. Open the privacy curtains.

    Prevents falls. Leaves patients with a means to communicate.

14. Place the towel in the laundry hamper. Remove and discard the disposable gloves in the waste container.

15. Clean and store the equipment for the next use.

16. Ask patients if anything else is needed. Follow through on their request if it is something you are permitted to do.

    Gives patients the opportunity to express other needs they might have.

Follow-Through

17. Wash hands.

    Prevents the spread of microorganisms.

18. Report to the nurse that the procedure has been completed. Report the patient's reaction to the procedure.

    The nurse is responsible for any decision based on an unusual reaction.

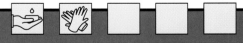

PROCEDURE

UNCONSCIOUS
unaware of the environment and not responsive to stimuli; unconsciousness occurs during sleep, fainting, and coma

TOOTHETTE
sponge on a stick; brand name

Cleansing the Oral Cavity of an Unconscious Patient

The inside of the oral cavity is cleansed to loosen and remove accumulated debris. Observe the condition of the mucous membranes during the procedure.

GATHER EQUIPMENT

Toothettes (brand name)
Solution of one-half hydrogen peroxide and one-half water
Emesis (kidney-shaped) basin

Disposable gloves
Moisturizer for the lips
Small towel

| **ACTION** | **RATIONALE** |

Procedural Steps

1. Follow steps 1–8 of the procedure for brushing the teeth of a conscious patient.

2. Moisten the Toothette in water or other solution. Put on the disposable gloves.

   To keep from injuring dry, cracked mucous membranes.

3. Clean the inside of the mouth. Be sure to cleanse all surfaces and beneath patients' tongue (Figure 13–31).

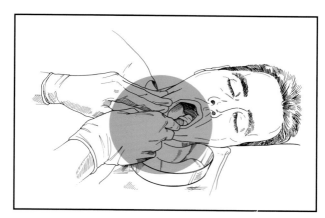

FIGURE 13–31

Cleansing the oral cavity of the unconscious patient. The side-lying position helps water and debris flow out of the mouth by gravity.

4. If secretions and debris are present, remove them with the Toothette.

   Prevents accumulation of debris. Adds to patient comfort.

5. Repeat the cleansing procedure until the mouth is clean.

6. Lower the bed, raise side rails, and open privacy curtain.

7. Follow steps 14 and 15, 17 and 18 of the procedure for brushing the teeth of a conscious patient.

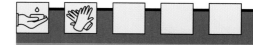

PROCEDURE

Flossing the Teeth

Flossing is performed as part of tooth care. It is done to remove debris from the surfaces of enamel between the teeth. Flossing can be performed at the same time the teeth are brushed.

GATHER EQUIPMENT

Dental floss   Disposable gloves
Glass of water with a straw   Small towel
Emesis (kidney-shaped) basin

| **ACTION** | **RATIONALE** |

Procedural Steps

1. Follow steps 1–7 of the procedure for brushing the teeth of a conscious patient.

Continued on following page

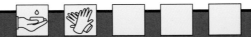

PROCEDURE

Flossing the Teeth *Continued*

2. Place the small towel across patients' chest.

3. Put on the disposable gloves.

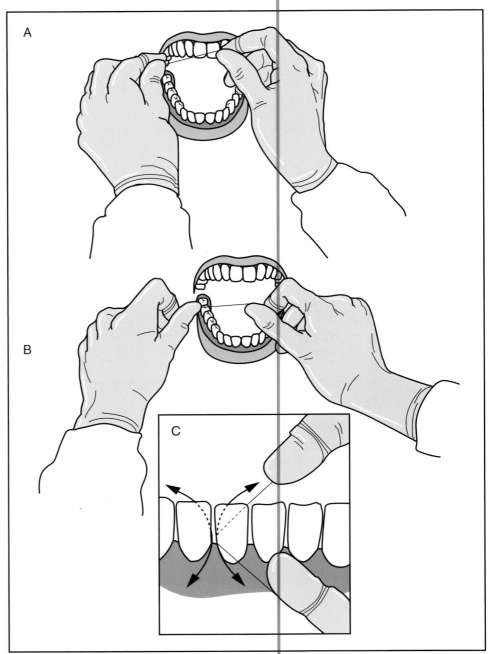

FIGURE 13–32

Using dental floss. Wrap floss tautly around the forefingers of both hands. A, Position of hands for flossing top teeth. B, Position of hands for flossing bottom teeth. C, Floss against sides of teeth. Floss to bottom of tooth and gum tissue.

4. Floss between the vertical edges of all teeth (Figure 13–32). (Do not force the dental floss below the gum line.)

Removes debris from enamel surfaces between the teeth.

5. Offer water so patients can swish it around in their mouth and loosen debris. Hold the emesis basin under patients' chin while they spit out water and debris.

6. Use the small towel to dry the lips and chin.

7. Continue with steps 13–18 of the procedure for brushing the teeth of a conscious patient.

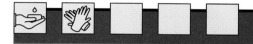

PROCEDURE

Cleaning Dentures

At bedtime, dentures are cleaned and stored in the denture cup overnight. Place the denture cup containing the dentures in a safe place during the night.

GATHER EQUIPMENT

Denture cup
Denture cleaner and brush
Dentures or other mouth appliances patients use

Emesis (kidney-shaped) basin
Three paper towels or a washcloth
Disposable gloves

ACTION	RATIONALE
Preparation	
1. Tell patients that you are going to clean their dentures.	An explanation helps gain patients' cooperation when a procedure is planned.
2. Identify yourself and the patient.	Verifies that the correct patient is receiving the procedure. Maintains patients' rights.
3. Provide privacy by pulling the curtains around the bed or closing the door.	Maintains patients' rights.
Procedural Steps	
4. Wash hands and put on the disposable gloves.	Prevents the spread of microorganisms.
5. Raise the head of the bed to a comfortable position for patients. Raise the side rails, and then raise the bed to a comfortable working position. Lower a side rail and ask patients to remove dentures and place them in the denture cup (Figure 13–33). **If you must remove the dentures:** Remove the top dentures first, then the lower dentures, and place them in the denture cup. Grasp the dentures firmly and give a slight tug downward to break the suction. Turn the denture slightly for ease in removing it from the mouth.	

Continued on following page

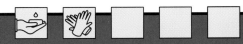

PROCEDURE

Cleaning Dentures *Continued*

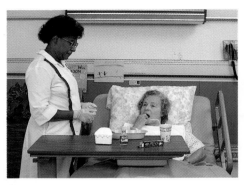
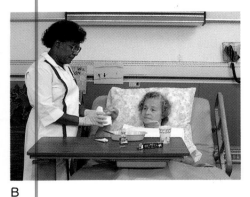

A   B

FIGURE 13–33

A, Ask the patient to remove dentures. B, Place dentures in a cup marked with the patient's name.

Note: An alternative way to remove dentures is to remove the lower denture first because it is smaller and therefore easier to remove. In addition, it "floats" on the lower jaw structure, whereas the upper denture can form a tight seal on the roof of the mouth. The tight seal must be broken before the upper denture can be removed.

6. Raise the side rail, take the dentures into patients' bathroom, and place them on a secure surface near the sink.

7. Place the emesis basin in the bottom of the sink and line it with paper towels or the washcloth, or fill it with water to cushion a falling denture.

    Lessens the chance of breakage should you drop the dentures during the cleaning procedure.

8. Clean dentures in either of two ways:
   • For patients who use a soaking solution, prepare the solution according to directions and soak the dentures for the appropriate amount of time.
   • For patients who use a denture cleanser that requires brushing, apply the cleanser as directed and brush the dentures to remove debris.

9. Adjust the water to a warm temperature.

    Very warm or hot water can change the shape of the denture material or cause cracking.

10. Brush the dentures under running water until debris is removed (Figure 13–34).

11. Rinse dentures and place them in the denture cup. Take them in the cup to patients.

    Do not carry dentures across the room in your hands.

12. Offer patients water, mouthwash, or a moistened Toothette to cleanse and remove debris from their mouth.

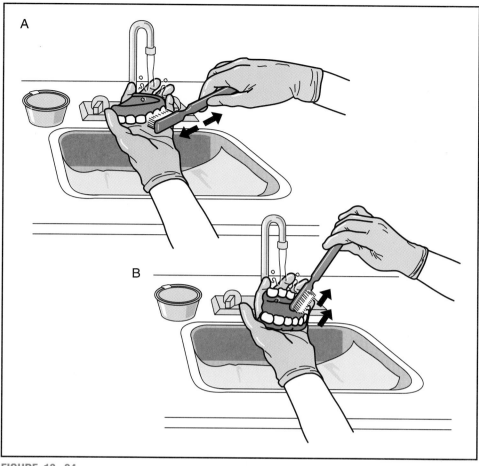

FIGURE 13–34

Cleaning dentures. Brush teeth and all other surfaces.

13. Offer patients their dentures.

Promotes independence.

14. If patients cannot place the dentures in their mouth, ask them to open their mouth. Insert upper denture first. Turn the denture at an angle, place it in the mouth, and straighten it. Affix the dentures to the roof of the mouth. Insert lower denture next and affix toward the bottom gums.

The upper denture is inserted first because it is larger and there is more room in the mouth without the presence of a lower denture.

15. Apply firm, even pressure so the dentures stay in place over the gums.

16. Remove and discard the disposable gloves in the waste container.

17. Place patients in a comfortable position and raise the side rails.

18. Lower the bed and place the call signal within reach.

Prevents falls. Leaves patients with means to communicate.

19. Clean and store the equipment for the next use.

20. Open the privacy curtains.

21. Ask patients if anything else is needed. Follow through on their request if it is something you are permitted to do.

Gives patients the opportunity to express other needs they might have.

Continued on following page

PROCEDURE

Cleaning Dentures *Continued*

Follow-Through

22. Wash hands even if you wore gloves.

Prevents the spread of microorganisms.

23. Report to the nurse that the procedure was completed. Report patients' reaction to the procedure if it was different from their usual response.

The nurse is responsible for a decision based on any unusual response.

GROOMING

GROOMING

making one's appearance neat and attractive

Grooming is the act of making one's appearance neat and attractive. The word *grooming* brings many ideas to mind. It is important to self-image. Self-image is individuals' mental picture of themselves.

Persons who are ill may not be able to follow their usual grooming routine. Care givers must provide the basic services that help patients look their best. Another consideration is how patients look to their loved ones. Loved ones may think the patient who has a 2-day growth of facial hair or oily, stringy hair is not being cared for properly.

When you finish with a patient's bath and oral hygiene, observe how the patient looks. The male patient should be shaved and his hair should be neatly combed. The female patient may desire makeup and ask to have her hair combed, brushed, or washed.

Grooming practices include

Shaving
Hair care
Makeup
Nail care
Dressing

SHAVING

Shaving is part of the daily routine for many men and women. Men shave facial and neck hair as part of their daily routine. A female who has facial hair growth may also choose to shave. A female may also ask to have her armpits, arms, and legs shaved. It is important that you check with the nurse before you shave the patient.

CARING COMMENT

In the following situations, the nurse must direct you in shaving patients:

- when the patient is receiving oxygen
- when the patient is taking certain medications (for example, an anticoagulant such as heparin or Coumadin)
- when the patient's religious beliefs prohibit shaving
- when the patient or family has a preference as to who shall shave the patient

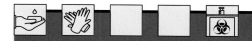

Shaving the Male Patient

The male patient can be shaved while lying in bed. You should plan to shave the patient when he cannot do so as part of his daily grooming. When the patient is able to shave himself but must remain in bed, provide all needed supplies within reach on the over-bed table.

GATHER EQUIPMENT

Rechargeable razor or disposable razor
Shaving cream or gel
Basin of water if shaving cream or gel is
  used

Bath thermometer
Bath towel and washcloth
Mirror
After-shave lotion if desired

ACTION	RATIONALE
Preparation	
1. Wash hands.	Prevents the spread of microorganisms.
2. Identify yourself and the patient.	Maintains patients' rights.
3. Provide privacy.	Maintains patients' rights.
4. Explain the procedure.	Informs patients what is happening.
Procedural Steps	
5. Position the over-bed table so needed items are within reach.	
6. Arrange supplies on the over-bed table in the order of use.	
7. Raise the bed to a comfortable working height. Keep all side rails up until you begin the procedure.	Working at waist level prevents strain or pull on your back muscles.
8. Place the patient in a comfortable position.	
9. **For a shave using an electric or rechargeable razor:**	A clean razor gives better performance.
• Check to see that the razor is clean and free of hairs from a previous shave.	
• Clean razor with a small brush if needed.	
• Place a small towel across patients' chest.	
• Turn on the razor and shave the areas of beard growth (don't forget the area under the chin). The skin around the mouth and the cheeks may need to be held taut during shaving.	

Note: If patients bring their own razor from home, it must be checked for safety by the appropriate department (engineering or maintenance) before it can be used.

For a shave using a disposable razor:	Warm water prepares the facial hair and skin to work with the shaving cream or gel and soften for a more comfortable shave. Encourage the patient to apply the shaving cream or gel if he is able. Shaving in the direction opposite of hair growth is not comfortable for the patient and can result in an uneven shave.
• Place the small towel across the patients' chest.	
• Dampen the area of facial growth with warm water.	
• Apply shaving cream or gel to the area.	

Continued on following page

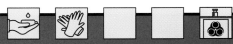

PROCEDURE

Shaving the Male Patient *Continued*

- Begin shaving in the direction in which the hair grows and continue shaving until the skin of the face is smooth (Figure 13–35).

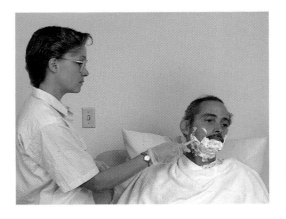

FIGURE 13–35

Shaving a male patient. Note the patient does not want his moustache shaved off.

Note: Be certain the razor is sharp.	A dull razor can damage the skin or make shaving uncomfortable.
When the razor collects the shaving cream or gel, rinse it in the basin of water before you continue.	The razor is more effective when not clogged by an accumulation of hair and shaving cream or gel.
10. When shaving is completed, use a warm, wet washcloth to remove excess residue. Hand the washcloth to the patient if he can assist by washing his face.	Encourages the patient to assist in the procedure if he is able.
11. To complete the procedure, use the palms of your hands to apply after-shave lotion to the area shaved. Or pour the lotion into the patient's hand if he can pat his face after the shave is complete.	Provides a cooling, soothing effect on the skin. Freshly shaved areas are tender and can sting.
12. Use the mirror to show the patient the results of the shave.	Involves the patient in the routine.
13. Place the patient in a comfortable position and raise the side rails.	
14. Lower the bed and place the call signal within patient's reach. Open the privacy curtains.	Prevents falls. Leaves patients with a means to communicate.
15. Clean and store equipment for next use. Place disposable razors in the appropriate sharps container. *Do not* place used razors in the waste basket.	Prevents injury to other health care givers.
16. Ask the patient if anything else is needed. Follow through on his request if it is something you are permitted to do.	Gives the patient a chance to express other needs he might have.

Follow-Through

17. Wash hands.   Prevents the spread of microorganisms.

18. Report to the nurse that the procedure has been completed. Report the patient's reaction to the procedure if it was different from usual.   The nurse is responsible for a decision based on an unusual reaction.

CARING COMMENT

Always check the nursing care plan or ask the nurse before shaving a man's beard to make sure that shaving is acceptable to him. He may not want it shaved for religious or other reasons.

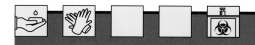

PROCEDURE

Shaving Female Underarms or Arms and Legs

Female patients may wish to have their underarms or arms and legs shaved. Underarms are shaved as part of a hygienic routine. Females in the North American culture accept this practice and find shaved underarms aesthetically pleasing.

When females have heavy hair growth on their arms or legs, they may choose to shave these areas. People inherit the tendency for heavy hair growth, or there may be an illness that causes excessive growth of hair.

GUIDELINES FOR SHAVING THE FEMALE PATIENTS' UNDERARMS OR ARMS AND LEGS

1. Check the care plan or ask the nurse if shaving underarms or arms and legs is permitted.
2. Follow the same preparation and follow-through as for any procedure.
3. A rechargeable razor or disposable razor is used.
4. Use a shaving cream or gel specifically made for use on female skin.
5. Place a towel under the body part before you begin shaving.
6. Support the body part while shaving if patients cannot help.
7. Shave in the direction the hair is growing.
8. The skin may need to be held taut while shaving.
9. Wash, rinse, and dry body parts when shaving is completed.

HAIR CARE

Brushing and combing the hair into a neat style are part of daily grooming. When the patient is on bed rest, the hair should be combed and brushed as often as needed. Try to arrange the patient's hair in an attractive style.

A shampoo can be given while a patient remains in bed. The patient may not be aware that the hair can be shampooed in this manner. Tell the patient that it can be done quite easily and explain how the procedure is done.

Special care is needed for the hair care of African Americans. Their hair tends to be dry, so special oils are available that are put in the hair to prevent damage and provide sheen. A large-toothed comb is more acceptable for use on the hair of an African-American person or anyone who has hair with tight curls and waves. Ask the patient or a family member for directions on hair care. Patients may prefer a member of the family to care for their hair. If a patient's hair is intricately braided, never remove the braids. The braids can remain for several months or however long the person wishes.

PROCEDURE

Combing or Brushing Hair

Patients' hair is combed or brushed as part of the morning care routine. If the patient wears a wig, it is combed (or brushed) and styled as needed.

GATHER EQUIPMENT

Comb or brush, as patients desire
Devices to secure the hair, such as small combs, barrettes, or elastic-covered rubber bands

Bath towel
Alcohol and cotton balls
Mirror

ACTION	RATIONALE
Preparation	
1. Wash hands.	Prevents the spread of microorganisms.
2. Identify yourself and the patient.	Maintains patients' rights.
3. Provide privacy.	Maintains patients' rights.
4. Explain the procedure.	Informs patients what is happening.
Procedural Steps	
5. Raise the bed to a comfortable working height. Keep all side rails raised until you begin the procedure.	Working at waist level prevents strain or pull on your back muscles.
6. Raise the head of the bed to a position that is comfortable for patients.	
7. Place the towel across the pillow under patients' head.	Keeps linen on the pillow clean.
8. Part the hair into 1- to 2-inch sections and comb or brush from the roots to the ends (Figure 13–36).	
9. If the hair is snarled or tangled, dab a small amount of alcohol on the snarled section.	Pulling can damage hair and cause patients discomfort during the procedure. Alcohol detangles the hair.
10. Continue combing or brushing until all sections of hair are completed.	
11. Arrange hair in the style patients desire (Figure 13–37).	Helps patients feel they are participating in their own care.
12. Remove the towel from under patients' head and discard in the laundry hamper. Discard cotton balls in the waste container.	
13. Place patients in a comfortable position and raise the side rails.	
14. Lower the bed and place the call signal within reach. Open the privacy curtains.	Prevents falls. Leaves patients with a means of communication.

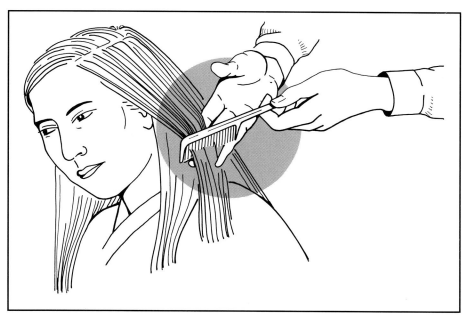

FIGURE 13–36

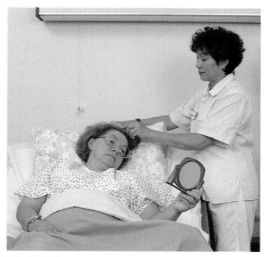

FIGURE 13–37

Use a mirror to show the patient how hair looks after combing.

15. Clean and store the comb or brush.

16. Ask patients if anything else is needed. Follow through on their request if it is something you are permitted to do.

Gives patients the opportunity to express other needs they might have.

Follow-Through

17. Wash hands.

Prevents the spread of microorganisms.

18. Report to the nurse that the procedure was completed. Report patients' reaction to the procedure if it was different from usual.

The nurse is responsible for a decision based on an unusual reaction.

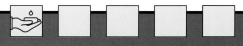

PROCEDURE

FRICTION
the rubbing of one object against another

VOID
to empty the bladder

Shampooing the Hair of Patients in Bed

A shampoo removes accumulated dirt and oil from the hair and scalp. The **friction** of the fingers stimulates the scalp. Patients can be given a shampoo while they remain in bed. An alternative is to place patients on a moveable cart and take them to the water source. Wherever you give the shampoo, keep the area private, warm, and free of drafts. Plan to dry, comb, and arrange the hair neatly as part of the shampoo. A shampoo can be included as part of the hygiene routine or can be arranged at the patient's and care giver's mutual convenience. The nurse tells you when a patient requires a shampoo.

GATHER EQUIPMENT

Shampoo
Conditioner if patients desire it
Small towel or washcloth
Two bath towels
Bath blanket
Waterproof bed protector
Water supply (large pitcher or shampoo attachment for water faucet)

Trough (device to drain the water)
Catch basin or pail
Comb
Hair dryer
Mirror
Bath thermometer

ACTION	RATIONALE
Preparation	
1. Tell patients what you are going to do. Offer the bedpan or urinal before you begin the procedure.	An explanation helps gain patients' cooperation when a procedure is planned. The sound and feel of water may activate the urge to **void.**
2. Wash hands.	Prevents the spread of microorganisms.
3. Identify yourself and patients. Call patients by name and check their identification band.	Maintains patients' rights. Verifies that the correct patient is receiving the procedure.
Procedural Steps	
4. If you are giving the shampoo to a patient who is in bed, pull the curtains around the bed or close the door. Close any windows.	Provides privacy and warmth.
5. Position the over-bed table so that needed items are within your reach.	Helps with your body mechanics.
6. Arrange supplies in order of use on the over-bed table.	Helps you work efficiently, thereby conserving (saving) your energy.
7. Raise the bed to a comfortable working height. Keep all side rails raised until you begin the procedure.	Working at waist level prevents strain or pull on your back muscles.
8. Place the bed in a flat position.	
9. Remove the pillow and place the waterproof bed protector and a towel under patients' head and shoulders (see Figure 13–38). Fanfold linens down and cover patients with the bath blanket.	
10. Arrange the trough to drain water into the catch basin or pail (Figure 13–38).	Provides drainage for water and rinse applications.

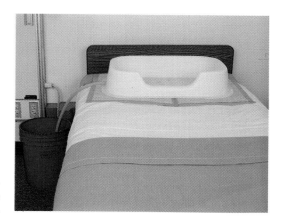

FIGURE 13–38

Place a shampoo trough under the patient's head. Arrange a basin or pail to catch the water that drains from the trough.

11. Comb and brush hair.

Removes snarls.

12. Place a folded washcloth or small towel across patients' forehead. Ask patients to hold it in place if they are able.

Keeps excess water out of patients' eyes.

13. Run water until warm. Using the bath thermometer, make the temperature of the water 110° F.

14. Wet hair thoroughly and apply a small amount of shampoo.

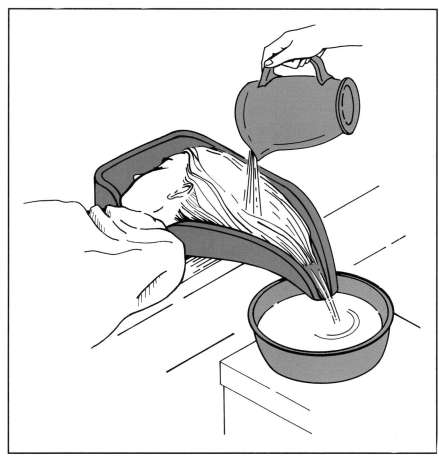

FIGURE 13–39

Continued on following page

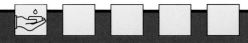

PROCEDURE

Shampooing the Hair of Patients in Bed *Continued*

15. Use both hands to work up a lather. Work from the hairline back to cover the entire scalp.

16. Use your fingertips to apply slight pressure in a circular motion over the entire scalp.

    Stimulates the scalp.

17. Rinse with water from the pitcher or shampoo attachment (Figure 13–39).

18. Repeat steps 14–17.

19. Apply a small amount of conditioner if patients desire it.

20. Work conditioner into the hair as directed on the container. Rinse thoroughly with warm water.

21. Wrap hair with the large towel.

    Prevents dripping of excess water and keeps in warmth.

22. Use the folded washcloth or small towel to dry patients' face, neck, and ears.

    As the water cools, discomfort and irritation can occur.

23. Dry the hair and scalp with the large towel.

24. Comb the hair until it is free of snarls. With one hand, hold hair close to roots (Figure 13–40). Female patients may use rollers to produce curls.

    Use a wide-tooth comb for longer hair to decrease breakage. Holding hair close to roots decreases pulling.

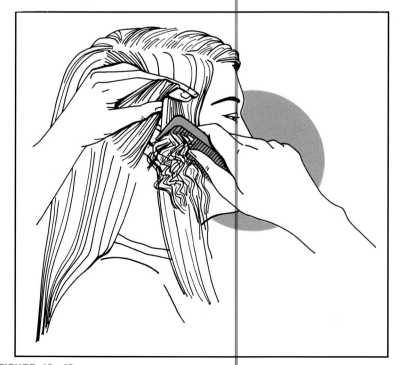

FIGURE 13–40
Fold a lock of hair over your fingers to reduce the discomfort of combing snarled hair.

25. Use the hair dryer on a low setting to dry hair quickly. Patients (male or female) may ask to have their hair styled during the drying process. Use the mirror to show patients the results.

Low heat decreases the risk of burns.

Note: If patients bring their own hair dryer from home, it must be checked for safety by the appropriate department (engineering or maintenance) before it can be used.

26. Place patients in a comfortable position and raise the side rails. Replace the pillow under patients' head. Unfold the bed linens and cover patients. Remove the bath blanket.

27. Lower the bed and place the call signal within reach. Open the privacy curtains.

Prevents falls. Leaves patients with a means of communication.

28. Clean and store the equipment properly. Discard disposables in the waste container. Place soiled linens in the laundry hamper.

Readies equipment for the next use.

29. Ask patients if anything else is needed. Follow through on their request if it is something you are permitted to do.

Gives patients the opportunity to express other needs they might have.

Follow-Through

30. Wash hands.

Prevents the spread of microorganisms.

31. Report to the nurse that the procedure was completed. Report patients' reaction to the procedure if different from usual.

The nurse is responsible for a decision based on an unusual reaction.

APPLYING MAKEUP

Applying makeup is an important part of many women's daily routine. When a patient is not able to apply makeup herself, you might be asked to help. The best rule is to ask the patient for directions and proceed accordingly. Women often use a moisturizing lotion, a foundation, and face powder, although some prefer to apply only a light dusting of face powder. Eye makeup, blush, and lipstick, if desired, can be applied. As part of this routine, a woman may desire jewelry for the day and an application of perfume or cologne. Applying makeup for your patients who wish it helps give them a good self-image.

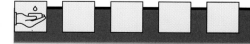

PROCEDURE

Assisting with Makeup Application

Makeup is applied to provide desired skin care for the face and neck. Use only the patient's own makeup. This prevents the spread of infection that could be caused by sharing personal supplies.

GATHER EQUIPMENT

Moisturizing lotion
Foundation
Facial powder

Lipstick
Blush
Eye makeup

Continued on following page

PROCEDURE

Assisting with Makeup Application *Continued*

ACTION	RATIONALE
Preparation	
1. Wash hands.	Prevents the spread of microorganisms.
2. Arrange makeup supplies in the order of use on over-bed table.	Helps simplify the procedure.
3. Check for odors among the supplies.	A foul odor may indicate that a cosmetic needs to be replaced.
Procedural Steps	
4. Use a cotton ball or makeup sponge to apply moisturizer, foundation, and facial powder as patient desires.	Provides for smooth, even coverage over the skin of the face and neck.
5. Apply eye makeup, blush, and lipstick if patient desires. Use cotton balls or appropriate makeup brushes.	Enhance self-image if patient desires them.
6. Ask the patient to close her eyes when you apply the eye makeup.	Prevents small particles from irritating the eye.
7. Apply a scent (perfume) of the patient's choice if desired.	Adds to the patient's positive self-image.
8. When the patient can apply some makeup herself, allow her to do so and help by opening and closing bottles and jars, if needed.	Encourages the patient to move the upper extremities.
9. Show the patient the finished results in a mirror.	Allows the patient to receive some feedback about her appearance.
Follow-Through	
10. Store makeup supplies.	
11. Wash hands.	Prevents the spread of microorganisms.

CARING COMMENT

If patients are not able to tell you how to apply makeup, a photo of them can assist you in applying makeup.

NAIL CARE

PERIPHERAL VASCULAR DISEASE
a disease caused by decreased blood supply to the extremities
DIABETES MELLITUS
a disorder that affects the body's ability to use glucose (sugar) because the body cannot produce or use insulin

The appearance of their fingernails is an important consideration to many individuals, both male and female. Nail care is performed as frequently as necessary. It may be a daily, weekly, or less often routine depending on the patient. As with makeup, patients may provide personal supplies. Before you give nail care, check the nursing care plan for information regarding care of patients' nails. Patients can also tell you what special routine has been followed in the past.

The toenails are a special area of concern for some patients. The patient with **peripheral vascular disease** (decreased blood supply to the extremities) or **diabetes** is usually referred to a **podiatrist**. Toenails are cut straight across without touching the flesh, because infection may occur if toe nails are rounded and shaped or if the skin is cut during care.

PODIATRIST

a doctor who treats diseases and conditions of the foot

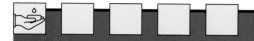

PROCEDURE

Assisting with Nail Care

Care is given to fingernails (and toenails) to keep nail edges smooth and short. Nail care also keeps the area under the nails free of debris (dirt).

GATHER EQUIPMENT

Cuticle stick (orange stick)
Emery board
Nail clippers
Small basin
Hand towel

Optional:
Nail polish
Nail polish remover
Cotton balls

ACTION	RATIONALE
Preparation	
1. Wash hands.	Prevents the spread of microorganisms.
2. Identify yourself and patients.	Maintains patients' rights.
3. Provide privacy.	Maintains patients' rights.
4. Explain the procedure.	Informs patients what is happening.
Procedural Steps	
5. Examine old nail polish to determine whether it is chipped and worn.	Harmful microorganisms may thrive in chipped nail polish.
6. If old polish is chipped, soak cotton balls in nail polish remover and use them to remove polish from each fingernail.	Old nail polish is removed before new polish is applied.
7. Place enough warm water in the basin so that all 10 fingers can soak. You may choose to soak one hand at a time. (A cuticle-softening agent may be added to the water or applied to each finger.)	Softening cuticles makes it easier to push them back.
8. Soak fingers for 2–4 minutes or until cuticles are softened. Remove hand from basin.	
9. Place the hand towel in front of patients. Use towel to dry the hand.	Provides a work area after fingers are dried.
10. Discard water and clean the basin.	
11. Use the cuticle stick to push back the cuticle gently.	Helps give shape to the nails and remove the excess growth of cuticle.
12. Use nail clippers (not scissors) to trim nails straight across and not close to the flesh (Figure 13–41).	Scissors are more likely to cut flesh. Trimming straight across encourages a neat appearance and discourages the formation of ingrown nails.
13. Use an emery board to file the rough edges and give a slightly rounded shape to each nail.	An emery board is gentler and causes less breakage than a nail file.

Continued on following page

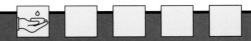

PROCEDURE

Assisting with Nail Care *Continued*

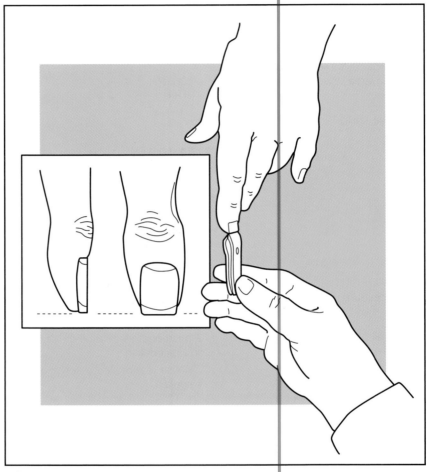

FIGURE 13–41

14. Use the pointed end of the cuticle stick to remove the debris from under each nail.

When debris accumulates, harmful microorganisms are encouraged to grow.

15. Wash patients' hands to remove debris. Rinse and dry.

Provides a clean surface for application of nail polish if desired.

16. Buff each fingernail or apply nail polish if patients desire. Allow polish to dry.

Nail polish needs time to harden. Otherwise it will smear.

17. Apply a second or third coat of nail polish if patients desire.

Follow-Through

18. Clean and store equipment.

Readies equipment for the next use.

19. Wash hands.

Prevents the spread of microorganisms.

Check with the supervisor or nurse *before* you trim patients' fingernails or toenails. The supervisor or nurse must make special arrangements with other professionals if patients have a medical condition that makes trimming or cutting fingernails or toenails dangerous.

DRESSING

The hospital gown is designed to be easy to put on and take off. Many patients feel exposed and awkward in hospital gowns and robes. They come in a one-size-fits-all adult size and in an extra-large size. In many institutions, bottoms are available and are located on the linen cart or other designated place. Child-size gowns and pajamas are also available. Because the back opening of the hospital gown may swing open, patients may prefer to wear their own clothing or sleep wear during the day.

Regardless of whether patients prefer to wear hospital or personal clothing, you need to know how to assist them in dressing. You should encourage independence in dressing when patients have the mobility and strength needed to complete this activity.

In a nursing home, most patients are encouraged to dress for the day. They may need help choosing an outfit for the day, or they may choose their own clothes. You should encourage patients to make choices whenever possible.

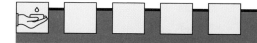

PROCEDURE

Assisting with Dressing

Dressing for the day is a part of the morning routine. Patients may also need a change of clothing at other times. Thus your assistance may be needed if clothing becomes soiled or a social event is scheduled. Be certain the clothing patients select is their own, fits them, and is in good condition.

GATHER SUPPLIES

Patients usually choose their clothes themselves. They may wish to wear nightclothes during the day if they have been ill over a period of time.

ACTION	RATIONALE
Preparation	
1. Wash hands.	Prevents the spread of microorganisms.
2. Check clothing for cleanliness and need for repair.	A change to fresh clothing that is in good condition helps boost patients' self-image and sense of dignity.
Procedural Steps	
3. Put on undergarments first. To assist with underpants, place patients in the supine (back-lying) position.	Undergarments are a basic part of dressing. Dressing the lower half of the body is more comfortable for patients in this position. Patients who have some ability to move can assist in dressing the lower part of the body while in this position.

Continued on following page

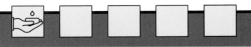

PROCEDURE

Assisting with Dressing *Continued*

4. Guide patients' feet through the appropriate leg openings. Bring the underpants up to the thighs and over the buttocks. The elastic waist band is positioned at the waist level.

Allows patients to take part in as much activity as permitted.

5. Repeat steps 3 and 4 when slacks, shorts, or panty hose are desired.

Slacks and panty hose provide extra warmth.

6. Apply socks one at a time. Make certain patients' toes are in alignment and put the sock over the toes; then pull the sock over the heel. Continue stretching the sock over the calf until it is in place.

Provides comfort and warmth when shoes are worn.

7. Put on shoes, nonslip slippers, or sneakers.

Provides a firm, safe support when walking. Shoes, slippers, or sneakers should be appropriate for patients' activity.

8. Put a brassiere on female patients. Guide the arms through the shoulder straps appropriately.

Provides support for breast tissue.

9. Adjust the brassiere cups to fit over the breasts.

Brassiere cups are designed to help support the breasts.

10. Adjust the straps over each shoulder.

The shoulders help support the weight of the breasts.

11. Close the hooks in the back, or put the brassiere on backwards if patients desire to adjust the closure themselves. (Note that patients may prefer a front-closing brassiere.)

When the back is closed, a brassiere is considered in place, ensuring proper comfort during daily wear. Allowing patients to close the hooks themselves permits them to assist in the dressing process. Patients may prefer to put on the undergarment in private.

12. An undershirt or T-shirt is put on male patients. (Female patients may also request an undershirt.)
    For patients who cannot dress themselves:
    Place the garment over patients' head and bring it down as far as the neck. Place one arm at a time through a sleeve and pull it through. *Remember this rule: Weak arm through first, strong arm follows. Reverse to undress: Strong arm out first, then weak arm.* Adjust the body of the garment over the chest, abdomen, and lower back.
    For patients who can dress themselves:
    Patients who are able can put their arms through the sleeve first, then pull the garment over the head.

An undershirt permits the skin to breathe and provides warmth and comfort next to the skin.

By dressing themselves or assisting in the dressing routine, patients maintain joint mobility and increase the circulation of the blood.

13. To assist a woman to put on a dress, put it on over the head first. Follow step 12.

14. Adjust dress over the hips and thighs. Finish by buttoning or zippering the garment. — Provides comfort and gives a finished look to dressing.

15. When the garment of choice is a blouse or shirt, guide the arms through the sleeves one at a time. Pull arms through and adjust garment.

16. Button or zip the garment or permit patients to do so whenever they are able.

17. Follow step 12 if patients desire a sweater. — Provides warmth and comfort.

Follow-Through

18. Wash hands. — Prevents the spread of microorganisms.

GROOMING AND SELF-IMAGE

When individuals are unable to follow an established grooming routine, a change in their self-image may occur. Patients may look and feel unhappy when such a change occurs. They may feel like a different person and lose interest in their appearance.

Grooming is a part of individuals' daily routine that helps boost their self-image. In addition, the movement of the arms to accomplish grooming tasks helps promote blood circulation, keeps the joints flexible, and helps patients feel better about themselves.

CARE OF PATIENTS WITH DISRUPTIONS IN SKIN

The lack of freedom of movement greatly affects the skin. Movement allows our body organs to work at a maximum efficiency. When movement is stopped or decreased, all body organs, including the skin, are affected.

When a patient lies or sits in one position for too long a time an increase in pressure results in the area of the body against the surface being lain or sat on (Figure 13–42). Because of the pressure, less blood circulates to the area. Blood brings **oxygen** and nutrients to tissues; reduced blood can cause the death of body tissue. When this occurs, a **decubitus ulcer** forms. You may hear this condition referred to as skin "breakdown" or "pressure sores." This can happen to *any* patient who lies or sits in one position too long, regardless of age.

The areas on the body where the body's weight can interfere with the right amounts of circulation of blood are called **pressure points**. The areas where the bone lies close to the skin are called **bony prominences**. Good examples of bony prominences for you to feel with your finger are the

- knob on the back of the neck
- elbows
- scapulas (shoulder blades), one on each side of the upper back
- hip bones on each side of the body
- tailbone
- ankles and heels

Other areas that are prone to the formation of decubitus ulcers are the ears, the skin under the breasts of the female, and the scrotum in the male. Warmth and moisture make the area under pendulous (sagging) breasts particularly prone to skin breakdown.

OXYGEN
a colorless, tasteless, odorless gas; the air we breathe is about 20% oxygen

DECUBITUS ULCER
a bedsore; a sore caused by continual pressure on the body parts of a patient who must stay in one place

PRESSURE POINTS
certain parts on the body where bone is located close to the skin, such as the elbow; also, various areas of the body where pressure is applied to control hemorrhage

BONY PROMINENCE
any area of the body where bone lies close to the skin (such as elbow or ankle)

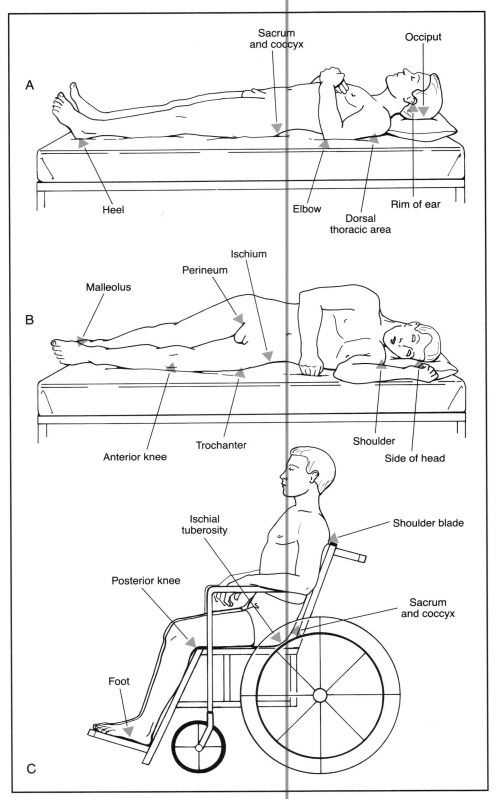

FIGURE 13–42

Pressure points in different body positions. A, Supine (back-lying) position. B, Side-lying position. C, Sitting position.

A decubitus ulcer begins as a small reddened area of the skin over one of the pressure points of the body. The area remains red or dusky even when the patient's position is changed. If you gently touch the reddened area with your fingers, you will observe a lighter, paler color followed by a quick return to the red or dusky color. You should report this observation to the nurse.

CARING COMMENT

Never put pressure on a reddened area. *Never* massage the reddened areas of skin. You can, however, massage the skin around the reddened areas to help increase circulation.

Once the top layer of skin is broken down and the layer underneath can be seen, the decubitus ulcer can progress from a very small area to a potentially large area that is difficult to heal. As the top layer of skin is lost, the body loses its protective shield. Harmful microorganisms can invade the area and cause an infection.

Because patients are already ill, their body may not be able to defend itself well against infection. In addition, the tissue under the open area may continue to break down. The decubitus ulcer can erode (eat away) deep into the body tissue and may reach bone.

The main defense against the formation of decubitus ulcer is to take the actions needed to prevent their occurrence (see Chapter 16). When the skin does break down, certain treatments performed by the nurse can help in the healing process. If the decubitus ulcer becomes large and infected, surgery and antibiotics may be indicated to help it heal.

CARING COMMENTS

With watchful attention from care givers, patients' skin can be kept intact (without breaks). When you care for a patient who cannot move or turn, think prevention. You can prevent the formation of decubitus ulcers.

Report any observation you make of a problem on the skin in any place on the body. Tell the nurse what you observe about the patient's skin and where the problem area is located.

CHAPTER WRAP-UP

- The skin protects the body in a variety of ways. Most important, it is the first line of defense against infection.
- Your effort to observe patients' skin during personal care is very important. It can contribute to early preventative action by all health care team members.
- Good hygiene plays a vital role in helping patients stay clean and comfortable.
- Performing or assisting with bathing, oral care, and grooming is part of giving personal care to your patients.

- Remember to observe the skin as well as the hair, mouth and teeth, and nails.
- Skin should be moist and warm to the touch.
- Observations you need to report are:
    reddened areas of the skin
    abraded, dry, or flaky skin
    rashes
    jaundiced skin
- Report and record any skin change and remember to note the location of the change.
- Certain steps should be followed by care givers whenever a procedure is done. You should:
    Wash hands.
    Gather supplies.
    Set up for the procedure.
    Provide for patient privacy.
    Complete the steps of the procedure in the correct order.
    Wear disposable gloves for any contact with body fluids.
    Note normal and unusual observations.
    Make patients comfortable.
    Restore order to the area.
- Along with reporting observations to the nurse, keep patients safe and warm, turn and position them at the scheduled times, and communicate with them.

REVIEW QUESTIONS

1. How does the skin help the body?
2. What are the normal observations of the skin that you can make during the bed bath? At what other times can you make observations of patients' skin?
3. Explain what you do for the patient during each of the following routines.
   AM:

   _____
   _____
   _____
   _____

   PM or HS:

   _____
   _____
   _____
   _____

4. What preparations are needed before you start bathing and grooming procedures for a patient?
5. Why do you use disposable gloves in any procedure in which you experience direct contact with patients' body secretions?

ACTIVITY CORNER

Look at the list of activities of daily living below. Think about a time you felt very ill and spent a day in bed. Check the column that corresponds to how you felt about caring for yourself on that day.

Activity	Felt Like Doing	Did Not Feel Like Doing	Would Have Liked Help With
Bathing/showering	_____	_____	_____
Brushing teeth	_____	_____	_____
Dressing	_____	_____	_____
Eating/cooking	_____	_____	_____
Using the bathroom	_____	_____	_____
Grooming (shaving, combing hair, etc.)	_____	_____	_____

How many activities did you feel like doing? _____

How did you feel when you did any of the self-care activities? Tired _____ Exhausted _____ Energetic _____

How would you have felt if someone had helped you? Better _____ More rested _____

Think about patients who need personal care help and how they might feel when personal care is given.

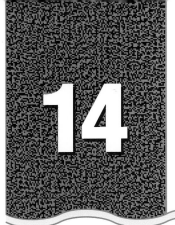

14 Making Beds

Objectives

AFTER YOU COMPLETE THIS CHAPTER, YOU WILL BE ABLE TO:

Make an occupied bed.
Make an unoccupied bed.
Define the terms *open bed* and *closed bed.*
Prepare a bed for the postoperative patient.

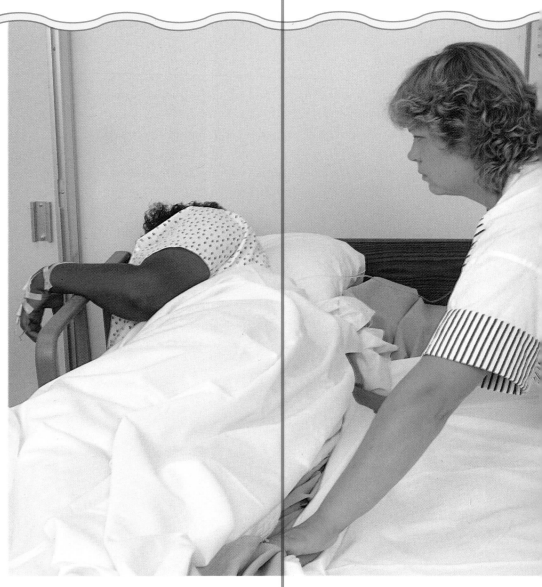

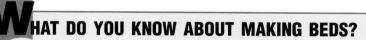

Overview Fresh linens are important to patient comfort. Linens should be kept clean, dry, and wrinkle free. You need to know how to make up a bed in a variety of ways and how to use good body mechanics when changing bed linens.

WHAT DO YOU KNOW ABOUT MAKING BEDS?

Here are four statements about making beds. Consider them to test your ideas about how and why beds are made in the health care institution. If you think the statement is true, circle the T; if you think the statement is false, circle the F. Change the false statements to make them true.

1. T F Bed linens are replaced every day.

2. T F Fresh linen can be put on the bed while the patient stays in the bed.

3. T F The patient's skin and ability to move and turn can be observed during a bed linen change.

4. T F Wrinkled sheets put pressure on the patient's skin and may cause skin breakdown.

ANSWERS

1. **False.** Bed linens *may* be replaced every day in some institutions. Your place of employment may have special rules about how often the linens should be changed.

2. **True.** The patient can be moved from one side of the bed to the other while you are changing the bottom linens.

3. **True.** You can observe patients' skin as well as watch them when they move and turn in the bed.

4. **True.** Blood circulation to the skin is slowed or stopped by the pressure wrinkles put on the skin. Lack of blood puts the skin at risk for breakdown.

BEDMAKING SCHEDULES

Making beds is a special part of giving patient care. A clean, dry bed without wrinkles is more comfortable for rest and sleep. Ask the nurse what rules you should follow when changing bed linens. For instance, in some health care institutions, bed linens are changed every other day unless they become soiled. If you are caring for infants or toddlers, linen changes are usually done much more often. Your health care institution may use fitted crib sheets. Fitted sheets stay on better and stay wrinkle free.

If you are employed at a long-term care setting or in the home, the linen may be changed

- once or twice a week unless something spills on the bed
- more often if the person becomes ill and stays in bed for long periods of time

The bed linens are also changed whenever they are soiled because patients were **incontinent** of **bowel** or **bladder** or because of an accidental spill or a procedure. The bedspread is replaced only if it is soiled. An ill patient may toss and turn all night, may sweat profusely (in great amounts), or drain body **secretions** on the linens. Any time linens are soiled, they must be replaced with clean linen.

INCONTINENT
unable to respond to the urge to eliminate the waste products of the body
BOWEL
the intestine
BLADDER
the elastic muscular sac that collects urine before it leaves the body
SECRETION
discharge; waste material that leaves the body through an opening

CARING COMMENT

Whenever you notice the linens are soiled, you should replace them with clean linens without being told. The patient should never lie on soiled bed linens.

If you notice the linens are wrinkled and not lying straight, you should smooth them out and straighten the bed. Smooth bottom sheets are more comfortable for patients. A neat bed also shows patients you care about how they look.

LINEN SUPPLIES

Linen supplies are usually found on a linen supply cart or in a special linen closet. If you notice the linen supply is getting low, notify the nurse or your supervisor.

Bed linens are usually replaced with fresh linens after the daily personal care routines are completed. The linens needed to make a bed include

DRAW SHEET
a piece of linen about half the size of a regular sheet, placed over a protector pad (rubber or plastic) for patient comfort; when edges are loosened from under the mattress, it can be used by two people to move a patient up in bed

- mattress pad
- protector pad
- two sheets (one may be a fitted sheet with elastic corners for the mattress)
- **draw sheet**
- pillowcase
- blanket
- bedspread

CARING COMMENT

A good way to know what linens are needed for your patient is to see what linens are on the bed before you go to the linen cart for supplies.

CARING COMMENT

Never return unused linens to the supply cart from the patient's room because you may be transferring **microorganisms** from one place to another. If the linens cannot be kept in the patient's room for future use, they should be placed in the laundry hamper.

MICROORGANISM

an organism so tiny it can be seen only under a microscope; capable of helping the body as well as causing disease

METHODS OF CHANGING A BED

A bed can be made up in several different ways:

- **occupied bed**—The bed linens are changed while the patient remains in it (after personal care or other procedures are completed).
- **unoccupied bed**—no one is in the bed when it is made. There are three ways to make an unoccupied bed:
  Closed bed
  Open bed
  Surgical bed

OCCUPIED BED

type of bedmaking in which the patient remains in the bed while linens are changed

UNOCCUPIED BED

type of bedmaking in which no one is in the bed while linens are changed

CLOSED BED

In the acute care setting, the bed is completely made up, with the bedspread and top sheet covering the entire bed. The pillow is covered with a clean pillow case and is placed at the head of the bed. The bed is left in a high position to signify that no patient is assigned to the room.

In the long-term care setting, the bedspread may be placed over the entire bed and tucked under the pillow and the bed placed in low position. The bed is "closed" during the day (Figure 14–1).

OPEN BED

In the acute care setting, the bedspread and top sheet are fanfolded to the bottom of the bed. The pillow is placed at the head of the bed. The bed is always placed in the lowest horizontal position so that the patient using the bed can get into and out of it safely (Figure 14–2). When patients return to bed, the bed linens are "open" and ready for them to lie down and pull up the linens over themselves. Unless your patient is scheduled for discharge, make an open bed.

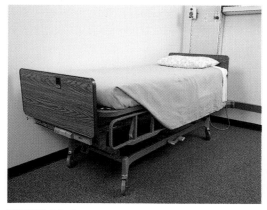

FIGURE 14–1
A closed bed.

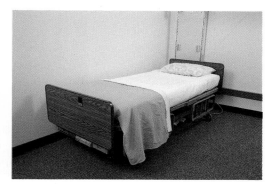

FIGURE 14–2
An open bed.

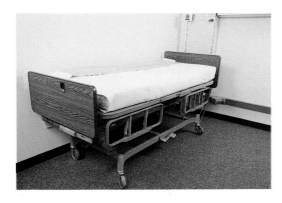

FIGURE 14-3
A surgical bed.

In the long-term care setting, the linens are fanfolded to the bottom of the bed at bedtime.

SURGICAL BED

In the acute care setting, a surgical bed is made up when your patient is in the operating room for scheduled surgery. It may also be called an OR (operating room) bed.

When the patient returns to the unit after surgery, a transfer to the bed can be easily accomplished because the linens are loose (not tucked under the mattress) and fanfolded to the side or foot of the bed so the patient can be covered quickly when transferred (Figure 14-3). The bottom corners of the bed are made after the patient is covered and positioned comfortably.

PROCEDURE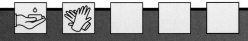

Making an Occupied Bed

When the patient is on bed rest or is too ill to get out of bed, the bed linens can be changed with the patient in the bed. The main concern during this procedure is the safety of the patient. Bed linens are changed after personal care is completed or whenever needed (for example, after spills, sweating, and incontinence of bowels or bladder).

GATHER EQUIPMENT

One or two pillowcases	Bed protector pad
One bedspread or blanket	Waterproof pad (if needed)
One top sheet	Mattress pad
One bottom sheet	Laundry hamper
One draw sheet	Disposable gloves (if body secretions are present)

ACTION

RATIONALE

Preparation

1. Arrange linens in the order they will be needed.

   Because you can remove each piece from the top, you are less likely to drop items on the floor.

2. After personal care is completed, tell patients you are going to change the bed linens. Let patients know they can

   An explanation helps gain patients' cooperation when a procedure is planned. Encouraging patients to assist in care

help by moving and turning while you change the linens. Remember that the patient is covered with a bath blanket when personal care is completed.

helps keep their muscles and joints flexible and helps their circulation.

3. Wash hands.

Prevents the spread of microorganisms.

4. Close curtain for privacy.

Maintains patients' rights.

5. Identify yourself and the patient. Call patients by name and check their identification band.

Maintains patients' rights. Verifies that correct patient is receiving the procedure.

Note: If blood or body fluids are present, you should put on disposable gloves for this procedure.

Procedural Steps

6. Raise the bed to a comfortable working height. Keep all side rails raised until you begin the procedure.

Working at waist level prevents strain or pull on your back muscles.

7. Place the bed in a flat position. Place the clean linens within your reach.

It is easier to change linens with the head of the bed down.

8. Ask patients to turn onto their side. Assist them or turn them yourself if necessary. Keep the pillow under patients' head. Keep patients covered with a bath blanket.

Patient comfort is an important consideration at this time.

9. Lower the side rail on the side at which you are working. Loosen the bottom linens on this side of the bed.

Keep patient safety in mind when the bed is raised to a comfortable working height.

10. Tell patient to hold onto the side rail.

Helps patient remain in side-lying position.

11. Fanfold the loosened linen toward patient's back. Tuck the linen as close to patient as possible. Your side of the bed is now stripped to the mattress (Figure 14–4).

Prepares the linen for easy removal when patients are rolled to the other side.

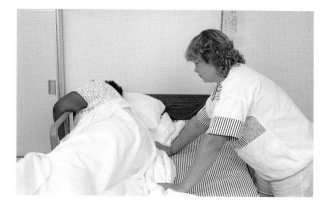

FIGURE 14–4

12. Unfold the mattress pad and place it on the side of the bed near you. Match the top edge of the pad with the top edge of the mattress. Smooth out toward the foot of the bed so there are no wrinkles.

13. Unfold the bottom sheet. (Use the center fold to guide placement of the

sheet.) Place the bottom hem of the bottom sheet even with the bottom edge of the mattress.

14. Smooth the bottom sheet toward the top of the mattress while keeping it centered so there are no wrinkles.

15. At the top of the mattress, tuck the edge of the bottom sheet under the mattress. Make a square corner and begin to tuck the sheet under the mattress (Figure 14–5).

A square corner anchors the linen securely and gives a finished look.

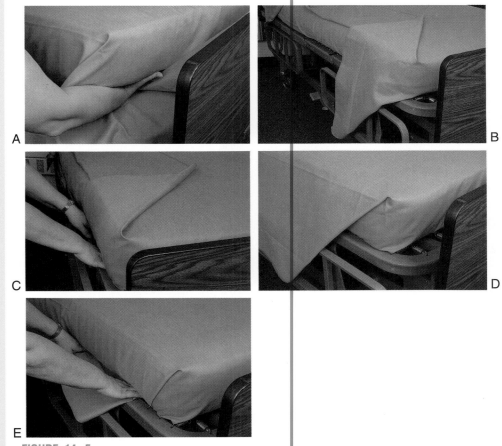

FIGURE 14–5

Making a square corner. A, Tuck the excess sheet under the mattress. B, Fold the top part of the sheet and lay it across the bed at a 45° angle. C, Tuck the excess under the side of the mattress. D, Bring the top part of the sheet down. E, Tuck the sheet under the mattress. Keep tucking the sheet under the mattress as you work your way to the bottom of the bed.

16. Keep tucking the bottom sheet under the mattress as you work your way to the bottom of the bed.

17. Unfold the protector pad and the waterproof pad and center them on the bed.

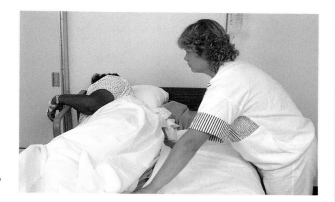

FIGURE 14-6
Tuck fanfolded linens close to patient's back.

18. Fanfold the edges of the bottom linens against patient's back. Repeat this with the draw sheet, if used (Figure 14-6).

19. Ask patients to turn toward you or assist them in turning. Make sure you tell patients to expect a "lump" made by the soiled and the clean linens when they roll toward you.

Prepares the patient to expect a lump when rolling over.

20. Keep patients covered with the bath blanket and make sure they are comfortable in the new position. Raise the side rails.

Protects patients' privacy, comfort, and safety.

21. Go to the other side of the bed and lower the side rails on that side. Grasp the soiled linens and roll them toward yourself. Place the soiled linens in the laundry hamper.

The soiled linens should always be placed in the laundry hamper. Never place soiled linen on the floor or on clean linen.

22. Grasp and then roll the clean linens from under patients toward yourself. Pull linens so they are taut and free of wrinkles. All linens should be in position to tuck in under the mattress (Figure 14-7).

Lying on wrinkled linens may cause skin problems for patients.

23. Repeat steps 15 and 16.

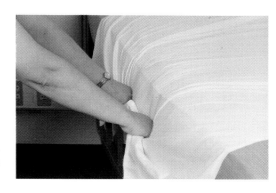

FIGURE 14-7
Grasp linens firmly and pull toward yourself to ensure that all linens are ready to be tucked under the mattress.

24. Patients can now be positioned on their back. Center the bath blanket and the pillow with patients in the supine (back-lying) or side-lying position.

25. Unfold the top sheet and place over the bath blanket. Place the hem at the top of the mattress or ask patients to hold the edge of the sheet if they are able. Pull the bath blanket out and place it in the laundry hamper.

26. Unfold and center the blanket or bedspread. Match the top edge of the blanket to the edge of the top sheet.

27. Smooth the sheet and blanket down

For comfort, try to place patients on their back or side as soon as possible.

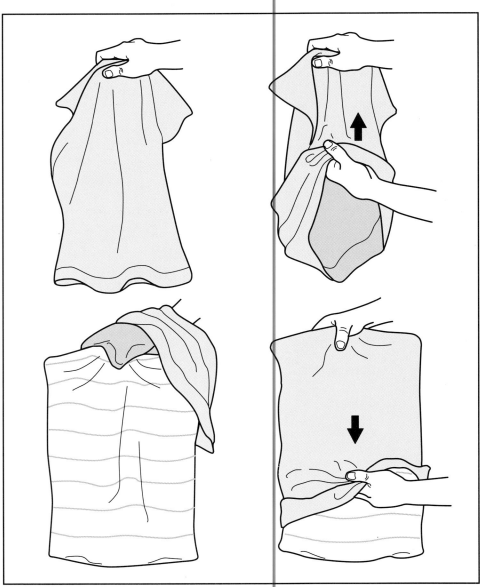

FIGURE 14–8

Putting on a clean pillowcase. Grasp the closed end of the pillowcase with one hand and invert pillowcase over your arm. Then grasp the narrow edge of the pillow with the same hand. While holding the pillowcase and pillow firmly with one hand, pull down the pillowcase over the pillow with the other hand.

toward the bottom of the bed. Tuck the sheet and the blanket or bed-spread under the bottom edge of the mattress.

28. Make a square corner to finish that side of the bed.

29. Raise the side rails and go to the other side of the bed. Repeat steps 27 and 28.

    Always keep patient safety in mind when doing a procedure.

30. Grasp the linens over patients' toes and give them a slight tug to loosen the top linens.

    Gives the patient room to move the toes freely and keeps the weight of the linens off the toes so that circulation is not slowed.

31. Go to the head of the bed and fold down the top edges about 6 inches across the bed.

    Gives linens a finished look.

32. Remove the pillow(s) from under pa-tient's head. Remove soiled pillow case. Put a clean pillowcase on each pillow (Figure 14–8) and position each pillow under the patient's head.

33. Lower the entire bed to the low posi-tion. Place the call signal within reach.

    Keeps patients safe. Leaves patients with a means to communicate.

34. Ask patients if anything else is needed. Follow through on their re-quest if it is something you are permit-ted to do.

    Gives patients a chance to express other needs they might have.

35. Place the laundry hamper in the soiled utility room.

36. Open curtain.

37. Wash hands.

    Prevents the spread of microorganisms.

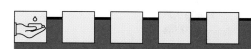

PROCEDURE

Making a Closed Bed

When a patient is discharged, a specific procedure is followed to clean the unit. Making a closed bed is the last step in the procedure. A closed bed signifies that the unit is ready for another patient.

GATHER EQUIPMENT

One or two pillowcases
One bedspread or blanket
One top sheet
One bottom sheet
One draw sheet

Bed protector pad
Waterproof pad (if needed)
Mattress pad

ACTION

RATIONALE

Preparation

1. Raise the bed to a comfortable work-ing position. The bed should be flat.

    Working at waist level prevents strain or pull on your back muscles.

Side rails can be lowered because there is no patient in the bed.

2. Wash hands.

3. Place clean linens within reach in the order they will be needed.

Prevents the spread of microorganisms.
Conserves (saves) your energy.

Procedural Steps

Important: apply all linens to one side of the bed, then complete the change on the other side of the bed.

4. Unfold the mattress pad and center it on the bed before spreading it out.

The center crease helps you keep an even amount of linen on each side of the bed.

5. Unfold the bottom sheet and center it on the bed. Place the bottom hem even with the mattress at the foot of the bed.

6. Smooth the bottom sheet toward the top of the mattress, using the center crease as a guide to keep the sheet centered on the bed.

7. At the top of the mattress, tuck the excess linen under the mattress. Make a square corner. (When you apply the bottom sheet, square corners are made at the top of the mattress only.)

The extra linen tucked under at the top helps keep the sheet in place more securely when a patient lies on the bed.

8. Tuck the rest of the bottom sheet under the mattress as you work toward the foot of the bed.

9. Unfold the protector and the waterproof pad and center them on the bed. Unfold the draw sheet and center it on the bed. Tuck the edge of the pads and the draw sheet under the mattress at the side of the bed.

10. Unfold the top sheet and use the middle crease to center it on the bed. Place the top hem of the top sheet even with the top edge of the mattress. Smooth the linen down toward the bottom of the bed. Make square corners with the top sheet only at the bottom of the mattress.

Square corners at the bottom of the bed help anchor the linens in place so patients can remain covered.

11. Unfold the blanket or bedspread and repeat step 10. The top edges of the top sheet and the blanket or bedspread can be folded if that is the policy of your institution.

12. At the bottom of the bed, tuck excess linen under the mattress. Make a square corner. Smooth linen to remove any wrinkles.

13. Go to the other side of the bed and repeat steps 4–12.

14. Grasp the pillow and put a clean pillowcase on it (see Figure 14–8). Center the pillow at the head of the bed.

15. **In the acute care setting:**
    Leave the bed in the high position. Report to the appropriate person that the closed bed is ready (see Figure 14–1).

    In the long-term care setting:
    Place the bedspread over the entire bed and tuck it in under the pillow. Place the bed in the low position (Figure 14–9).

The closed bed means that the unit is ready for a new patient.

The closed bed means the patient is up for the day. It helps provide a more home-like setting.

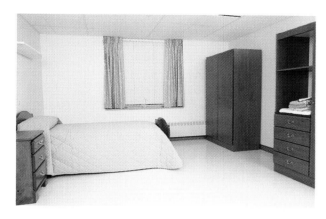

FIGURE 14–9
A closed bed in a nursing home.

Follow-Through

16. Report to the appropriate person that the closed bed is ready.

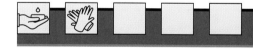

Making an Open Bed

When patients are allowed out of bed, the linens can be changed once the patients are up and sitting in a chair. The open bed signifies that the patients can return to bed when they desire.

GATHER EQUIPMENT

One or two pillowcases
One bedspread or blanket
One top sheet
One bottom sheet
One draw sheet

Bed protector pad
Waterproof pad (if needed)
Mattress pad
Laundry hamper
Disposable gloves (if body secretions are present)

ACTION

RATIONALE

Preparation

1. Take a laundry cart to patient's room.

Provides a container in which to place soiled linen.

Procedural Steps

2. Follow steps 1–13 of the procedure for making a closed bed.

3. Go to the head of the bed and grasp

the folded top edges of the linens. Lift the linens and fanfold them to the bottom of the bed. The top sheets should all be folded at the bottom of the bed.

4. Replace the used pillowcase with a clean one. Center the pillow at the top of the bed.

5. Place the bed in the lowest horizontal position and raise the head of the bed as patients desire.

6. Tell patients that the linen change is complete. Patients can return to bed if they desire. Ask patients if they need assistance in returning to bed.

7. Place the call signal within reach before you leave patient's room.

Leaves patients with a means to communicate.

8. Ask patients if anything else is needed. Follow through on their request if it is something you are permitted to do.

Gives patients a chance to express other needs they might have.

Follow-Through

9. Take the laundry hamper to the soiled utility room.

The laundry hamper is kept in the soiled utility room until soiled linens are sent to the laundry.

10. Wash hands.

Prevents the spread of microorganisms picked up while handling soiled (dirty) linens.

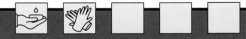

PROCEDURE

Making a Surgical or an OR Bed

The surgical bed is made up after the patient has left for the operating room (see Figure 14–3). The top sheet and blanket or bedspread are folded in a way that allows for easy transfer of the patient back to bed after surgery. After the transfer, the patient can be quickly covered up and made comfortable.

GATHER EQUIPMENT

One or two pillowcases
One bedspread or blanket
One top sheet
One bottom sheet
One draw sheet

Bed protector pad
Waterproof pad (if needed)
Mattress pad
Laundry hamper
Disposable gloves (if body secretions are present)

ACTION   **RATIONALE**

Procedural Steps

1. Follow steps 1–13 of the procedure for making a closed bed.

2. Remove the used pillowcase and replace it with a clean one. Place the pillow on the over-bed table.

3. Fold the top linens as shown in Figure 14–3 or according to your institutions preference.

4. Leave the bed in the high position.

The patient will return from the operating room on a cart or **gurney.** The high bed position matches the height of the cart and makes for ease in transfer.

GURNEY
stretcher on wheels

Follow-through

5. After you make an OR bed, make sure the following items are in the room:
   * A **stethoscope** and **sphygmomanometer** are on the bedside stand.
   * An **intravenous (IV)** pole is placed in a hole in the headboard or, if portable, is placed next to the head of the bed.
   * A box of tissue and an **emesis** basin are on the bedside stand.
   * A special flow sheet and pen for recording vital signs are on the bedside stand. (Make sure the sheet is stamped with the correct patient's name.)

6. Wash hands.

At the end of this procedure, the unit should be ready to receive the patient from the operating room.

Prevents the spread of microorganisms.

STETHOSCOPE
an instrument used to hear and amplify the sound of an internal organ (heart, lungs, or bowels)

SPHYGMOMANOMETER
the instrument used to measure the arterial blood pressure

INTRAVENOUS
through the vein

EMESIS
stomach contents (digested particles) brought up and expelled from the mouth; vomitus

GUIDELINES FOR HANDLING LINENS

By following special guidelines for handling linens you will be creating a safer environment:

* Roll soiled linen gently and be on the lookout for personal items such as dentures, wallets, and pajamas.
* Never carry soiled linens against your body. Hold them away from you so you do not spread microorganisms.
* Always place soiled linen in the laundry hamper or other appropriate containers.
* Keep all containers holding soiled linen covered at all times.
* Never put soiled linen on the furniture in the room or on the floor.
* Never return unused linens to the linen supply cart.
* When you notice that the laundry hamper is full but not overflowing, remove it from the cart and take it to the place from which it will be picked up and taken to the laundry. Place a fresh laundry hamper in the cart.
* If a personal item is lost and you must sort through soiled linens in the laundry hamper, you should wear gloves and not let any soiled linen touch your uniform.

CARING COMMENT

After you complete personal care and linen changes, take a few moments to tidy up the patient's unit so it looks neat and organized.

CHAPTER WRAP-UP

- A bed can be made as an
  Occupied bed
  Unoccupied bed (a closed, open, or surgical bed)
- A closed bed means that the bed is clean, has fresh bed linens, and is ready for a new patient.
- An open bed means that the bed is ready for a patient who wishes to return to it.
- A surgical bed is prepared so that the patient who returns from the recovery room can be transferred in the most comfortable way.
- Soiled linens must be handled in a safe way so that harmful microorganisms are not spread to yourself and others.

REVIEW QUESTIONS

1. How can you tell whether a bed is a closed bed, an open bed, or a surgical bed?
2. Name three reasons for changing the bed linens.
3. What kind of bed describes the situation in which the patient cannot leave the bed while the linens are changed?

ACTIVITY CORNER

The next time you give a patient care, keep track of how many times the patient's bed needed to be changed. What were the reasons the bed needed to be changed?

_____ Patient was on bed rest.

_____ Patient returned from surgery.

_____ Patient was sweating a great amount.

_____ Patient was incontinent of bowels and/or bladder.

_____ Bath water was spilled on the bed.

_____ Other fluids (coffee, tea, etc.) were spilled on the bed.

_____ Other _____

Should you use the problem-solving technique to help you make the decision to change the bed linens? Yes _____ No _____

Making Patients Comfortable 15

15 Making Patients Comfortable

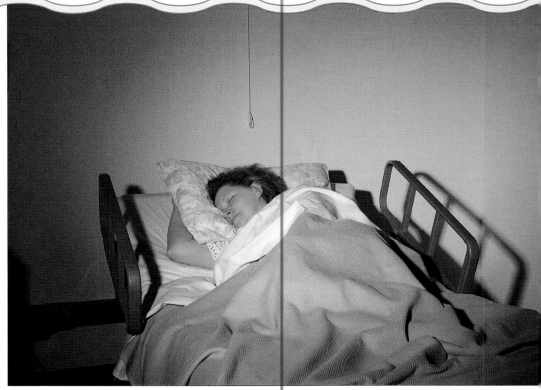

Objectives

AFTER YOU COMPLETE THIS CHAPTER, YOU WILL BE ABLE TO:

Define the terms *comfort, rest,* and *sleep.*

Describe the need for comfort, rest, and sleep.

Describe pain.

List observations of the patient in pain.

Provide care for the patient in pain.

List observations of the sleep-deprived patient.

Describe the care of the patient with sleep disruptions.

Overview All humans need comfort, rest, and sleep. These states provide the body time to prepare for the stresses of everyday life. In addition to refreshing the mind and body, these states help the body with healing. When people become ill, their need for comfort, rest, and sleep increases. If this need is not met, the body and mind react in various ways.

WHAT DO YOU KNOW ABOUT COMFORT AND SLEEP?

Here are eight statements about comfort, rest, and sleep. Consider them to test your current ideas about these states. If you think the statement is true, circle the T; if you think the statement is false, circle the F. Change the false statements to make them true.

1. T F The average person does not rest during the day.
2. T F Rest and sleep mean the same thing.
3. T F Pain cannot be seen.
4. T F A person is most comfortable sleeping in a high Fowler's position.
5. T F The environment in a hospital or long-term care facility can disturb sleep.
6. T F Many people follow a bedtime ritual as they prepare for sleep.
7. T F The person who is not able to sleep has a condition known as sleepwalking.
8. T F A sleep cycle lasts about 8 hours.

ANSWERS

1. **False.** People do rest during the day. Each person's mode of rest is individual.
2. **False.** Rest is a time of freedom from activity and labor. It is not necessarily sleep. Sleep is the natural suspension of consciousness during which the powers of the body are restored.
3. **True.** One can observe the behavior of a person in pain, but one cannot actually see pain.
4. **False.** This almost upright position is comfortable only for persons who have chronic breathing problems, because it helps them breathe better.
5. **True.** Undesirable sights, sounds, and smells can easily disturb sleep. Because patients are not able to control the distractions, they can become frustrated.

6. **True.** Although it is especially important to children, people at all ages practice some type of bedtime ritual. A bedtime ritual provides comfort, security, and ease in falling asleep.
7. **False.** A person who walks while sleeping is sleepwalking; the person who cannot sleep is an insomniac.
8. **False.** A sleep cycle normally lasts about 90–100 minutes.

COMFORT

COMFORT
a sense of contented well-being

DISCOMFORT
distress; mental or physical uneasiness

PAIN
a feeling of discomfort, suffering, or agony

The person who is comfortable is in a state of contented well-being. **Comfort** promotes health. When persons feel mental or physical uneasiness, they may be experiencing **discomfort** or **pain.**

PAIN

Pain is a feeling of discomfort, suffering, or agony (Figure 15–1). Pain is a universal experience, and people of all ages experience it. There are a number of theories about how pain occurs, but experts are not certain of any one explanation. Pain serves as a warning signal; it is how the body alerts a person to danger (Figure 15–2). Report patients' comments about pain to the supervisor or nurse.

Recognizing a Patient in Pain

SUBJECTIVE OBSERVATION
information gathered through the statements of another person, for example, "I am cold"

SUBJECTIVE OBSERVATIONS Each person feels pain differently. It is a subjective experience that no one can see. Only the person who is having the pain can describe it. H*urt* and *ache* are words often used to indicate pain. When patients tell you they have pain, listen for descriptive words that they use and make **subjective observations.** Use patients' own words to report and record the presence of pain. Subjective words patients may use to describe their pain or discomfort include

ache   *cramping*
dull   *crushing*
sore   *piercing*
sharp   *pressure*
tender   *stabbing*
burning   *squeezing*
gnawing   *throbbing*
constant   ***excruciating***

EXCRUCIATING
very intense

In addition to asking for a description of how the pain feels, you can ask patients the following questions about their pain:

- When did the pain start?
- Describe what the pain feels like.
- Can you tell me what you think might be causing the pain?
- Where is the pain located?
- Did you ever have pain like this before?
- How long did it last?
- What helped the pain?
- On a scale of 1 to 10, how much pain do you have?

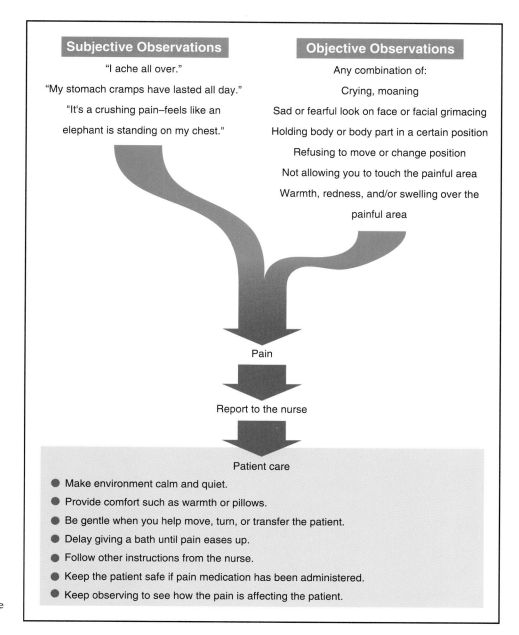

Subjective Observations

"I ache all over."

"My stomach cramps have lasted all day."

"It's a crushing pain–feels like an elephant is standing on my chest."

Objective Observations

Any combination of:

Crying, moaning

Sad or fearful look on face or facial grimacing

Holding body or body part in a certain position

Refusing to move or change position

Not allowing you to touch the painful area

Warmth, redness, and/or swelling over the painful area

Pain

Report to the nurse

Patient care

- Make environment calm and quiet.
- Provide comfort such as warmth or pillows.
- Be gentle when you help move, turn, or transfer the patient.
- Delay giving a bath until pain eases up.
- Follow other instructions from the nurse.
- Keep the patient safe if pain medication has been administered.
- Keep observing to see how the pain is affecting the patient.

FIGURE 15–1

Flow chart for pain and what the nursing assistant needs to do.

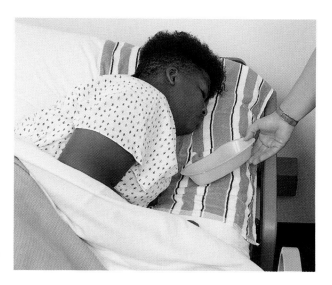

FIGURE 15–2

Observe the patient's behavior for signs of pain or discomfort.

CARING COMMENT

If a patient tells you, "I hurt all over," ask the patient to point to the spot where it hurts the most.

OBJECTIVE OBSERVATIONS   Observe the behaviors of patients in pain. Although you cannot see patients' pain, you can observe the way they react to it. This is known as **objective observation.** The following are behaviors that may indicate a patient is in pain (Figure 15–2):

OBJECTIVE OBSERVATION
information gathered by using the five senses: sight, hearing, smell, taste, and touch

- crying
- moaning
- sad or fearful facial expression
- facial grimacing
- clenched fists
- holding the body or body part in a certain position
- not allowing anyone to touch the painful area
- refusing to move
- warmth, redness, or swelling over the affected body part

You may observe changes in the body that occur as a response to pain. These changes include

- increased pulse rate
- increased respiratory rate
- increased systolic blood pressure
- pallor (paleness of the skin)
- diaphoresis (sweating)
- pupil dilation (pupils become larger)
- nausea and vomiting

Again, report any behaviors you observe about patients' pain to the nurse or supervisor. The nurse or supervisor is responsible for assessing patients further to determine whether a medication to decrease pain is needed.

CARING COMMENT

Remember that people of certain cultures do not always express pain verbally. It is all right to ask your patient, "Are you in pain?"

It is especially important to observe for comfort or discomfort in patients who cannot tell you verbally about pain. Infants and young children are unable to tell you they have pain, so you must be a keen observer of these patients. A child who is of preschool age (3–5) can usually tell you when something hurts. You might try drawing three circles in a row. In the circle at one end, draw a smiley face and in the circle at the other end draw a very sad face. In the middle circle, draw a wavy line for the mouth. Ask the child to point at the face that shows how much pain there is. Children closer to the age of 5 may be able to draw a face showing how the pain is making them feel. You might also ask children to squeeze your hand as hard as the pain feels. Slight pressure might mean slight pain while a harder, firm pressure might mean more pain is present.

The elderly person with a chronic disease may have pain or discomfort. Older persons may not tell you that they have pain because they believe nothing can be done or no one cares. In a long-term care setting such as the nursing home, you learn about your patients' reactions to pain over a longer period of time. You may be the first to observe some of the effects of pain listed above on your patients' behavior. In addition to the observations already discussed, look for these other signs:

- change in appetite
- increased need for sleep and rest
- decreased ability or desire to perform activities of daily living
- changes in behavior such as anxiety, withdrawal from activities and socializing, or depression

CARING FOR THE PATIENT IN PAIN

Observe patients for the signs and symptoms of pain discussed in the preceding section and report your observations to the nurse or supervisor. When patients tell you they are in pain, report this information to the nurse or supervisor. The nurse is responsible for giving medication to relieve pain.

There are some things you can do to make patients in pain as comfortable as possible:

- Provide a calm, quiet environment.
- Darken the room by shutting off lights or pulling blinds or draperies closed.
- Respond to patients' needs, for example, by providing ice water or an extra blanket or pillow.
- Offer a back rub.
- Help patients change position.
- Adjust the room temperature when requested.
- Use the most gentle touch possible when handling or moving a painful body part.
- Wait until the pain has decreased to perform procedures such as giving a bath or performing range of motion exercises.
- Elevate the painful body part when this has been ordered by the physician. (Follow instructions from the nurse.)
- Apply warmth or cold to the painful areas when this has been ordered by the physician. (Follow instructions from the nurse.)

REST

Rest is the condition in which a person is free from activity and labor. It can involve the entire body or a part of the body. People can rest while they are awake or asleep. The need for rest is very individual. People do many things that help them rest. Examples of resting activities are

REST
freedom from activity and labor

- sunbathing
- watching TV
- listening to soft music
- resting in bed (Figure 15–3)
- reading a book or magazine
- doing a craft (such as knitting or painting)

Rest produces muscular relaxation and a calm mental attitude and prepares the person for sleep. Even 15 minutes of rest can relieve stress. Rest clears the mind and relaxes the body so individuals are better able to face the demands of their day. Rest allows the body to repair itself, remove wastes, and restore tissue.

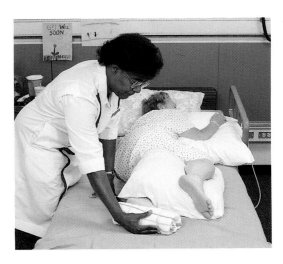

FIGURE 15-3
Physical comfort enhances the rest period.

SUBJECTIVE OBSERVATIONS

Your patient may tell you, "I need to rest." After a period of rest, the patient might say, "That was a good rest!" These comments, in which patients tell you their feelings about rest, are examples of subjective observations of resting. Use patients' own words to report and record how they feel after resting.

You can ask patients the following questions about their resting habits:

- How often do you take a rest?
- Do you think that rest periods are important?

After a rest period, you can ask them

- How do you feel now that your rest period is over?
- Did the rest period help you?

OBJECTIVE OBSERVATIONS

You can observe patients objectively during periods of rest. You may observe the following in the patient who is resting:

- closed eyes
- decreased rate of breathing
- decreased response to outside stimulation (for example, may not answer to name when called)

WHEN IS REST NEEDED?

Patients who are rested look relaxed whether they are walking, sitting, or lying in bed.

In the hospital setting, patients may need several rest periods scheduled throughout the day. Very ill persons may need to rest in between or during activities of daily living (bathing, toileting, dressing, and grooming). Remember that very ill or recovering patients may not have the strength to complete their activities of daily living unless rest periods are provided by the care giver. For example, after the bath has been completed, you should provide the very ill patient with a rest period before you change the bed linens. A 20- to 30-minute rest period helps the patient gather strength and energy for the next activity.

In the long-term care setting, a rest period may be scheduled for all patients at the same time. The rest period is usually scheduled after the noon meal. Ill patients are scheduled rest periods more often until they regain their usual level of functioning.

In both the hospital and long-term care settings, a rest time is usually scheduled for children after the noon meal. Curtains are closed and TV sets and radios are turned off or put on low volume to help the children relax and gain some rest.

SLEEP

Sleep is a state of unconsciousness. It is the natural periodic suspension of consciousness during which the powers of the body are restored. When asleep, people have a decreased perception of their surroundings. A person can be wakened by sleep by an appropriate **stimulus.** A ringing alarm clock, a baby's cry, and calling them by name are stimuli that can wake up sleeping persons.

Sleep is needed for mental and emotional balance. It eases stress and tension and helps people regain energy. People's requirements for sleep and rest vary according to their individual needs. People who are ill need more rest and sleep than healthy people.

SLEEP
the natural periodic suspension of consciousness during which the body's mental and physical powers are restored

STIMULUS
something that causes an activity to start

SLEEP CYCLE

Humans function according to a sleep cycle in which a certain amount of sleep and rest is needed every 24 hours. The sleep cycle is influenced by a 24-hour cycle called the **circadian** rhythm. The circadian rhythm is like a built-in biologic clock. These biologic clocks are found in plants, animals, and humans. The events in the environment, such as light and darkness, regulate the biologic clock. For example, flowers open in response to daylight and close when darkness falls.

CIRCADIAN
occurring about every 24 hours

The need for sleep is a common example of the biologic clock at work in the human body. Most people average about 8 hours of sleep during every 24-hour period. However, some can function on less sleep and others may require more.

People also have a period of increased activity during every 24-hour period. During this time, a person is more energetic and is able to think better. This energetic period in the 24-hour period is different for everyone. A person who is awake and alert at or before sunup is called a "lark." The lark functions best physically and emotionally during the early daylight hours. "Owls" are people who come alive after the sun goes down. For them, the night hours are the most productive time to be awake.

STAGES OF SLEEP

Two kinds of sleep occur in each individual:

rapid eye movement (REM) sleep
nonREM sleep

Key points about REM and nonREM sleep are as follows:

- REM sleep and nonREM sleep occur in a series of stages during the night.
- Very distinct changes occur during each stage.
- A person must go through each stage in a certain sequence to gain the benefits of sleep.
- Each cycle of sleep lasts about 90 minutes.
- A person has four to six of these cycles each night.

REM Sleep

**RADID EYE MOVEMENT
(REM) SLEEP**
the active stage of sleep, in which
the eyeballs move rapidly

Rapid eye movement (REM) sleep is an active sleep. During this stage, people move their eyeballs rapidly. Their dreams are colorful, exciting, and busy. The muscles are very relaxed, and the heart rate may be irregular and faster than normal. The amount of REM sleep affects the quality (restful or restless) of sleep. The quantity of sleep is the length of time a person sleeps. During REM sleep, people review the events of the day and store this information. REM sleep refreshes and restores the *mental processes* of the individual.

NonREM Sleep

NONREM SLEEP
the deep, restful stage of sleep, in
which eyeball movement is slow and
rolling

NonREM sleep is a deep, restful sleep. People become more relaxed during this stage. Their eyeball movements are slow and rolling. They may have simple, ordinary dreams or no dreams at all in this stage. All the body's vital signs are decreased at this time. NonREM sleep restores the person *physically*.

FACTORS THAT AFFECT SLEEP

Factors that can affect a person's sleep requirements include

    Age
    Eating
    Environment
    Exercise
    Hormonal changes
    Illness
    Medications

Age

About 50% of newborns' sleeping is REM sleep. In contrast, only about 15% of elderly persons' sleeping is REM sleep. Newborns often sleep 16–20 hours of every 24-hour period. As they age, humans generally need less sleep. During school age (ages 6–12), children need only 10–12 hours of sleep. Elderly persons usually require only about 6 hours of sleep each night.

Eating

CAFFEINE
a substance in coffee, tea, colas,
and chocolate that acts as a
stimulant and diuretic

Caloric intake (eating) before bedtime interferes with sleep. When a person digests food, energy is produced. This causes a person to become too alert and energetic to sleep. **Caffeine** in certain beverages and food (coffee, tea, soda pop, and chocolate) gives a quick boost to the mind and body so the person cannot relax enough to fall asleep.

Environment

ENVIRONMENT
the conditions, circumstances, or
objects that surround a person

One's **environment** can help or hinder sleep. A comfortable room temperature and a quiet atmosphere help persons to rest and fall asleep according to the routine of their choice (Figure 15–4). Distracting noises or light, whether at home or in a health care institution, can interfere with an individual's sleep routine.

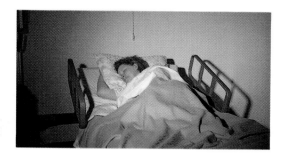

FIGURE 15-4
A comfortable environment free of distractions can help the patient get the rest and sleep needed for healing.

Exercise

A baby or young child who is "fighting" sleep may have had a busy, overactive day with a lot of **exercise.** This can result in a feeling referred to as being "too tired to fall asleep."

Moderate exercise helps a person to relax and fall asleep much easier. Strenuous exercise just before bedtime can activate the body's functions and keep persons awake and alert long after their usual bedtime.

EXERCISE
the performance of physical activity to improve health

Hormone Changes

Hormonal changes in the body can affect an individual's pattern of sleep. For example, the changes caused by pregnancy increase the need for sleep in the pregnant woman. Hormonal changes also occur during periods of active growth, and therefore teenagers require extra sleep to remain healthy.

HORMONE
a substance that endocrine glands secrete directly into the blood; the hormone travels to a designated place in the body where it is used in a chemical action

Illness

Illness disrupts an individual's normal pattern of sleep. More sleep than usual is needed. Pain can prevent sleep or actually wake up a patient, however.

Medications

Certain medications interfere with an individual's REM sleep needs and result in a poor quality of sleep. Medications may contain caffeine, a stimulant that can prevent rest and sleep.

Sleep Patterns

Sleep patterns govern how, when, and where a person sleeps. Most people adjust to the rhythm that is most comfortable and convenient for them. Health care givers, police officers, factory workers, and other night shift employees may find that shift work interferes with the natural circadian rhythm of their body. Disrupted sleep patterns result in lack or loss of sleep.

OBSERVING A SLEEPING PATIENT

If you are assigned to care for patients during the night shift, you are expected to observe the patients as they sleep. A comfortable, relaxed position and quiet, even breathing are the most noticeable observations of sleeping patients. Patients who sleep well look rested in the morning and often tell you that they had a good night's sleep. Patients who cannot sleep may toss and turn in bed. They may get out of bed and pace, watch TV, or read. These patients probably will not look or feel rested in the morning. Puffy eyes and dark circles below the eyes are signs of disrupted sleep.

CARING COMMENT

Use a flashlight when you check patients during the night. Point the flashlight at the floor to light the way. Then direct the beam of light toward the patient. Observe that the patient is breathing.

The flashlight is also used to check any equipment in the room, such as an intravenous line or oxygen equipment, at night. The nurse or supervisor tells you what observations you need to make at night.

OBSERVING A PATIENT WITH SLEEP DISRUPTIONS

The lack of sleep may result in physical and mental changes in an individual. Below are observations you may make about patients with sleep disruptions:

- Acting fatigued when they awaken
- Frequent yawning and dozing during the daylight hours
- Puffy eyes and dark circles under them
- Saying that they did not sleep well (even if you thought they looked asleep when you checked on them, you should believe the patients because each individual is the best judge of benefit of a good night's sleep)
- Shortened attention span
- Change in attitude (for example, a normally cheerful individual may become irritable and easily frustrated by a lack or loss of sleep)

THE HOUR-OF-SLEEP ROUTINE

Each individual has a routine at bedtime. Some people may think of a bedtime routine (or ritual) as something practiced by babies and young children. However, people of all ages keep an hour-of-sleep routine for much the same reasons as babies and children do (Figure 15–5). A routine provides a comfort-

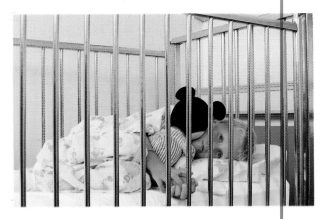

FIGURE 15–5
A favorite stuffed toy or a special blanket offers a feeling of comfort and security as the child falls asleep.

able, secure feeling (Figure 15–5). It is also a signal to the mind and body to prepare for a good night's sleep.

Ask patients about their hour-of-sleep routine. For child patients, you may have to ask their parents what the bedtime routine is. Do your best to help patients or children maintain the same routine. Try to reduce extra lights and noises to provide a comfortable environment for patients. Plan your activities so that patients are not awakened unnecessarily. For example, you can measure vital signs and turn and position the patient at the same time, disturbing the patient only once instead of twice.

CARING COMMENT

You may need to take vital sign measurements during the night or turn and position your patient. It is a good idea to tell the patient this will happen. Patients do not need to be awake for most nighttime procedures and can continue to sleep if they desire.

You can suggest a glass of milk at bedtime to increase the chances of falling asleep. A back rub often helps relax a patient of any age.

If you know a patient's sleep is disturbed by drinking caffeinated beverages (coffee, tea, and colas), offer a substitute beverage. Remember that coffee, tea, and colas are available in decaffeinated forms. In some instances, you may observe that a patient who is receiving **diuretics** (also called water pills) or who drinks a lot of fluids just before bedtime will awaken during the night one or more times for toileting. Always record and report this observation to the supervisor or nurse.

DIURETIC
a substance that causes an increase in urination

For patients who nap or doze during the day, an increase in daytime activities is important so that they will be able to sleep at night. If able, these patients should walk a little more and try to limit the number of naps they take during the day. You can add to the usual bedtime routine by giving the patient a warm bath and a back rub. Soft music and lighting may also help some patients fall asleep.

Children need special attention to their bedtime routine. Children may become frustrated if their routine is not followed in the order to which they are accustomed. In most health care institutions, parents are encouraged to stay and assist in the care of their child. The presence of one or both parents provides security for the ill child. When a parent is unable to remain during the night, the child may experience a sense of abandonment. Children often have vivid nightmares and are fearful in strange environments. Spend extra time with young patients so they become comfortable with you as well as the health care setting.

CARING FOR PATIENTS WITH COMMON DISRUPTIONS IN SLEEP

INSOMNIA

Insomnia is the inability to fall asleep easily or to remain asleep throughout the night. The person with insomnia is called an insomniac. Another problem of insomniacs is that they can awaken earlier than usual and cannot

INSOMNIA
the inability to fall asleep easily or remain asleep throughout the night

fall back to sleep again. This is considered an abnormal sleep pattern. No one understands why insomnia occurs.

The nursing assistant can help the insomniac by encouraging a quiet atmosphere before bedtime. The patient should go to bed for the night only when sleepy or tired. If the patient is unable to sleep, provide reading material or music, or you can offer to stay and talk with the patient. Some patients are more willing to talk about their fears and concerns during the night. Patients may ask you if they can have something to help them sleep. Report your observations and the patient request to the nurse or your supervisor. Only the nurse can give patients something to help them sleep.

SLEEP DEPRIVATION

SLEEP DEPRIVATION

a prolonged loss of sleep that occurs when rapid eye movement sleep is interrupted over a long period of time

Sleep deprivation is a prolonged lack of sleep. It occurs when a person's REM sleep is frequently interrupted over a long period of time. Patients in the intensive care unit often experience sleep deprivation. Whenever pain, anxiety, or medications interfere with sleep and rest, sleep deprivation can occur. Patients may be irritable and doze throughout the day. You might notice that they are unable to concentrate long enough to answer brief questions appropriately. Over a period of time, the patients begin acting fatigued, sleepy, and restless. Confusion, depression, disorientation, and lack of coordination can follow. The best ways to help sleep-deprived patients are to

- make them as comfortable as possible
- arrange your care so that they can sleep for longer periods at a time.

SLEEPWALKING

SLEEPWALK

to rise from bed and walk in an apparent state of sleep

The person who **sleepwalks** arises from bed and walks in an apparent state of sleep. A person does not remember sleepwalking. If a patient has a known history of sleepwalking, you will receive this information during the change of shift report. The greatest danger to patients who sleepwalk is injury. Sleepwalkers may attempt to climb over the side rails during the night and hurt themselves. If an intravenous solution is infusing (running), it can be dislodged when the patient gets up to sleepwalk.

It is important for you to know what to do for patients who sleepwalk. If you know that a particular patient sleepwalks, be especially observant of the patient during the night. Keep floors clear and uncluttered. Sleepwalkers should be awakened gently and helped to orient themselves to what has happened. Assure patients that they are safe and that you will keep a closer watch over them during the night.

THE CARE GIVER AND SHIFT WORK

Remember that care givers who lack sleep can experience the same effects as a patient who lacks sleep. Not all persons fall asleep when they arrive home from work, no matter what shift they work. If you work the night shift (11 p.m.– 7 a.m.), the following hints may help you establish a routine and get to sleep:

- Plan time to relax and unwind. Will a shower and change of clothing help you relax? Will an exercise class help you unwind? What do you do when you come home from other shifts you work? Can some of the same activities be done in the early morning?

- Plan what meals you will eat that day. If you ate one meal at work, at what times will you eat two other meals? Will you be able to prepare meals for others in the family if you need to and eat with them?
- Plan what chores need to be done and when you will do them. Do the children need help getting ready for school? Do you have the energy to clean house or run errands early in the morning, or is early afternoon best for you?
- Attend to the needs of your family if you are a parent. When can you be available for them? When is it best for you to schedule appointments (doctor's, teacher's, music lessons, etc.)? If you have small children, can you make arrangements for their care while you sleep?
- You may need to adjust your social life for the period you are scheduled to work the night shift. When is the best time for you to call or visit friends and relatives?
- Give yourself and your family time to adjust to your routine of working nights or rotating shifts.
- Determine what block of time (usually about 8 hours) you will set aside to sleep. You will find this is very individual. You may need to experiment with different blocks of time until you find the one that is best for you.
- Establish a special hour-of-sleep routine and follow it. Does reading help you fall asleep? Will a quiet, darkened room encourage sleep? Remember that some of the measures that help patients relax and fall asleep may help you get a good night's sleep too.

CHAPTER WRAP-UP

- The need for comfort, rest, and sleep is universal. All individuals have certain requirements for each.
- Comfort is a sense of well-being.
- Discomfort and pain interfere with a person's sense of well-being.
- Rest and sleep allow the body time to heal and the mind time to refresh itself.
- Rest and sleep can be disturbed by changes in the body and in the environment.
- The amount of sleep people need averages about 8 hours a night.
- Patients who are sleeping restfully look comfortable while sleeping and turn and position themselves with slow, relaxed movements.
- Insomnia is the inability to fall asleep or stay asleep.
- Insomniacs toss and turn frequently and appear to be fighting with the linens.
- Puffiness and black circles under the eyes can indicate lack of restful sleep. You may also observe the patient dozing and napping during the day.
- Activities that help patients sleep include a nap before lunch, a back rub, hot decaffeinated tea or warm milk (if allowed) before bedtime, and encouragement to follow their usual routine.
- A night shift (11 p.m.–7 a.m.) worker should plan a routine that allows regular sleep.

REVIEW QUESTIONS

1. Describe what you would observe in a patient who is experiencing pain or discomfort.
2. How will you comfort the patient who is experiencing pain?
3. What are the benefits of sleep?
4. List the factors that affect sleep.

ACTIVITY CORNER

Ask two people to think about a time they were in pain. Then ask them the following questions and place their answers in the appropriate column. Think about a time you were in pain and place your own answers in the last column.

Question	First Person	Second Person	Yourself
What kind of pain was it (throbbing, sharp, etc.)?			
How did you react to the pain (cry, grit your teeth, etc.)?			
Who listened when you had pain (spouse, friend, etc.)?			
What did people do to help you (talked softly, made the room quiet, etc.)?			
What made you comfortable (lying still, not thinking about it, etc.)?			

Compare the answers. Realize there are important differences in how people react to pain and what helps them feel better.

Ask people from three different age groups the following questions about their sleep patterns and routines. Place their answers in the appropriate column.

Question	Person Aged 13–21	Person Aged 21–55	Person Aged 56–85+
What is your usual bedtime routine?			
How many hours do you sleep each night?			
Is it easy or difficult for you to fall asleep?			

Is it easy or difficult for you to wake up? _____ _____ _____

Do you take daytime naps? _____ _____ _____

Do you feel rested with the amount of sleep you get? _____ _____ _____

Compare the answers. Are any answers the result of the person's age or life-style?

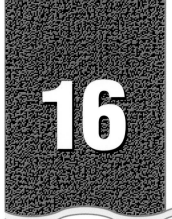

16 Helping with Activity and Mobility

Objectives

AFTER YOU COMPLETE THIS CHAPTER, YOU WILL BE ABLE TO:

Describe the structure and function of the muscles and bones of the body.

Move and turn patients.

Describe complications that can occur when a patient is inactive and immobile.

Describe measures taken to prevent complications in the patient who is inactive and immobile.

Perform range of motion exercises on all extremities.

Apply an elastic bandage.

Define the term *bone fracture*.

Discuss the care of a patient with a hip fracture.

Discuss the care of the patient with a cast.

List the observations of a patient with a cerebrovascular accident.

Care for a patient with a cerebrovascular accident.

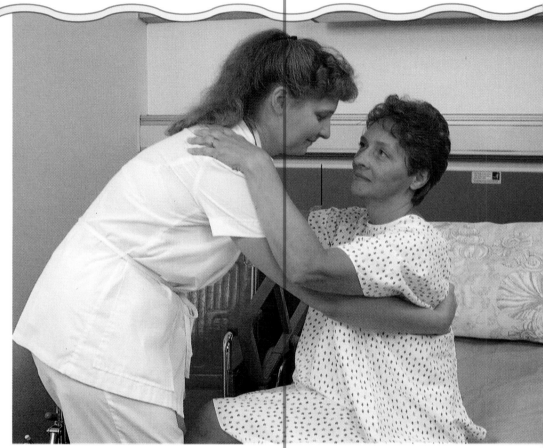

Overview   Due to broken bones, injuries, strokes, and other illnesses, many patients are not able to move or be as active as they are used to being. This may affect their outlook on life and their physical health. Your assistance can be invaluable in helping these patients return to the point where they are feeling and moving well and can do most things for themselves again.

WHAT DO YOU KNOW ABOUT ACTIVITY AND MOBILITY?

Here are 11 statements about activity and mobility. Consider them to test your current ideas about activity and mobility. If you think the statement is true, circle the T; if you think the statement is false, circle the F. Change the false statements to make them true.

1. T   F   The nerves help regulate the movement of muscles and bones.
2. T   F   Middle age is the most energetic time of life.
3. T   F   Exercise increases the circulation of blood through all the body tissues.
4. T   F   A patient can lose weight while on bed rest.
5. T   F   Secretions of the body are loosened by movement and activity.
6. T   F   Many patients on bed rest develop diarrhea.
7. T   F   Sitting up in a chair contributes to a patient's mobility.
8. T   F   A change in activity and mobility affects a person's self-image.
9. T   F   Passive range of motion exercises are done by the patient alone, with no help.
10. T   F   Surgery is needed to help broken bones heal.
11. T   F   A stroke (cerebrovascular accident) always leaves a patient paralyzed.

ANSWERS

1. **True.** Muscle and bone cannot work together unless they are stimulated by the nerves.
2. **False.** The most energetic time of life occurs during infancy and toddlerhood.
3. **True.** Blood carries fresh oxygen to the body tissues, and exercise causes more blood to be delivered.

4. **True.** If a patient is not able to eat or experiences a loss of appetite, weight loss can occur.
5. **True.** When a person lies in one spot, secretions become thicker and remain in place (especially in the lungs).
6. **False.** Because the activity of the intestines slows down during bed rest, more patients experience constipation.
7. **True.** Sitting provides a change in position. It also provides an increase in sensory stimulation (seeing and hearing).
8. **True.** Patients who lose the ability to move and walk unassisted may feel powerless and without control. They may value themselves less and become depressed.
9. **False.** Active range of motion exercises are done by the person. You will perform passive range of motion exercises for patients who are unable to do the exercises themselves.
10. **False.** A simple, closed fracture can heal with the support of a cast. If the bone fragments pierce the skin, or other major repair is needed, surgery is performed.
11. **False.** Paralysis is only one possible result of a stroke. The results of a stroke vary from person to person.

STRUCTURE AND FUNCTION OF BONES AND MUSCLES

MOBILITY
ability to move or be moved
MUSCULOSKELETAL
referring to muscle and skeleton

The activity and **mobility** of the body are provided by the muscles and bones. Muscles and bones are part of the **musculoskeletal** system (Figures 16–1 and 16–2). These muscle and skeletal systems are often linked together because they work in harmony to provide movement. The nervous system also plays a role in mobility, by regulating movement. The brain sends messages along nerves to each muscle to produce movement.

BONES

BONE
the hard, rigid connective tissue that makes up most of the skeleton

The 206 bones of the body make up the skeletal system. **Bone** is a hard tissue that is constantly created. Special cells are responsible for bone creation. The size and strength of a bone are determined when the bone is created. The bone has a blood supply, and a network of sensory nerves regulates its movement.

Function of Bone

The bones of the skeletal system function to

LEVERAGE
mechanical advantage gained by using a lever

- Support surrounding tissue and provide a framework for the entire body.
- Protect the vital organs (heart and lungs) and the soft tissues of the body (liver).
- Assist with movement (by providing **leverage** and a place of attachment for muscles).
- Manufacture red blood cells in the marrow.
- Store mineral salts like calcium and phosphorus.

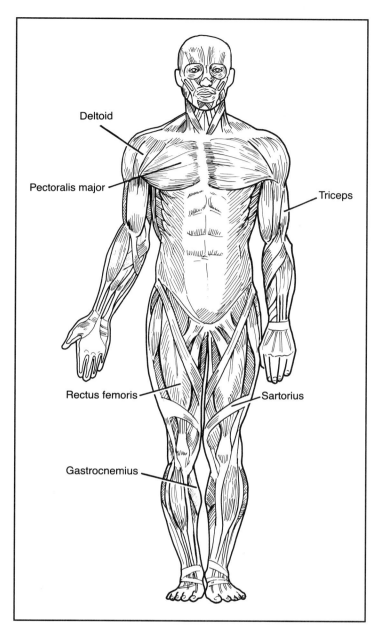

FIGURE 16-1
The muscles of the body.

Classification of Bone

Bones are classified according to their shape. There are four types of bones in the human body.

LONG BONES Long bones are found in the long parts of the body, such as the arms and legs. The thigh bone is the longest bone in the body. It supports the weight of the body.

SHORT BONES Short bones are located in the hands, fingers, and feet.

FLAT BONES Flat bones make up the rib cage, which protects the heart and lungs, and the skull, which protects the brain.

IRREGULAR-SHAPED BONES Irregular-shaped bones include the bones of the spinal column and the small bones of the ear.

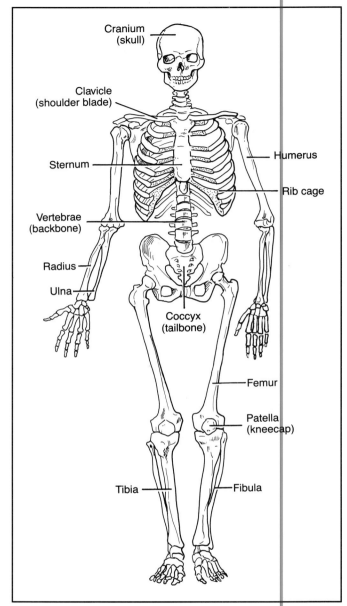

Cranium
(skull)

Clavicle
(shoulder blade)

Sternum

Humerus

Rib cage

Vertebrae
(backbone)

Radius

Ulna

Coccyx
(tailbone)

Femur

Patella
(kneecap)

Tibia

Fibula

FIGURE 16—2
Anterior (front) view of the bones of the body.

JOINTS

JOINT

the place where two or more bones
meet

A **joint** is the area of contact between two bones. Joints are classified according to how much they move. The three main types of joint are

Moveable
Partially moveable
Immobile

The moveable joints are the most common joints in the body. When you sit down, you flex (bend) your hips and knees. When you open a jar, you use your fingers. These are examples of moveable joints in action. Most joints in the body are moveable. The other joints are much fewer in number. The area where the ribs attach to the spine is an example of a partially moveable joint. The bones that **fuse** together in the skull are examples of immovable joints.

The moveable joints permit the body to make changes in its position and motion. No direct contact of bone occurs when two bones meet in a moveable joint (for example, in a finger), because the ends of the bones are covered by a substance called the **articular cartilage.** This cartilage acts like a shock absorber when the bones are jolted or used for leverage.

The place where two bony surfaces meet is enclosed by a tough connective tissue called the articular capsule. A membrane inside the capsule secretes synovial fluid. The **synovial fluid** acts like a **lubricant** and reduces friction when the joints are moved.

Joints deteriorate (wear down) to some degree as people age. Less synovial fluid is secreted in articular capsules. The articular cartilage at the ends of bones ossifies (becomes bone), causing stiffness, **inflammation,** and pain. As a result, the person experiences decreased mobility.

MUSCLES

The **muscles** of the body produce movement or motion by contracting (shortening) and relaxing (lengthening). The nerves of the body tell muscles to contract and relax to produce movement. Muscles contain a rich blood supply and need oxygen to function. Muscles make up 40–50% of the body's weight.

Muscles that are attached to bone are called skeletal muscles. They are usually long, slender bundles of muscle fibers. The nervous system maintains skeletal muscle tone by keeping muscles partially contracted and ready for movement. This is called muscle tone. The person who exercises on a regular basis has good muscle tone. If a person is ill and does not exercise regularly, muscle tone can be lost.

ACTIVITY AND MOBILITY

Activity is some type of action taken by a person. Mobility is the ability to move about (Figure 16–3). Activity and mobility are accomplished by muscles and bones that are directed by the body's nervous system.

People seldom think of their activities as something that contribute to their **health** and well-being. However, activity has a positive effect on the mind and body, just as lack of activity and mobility has a negative effect.

FUSE
to blend or join together
ARTICULAR
pertaining to a joint
CARTILAGE
a fibrous semi-rigid tissue found in adults

SYNOVIAL FLUID
a fluid that lubricates joints to reduce friction when they move
LUBRICANT
a substance that reduces friction
INFLAMMATION
a painful red swelling; the body's response to illness or injury

MUSCLE
fibrous tissue that expands and contracts to allow the body to move

ACTIVITY
an action or function

HEALTH
any state of physical, emotional, and social well-being felt by an individual

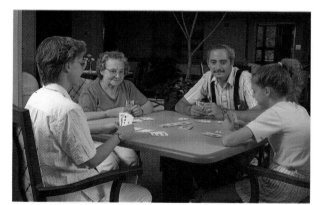

FIGURE 16–3
Performing everyday activities depends on a person's ability to move about.

POSITIVE EFFECTS ON THE MIND

STRESS
pressure caused by something in the internal or external environment
DEPRESSION
sadness and a decrease in the usual behaviors associated with daily functioning

Activity helps the body and mind reduce tension and relieve **stress.** Persons who are experiencing stress may keep their feelings bottled up. Physical activity provides a release for this kind of energy. A person who is not able to move and be active can feel useless, helpless, and **depressed.**

POSITIVE EFFECTS ON THE BODY

OXYGEN
a colorless, tasteless, odorless gas; the air we breathe is about 20% oxygen
CIRCULATION
the movement of blood through the body caused by the heart's pumping action
GASTROINTESTINAL TRACT
the small and large intestines
URINARY
pertaining to urine
ELIMINATION
the way the body rids itself of unusable food and fluid; the discharge of the waste products created by the body's metabolism
CONTRACTION
shortening or tightening of a muscle
RELAXATION
easing of tension, resting

Each area of the body function benefits by activity and mobility. Physical activity:

- Helps the musculoskeletal system increase or maintain joint mobility. Weight-bearing exercise such as walking helps keep bones strong (Figure 16–4).
- Helps the heart and lungs function more efficiently. The lungs develop a better capacity to take in **oxygen.** They complete the oxygen–carbon dioxide exchange more efficiently and send more oxygen-rich blood to the cells. The heart muscle becomes stronger with exercise, so each beat pumps more blood, making fewer beats necessary.
- Improves the **circulation** of the blood, so more oxygen is delivered to the body's tissues. The improved circulation of blood to the skin produces a healthy pink color and strengthens skin tone.
- Improves the appetite and strengthens the tone of the **gastrointestinal tract.**
- Improves **urinary** function. More blood flows to the kidneys. This results in more efficient **elimination** of the body wastes.
- Helps the colon eliminate stool by assisting in **contraction** and **relaxation** of the colon.
- Stimulates the senses of seeing, hearing, and touching. A person is more alert and responsive to the environment when physical activity is maintained.

FACTORS THAT INFLUENCE ACTIVITY AND MOBILITY

People differ in their levels of activity and mobility. Factors that influence a person's level of activity and mobility include

Health status
Age
Energy level

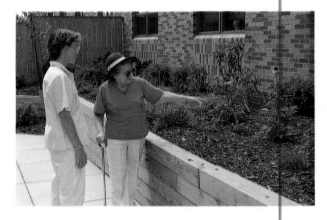

FIGURE 16–4
Walking is a safe exercise for people of all ages.

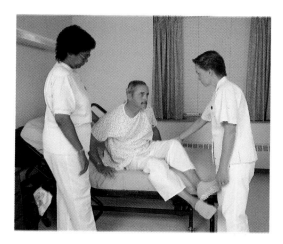

FIGURE 16-5
Activity and mobility are important for patients. They should be encouraged to do as much as possible for themselves.

> Life-style
> Attitude
> Injury and illness

HEALTH STATUS Individuals have their own concepts of what health means to them. Our concepts of health care often based on our

> Culture
> Education
> Family history
> Personal needs

AGE The periods of rapid growth in a human are

> Infancy
> Childhood
> Adolescence

During these periods, the body produces so much energy that the days are never long enough for all there is to accomplish. The decline in activity and mobility begins in adults during middle age. Barely noticeable at first, the body continues slowing down throughout the life span.

ENERGY LEVEL Energy level varies from person to person. It may also vary from one time to another in a person.

LIFE-STYLE AND ATTITUDE People learn the value of activity early in life. Activity is important to maintaining good health at all stages of life.

INJURY AND ILLNESS Many people who are injured or ill experience a reduction in their level of activity and mobility (Figure 16-5).

EFFECTS OF INACTIVITY AND IMMOBILITY

NEGATIVE EFFECTS ON THE MIND

Inactivity and **immobility** may produce profound changes in a patient's emotional status. Patients who are unable to **interact** with their **environment** can experience loneliness and a sense of **isolation.** A sense of worthlessness, a decreased self-concept, and a change in **self-image** can occur.

IMMOBILITY
the inability to move; loss of freedom of movement
INTERACT
to communicate with
ENVIRONMENT
the conditions, circumstances, or objects that surround a person
ISOLATION
being separated
SELF-IMAGE
your idea of who you are and what your role in life is

ILLNESS
sickness; a condition different from the normal health state; any change, temporary or long-lasting, in a person's physical, mental, emotional, or spiritual health and well-being

ATROPHY
to waste away or decrease in size

CONTRACTURE
a shortening of muscle that causes the permanent disability of an extremity; the extremity loses flexibility and freezes in position

MICROORGANISM
an organism so tiny it can be seen only under a microscope; capable of helping the body as well as causing disease

BONY PROMINENCE
any area of the body where bone lies close to the skin (such as elbow or ankle)

DECUBITUS ULCER
a bedsore; a sore caused by continual pressure on the body parts of a patient who must stay in one place

URINARY TRACT INFECTION
infection of the urinary tract, especially the bladder and urethra

CALCULI
stones in the body made up of mineral salts

PERISTALSIS
alternate contraction and relaxation of the esophagus and intestines

DISRUPTION
an interruption of normal function or activity

NEGATIVE EFFECTS ON THE BODY

Just as each area of body function is benefited by activity and mobility, it is affected by inactivity and immobility, for example, during disease or **illness**:

- Muscles **atrophy.**
- Muscles in the limbs or extremities may contract permanently, causing a **contracture** of a limb or extremity
- The heart begins to work harder, and a thrombus (blood clot) could form.
- Secretions remain in the lungs, providing an ideal growing place for harmful **microorganisms.**
- The skin over the **bony prominences** is affected. At first the pressure causes a reddened area. If action is not taken to prevent further pressure, the reddened area can develop into an open **decubitus ulcer.**
- Patients' nutritional status is often affected. They may experience loss of appetite and thus loss of weight. Or they may eat out of boredom and experience a weight gain.
- When a patient remains bedridden, the urine stays in the bladder, providing harmful microorganisms with a place to thrive. A **urinary tract infection** can result. Over a period of time, the urine can form into **calculi.** They can form in the bladder and in the kidneys.
- **Peristalsis** decreases, causing a slowing of intestinal activity and consequently constipation.
- The senses may dull because of the decrease in stimulation. Patients' degree of awareness changes. They might lose track of time, take longer to react to a simple question, and become less alert. The patient may need more time to react to the environment and process information.

COMPLICATIONS ASSOCIATED WITH INACTIVITY AND IMMOBILITY

Disruptions in activity and mobility can affect each area of human functioning (see Complications of Inactivity and Immobility chart). Individuals are affected in their own unique way. Remember that very young and elderly persons are often more affected than others by lack of activity and mobility.

COMPLICATIONS OF INACTIVITY AND IMMOBILITY	
Function	**Complication**
Sensory and perceptual	Sensory deprivation (senses are not stimulated)
	Sensory overload (senses are stimulated too much)
Oxygenation	Hypostatic pneumonia (lung infection caused by long-term bed rest)
	Orthostatic hypotension (dizziness)
	Thrombophlebitis (inflamed blood clot)
Nutrition	Decreased appetite
	Weight loss
Elimination	
Kidneys and bladder	Urinary retention
	Urinary tract infection
	Calculi

	Bladder incontinence
Intestines	Constipation
	Bowel incontinence
Protective	Decubitus ulcer
Comfort, rest, and sleep	Sleeplessness
Activity and mobility	Muscular atrophy
	Contracture
Psycho-socio-cultural	Depression
	Change in self-image

SENSORY AND PERCEPTUAL FUNCTIONS

The brain in immobile patients may misinterpret or not be able to interpret incoming **stimuli** such as light or noise. Also, patients in an intensive care unit (ICU) may not be able to tell night from day because the ICU is usually well lighted. Patients may not respond to harmful stimuli because their nerves do not carry a message of pain to their brain. Pain is the usual warning signal of harm.

OXYGENATION FUNCTIONS

In immobile patients, the lungs may not expand enough for the good oxygen–carbon dioxide exchange that is necessary for breathing. Lying in one position causes an accumulation of secretions in the lungs. In a short period of time, **pneumonia** can develop as a **complication.** This kind of pneumonia is called **hypostatic pneumonia.**

When the lungs are infected or inflamed, they cannot perform as efficiently as they normally do to rid the body of carbon dioxide and take in a fresh supply of oxygen. When a person moves and walks, lung secretions are loosened. They are then brought up to the mouth and coughed out. Thus movement and walking help prevent pneumonia from developing.

When a person lies in bed for a long period of time, the force of gravity and the position of the chest interfere with the exchange of oxygen and carbon dioxide. When the lungs cannot expand enough, less oxygen is delivered to the brain, heart, and other major organs of the body. Remember how important oxygen is to each of the body's tissues (See Chapter 10).

The heart has to beat more often because the blood pumped by each beat contains less oxygen. The heart has to work harder to get oxygen to the tissues of the body. If a person remains inactive, the valves in the veins do not help return the blood to the heart. When this happens, not only is there less blood returned to the heart, but blood can pool (stay) in the lower extremities and cause a **thrombus.**

A thrombus can become loose and travel in the bloodstream until it reaches the lungs or brain. When the thrombus travels, it is called an embolus. The area where it stops does not receive any blood supply and death of tissue occurs. The brain, for example, cannot survive for long without a supply of oxygenated blood. **Thrombophlebitis** is an inflammation of the vein where the clot is formed.

Another condition that may result is orthostatic hypotension. **Orthostatic hypotension** is a dizzy feeling caused by a fall in blood pressure. It occurs when the patient sits or stands up quickly. When patients tell you they feel dizzy as they're standing up or sitting down, let them rest a moment until the blood circulates enough to get rid of the feeling of dizziness.

STIMULI
something that causes an activity to start

PNEUMONIA
acute inflammation or infection of lung tissue
COMPLICATION
the occurrence of another disease or problem in addition to the original disease or problem
HYPOSTATIC PNEUMONIA
infection of the lung that occurs as a result of lying on the back for a long period of time

THROMBUS
a blood clot

THROMBOPHLEBITIS
inflammation of a vein where a clot is formed
ORTHOSTATIC HYPOTENSION
a dizzy feeling caused by a fall in blood pressure; occurs when a person sits or stands too quickly

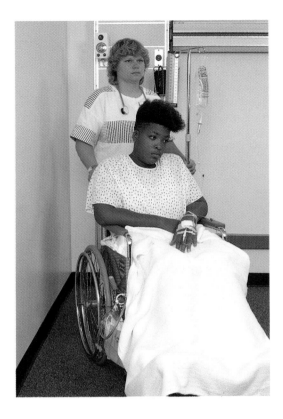

FIGURE 16–6
A patient receiving fluids through a vein in her hand can still be active and get out of bed.

NUTRITION
the study of food's relationship to health; the act of providing food to nourish the body

FLUIDS
liquids

NUTRIENT
a chemical substance that helps the body break down, absorb, and use foods and fluids

CALORIE
a measure of energy produced by the breakdown of food in the body

VITAMIN
an organic substance that is essential in small amounts to the body's health

MINERAL
an inorganic (neither animal nor vegetable) substance needed for health

BACTERIA
microorganisms that reproduce by cell division; also called germs

CONSTIPATION
inability to have or difficulty in having a bowel movement

NUTRITIONAL FUNCTION

The body needs proper **nutrition** and **fluids** to heal and regain strength. Eating and drinking are not possible for an unconscious patient. Other patients may experience a loss of appetite. The presence of loose-fitting dentures may also decrease a patient's appetite because it lessens the ability to enjoy foods.

Fluids and **nutrients** can be given through an intravenous line (Figure 16–6) or through a special tube that is inserted into the stomach. Special formulas that provide extra **calories, vitamins,** and **minerals** are available. The lack of proper nutrition causes weight loss and decreases the body's ability to heal.

ELIMINATION FUNCTIONS

Urine may stay in the bladder longer when patients cannot toilet themselves. If the patient is unable to move, the urine stays in the bladder and provides an ideal environment for **bacteria** to grow. The result is a urinary tract infection. Over a period of time, the urine crystallizes into calculi. Calculi can block the kidneys or ureters (the tubes leading from the kidney to the bladder) and cause severe pain. It is important for patients to take in enough fluids to keep the kidneys flushed.

Constipation is a common complication of disruption in activity and mobility. When patients are inactive and immobile and do not have a sufficient amount of fiber and fluids in their diet, the intestines react by decreasing their peristalsis. When the fecal material is not moved along the intestines as normal, water is reabsorbed back into the body. Thus, the fecal material becomes harder and drier and more difficult to pass.

The patient on bed rest may lose control of the muscles that respond to the brain's signal to empty the bladder and bowels. When these muscles lose their tone, the patient may become **incontinent.**

PROTECTIVE FUNCTION

The skin is a major area of concern in the patient. Lying for a long period in one position puts pressure on areas of skin located over bony prominences. The result is less circulation of blood to the skin surface. Without blood, the skin tissue begins to die and decubitus ulcers form. Remember that the skin functions to protect the tissues of the body. Action must be taken to prevent the breakdown of the body's first line of defense against harmful microorganisms. A turning and positioning schedule is followed to prevent skin breakdown. Good hygiene and nutrition also help keep the skin in good, intact condition.

COMFORT, REST, AND SLEEP FUNCTIONS

Patient **comfort** is affected by inactivity and immobility (Figure 16–7). The freedom to move and change position as desired may be restricted. The ability to **sleep** well is also disturbed. Lack of sleep makes a person irritable and restless. A person needs a good night's sleep to rest the mind as well as the body.

ACTIVITY AND MOBILITY FUNCTIONS

Lack of movement causes muscles to lose their tone (their ability to contract normally) and to atrophy. The patient also loses strength and mobility in the joints of the body. If passive range of motion exercises (see Range of Motion) are not performed consistently, a contracture of the joint can develop, in which the joint "freezes" permanently in a flexed (bent) position.

When you flex your hand at the wrist or bend your leg at the knee, your flexor muscles are acting. Because the flexor muscles are so strong, permanent flexion can result if they stay in one position for too long. The joint must be put through passive range of motion exercises on a regular basis.

Patients on bed rest for a period of time may not stand long enough to put the full weight of their body on the legs. This causes **calcium** to leave the bones and enter the bloodstream. Bone without enough calcium is no longer strong and is prone to break easily. Most patients in the acute care setting are

INCONTINENT
unable to respond to the urge to eliminate the waste products of the body

COMFORT
a sense of contented well-being
SLEEP
the natural periodic suspension of consciousness during which the body's mental and physical powers are restored

CALCIUM
the chemical element that is important to bone and tooth formation

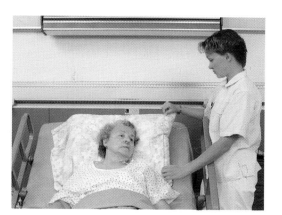

FIGURE 16–7
When the patient has difficulty moving, you can adjust the pillows and blankets to add to the patient's comfort.

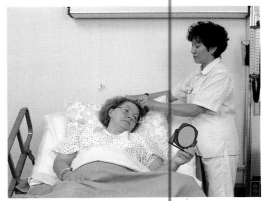

FIGURE 16-8

Make positive comments about patients' appearance to help increase their self-image.

encouraged to stand and walk as soon as they are able to prevent this complication. In the long-term care setting, each patient is helped to achieve and maintain the best possible level of activity and mobility. Whenever possible, weight-bearing activity should be maintained so that the bones do not lose their calcium.

PSYCHO-SOCIO-CULTURAL FUNCTIONS

Patients who are unable to move or get out of bed may become depressed. Their self-image changes as they discover how little they can do for themselves. Patients may feel powerless. They should be allowed to make choices whenever possible. It often helps when words of praise and encouragement are offered during the process of getting well (Figure 16-8).

PREVENTING COMPLICATIONS ASSOCIATED WITH INACTIVITY AND IMMOBILITY

The complications that can occur as a result of inactivity and immobility can be prevented. Your supervisor or nurse will direct you in the activities that help prevent complications in body functioning (see Ways to Prevent Complications Associated with Inactivity and Immobility chart).

WAYS TO PREVENT COMPLICATIONS ASSOCIATED WITH INACTIVITY AND IMMOBILITY

Complications	Action	Rationale
Hypostatic pneumonia	Offer fluids every 2 hours, when permitted	Thins secretions
	Ask the patient to move and turn every 2 hours	Helps loosen secretions
	Encourage the patient to cough and deep breathe every 2 hours	Expands the lungs

Thrombo-phlebitis	Encourage the patient to move all extremities every 2 hours	Increases the circulation of blood
Orthostatic hypotension	Tell patient to change positions slowly (from lying to sitting or sitting to standing)	Prevents the decrease in blood circulation to the brain
Weight loss, poor healing	Feed patients if they are not able to feed themselves	Provides calories and vitamins
	Encourage patients to eat all meals and supplements	
Urinary tract infection, calculi	Offer fluids every 2 hours, when permitted	Keeps kidneys and bladder flushed
	Move and turn the patient every 2 hours	Prevents urine from staying in one place
Constipation	Offer fluids every 2 hours, when permitted	Encourages formation of a soft, easily passed stool
	Encourage dietary fiber and exercise as permitted	
Muscle atrophy, contracture	Encourage active range of motion exercises	Helps muscles keep strength
	Perform passive range of motion exercises	Keeps joints flexible
	Encourage patient to do as many of own activities of daily living as possible	Keeps muscles and joints in use
Decubitus ulcer	Turn and position every 2 hours; have patient stand if in a chair, if permitted	Relieves pressure from the skin
	Perform skin care as needed	Removes harmful microorganisms from the skin
	Use special mattresses, as ordered (eggcrate, air mattress, etc.)	Relieves pressure on the skin
	Provide nutrition and supplements if ordered	Helps tissues heal
	Provide fluids	Helps cells function
Depression	Encourage patients to talk and express feelings	Lets them know you care

OBSERVATIONS OF ACTIVITY AND MOBILITY FUNCTIONING

Normally, people pay little attention to their movement, strength, and muscle condition. When observing patients, ask them several questions to determine whether they are experiencing pain, stiffness, or swelling of a joint. Gaining background information about patients' ability to perform **activities of daily living (ADLs)** is important. Determine the daily activity pattern of each patient.

Gather objective data about the range of motion in your patients' extremities:

- Is there enough muscle strength and mobility to comb the hair and wash the feet?
- Can patients walk unassisted?
- When patients walk, are they standing tall or stooping over?
- Do patients walk smoothly and evenly?
- How far do patients walk?

OBSERVATIONS OF DISRUPTIONS IN ACTIVITY AND MOBILITY

All patients who need assisted care are encouraged by health care givers to perform their ADLs themselves as soon as possible. However, a partial disruption in activity and mobility can occur, limiting patients' ability to participate in their care. These patients need partial assistance for their ADLs from a nurse or nursing assistant (Figure 16–9). Some patients have a total disruption in their ability to move and require complete assistance from you to meet their daily needs.

If patients cannot move the extremities freely and without pain, you might observe a decreased **range of motion** in these extremities. Note whether the patient wears a **prosthesis** (artificial replacement for a missing body part). If a cast is present, it can limit the range of motion of a body part. A patient who is paralyzed might not be able to use the arm and leg on one side of the body.

Ask yourself the following questions after observing the patient.

- Is the patient weak?
- Does the patient have the strength and coordination to feed, dress, and toilet independently?
- How much is the patient able to contribute to meeting personal needs?
- How much assistance does the patient need to complete care?

Check the joints of the fingers, elbows, and knees, comparing their size

ACTIVITIES OF DAILY LIVING
actions used to accomplish tasks such as toileting and grooming on a daily basis

RANGE OF MOTION
the range, measured in degrees like a circle, through which a joint can be extended and flexed (bent)

PROSTHESIS
an artificial replacement for a missing part of the body

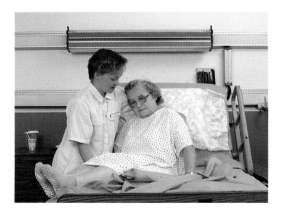

FIGURE 16–9
The care giver and patient work together to move the patient into a sitting position.

and shape. Joints should be similar in size and shape on both sides of the body. Report the following to the nurse:

- changes in the range of motion of any extremity
- the lack of strength and range of motion to perform ADLs
- the lack of desire or unwillingness to move or **ambulate**
- redness, warmth, or swelling over a joint
- any pain or stiffness the patient reports to you
- the use of a prosthesis, such as an artificial limb or a brace, if one has been prescribed

AMBULATE
walk

CARE OF PATIENTS WITH A DISRUPTION IN ACTIVITY AND MOBILITY

Patients who are not able to take part in their own care or move without help have many needs. You are responsible for helping them with their ADLs. As patients grow stronger, they can begin to participate in their own care.

The nurse tells you how much assistance a patient needs. You should help the patient become as independent as possible in self-care activities. Follow these guidelines to help your patient:

- Follow the nurse's direction regarding the patient's needs for care.
- Encourage the patient to perform ADLs.
- Allow time for the patient to perform an ADL.
- Praise the patient for any success in completing an ADL.
- Report and record the patient's ability to participate in self-care.

The physician or surgeon writes a series of activity orders for each patient. The activity orders allow patients to progress to complete self-care, or at least to the highest level possible for them, as their condition improves. As a nursing assistant, you care for patients with various degrees of mobility. Patients may be

- on complete **bed rest**
- on bed rest with bathroom privileges
- able to ambulate with assistance
- allowed to sit up in a chair
- allowed to ambulate in the room
- allowed to be up ad lib (as often as wanted)

BED REST
the physician's order that the patient stay in bed

Complete Bed Rest

The physician orders complete bed rest to allow the patient's body to use its energy for healing. Bed rest is usually ordered for the shortest amount of time possible. The longer the patient remains on bed rest, the higher the risk of complications.

Patients for whom complete bed rest has been ordered are not permitted to do anything for themselves. Care givers perform all ADLs for patients on bed rest. An order for complete bed rest might be written for a patient who

- is awake and alert but unable to move due to **paralysis** or other injury
- has experienced a heart attack (to allow the heart muscle to begin healing)
- is unconscious and unable to move

PARALYSIS
loss of feeling in a body part and the inability to move that body part

For most patients, the length of time bed rest is ordered is related to the nature of the disease or injury. The order can be short (as little as 6 or 12 hours) or can extend for any length of time the physician deems necessary. As soon as possible, the order includes patient participation in ADLs. The patient may require a set-up of supplies in order to perform bathing, grooming, and dressing activities, but each day the patient is encouraged to perform ADLs as independently as possible.

Bed Rest with Bathroom Privileges

Patients who have been ordered bed rest with bathroom privileges are permitted to leave their bed to attend to toileting needs. Ask your supervisor or nurse whether the patient requires assistance to walk to the bathroom.

Patients may be permitted to wash their face, neck, ears, and **perineal area.** They may be allowed to move and turn in bed. (After a while they may be allowed to sit in a chair; see below.)

Your responsibility is to perform ADLs so patients can rest. As their condition improves patients become strong enough to perform their own self-care.

Walking with Assistance

Patients may be allowed to ambulate in the room or the hallway with assistance (Figure 16–10). Find out from the nurse whether the patient can walk with the assistance of one person. If patients are alert, they may be able to tell you how much help is needed. If more than one person is needed, be sure to arrange for help. Keep safety a top concern, because a fall is likely to cause injury. Help patients to walk as long a distance as permitted by physician's orders.

Sitting in a Chair

Sitting in a chair and walking are ordered in progressive stages. At first, the patient may be permitted to sit in a chair for 10 or 15 minutes. Over a period of days, this time is extended according to the patient's comfort and ability to remain seated. The patient may be permitted to walk from the bed to the chair or from the bed to the bathroom and back. When strength and the ability to walk return, walking in the corridors is permitted.

PERINEAL AREA
the area between the legs, including the genitals and anus

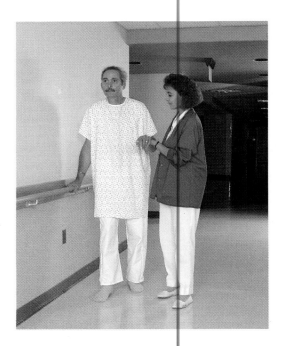

FIGURE 16–10
A patient may be able to walk by using a handrail for support on one side and the help of a care giver on the other side.

Walking in the Room

When patients are stronger, walking around the room is permitted. As their health and strength return, patients are encouraged to complete their own ADLs.

If a patient uses an assistive device (a walker or cane), be sure it is in good repair and located nearby. These devices are measured to fit the patient using them. The care giver is responsible for helping restore the patient to activity and mobility as soon as possible.

Up Ad Lib

The term used to describe a self-care patient is "up ad lib." The patient paces him or herself, and performs all tasks associated with daily living. The periods of rest and activity are balanced. The patient with an "up ad lib" order is a patient preparing for discharge from the hospital. In the nursing home, you will help your patients maintain or reach independence by encouraging and/or assisting them to be active.

CARING COMMENT

Some patients in a wheelchair may be assigned up ad lib status, because many activities can be done while seated.

ACTIVITIES OF DAILY LIVING

The ADLs are all the activities required to prepare for each day. These include

Hygiene
Grooming
Dressing
Preparing and eating meals

Patients may not be able to do these activities for themselves if they are

Bedridden
Ill
In pain
Paralyzed (have loss of movement or feeling in a body part)

As discussed earlier, **hygiene** is the practice of cleanliness. Good hygiene results in a feeling of well-being and comfort. It also helps prevent skin problems. The hygiene practices of oral care, bathing, back care, grooming, and dressing are discussed in Chapter 13. By participating in self-care activities, patients maintain or strengthen their muscles and joints in addition to keeping as independent as possible.

HYGIENE
the practice of cleanliness to promote health

When patients need assistance with moving their arms, legs, and body you are expected to do the following:

- Keep patients in good **body alignment.**
- Turn and position patients.
- Use special devices that help turn and support patients.
- Transfer patients.
- Perform range of motion exercises for patients.

BODY ALIGNMENT
the body's correct, straight position

While assisting patients with movement, the first thing you must remember is to use good body mechanics.

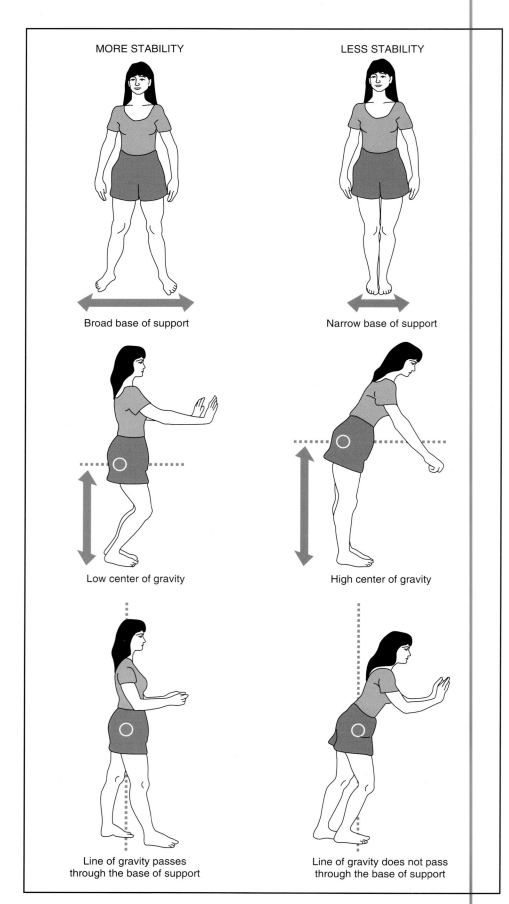

MORE STABILITY

LESS STABILITY

Broad base of support

Narrow base of support

Low center of gravity

High center of gravity

Line of gravity passes
through the base of support

Line of gravity does not pass
through the base of support

FIGURE 16–11

Factors that affect stability. (Modified from Sorensen KC, Luckmann J: Basic Nursing: A Psychophysiologic Approach, 2nd ed. Philadelphia, W. B. Saunders Company, 1986.)

BODY MECHANICS

Body mechanics is the art of using the body efficiently. When you push, pull, or lift, appropriate body mechanics can work for you. The principles of body mechanics will help your muscles and the motion of your body work for you when you are lifting or turning patients and making beds.

Every activity has the potential to put stress and strain on the muscles of the body. You can avoid injury by paying attention to the following important principles about body mechanics.

Center of Gravity

The center of gravity of an object is the point where the most weight is centered. When you stand, your center of gravity is located in the center of the pelvis (the lowest part of the trunk) about midway between the umbilicus (naval) and the symphysis pubis (the area of the pubic bones). When you are standing straight, a vertical (up and down) line passes through the center of gravity.

Base of Support

The base of support is like a foundation. It gives your body a sense of stability. When a person uses a wide base of support and a low center of gravity, the body is more stable (Figure 16–11).

Image a tug-of-war at a summer picnic. The members of the winning team spread their legs apart. Their legs look planted against the ground. This offers a wide base of support. The players flex (bend) their knees and hips; by doing this, they lower their center of gravity. A lower center of gravity gives more leverage. The losing team's poor performance is caused by poor use of body mechanics. Their feet are too close together, giving them no broad base of support. When the people on the losing team pull on the rope, their bodies tilt backwards and become unstable because the vertical line of gravity is off center. Because their legs are straight, not flexed, their center of gravity is too high, preventing them from getting the leverage they need to use their body most efficiently.

The winners in the tug-of-war use the major muscle groups of the body to work for them. They use the strong muscles of the body to provide necessary coordination and leverage. The losers work against the major muscle groups. This can result in stress and strain of the muscles because the use of poor body mechanics increases stress on the back muscles.

The Levers and Fulcrums of the Body

A **lever** provides a mechanical advantage to the action of moving or lifting (Figure 16–12). A **fulcrum** is a type of support for a lever (see Figure 16–12). When you lift a heavy object, the weight of your arms and the object you are lifting provide the leverage needed to lift efficiently. The elbow joint is the fulcrum; it works like a hinge when you actually lift a heavy object. You can lift and move patients easily and safely by

- Standing with a wide base of support.
- Lowering your center of gravity.
- Using the large, strong muscles of your body.
- Using the natural levers and fulcrums of your body.

When you need to move a patient on bed rest toward you, remember to use good body mechanics. It is easier to pull an object than to push it.

BODY MECHANICS
the use of the body to push, pull, or lift objects

LEVER
an object that moves or raises another object
FULCRUM
a support for a lever

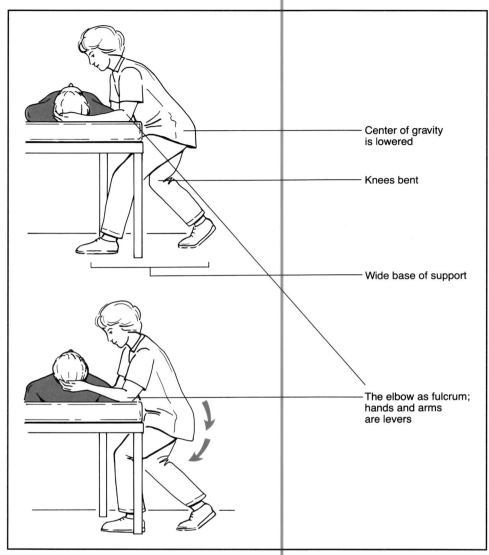

FIGURE 16–12
Levers and fulcrums of the body.

CARING COMMENT

You can use good body mechanics in everyday life. Carrying laundry or grocery bags and lifting children are easier and cause less discomfort when you use good body mechanics.

BODY ALIGNMENT

Body alignment is the correct positioning of patients' head, spine, and extremities. You should observe for correct body alignment in all patients, regardless of whether they are lying, sitting, or standing. To check on body alignment do the following (Figure 16–13):

1. Stand at the foot of the bed.
2. Draw an imaginary line from the top of patients' head to a spot between their feet.
3. Make certain the line is straight.

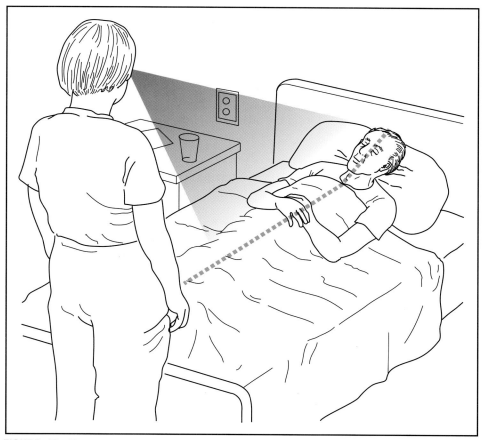

FIGURE 16-13

Checking for straight body alignment. I. Stand at the foot of the bed. 2. Draw an imaginary line from the top of the patient's head to a spot between the feet. 3. Make certain the line is straight.

You are responsible for keeping patients in good body alignment when they cannot do so themselves. Body alignment is important because it

- Promotes patient comfort.
- Allows blood to flow to all body parts.
- Decreases aches and pains.
- Prevents **deformities**, such as contractures.

DEFORMITY
abnormal part

TURNING AND POSITIONING THE PATIENT

The purposes of turning and positioning are to

- Relieve pressure on the skin.
- Prevent the formation of decubitus ulcers.
- Provide comfort.
- Loosen secretions that encourage growth of bacteria.

Turning and positioning are performed according to a turning schedule set by the nurse. The schedule may be posted in the patient's room. Turning and positioning are performed at least every 2 hours. Remember to check patients' skin every time you turn and position them. Pay particular attention to the bony prominences.

PROCEDURE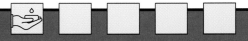

Moving and Turning Patients

When you use the draw sheet to move or turn patients, good body mechanics come into play. The draw sheet makes the turning and moving procedures easier for both the patient and you. Moving and turning are usually performed by two care givers.

GATHER EQUIPMENT

Draw sheet   Extra pillows

ACTION	RATIONALE
Preparation	
1. Wash hands.	Prevents the spread of microorganisms.
2. Identify the patient. Call the patient by name and check the identification band.	Maintains patients' rights.
Procedural Steps	
3. Tell patients that you are going to move them up in bed or turn them on their side. Ask patients if they are able to help in moving or turning.	Informs patients what is happening.
4. Raise the bed to a comfortable working height and place it in a flat (horizontal) position.	Prevents strain and pull on your back muscles.
Moving patients up in bed	
5. A care giver stands at each side of the bed and lowers the side rails.	Helps distribute patients' weight more equally.
6. Place the pillow against the headboard.	Acts as a cushion to prevent patients' head from hitting the headboard.
7. Each care giver should loosen the draw sheet from under the mattress.	
8. Place patients' arms across their chest or ask them to do so.	Patients should participate in care whenever possible.
9. Each care giver should then roll the draw sheet toward patients.	
10. Ask patients to bend their knees. Position patients' legs with knees bent if they cannot do so independently.	Prevents patients' heels from dragging against the sheets and causing friction against the skin.
11. Tell patients you will move them up in bed on the count of three. Ask them to push with their feet on the count of three.	
12. Stand with your legs wide apart and grasp the draw sheet firmly.	
13. On the count of three, both care givers lift and move the patient toward the head of the bed. The patient can push to help in the moving procedure (Figure 16–14).	Patients can make the move more comfortable for themselves.
14. Adjust the linens and the pillow under patients' head and ask if they are comfortable.	
15. Tuck in the ends of the draw sheet on each side of the mattress.	

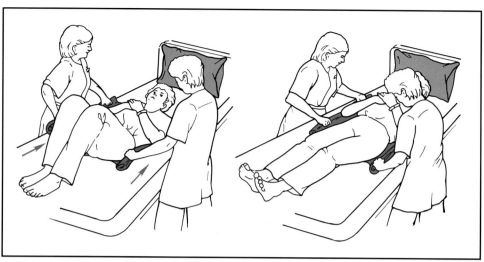

FIGURE 16–14
Moving a patient up in bed.

16. Roll up the head of the bed as the patient wishes.

Turning patients on their side

17. A care giver stands at each side of the bed and lowers the side rails.

18. Place patients' arms on their chest. Cross their feet at the ankle, in the direction of the turn. For example, place the right leg on top if moving patients toward the right.

19. Loosen the draw sheet on one side of the mattress.

20. Roll the sheet toward patients and hand the rolled draw sheet to the care giver on the opposite side of the bed (Figure 16–15).

Adds to patient comfort.

Helps the body turn as one unit.

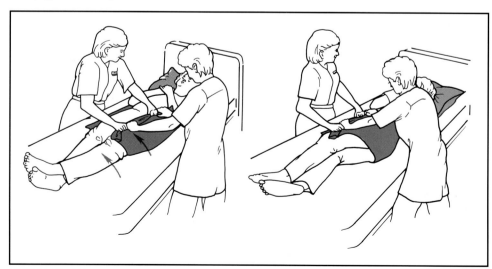

FIGURE 16–15
Turning a patient onto the side.

Continued on following page

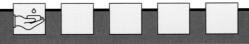

PROCEDURE

Moving and Turning Patients *Continued*

21. On the count of three, the care giver holding the rolled draw sheet begins pulling the draw sheet toward him- or herself while the other care giver reaches under patients' buttocks and uses both arms to pull patients toward the middle of the bed.

22. Tuck the loose end of the draw sheet back under the mattress.

23. Use extra pillows to support patients' back. Place pillows where bony areas touch each other.

    Without support, patients may not remain in the side-lying position.

24. Place arms and legs in a position of comfort and correct body alignment.

Moving patients to the side of the bed

25. Raise the side rails on one side of the bed. Lower the side rail on the side of the bed where you will be standing.

    Ensures safety if you are working alone.

26. Start at the head of the bed. Place your arms under patients' head and shoulders and slide the upper portion of the body toward you (Figure 16–16).

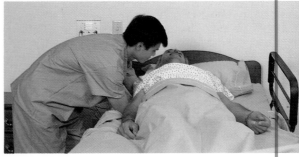

FIGURE 16–16

Support the head and shoulders and move them toward you.

27. Pull your arms out and place them under patients' middle and lower back. Slide this portion of the body toward you (Figure 16–17).

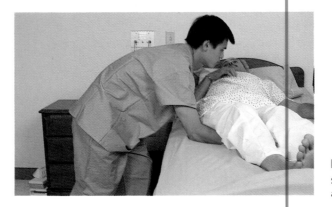

FIGURE 16–17

Support the middle of the body and slide it toward you.

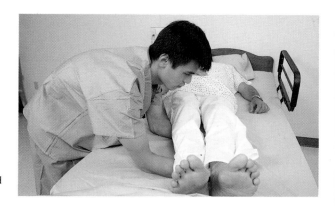

FIGURE 16–18
Support the thighs and legs and slide them toward you.

28. Pull your arms out and place them under patients' thighs and lower legs. Slide this portion of the body toward you (Figure 16–18). Patients are now in a position near the edge of the bed nearest you.

Follow-Through

29. Raise the side rails and lower the bed to the low position.

Promotes patient safety.

30. Place the call signal within patients' reach.

Leaves patients with the means to communicate.

31. Ask patients if anything else is needed. Follow through on their request if it is for something you are permitted to do.

Gives patients a chance to express other needs they might have.

32. Wash hands.

Prevents the spread of microorganisms.

Protective Positioning

Protective positioning and support are used to support the extremities and keep the body in good body alignment. You need to know what positions to use and how to use pillows to support the patient in that position. A patient may be placed in the following protective positions

Prone (Figure 16–19A)
Supine (Figure 16–19B)
Fowler's (Figure 16–19C)
Semi-Fowler's (Figure 16–19D)
Side-lying (Figure 16–19E)
Sims' (Figure 16–19F)
Trendelenburg (Figure 16–19G)

When a patient needs to be turned so that the spinal column (the back) is kept straight, a method called **log-rolling** is used (Figure 16–20). Log-rolling is usually ordered when the patient has had a severe back injury or spinal surgery.

LOG-ROLLING

moving a patient's body as one unit

USING SPECIAL DEVICES TO TURN AND SUPPORT PATIENTS

A contracture occurs when a joint stiffens and freezes in one position. Patients who use their joints to move do not develop contractures. When you do

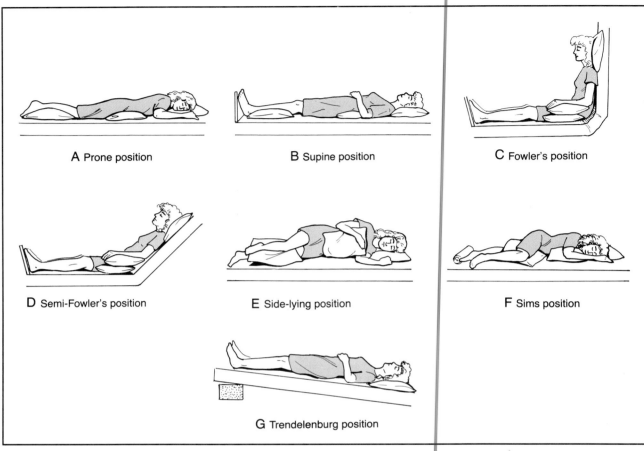

FIGURE 16–19
Protective positions.

passive range of motion exercises for the patient, contractures are less likely to occur (see Range of Motion).

Handrolls

A handroll is placed in the palm of the hand to prevent the hand and fingers from contracting in a flexion (bent) position. Handrolls are commercially available (Figure 16–21) or can be made by rolling a washcloth and placing it in the palm of the patient's hand.

Footboards

DORSIFLEXION
bending backwards
ANATOMIC
pertaining to body structure

For the patient who is inactive and immobile, it is important to keep the feet in a position called **dorsiflexion**. A footboard helps keep the feet in correct **anatomic** position and prevents external rotation of the hips (Figure 16–22). Some health care institutions, especially rehabilitation centers, ask their patients to wear high-top sneakers for support. These measures prevent the formation of foot contractures.

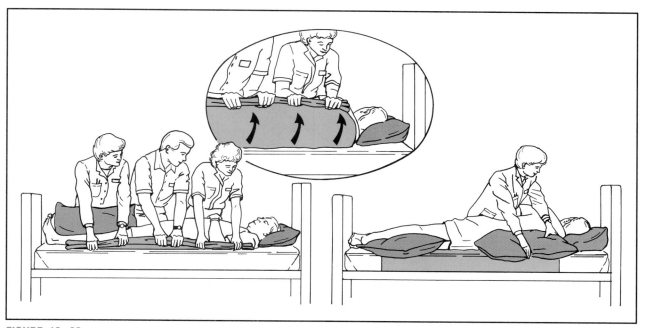

FIGURE 16-20

Log-rolling the patient. The care givers work together to turn patients onto their side with one motion.

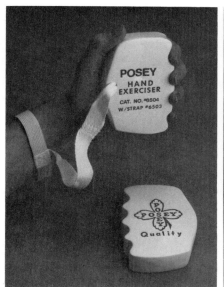
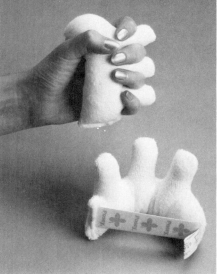
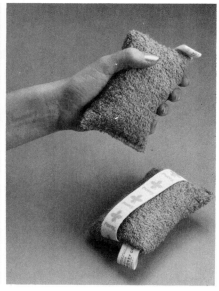
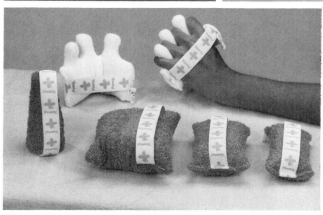

FIGURE 16-21

Devices used to prevent contractures of the hands and fingers. (Courtesy of J. T. Posey Company, Arcadia, CA.)

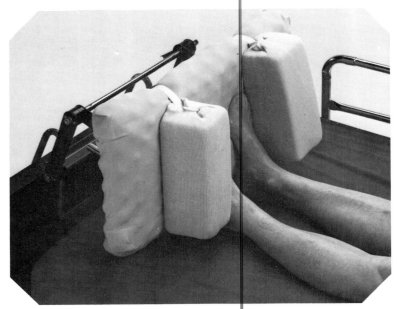

FIGURE 16-22

Adjustable footboard, used to keep the patient's feet in dorsiflexion. (Courtesy of J. T. Posey Company, Arcadia, CA.)

Splints

A splint can also be used to provide support and keep a body part in proper alignment. A splint is made of plastic or metal and padded with foam. This type of splint is made for the hand or the foot and is kept in place by Velcro strips.

Pillows

Pillows help support body parts as well as provide padding to prevent body parts from rubbing against each other and causing skin breakdown.

Sandbags

Bags of sand are placed against extremities to help keep them in a certain position. They can be padded for comfort. They are placed against the soles of the feet to keep them at a 90° angle and thus prevent "foot drop."

ROTATION

the process of turning on an axis, for example, turning the head from side to side

Trochanter Rolls

The ends of a towel or blanket are rolled under until they fit snugly against the patient's thighs. Trochanter rolls prevent the external **rotation** of the hips (Figure 16-23).

USING SPECIAL DEVICES TO PREVENT DECUBITUS ULCERS

Bed Cradles

Special equipment placed at the foot of the bed keeps the covers off the patient's feet (Figure 16-24). The patient's feet can be placed against a footboard placed under the bed cradle.

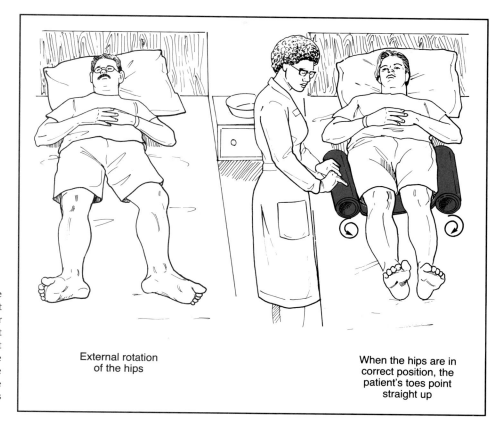

FIGURE 16–23
Making a trochanter roll. Place the patient on a folded blanket or towel. Position the blanket or towel so that the edges are at the patient's hips and about one-third of the way down the thighs. Roll the edges of the blanket or towel *under* until the roll is snug against the patient's hips.

External rotation of the hips

When the hips are in correct position, the patient's toes point straight up

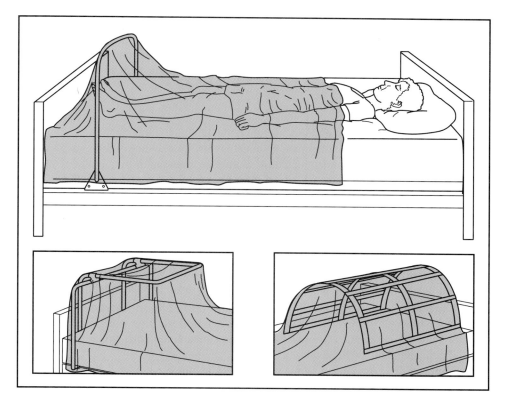

FIGURE 16–24
A bed cradle.

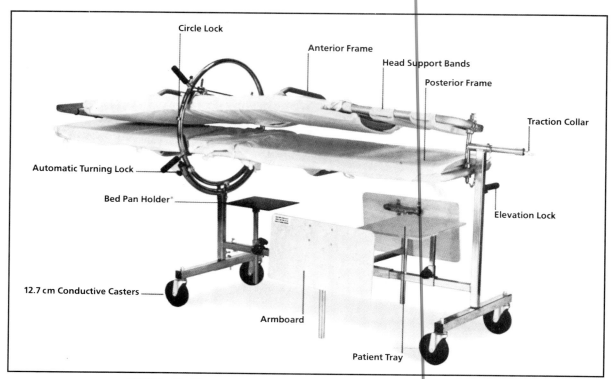

Circle Lock

Anterior Frame

Head Support Bands

Posterior Frame

Traction Collar

Automatic Turning Lock

Bed Pan Holder

Elevation Lock

12.7 cm Conductive Casters

Armboard

Patient Tray

FIGURE 16–25

Stryker Wedge Turning Frame. (Courtesy of Stryker, Kalamazoo, MI.)

Special Beds

Special beds, like the Stryker Wedge Turning Frame (Figure 16–25) and the Stryker CircOlectric bed (Figure 16–26) are made so that the patient is kept in good body alignment while the bed is turned. The bed can be rotated in many positions. The Clinitron bed is another special bed. The patient floats on a Clinitron bed because air is circulated through specially made particles in the bed. The bed also has a filter system that carries body fluids such as urine away from the patient's skin and keeps it dry.

Special Mattresses

Special mattresses relieve pressure caused by the body's weight. An air mattress may be placed under the patient. Some mattresses may be filled with a gel-like substance or water. An alternating-pressure air mattress deflates and inflates selected parts of the mattress to relieve pressure on the patient's skin (Figure 16–27).

Special Padding

Pads placed under the patient help reduce pressure when the patient is not able to move. Two common pads are the eggcrate and the sheepskin:

- **Eggcrate**—The eggcrate is made of foam and shaped like an egg holder. It is placed under the bottom sheet. If soiled, the eggcrate mattress should be discarded because laundering interferes with the fire-retardant characteristics of the eggcrate foam.
- **Sheepskin** (also called lamb's wool)—The sheepskin is a large piece of

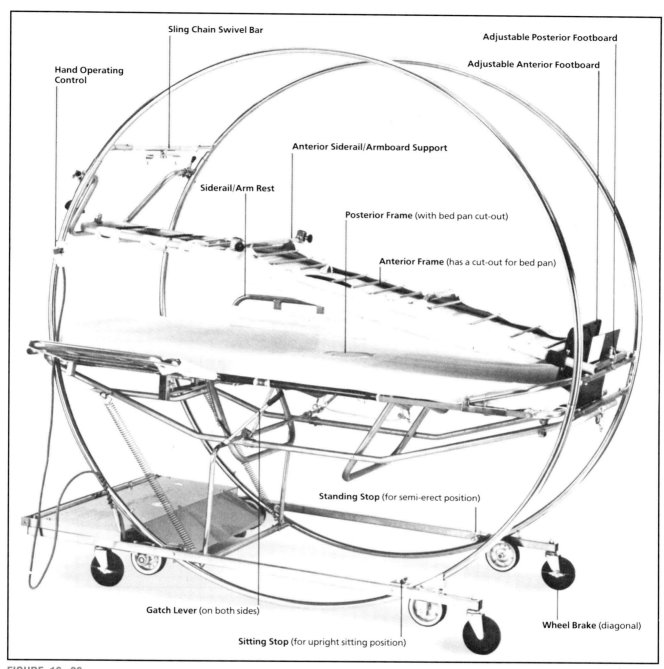

FIGURE 16–26

Stryker CircOlectric Bed. (Courtesy of Stryker, Kalamazoo, MI.)

soft, thick material that is placed directly beneath the patient. If soiled, the sheepskin can be washed, fluffed, and used again. If the sheepskin becomes lumpy, do not use it.

Certain pads are made to help protect the immobile patient's elbows and heels, which are prone to breakdown and decubitus ulcers. A commercial pad, made of a soft, stretchable material, may be slipped over the elbow or foot. Another type of heel protector is more sturdy and also helps prevent foot drop, because it keeps the foot in dorsiflexion (Figure 16–28).

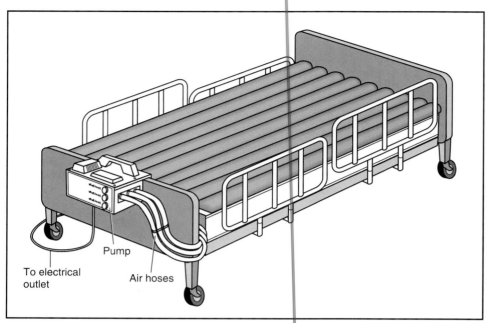

FIGURE 16–27

An alternating-pressure mattress.

CARING COMMENT

Before you care for a patient in any special bed, you need to learn how to operate it and to practice using it so that you become comfortable with the procedure. Follow your institution's procedure when you work with special beds.

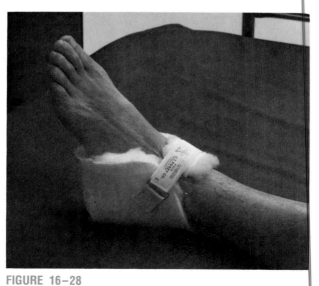

FIGURE 16–28

Heel protector. Note the soft padded lining. (Courtesy of J. T. Posey Company, Arcadia, CA.)

TRANSFERRING PATIENTS

It is necessary for you to use good body mechanics when you transfer a patient from one place to another. You can plan how to transfer a patient safely by asking yourself the following questions:

- What kind of transfer are you about to perform?
- Is the proper equipment available in the room?
- What special equipment is needed to accomplish the transfer?
- What is patients' size in relation to their weight?
- How much can patients assist you?
- How much assistance do you need from others?

Use your answers to plan a safe transfer that causes no muscular stress or strain. The most common transfers are (a) from the stretcher to the bed and back and (b) from the bed to chair (or wheelchair) and back.

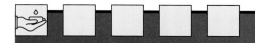

PROCEDURE

Transferring Patients from Stretcher to Bed

If patients are not able to assist in the transfer, there should be at least three care givers to help. Fold the linens down to the foot of the bed. Place the bed in high position. Check that the brakes are on.

ACTION	RATIONALE
Preparation	
1. Wash hands.	Prevents the spread of microorganisms
2. Provide for privacy by closing the door or the privacy curtains around the bed.	Maintains patients' rights.
Procedural Steps	
3. Position the stretcher next to the bed and lower the side rail nearest to the bed (Figure 16–29).	
4. Stabilize the stretcher by applying the brakes.	Prevents the stretcher from moving during the transfer.
5. Position one care giver at the head of the bed, one at the foot of the bed,	Helps distribute the weight equally. One care giver moves patients' head and

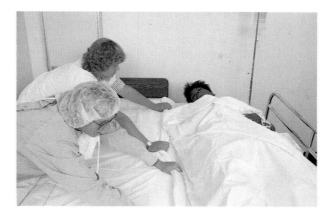

FIGURE 16–29
Transferring the patient from stretcher to bed.

Continued on following page

PROCEDURE

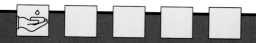

Transferring Patients from Stretcher to Bed
Continued

and one at the middle of the bed. Other care givers can remain on the side of the stretcher with the side rails up. The side rail can be lowered when the transfer begins and care givers assist with the transfer.

shoulders, another the torso, and the third the lower extremities.

6. Loosen the sheet on the stretcher and roll the loose edges toward patients.

7. Ask patients to place their arms across their chest.

8. Tell patients you are going to move them toward you on the count of three. Count to three.

Alerts patients to get ready for the transfer.

9. All three care givers should use a smooth motion at the same time to pull the patient toward you in the bed. Move at a slow, even pace.

Transfer with a single motion is more comfortable for the patient.

10. Raise the side rails on the bed and remove the stretcher from the room.

Ensures patient safety. There is more room when the stretcher is removed.

11. Lower one side rail and help patients roll toward you. One care giver can fanfold the sheet under patients' side after lowering the opposite side rail.

A loose piece of linen under the patient can cause discomfort.

12. Help patients roll to their other side and remove the sheet used in the transfer.

13. Position patients on the pillow.

14. Cover patients with the sheet and blanket or spread folded at the foot of the bed.

15. Raise the head of the bed if this is permitted and desired by patients.

Shows your concern for patients' comfort.

16. Lower the bed and open the door or privacy curtains.

17. Place the call signal within patients' reach.

Leaves patients with a means to communicate.

18. Ask patients if anything else is needed. Follow through on their request if it is for something you are permitted to do.

Gives patients a chance to express other needs they might have.

Follow-Through

19. Wash hands.

Prevents the spread of microorganisms.

UNCONSCIOUS

unaware of the environment and not responsive to stimuli; unconsciousness occurs during sleep, fainting, and coma

The same procedure is used to transfer the patient from the bed to the stretcher.

The patient being transferred may be awake and alert or may be **unconscious.** When transferring unconscious patients from the stretcher to the bed or vice versa, follow the procedure for transferring and

• Use four or more care givers to perform the transfer.

- Cross patients' arms across their chest since they cannot do so.
- Use extra caution in the transfer to prevent patient injury.
- Continue to talk to patients and explain what you are going to do, during the transfer.
- Roll patients toward yourself and ask another care giver to place the transfer sheet (before transfer) or remove it (after transfer).
- Place patients on their back (or other protective position as indicated on schedule) and make them comfortable.

Stretcher or Cart

A stretcher is used to transport patients off the unit when they need to go to the operating room or to other departments for diagnostic studies. A stretcher may also be called a cart or a gurney. All stretchers are supplied with side rails that should be raised during transport of a patient. The brakes on the wheels should always be locked for safety during patient transfers. If belts are attached to the stretcher, they should be secured over the patient's body.

Chairs

Each patient's room is furnished with some type of chair. An important step is reached when a patient is allowed out of bed. The activity and motion generated by movement during a transfer are beneficial to the patient. Sitting up in a chair

- Increases the circulation of the blood.
- Increases lung expansion so breathing is easier.
- Increases the use of the muscles that help patients stand, **pivot**, and sit.
- Allows better interaction with the environment.
- Provides contact with stimulating sights and sounds in the environment.
- Shows patients that progress is being made.
- Provides a better position for eating and eliminating body wastes.

PIVOT
turn

Special chairs are available to serve specific purposes. These special chairs are the

Geri-chair
Recliner
Lift chair
Wheelchair

GERI-CHAIR   A geri-chair is a padded chair on wheels; it may have a recliner feature (Figure 16–30A). It is equipped with a detachable tray on which food or personal items can be placed. A seat belt helps secure the patient in the geri-chair.

RECLINER   In some instances, a recliner is ordered so that a patient can sit in a chair and keep the lower extremities (legs) elevated and supported comfortably (Figure 16–30B).

LIFT CHAIR   A lift chair is similar to a recliner. It has a special **apparatus** that allows a patient to get out of the cushioned chair safely (Figure 16–30C). A mechanism is built into the chair that, when activated by a button, slowly raises the patient to an upright, almost standing position. The lift chair is used for arthritic patients or patients who are not strong enough to lift themselves out of a chair unassisted.

APPARATUS

equipment designed for a particular use

WHEELCHAIR   A wheelchair is a chair mounted on wheels (Figure 16–31). The patient can use both hands to move the wheelchair. The movement of the hands on the wheels causes the chair to go forward or backward and to turn.

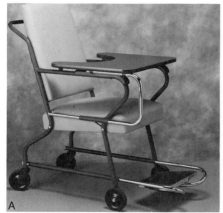
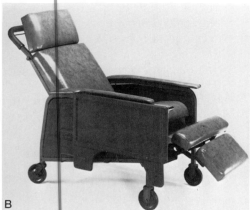
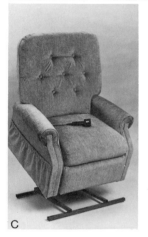

FIGURE 16–30
Special chairs for patient comfort. A, Geri-chair. B, Recliner chair. C, Lift chair. (Courtesy of Graham-Field Inc., Hauppauge, NY.)

For patients who are unable to use their hands to manipulate the wheelchair, battery-powered chairs are available.

Everyone, from the patient to visitors to staff, should practice wheelchair safety. The following are the basic rules of wheelchair safety:

- Check that there are no missing parts and all parts of the wheelchair are firmly attached.

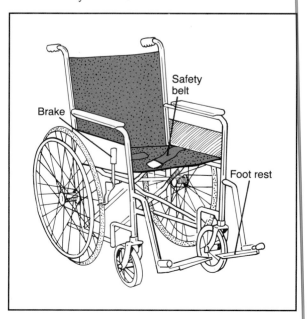

FIGURE 16–31
Wheelchair.

- Always set both brakes before transferring a patient to or from the wheelchair.
- Use the seatbelt (when provided) to prevent accidental falls.
- Use leg supports properly.
- Use the right size wheelchair for the patient (adult, large, or child).

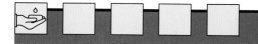

PROCEDURE

Transferring Patients from the Bed to a Wheelchair or Chair and Back to the Bed

GATHER EQUIPMENT

Patient robe
Nonslip shoes or slippers
Sheet or blanket

Paper or pad to protect the bed linens
Wheelchair or sturdy chair with side arms

ACTION	RATIONALE

Preparation

1. Wash hands.	Prevents the spread of microorganisms.
2. Identify yourself and the patient.	Maintains patients' rights.
3. Provide privacy.	Maintains patients' rights.
4. Explain the procedure.	Informs patients what is happening.

Procedural Steps

5. Place wheelchair at the side of the bed on the strong, not weak, side of patients.	
6. Lock the wheelchair brakes and open the footrests or remove the footrest closest to the bed.	Prevents injury and allows for easier transfer.
7. Raise the bed to your waist level or to the high position that enables you to use good body mechanics.	Makes your job easier and safer.
8. Lower the side rail nearest you.	
9. Fanfold the top bed linens down to the foot of the bed.	
10. Ask or assist patients to move toward you.	
11. Place the paper or pad protector under patients' feet.	Keeps the linens clean.
12. Place nonslip shoes or slippers on patients' feet.	Decreases the chance of slipping.
13. Assist patients to a sitting position: • Raise the back of the bed to the high position. Remain at patients' side to protect them from a fall. • Ask patients to bend their knees or assist them to do so. • Grasp the shoulder that is farthest away from you. • Place your arm under patients' knees and grasp the knee farthest away from you.	Makes transfer easier.

Continued on following page

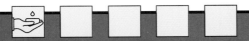

Transferring Patients from the Bed to a Wheelchair or Chair and Back to the Bed
Continued

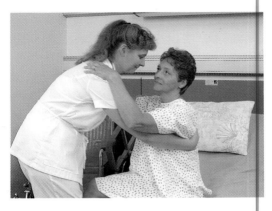

FIGURE 16–32
Patients' arms should rest on your shoulders; their hands should not lock together behind your neck.

- Spread your legs about 12 inches apart with one foot 6–8 inches in back of the other. Flex your knees.
- Swing your body a quarter turn backward and bring patient's legs toward you. The patient is now sitting up.
- Ask patients to push both fists into the mattress.
- Stand in front of patients and lower the bed to its lowest position (when controls are located at the side).
- Allow patients to rest for a few moments while you count their pulse.

The weight of the legs coming down off the edge of the bed helps the patient to sit upright.

Helps them support themselves in the sitting position.

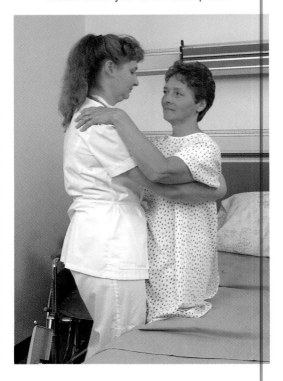

FIGURE 16–33
Placing your knees against patients' knees gives you leverage when you help them to stand.

14. Ask patients to place one arm on each of your shoulders (Figure 16–32).

Be sure the patients do not put both hands together around your neck. (Prevents injury because patients' body weight is more evenly distributed.)

15. Place your arms under patients' shoulders, reach around patients' back, and grasp both of your wrists.

16. Position your feet apart and lower your pelvic area.

Broadens your base of support.

17. Place your knees against patients' knees (Figure 16–33).

18. Tell patients to stand on the count of three.

Patients cooperate more when told what to expect.

19. Use a rocking motion when you begin to count.

20. On the count of three, rock backward and use the momentum of your body to bring patients to a standing position.

21. Ask patients to pivot on the foot farthest away from the wheelchair.

22. Tell patients to lower an arm to grasp the side of the wheelchair (Figure 16–34).

Helps patients steady themselves before sitting down.

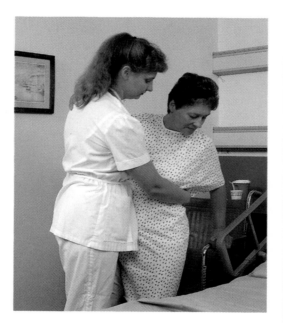

FIGURE 16–34
Patients can use their arm for support during transfer.

23. Help patients lower themselves into the wheelchair (Figure 16–35).

24. Secure the seatbelt.

25. Lift patients' legs one at a time, reposition the footrests, and place the legs on the footrests (Figure 16–36).

26. Make patients comfortable and be sure their body is in good alignment.

27. Place a sheet or blanket across patients' lap (Figure 16–37).

Provides modesty, privacy, and warmth.

Continued on following page

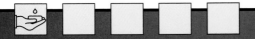
Transferring Patients from the Bed to a Wheelchair or Chair and Back to the Bed
Continued

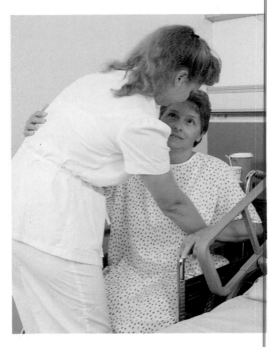

FIGURE 16-35

Be sure the patient is seated securely in the wheelchair.

28. Open the privacy curtains.
29. Release the wheelchair brakes and position wheelchair where patients desire.
30. Remove the paper or pad from the bed and discard. Straighten the bed linens and fanfold them to the bottom of the bed.

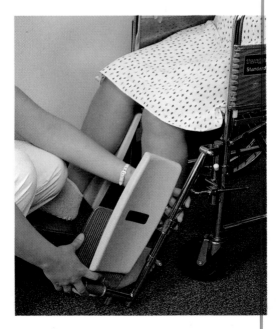

FIGURE 16-36

Footrests are important for patient safety and comfort.

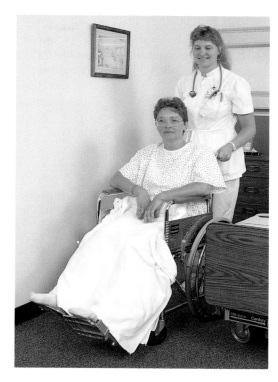

FIGURE 16–37
Cover the patient before you leave the room.

31. To return patients to bed, reverse the procedure.
32. Cover patients with the bed linens.
33. Lower the head of the bed to a position of comfort for patients.
34. Raise the side rails if this is the policy of your institution.
35. Place the call signal within patients' reach.
36. Put robe and shoes or slippers away in patients' closet.
37. Ask patients if anything else is needed. Follow through on their request if it is something you are permitted to do.

Leaves patients with the means to communicate.

Gives patients a chance to express other needs they might have.

Follow-Through

38. Wash your hands.

Prevents spread of microorganisms.

39. Report the following to the nurse or supervisor:
   • How well patients tolerated the procedure
   • Patients' pulse and respiratory rates
   • The amount of help patients required
   • How much patients assisted in the activity
   • The length of time patients were able to sit
   • Other patient observations
   • Comments patients made about the transfer

Special Lifting Devices

A special mechanical device may be available to help you transfer a patient. Most long-term care institutions have them. The Hoyer lift and Versa lift are two pieces of equipment designed to help move a patient who is unable to assist in the transfer (Figure 16–38). You can use them to transfer a patient to a wheelchair or a geri-chair. These special lift devices may also be used to lift patients off a bed and transport them to another room for a treatment or procedure, such as a tub bath. The following are safety guidelines for using a lift device:

- Make sure equipment is properly functioning.
- Apply the device correctly.
- Follow the manufacturer's directions.

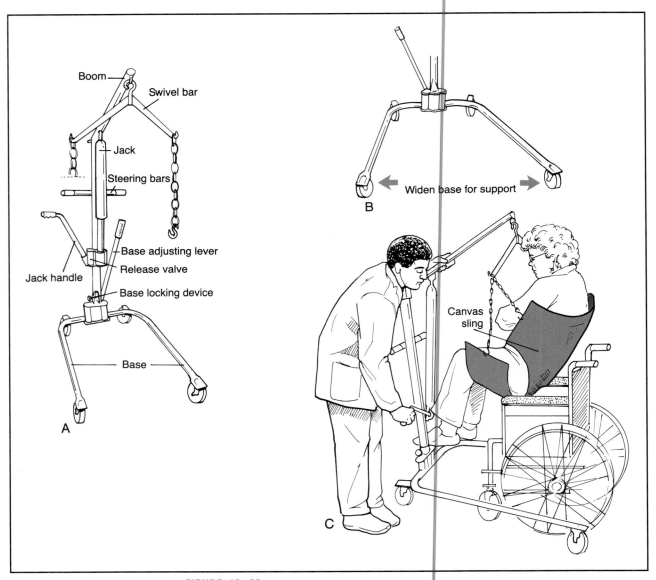

FIGURE 16–38

Using a mechanical lift. A, Parts of a Hoyer lift. B, Use the base adjusting lever to broaden the base before attaching the lift to the canvas. C, Be sure to support the patient's head and/or legs when needed.

Transfer Belts

A transfer belt (also called a safety or ambulation belt) is used during transfer of patients who are weak or uncoordinated. It is made of a heavy material such as canvas and is placed over patients' clothing at the waistline. It should be adjusted for a snug fit around the waist.

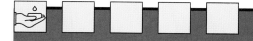

PROCEDURE

Using a Transfer Belt

The transfer belt is used by care givers to assist the patient to walk safely.

GATHER EQUIPMENT

Transfer belt

ACTION	RATIONALE
Preparation	
1. Wash hands.	Prevents the spread of microorganisms.
2. Identify yourself and the patient.	Maintains patients' rights.
3. Provide privacy.	Maintains patients' rights.
4. Explain the procedure.	Informs patients what is happening.
Procedural Steps	
5. Place the transfer belt around patients' waist and adjust (Figure 16–39).	Provides a firm area for you to hold patients.
6. Help patients to a standing position.	Allows you to observe patients' strength.

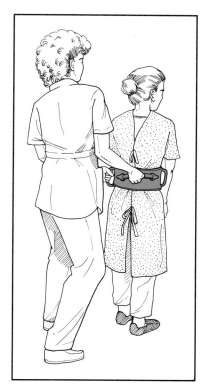

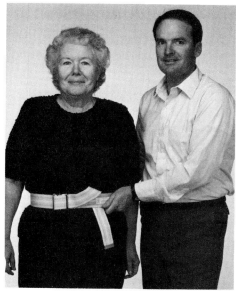

FIGURE 16–39

Using a transfer belt is safer for the patient and the care giver. (Courtesy of J. T. Posey Company, Arcadia, CA.)

Continued on following page

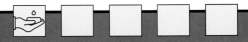

PROCEDURE

Using a Transfer Belt *Continued*

7. Stand behind and to the side of patients while using the belt to support them.

8. For patients who are weak on one side,
   • Stand on the weak side.
   • Place the hand closest to patients around their waist and grasp the transfer belt.
   • Use your other hand to support patients' arm on their weak side.

9. Walk with patients for the desired distance and observe their strength while walking.

10. Assist patients to a chair or bed if they become weak or dizzy.

11. If patients begin to fall, do the following:
    • Stand with your legs far apart and one foot forward.   Provides a good base of support.
    • Bring patients' body close to you.   Your body supports patients' body and helps break the fall.
    • Lower patients to the floor while you support their body.   Helps prevent patient injury.
    • Seek assistance from other care givers to return patients to bed. When patients are in bed, take their vital signs.
    • Report the fall to the supervisor or nurse.

11. At the end of the walk, assist patients to a bed or chair and remove the transfer belt.   The belt is not needed while patients are sitting or lying in bed.

Follow-Through

12. Store the belt in the proper place.

13. Record and report the following to the supervisor: Provides a legal record of the activity.
    • How far and how long patients walked
    • How much assistance patients needed
    • That a transfer belt was used
    • Patients' comments about the walk
    • Any falls (Report immediately. Fill out your institution's accident/incident form.)

RANGE OF MOTION

FLEXIBLE
bendable

Range of motion is the range through which a joint can be extended (straightened) and flexed (bent). Range of motion exercises are carried out to keep the joints **flexible**. Range of motion exercises may be either active or passive.

- **Active range of motion (AROM) exercise** is performed by patients without assistance. When the patients are able to move the extremities (as determined by the physician), you need to encourage them to continue to do so. When patients move and turn in bed, perform self-care activities, and walk when allowed, they are performing AROM exercises.
- **Passive range of motion (PROM) exercise** is performed by the care giver for the patient (Figure 16–40). When the patient cannot move, PROM exercises are started on the affected extremity or extremities. You should be certain to perform PROM exercises for your patient at least once a shift. Each exercise should be repeated five times or as indicated by the policy of your health care institution.

Your supervisor or the nurse tells you the degree of your patients' range of motion and the need for AROM or PROM exercises. This information can also be found on patients' chart or care plan. The words you need to remember about range of motion are included in the chart below.

RANGE OF MOTION TERMINOLOGY

Flexion—bending
Extension—straightening of a flexed (bent) limb
Hyperextension—overextension of a limb or part
Eversion—turning outward
Inversion—turning inward
Abduction—moving a body part away from a center or middle line
Adduction—bringing a body part back to a center or middle line
Dorsiflexion—bending a part backwards
Plantarflexion—bending the sole of the foot
Pronation—turning the palm downward
Supination—turning the palm upward
Rotation—the process of turning on an axis, for example, turning the head from side to side
Circumduction—circular movement of a limb or eye
Lateral—referring to the side

When you help a patient with PROM exercise, you should
- Support the body part being exercised by holding or cradling it at the joint (Figure 16–41).
- Repeat each exercise slowly.
- Try to perform PROM exercises during patient care.
- Feel for muscle resistance or limitation in movement.
- Report and record that the exercises were done, identify the body part exercised, and note the time.
- Report and record any patient statements that indicate there is a problem.

Patients may have some degree of AROM. For example, they may be paralyzed on one side of the body but be able to use body parts on the other side of the body. They may have difficulty moving and turning or holding an object. In another instance, a patient may have a cast applied that can interfere with full range of motion but allows some ROM. When patients can help with some of their care, you should encourage them to do as much as possible for themselves.

- If you are assisting with a partial bath, encourage patients to bathe the body parts they can reach.
- Patients may be able to feed themselves if you open containers and packages, pour liquids, and cut food into bite-sized pieces.
- The nurse or physical therapist teaches patients exercises they can do

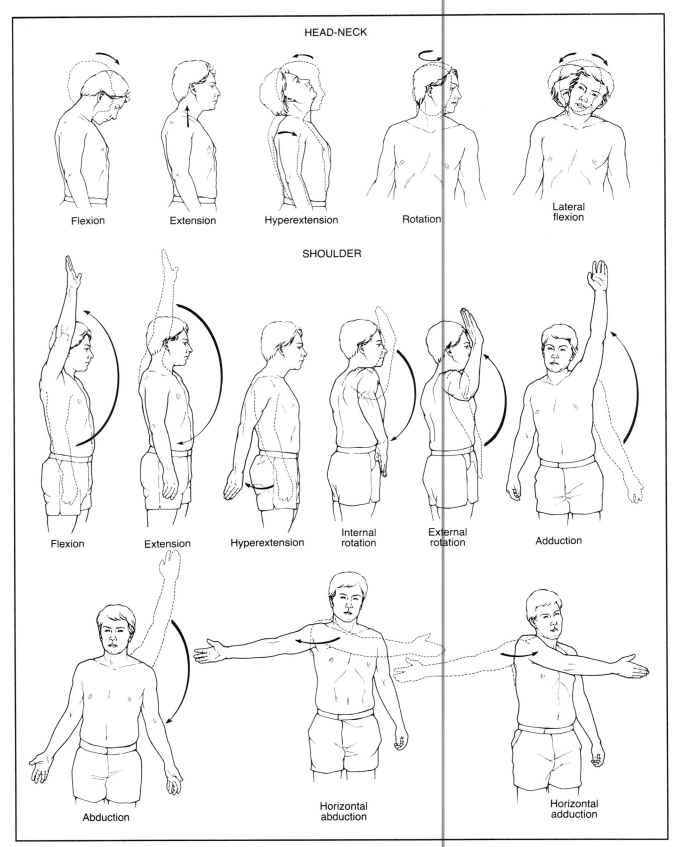

HEAD-NECK

Flexion   Extension   Hyperextension   Rotation   Lateral flexion

SHOULDER

Flexion   Extension   Hyperextension   Internal rotation   External rotation   Adduction

Abduction   Horizontal abduction   Horizontal adduction

FIGURE 16–40

Passive range of motion exercises. (Redrawn from Bolander VB: Sorensen and Luckmann's Basic Nursing: A Psychophysiologic Approach, 3rd ed. Philadelphia, W.B. Saunders Company, 1994.)

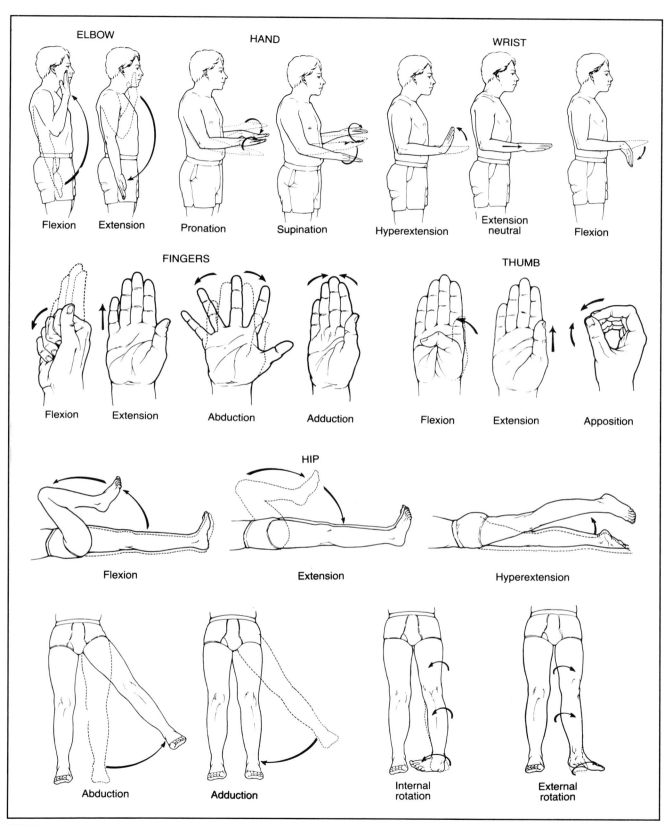

ELBOW

Flexion   Extension

HAND

Pronation   Supination

WRIST

Hyperextension   Extension neutral   Flexion

FINGERS

Flexion   Extension   Abduction   Adduction

THUMB

Flexion   Extension   Apposition

HIP

Flexion   Extension   Hyperextension

Abduction   Adduction   Internal rotation   External rotation

FIGURE 16−40
Continued

Continued on following page

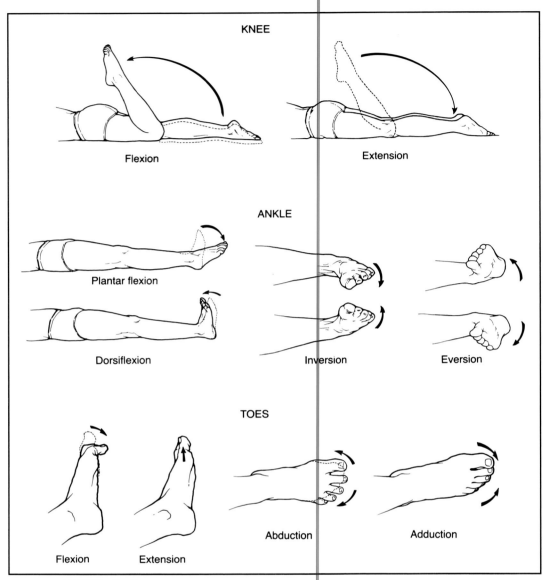

KNEE

Flexion   Extension

ANKLE

Plantar flexion   Inversion   Eversion

Dorsiflexion

TOES

Flexion   Extension   Abduction   Adduction

FIGURE 16–40
Continued

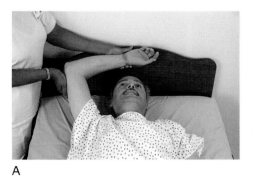

A

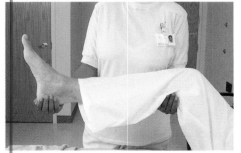

B

FIGURE 16–41
Support the extremities appropriately during passive range of motion exercises. A, Hold the patient's arm at the elbow and wrist. B, Hold the leg at the knee and ankle.

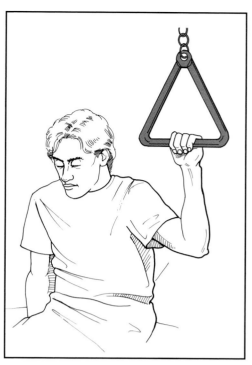

FIGURE 16–42

Trapeze bar. When patients use a trapeze bar, they are giving active exercise to the upper part of their body.

while in bed or sitting in a chair. The nurse or supervisor informs you which exercises patients have been taught. A simple exercise might be to squeeze a small ball to strengthen the muscles and move the joints of the hand. Another simple exercise is to have patients tighten and loosen their muscles.

- Patients may be able to help in moving and turning themselves. Encourage patients to help because this activity exercises the muscles and moves the joints.
- Encourage patients to use a trapeze bar (also called a patient helper) if one has been ordered (Figure 16–42). A trapeze is a piece of metal shaped like a triangle. It is suspended over patients' bed. Patients use the trapeze bar to raise their torso (trunk) to change position and help in moving.

COMMON CAUSES OF A DISRUPTION IN ACTIVITY AND MOBILITY

There are many causes of a disruption in activity and mobility. Most disruptions are short term and temporary. For example, a burst of energy and exercise in an unconditioned person can result in a sprained ankle or sore muscles. A few days of rest often brings relief. An accident often results in a bone fracture. This is a temporary disruption; most bone fractures heal over a period of 4 weeks or more.

On the other hand, a disruption caused by illness can be long term. It may affect activity and mobility for a lifetime. Patients who have experienced a cerebrovascular accident (stroke) are affected in varying degrees. Following

REHABILITATION
a program that helps a patient
return to as normal a life as possible

rehabilitation, some patients can walk again with the assistance of a cane or walker. Other patients remain weak and need more assistance to move about and perform their ADLs.

CARING COMMENT

When you give care to children or elderly patients, use extra measures to keep them safe from a fracture injury.

THE PATIENT WITH A BONE FRACTURE

FRACTURE
a break in the bone at any point or place

OSTEOPOROSIS
disease in which calcium leaves the bones and enters the bloodstream

DEMINERALIZE
to lose minerals or organic salts

A **fracture** is a break in the bone at any place. It may be caused by disease, stress, or trauma.

    Osteoporosis is a disease in which the bone **demineralizes** and becomes weakened and brittle. Demineralized bones break with little stress or trauma. A direct blow to the bone can cause enough stress to fracture the bone. Torsion (a twisting motion) or a severe muscle contraction (tightening) can also cause a bone fracture.

Classification of Fractures

Fractures are first classified by whether or not the bone pierces the skin (Figure 16–43):

- In a **closed fracture**, the bone is broken but does not break through the skin.
- In an **open fracture**, the bone breaks and pierces the skin.

Because a bone or the end of a bone is exposed through the skin in an

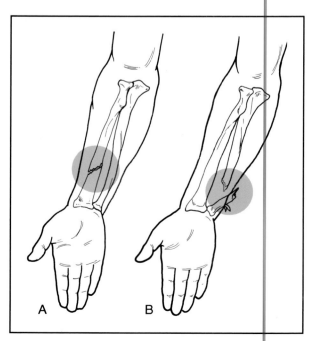

FIGURE 16–43

Closed and open fractures. A, Closed fracture: the bone does not pierce the skin. B, Open fracture: the bone or bone fragments pierce the skin.

open fracture, surgical repair is necessary. An open fracture also exposes the patient to potential infection during the healing process.

Types of Fractures

A fracture (break in **continuity**) is described by the line of the break (the direction it takes). The following are five types of bone fractures:

- **comminuted**—three or more fragments are present.
- **oblique**—the break slants in the direction of the bone.
- **spiral**—the break goes around the bone.
- **segmented**—a piece of the bone is broken off the bone.
- **transverse**—the break travels across the bone.

An additional way to describe a fracture is according to the relationship of the break to the bone. There are the four ways to describe this type of a fracture:

- **compression**—the bone is crushed.
- **depressed**—fragments of bone are pushed inward.
- **impacted**—the bone ends are pushed or shoved into each other.
- **longitudinal**—the break runs the length of the bone rather than across the bone.

The orthopedic physician, a specialist in the treatment of bone and joint diseases, uses these terms to describe a fracture. The anatomical location (place in the body) of the fracture is also described.

A fractured bone requires about 4–6 weeks or more to heal. The amount of time required depends on the nature of the break, the kind of bone that has been fractured, and the patient's age and health status.

Treatment of Fractures

The orthopedic physician applies a cast, **sling,** or **brace** at the site of the break. An x-ray shows the exact location and nature of the break. A pain reliever may be ordered. A serious fracture may require a bone graft, a pin, wires, or a plate to help the bone ends remain stable enough to begin the healing process. A bone graft or the insertion of a pin, wires, or a plate requires surgery.

The common treatment of a closed fracture is application of a cast to the fractured extremity. A cast is made of plaster or fiberglass. It must be strong enough to support the body part until the bone heals, yet light enough that the person can continue with daily activities.

When a new cast is applied, remember to prevent any pressure on the wet cast. The pressure may cause a dent that rubs against the skin under the cast and causes injury. The patient may tell you that there is a warm feeling under the cast. This sensation may last until the cast is dry. In patients who have a cast applied, you are expected to:

- Elevate the extremity as directed.
- Keep the cast clean and dry.
- Check for swelling, skin discoloration, odor, or loss of sensation.
- Ask about pain or itching at the site.

If you observe swelling, skin discoloration, odor, or loss of sensation, promptly report your observations to the nurse.

When you care for a patient who is wearing a cast, sling, or other appliance to support bones and muscles, you should check for color, sensation, and movement (CSM) by comparing the injured extremity with the uninjured extremity. You should also observe for **edema.** Follow these steps to check for CSM and edema in patients with a fracture:

- Look at both extremities. They should be the same in color. (Color)

CONTINUITY

condition of having no breaks or interruptions

SLING

a bandage hanging from the neck that supports an injured arm or hand

BRACE

a metal or plastic appliance that supports or protects a weakened body part

EDEMA

an abnormal accumulation of fluid between cells

- Touch both extremities while asking patients if they can feel your touch. Patients should be able to feel you touching both extremities. (Sensation)
- Ask patients to move their fingers or toes. They should be able to do this. (Movement)
- Compare the extremities for the presence of edema.

Traction

TRACTION

application of a pulling force to a fractured bone or a dislocated joint

Traction is the application of a pulling force to a fractured bone or a dislocated joint. It helps the bone maintain proper position while healing. Traction can be applied to the skin or directly to bone. A variety of traction methods are used in a hospital orthopedic unit. The nurse has the responsibility for maintaining correct traction. If the patient tells you about pain or anything unusual, such as a prickling sensation, report the information to the nurse.

Elastic Bandages

ELASTIC BANDAGE

an elasticized material that provides support and even pressure when wrapped over the site of injury

An **elastic bandage** provides support and equal pressure over the site of injury. Elastic bandages are made of an elasticized cotton material. They come in rolls of different sizes. A metal clip, safety pin, or a piece of adhesive tape keeps the bandage in place. An elastic bandage may also be used to hold a dressing in place. When wrapped correctly, an elastic bandage helps the circulation of blood. In some health care institutions, you may be asked to wrap an extremity with an elastic bandage, a sling, or a brace.

PROCEDURE

Applying an Elastic Bandage

Elastic bandages are applied to give a firm, equal pressure; to provide support; and to help the circulation of the blood. They may also be used to hold a dressing in place.

GATHER EQUIPMENT

Required number of bandages of proper size (determined by the location of the injury)

Metal clips or
Safety pins or
Adhesive tape

ACTION	RATIONALE
Preparation	
1. Wash hands.	Prevents the spread of microorganisms.
2. Identify yourself and the patient.	Maintains patients' rights.
3. Provide privacy when you apply an elastic bandage. You can ask visitors to leave for a short time and pull the curtains around the bed for privacy.	Maintains patients' rights.
4. Explain the procedure.	Informs patients what is happening.
Procedural Steps	
5. Raise the bed to a comfortable working height.	Reduces strain on your muscles.
6. Place the patient in a position of comfort. Expose the part to be wrapped.	

7. Examine the skin after you remove the old bandage and before you put on the new one. Check for CSM and the presence of edema.

Makes certain that skin changes are noted.

8. Face the body part you will bandage. Extend it and support it at the large joints (the elbow or knee).

Provides comfort when patient cannot extend body part without pain.

9. Hold the elastic bandage and place the loose end against the skin. Begin by taking two turns around the limb to anchor the bandage (Figure 16–44).

Anchors bandage in place.

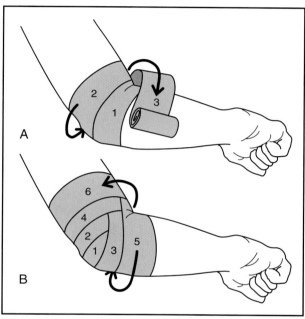 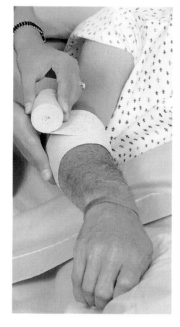

FIGURE 16–44

10. Begin to wrap the bandage from the outermost part of the body part and continue wrapping toward the trunk of the body.

11. Continue to wrap around the limb while you unroll the bandage.

12. Overlap the edges about one-half the width of the bandage as you wrap upward.

No skin should be visible between the spiral turns.

13. Wrap the bandage snugly.

Wrapping it too tightly may cut off circulation to the body part.

14. Keep an even, light pressure while you continue to roll the bandage.

15. When permitted, leave fingers or toes uncovered.

Extremities can be examined for circulation.

16. If more than one bandage is needed, overlap them.

Secures the bandage.

17. Secure the end of the bandage with small metal clips, pins, or adhesive tape (Figure 16–45).

Continued on following page

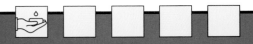

Applying an Elastic Bandage *Continued*

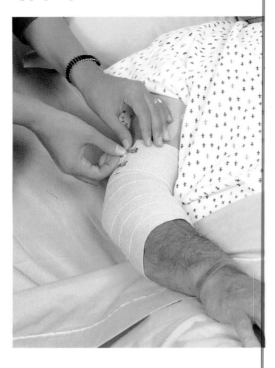

FIGURE 16–45

18. To remove an elastic bandage, remove the fastener and unwind. Remove loosely by passing the bandage from hand to hand.

19. If the bandage is soiled heavily, it may be necessary to discard it. If it is not soiled, reroll it.

    Readies the bandage for reapplication.

20. An elastic bandage may be washed by hand. It should be laid flat to dry.

    Hand care preserves the elastic quality of the bandage.

21. Make the patient comfortable.

22. Lower the bed and raise the side rails.

    Ensures patient safety.

23. Place the call signal within reach of the patient.

    Leaves patient with a means to communicate.

24. Open the curtains and invite the family or visitors back into the room.

Follow-Through

25. Wash your hands.

    Prevents the spread of microorganisms.

26. Report the following information to the supervisor or nurse:
    • The time the bandage was applied or removed
    • The area of application
    • How the patient tolerated application of the bandage
    • Any unusual observations of the skin or body part

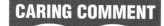

An elastic bandage should be applied so that it is snug but not tight. When the bandage is applied too tightly, the circulation of the blood is affected and edema can result.

Slings

A sling is a device that supports and helps stabilize and injured arm. A common sling is made of a large square of muslin (a type of cloth). Specialized splints may be made of a commercial material and feature special padding and straps for comfort. You may be expected to apply a sling in special circumstances.

Braces

A brace is designed to support or protect a weakened extremity. It is usually custom-designed for the patient. Braces are available in a combination of metal and plastic; they are often cushioned with foam for comfort and to prevent skin breakdown. They are applied daily to help the patient function. When patients are unable to apply the brace themselves, they can often tell you how to proceed.

Some persons need to wear a brace all their life (for example, a child who is born with certain musculoskeletal defects). A brace may be needed for a while after an illness such as a stroke or after an accident.

Canes and Walkers

Canes and walkers are supportive devices that help a person walk (Figure 16–46). A nurse or **physical therapist** teaches a patient how to walk with these aids. Canes are available in wood and metal. A cane should have a rubber cap on the bottom to prevent slippage. (Figure 16–47). A quad cane is made with four shorter pieces that stick out from the bottom and stabilize it. Because the four pieces offer a broad base of support, the quad cane is considered the safest for patients to use.

PHYSICAL THERAPIST
professional who helps ease the pain of muscle, bone, nerve, and joint injury or disease

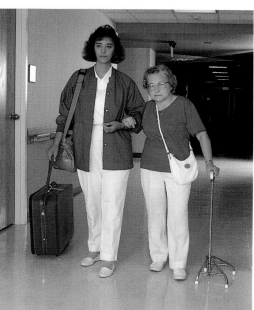

FIGURE 16–46
The quad cane offers a broad base of support. Notice the position of the care giver who provides patient support on the other side.

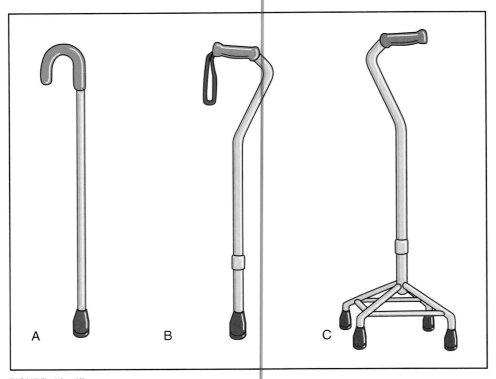

FIGURE 16-47

A, non-adjustable cane. B, Adjustable cane with wrist strap. C, Adjustable quad cane. Metal canes are adjustable.

Walkers are made of a lightweight metal (Figure 16-48). They also provide a broad base of support. A patient who needs more support than a cane offers can move about with a walker because it is light and can be easily lifted. Some walkers may be equipped with wheels and seats; these features make mobility available to certain patients. Walkers come in a range of sizes to fit children and adults.

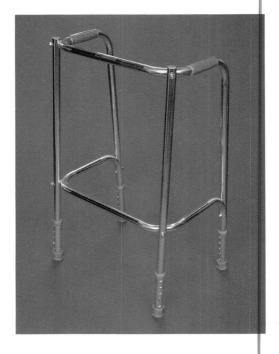

FIGURE 16-48
An adjustable metal walker.

The patient who requires a cane or walker to assist in ambulation (walking) is at risk for injury from falling. To prevent a fall, practice the following safety measures:

- Bring the cane or walker within the patient's reach.
- Help the patient put on sturdy shoes.
- Help the patient to a standing position.
- Walk with the patient if extra support is needed.

Crutches

Crutches are used in the event of injury to the lower extremities. Made of wood or aluminum, crutches are adjustable and are available in many sizes. The ends of crutches are capped with rubber to prevent slipping. The top of crutches may be padded. A nurse or a physical therapist teaches the patient to walk with crutches.

Patients must possess enough strength in their arms and hands to carry the weight of their body. Crutches are adjusted to fit individual patients. The most important consideration regarding fit is the length. The most important thing to check when you watch patients using crutches is that patients support their body with their hands. If patients support themselves by resting on the arm rests (on the top of the crutch), they risk permanent injury to the nerves that serve the arm and hand.

THE PATIENT WITH A HIP FRACTURE

Because the population of elderly persons is increasing, there are many patients in hospitals as well as nursing homes who have experienced hip fractures. The elderly are at a high risk for hip fractures. Some elderly people become weak and undernourished and fall easily. Persons who do not use an aid such as a cane, walker, or wheelchair when they should be using one risk a fracture of the hip, the healing of which may be poor. Falls are a common cause of hip fracture in the elderly population. Even a fall from a bed or sofa can cause a hip fracture.

Older persons can practice some safety measures to prevent hip fracture. The best method to prevent a hip fracture is a combination of diet and exercise. All persons need calcium to form strong, dense bones. As discussed earlier, in order for the body to use the calcium, the person needs to be able to bear weight on the bones of the legs when walking. You can remind patients that walking is the best exercise for people of all ages. If a device is prescribed to assist in walking, the patient should be taught the correct use of the equipment. Patients should be encouraged to use the device for as long as necessary.

Most patients with hip fractures are treated with surgery. The patient's age, physical and emotional conditions, and response to surgery and healing are important considerations in caring for a patient with a fractured hip. When you care for a patient who has had a surgical repair of a fractured hip, you give good care when you

- Follow any restrictions on flexion (Figure 16–49). These may include the prevention of bending at the hip by not elevating the head of the bed or allowing the patient to sit in a chair (the hip is flexed while in the sitting position).
- Follow restrictions on the position of the affected leg. The leg is maintained in an abducted position (Figure 16–50).
- Follow restrictions on rotating (turning) the leg inward or outward.
- Keep the patient in proper anatomical alignment while in bed.

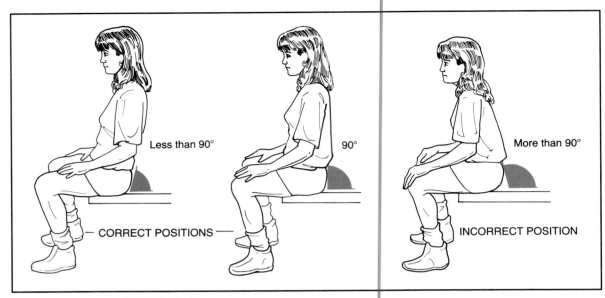

Less than 90°   90°   More than 90°

— CORRECT POSITIONS —   INCORRECT POSITION

FIGURE 16–49

Correct and incorrect sitting positions for the patient who has had total hip replacement surgery.

- Assist patient during ambulation, which is allowed after the third or fourth postoperative day.
- Report any pain the patient expresses to the supervisor or nurse.

The ADLs performed by the patient with a hip fracture provide the movements needed to keep the joints moveable and help the circulation of the blood. Encourage patients to use their unaffected extremities as much as possible. The nurse or physical therapist performs the prescribed range of motion exercises for the patient.

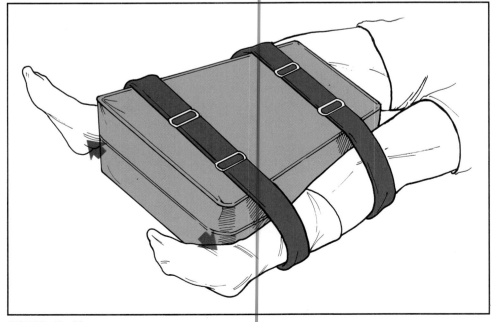

FIGURE 16–50

Legs are held in abduction (apart) by placing an abductor pillow between the legs.

THE PATIENT WITH A CEREBROVASCULAR ACCIDENT

A **cerebrovascular accident** (CVA) is the death of brain tissue that occurs from a lack of blood supply to part of the brain. The word **"stroke"** is the everyday word for a CVA. A CVA can affect a person at any age. It commonly affects people between 75 and 85 years of age.

A CVA is caused by a blockage of blood supply to a part of the brain. The blockage can be caused by a **thrombosis** or an **embolism**. A thrombosis occurs when blood clots form inside a blood vessel or a chamber of the heart and block or interfere with the flow of blood. When the thrombosis occurs in the brain, it is called a cerebral thrombosis.

An embolism occurs when a blood clot travels in the bloodstream until it stops somewhere and blocks the flow of blood. Remember that when the flow of blood is blocked, **necrosis** results. When an embolism travels in the blood vessels of the brain and results in necrosis, it is called a cerebral embolism.

A CVA occurs when part of the brain is deprived of oxygen, which is carried by blood. This lack of oxygen causes death of the brain tissue that controls a certain body function. This may result in paralysis. The paralysis usually occurs on one side of the body from head to toe. The term for this kind of paralysis is **hemiplegia.** Other types of paralysis that can occur include **quadriplegia,** in which all four limbs are paralyzed, and **paraplegia,** in which the legs or the lower part of the body is paralyzed.

The person who is paralyzed is not able to feel anything that touches the paralyzed area. The person may lose the ability to feel the sensations of hot or cold. The speech center in the brain may also be affected by the lack of oxygen. The patient may

- not be able to speak at all
- may slur or garble words
- may use words inappropriately

A **transient ischemic attack** (TIA) is a warning sign that a CVA may occur. Ischemia is the lack of blood in any part of the body due to blockage of a blood vessel. A TIA is a *temporary* lack of oxygen to the brain tissue that can last a period of days, weeks, or even months.

During a TIA, there is a momentary lack of oxygen to the brain. Any lack of oxygen to the body's tissue causes necrosis. The person may experience weakness or some loss of movement in an extremity when the brain tissue that controls the extremity is deprived of oxygen.

TIAs are a warning because they happen before a CVA occurs. The person who has TIAs needs treatment to prevent a CVA from occurring.

Preventing a Cerebrovascular Accident

The best way to prevent a CVA is to adopt healthy living habits and practice them for life. Daily exercise, like walking, and three well-balanced meals a day are suggested. The amount of fat in the diet should be reduced. A person may be under the care of a physician. The physician uses a combination of the following to decrease the likelihood of a CVA:

Diet
Exercise
Blood tests for **cholesterol**
Medication

Care of the Patient with a Cerebrovascular Accident

Rehabilitation is the process of restoring a person's ability to perform ADLs and to function as normally as possible after a CVA. Rehabilitation begins immediately after a person experiences a CVA. The rehabilitation team consists of

- patient

CEREBROVASCULAR ACCIDENT when the blood stops going to the brain, causing brain tissue to die; a stroke
STROKE cerebrovascular accident; when blood stops going to a part of the brain
THROMBOSIS formation or presence of a thrombus (blood clots inside a blood vessel)
EMBOLISM the sudden blocking of an artery by an embolus (traveling blood clot)
NECROSIS death of tissue
HEMIPLEGIA paralysis of one side of the body
QUADRIPLEGIA paralysis of all four limbs
PARAPLEGIA paralysis of the legs or the lower part of the body
TRANSIENT ISCHEMIC ATTACK temporary lack of oxygen to brain tissue
CHOLESTEROL fatty substance that attaches to the lining of arteries; comes from animal fats and oils

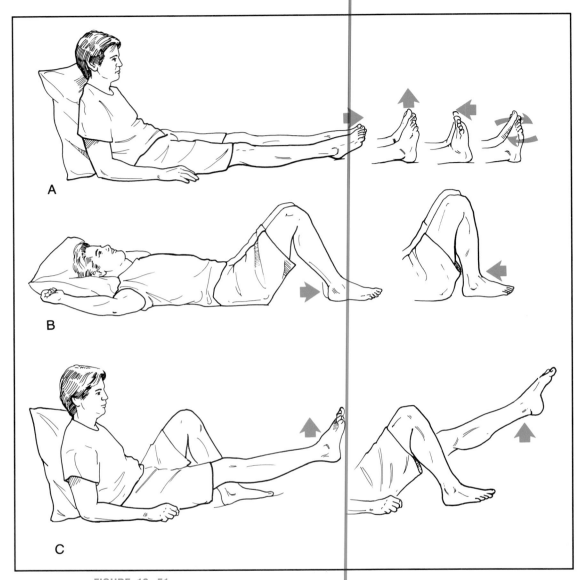

FIGURE 16–51

Leg exercises. To improve circulation, each exercise should be repeated three times. A, Point toes toward the foot of the bed; point them toward the ceiling; relax. Repeat. With both ankles, make circles in one direction and then the other. B, Bend at the knee and keep feet flat on the bed. Slide feet back and forth as far as possible. C, Alternate raising and lowering one leg while keeping the other leg flexed at the knee.

PHYSIATRIST

physician who specializes in physical therapy

PSYCHIATRIST

physician who helps people with mental, emotional, and behavioral disorders

PSYCHOLOGIST

professional who helps people with mental, emotional, and behavioral problems

OCCUPATIONAL THERAPIST

professional who helps patients relearn self-care, work, or leisure activities when illness or injury has made them incapable of performing these activities

- **physiatrist**
- nurses and other care givers
- social worker
- **psychiatrist** and **psychologist**
- physical therapist
- **occupational therapist**

Any other health care professional who can help the person return to normal function is also consulted.

You may be assigned to care for a patient who has had a CVA. The patient may report

- headache
- lack of sensation in a body part
- problems with vision (blurred or double vision)

You may observe the following:

- lack of movement of the affected extremity
- changes in or loss of speech
- change in level of **consciousness** and ability to think clearly

CONSCIOUSNESS
state of being awake, alert; not sleeping

Your role in the care of patients who have had a CVA is to help prevent any complications associated with inactivity and immobility. As discussed previously, you should encourage the patient to perform as much AROM exercise as possible to help strengthen muscles and keep joints flexible. The patient may also be taught leg exercises to improve circulation (Figure 16–51).

You also need to provide emotional support and encouragement to help CVA patients to do as much as possible for themselves. Since rehabilitation begins immediately, you become a member of the rehabilitation team.

CHAPTER WRAP-UP

- Activity and mobility have positive effects on the mind and body. Inactivity and immobility have far-reaching negative effects on the mind and body.
- The skeletal system consists of a framework of bones that support the soft tissues of the body. The bones provide protection for the brain, heart, lungs, and kidneys.
- The nervous system stimulates the muscles to contract and relax to produce movement.
- Individuals have their own normal level of activity and mobility. Ambulating, moving all extremities, and performing activities of daily living are indicators of a person's normal level of activity and mobility.
- Illness and weakness affect activity and mobility. You should keep the patient's body in proper alignment. Perform or assist with range of motion exercises when patients are unable to do so for themselves. Transferring patients from the bed to a chair helps them maintain a degree of activity and mobility. Use good body mechanics in all your procedures involving patient mobility.
- Disruptions in activity and mobility range from minor, short-term disruptions to permanent disruptions in function. Events such as fractures and strokes cause varying degrees of disruptions of activity and mobility. Problems with medications can also affect a person's level of activity and mobility.
- Each body system can be affected by a disruption in activity and mobility. Over a period of time, complications like decubitus ulcers, muscle atrophy, or contractures can occur. As a nursing assistant, you take action to prevent the complications associated with these disruptions. Giving fluids (when permitted), performing range of motion exercises, turning and positioning the patient, and giving good hygiene care are important preventive actions.
- A fracture is a break in the bone that heals over a period of time extending from 4 weeks to 6 weeks or more. A fracture is either open or closed.
- Most closed fractures are treated by immobilizing the body part until the bone heals. Casts and supportive devices are used to maintain and support the body part in a position necessary for healing to occur.
- An open fracture is treated surgically, after which a cast or other stabilizing device such as a pin, screw, plate, or nail is inserted.
- A cerebrovascular accident, also called a stroke, occurs if the blood supply to any part of the brain is interrupted. When the blood supply to

the brain is interrupted, brain tissue dies, and thus the body function that is controlled by that brain tissue is lost. During the early part of treatment, you are responsible for helping prevent the complications of inactivity and immobility. In the rehabilitation phase, you help the patient regain some degree of activity and mobility.

REVIEW QUESTIONS

1. Why is the use of good body mechanics so important?
2. What can you do to help a patient maintain activity and mobility?
3. Name the complications that occur in each body system as a result of a disruption in activity and mobility.
4. What actions help prevent complications associated with inactivity and immobility?
5. Explain the care of a patient in a cast.
6. Describe the care of a patient on bed rest.

ACTIVITY CORNER

Using good body mechanics prevent injury to yourself and your patients. The next time you perform the following activities, pay attention to your body mechanics. Are you using the rules of good body mechanics when you

Transfer patients from the bed to a chair?	Yes _____	No _____
Help patients to the bathroom?	Yes _____	No _____
Carry supplies to patients' room?	Yes _____	No _____
Make up a bed with clean linens?	Yes _____	No _____

Observe one other person perform the above activities. Are good body mechanics being used?   Yes _____ No _____

What can you or the other person do to improve your body mechanics? _____

_____

Range of motion is something each of us does when we move our extremities. Stand facing a mirror and do the following motions. With each movement you make, name the range of motion (answers below).

Movement	**Name**
Bend your head to look down at the floor	_____ of the head
Look up at the ceiling	_____ of the head
Touch your fingers to your shoulder	_____ of the elbow
Raise your arm away from your body at the side and return	_____ of the arm, followed by _____
Bend your fingers toward the palm of your hand and then straighten them out	_____ of the fingers, followed by _____
Raise one leg up by bending it at the knee and then return the leg to the straight position	_____ of the hip and knee, followed by _____ _____
Swing one leg away from your body toward the side and bring it back	_____ of the leg, followed by _____ _____

Spread your toes apart and bring   _____ of the toes,
   back together   followed by _____

(*Answers:* hyperflexion; extension; flexion; abduction, adduction; flexion, extension; flexion, extension; abduction, adduction; abduction, adduction.)

A good way to learn range of motion is to practice doing the range of motion movements. This will give you confidence when you perform range of motion exercises for your patients.

UNIT FIVE

Learning About Body Functions and Patient Care

17 Learning about Body Structure and Function

Objectives

AFTER YOU COMPLETE THIS CHAPTER, YOU WILL BE ABLE TO:

Define *anatomy* and *physiology*.
List the functions of each of the body systems.
Locate the cavities of the body.
Locate different areas of the body.

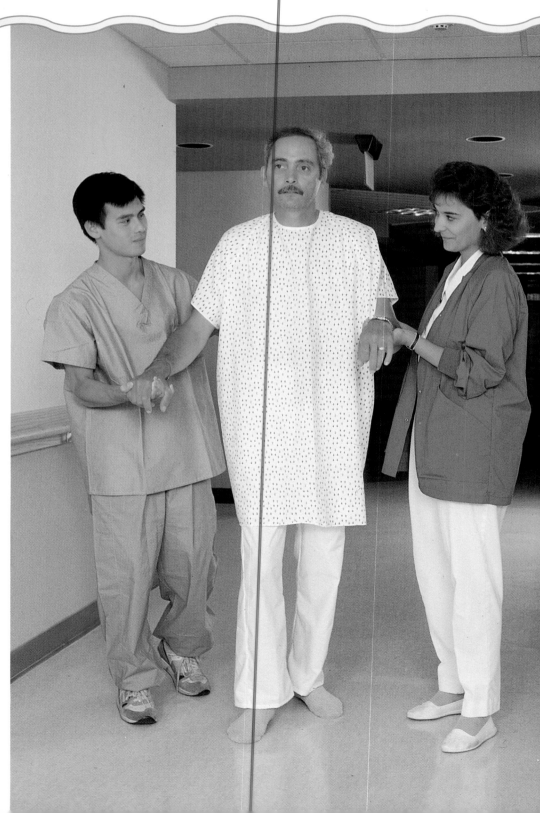

Overview The human body is organized into many systems. These systems are designed to work together. When one or more body systems are affected by disease or illness, the body may not function as it usually does. Having a basic understanding of how the body is built and how it functions will help you give safe and efficient care to your patients.

WHAT DO YOU KNOW ABOUT THE HUMAN BODY?

Here are five statements about the human body. Consider them to test your current ideas about the structure and function of the human body. If you think the statement is true, circle the T; if you think the statement is false, circle the F. Change the false statements to make them true.

1. T F Physiology is the study of how the body is built.
2. T F Muscle tissue has the ability to expand and contract.
3. T F Cells need only food and water to survive and grow.
4. T F The human body has two major cavities.
5. T F The skin, hair, nails, and sweat glands make up the smallest body system.

ANSWERS

1. **False.** Physiology is the study of how the parts of the body work.
2. **True.** Muscle tissue is specifically designed to expand and contract to allow the body to move.
3. **False.** The cell needs food, water, and oxygen to survive and grow.
4. **True.** The human body has two major body cavities: the dorsal and ventral cavities.
5. **False.** The skin, hair, nails, and sweat glands make up the largest body system.

ANATOMY
the science of body structure
PHYSIOLOGY
the study of body function

CELL
the basic unit of any living organism
WATER
clear, odorless, tasteless, colorless
fluid
OXYGEN
a colorless, tasteless, odorless gas;
the air we breathe is about 20%
oxygen
MEMBRANE
a layer of tissue that acts as a
covering or lining
NUCLEUS
a small body inside the cell that acts
as the control center; also contains
chromosomes
CYTOPLASM
the substance surrounding the
nucleus; contains smaller bodies
that do the work of the cell

Two important fields of study of the human body are anatomy and physiology. **Anatomy** is the science of body structure; when you study anatomy you learn how the parts of the body are built. **Physiology** is the study of body function; when you study physiology you learn how the parts of the body work.

THE CELL

The **cell** is the basic unit of any living organism (Figure 17–1). It is so small it can be seen only under a microscope. Each cell is designed to perform a specific task. Cells vary in shape, size, and function. In order to function, all cells need

    Food
    Water
    Oxygen

Food is needed because it contains energy. Oxygen helps cells break down the food to get to the energy, which they need to grow. Water provides cells a way to move substances from one place to another.

The basic parts of the cell are the

    Cell membrane
    Nucleus
    Cytoplasm

The cell **membrane** is the outer covering of the cell. This thin membrane protects the cell but allows substances to pass in and out. The **nucleus** is a small body inside the cell that acts as the control center. The **cytoplasm**

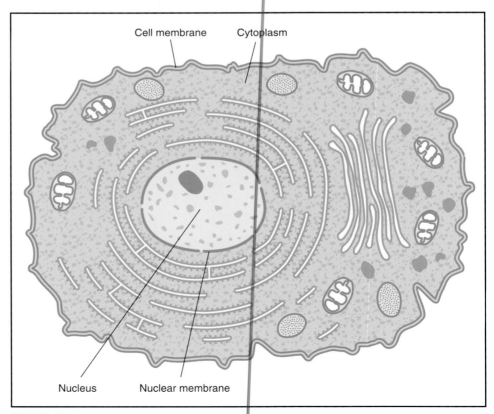

FIGURE 17–1
The cell.

surrounds the nucleus and contains other small cell parts that do the work of the cell.

The nucleus contains the **chromosomes.** Each chromosome contains special threads that carry genetic information. The **gene** is the biologic unit of **heredity** and is located in the chromosome. The gene carries information the cell needs when it reproduces.

The cell reproduces by division. The nucleus ensures duplication when pairs of chromosomes pull apart during cell division. When cell division is complete, two new cells exist that are identical to the original cell.

CHROMOSOME
the part of the cell that contains genetic information
GENE
biologic unit of heredity located in the chromosome
HEREDITY
the physical and mental traits you receive from your ancestors; inheritance

CARING COMMENT

The cell can be seen only under the microscope. However, tissue—cells joined together—may be seen by the human eye. For example, the cells that join to form the skin can be seen. The skin that covers the outside of the body is a large organ protecting the body from invasion by harmful microorganisms.

TISSUE

Tissue is a group or layer of cells that all perform the same function (Figure 17–2). There are four main types of tissue in the body:

- **Connective tissue**—Connects and holds parts of the body together. Ligaments and tendons are connective tissues in the body.
- **Epithelial tissue**—Covers the internal and external surfaces of the body. An example of internal epithelial tissue is the tissue that lines the gastrointestinal system (mouth to anus). An example of external epithelial tissue is the skin.
- **Muscle tissue**—Expands (becomes larger) and contracts (becomes smaller). It allows the body and its parts to move.
- **Nervous tissue**—Sends and receives messages, permitting different parts of the body to communicate with one another.

TISSUE
a group or layer of cells that all perform the same task

CONNECTIVE TISSUE
tissue that connects and holds parts of the body together
EPITHELIAL TISSUE
tissue that covers the internal and external surfaces of the body
MUSCLE TISSUE
fibrous tissue that expands and contracts to allow the body to move
NERVOUS TISSUE
tissue that sends and receives messages

ORGANS

Groups of tissues combine to form organs. An **organ** is a body part that performs a specific function or functions (Figure 17–3). The heart, lungs, brain, liver, and kidneys are examples of organs.

ORGAN
a body part that performs a specific function or functions

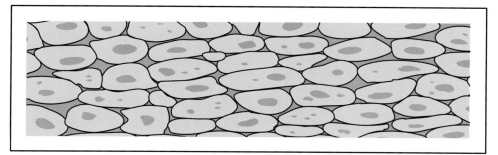

FIGURE 17–2
Tissue.

BODY SYSTEM

a group of organs that work together to perform one or more body functions (for example, in the urinary system, the kidneys produce urine and the bladder stores urine)

HOMEOSTASIS

a state of balance

CAVITY

a hollow or a space

DORSAL

toward the back

VENTRAL

toward the front

CRANIAL

inside the skull

SPINAL

pertaining to the spine (backbone)

THORACIC

pertaining to the chest

ABDOMINAL

pertaining to the abdomen

DIAPHRAGM

the muscular membrane that separates the thoracic and abdominal cavities

HEART

the hollow muscular organ located in the left side of the chest that is an electrical pump that controls the flow of blood

LUNGS

the two main organs of respiration

ESOPHAGUS

a muscular tube from the pharynx to the top of the stomach

STOMACH

a pouch-like organ located on the left side of the abdomen; the widest part of the gastrointestinal system

LIVER

the largest organ in the body; stores red blood cells and secretes bile

PANCREAS

located behind the stomach; secretes insulin

GALLBLADDER

a small pear-shaped sac located under the liver; concentrates and stores bile

SPLEEN

an abdominal organ that stores red blood cells and helps keep the blood free of waste material

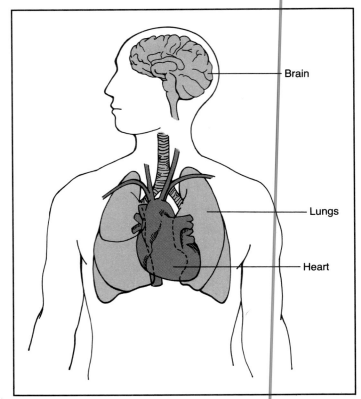

FIGURE 17-3
Organs.

BODY SYSTEMS

A system is a set of things that act together to produce results that each thing cannot produce alone. A **body system** is a group of organs that work together to perform one or more body functions (Figure 17–4). Body systems work together to keep the body in a balanced state. The term **homeostasis** is used to refer to the body's balanced state.

The body systems, their parts, and their functions are listed in Table 17–1.

BODY CAVITIES

The body has two major **cavities** (Figure 17–5):

- the **dorsal** cavity—located toward the back of the body
- the **ventral** cavity—located toward the front of the body

The dorsal cavity includes the **cranial** and **spinal** cavities. The cranial cavity contains the brain and its covering membranes, blood vessels, and nerves. The spinal cavity contains the spinal cord.

The ventral cavity includes the **thoracic** and **abdominal** cavities. The **diaphragm** is a muscle that separates the thoracic and abdominal cavities. The thoracic cavity contains the **heart, lungs,** and major blood vessels. The **esophagus** begins in the thoracic cavity, passes through the diaphragm, and ends at the stomach. The **stomach** is located in the abdominal cavity, along with the **liver; pancreas; gallbladder; spleen;** small and large **intestines;** the urinary **bladder;** and, in females, the **ovaries** and **uterus.** These organs are enclosed in

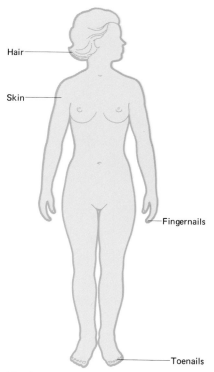

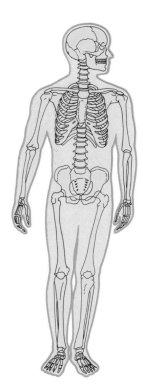

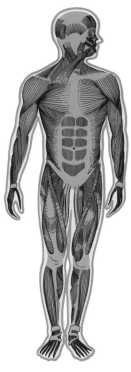

(*a*) The integumentary system consists of the skin and the structures derived from it. The integumentary system protects the body, helps to regulate body temperature, and receives information about touch, pressure, pain, and temperature.

(*b*) The skeletal system consists of bones and cartilage. This system helps to support and protect the body.

(*c*) The muscular system consists of the large skeletal muscles that enable us to move, the cardiac muscle of the heart, and the smooth muscle of the internal organs

FIGURE 17–4

Body systems. (From Solomon EP: Introduction to Human Anatomy and Physiology. Philadelphia, W. B. Saunders Company, 1992.)

Illustration continued on following page

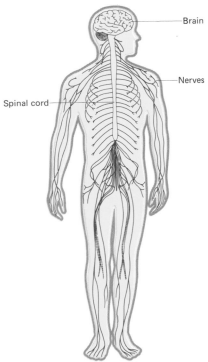

(d) The nervous system consists of the brain, spinal cord, sense organs, and nerves. The nervous system regulates other body systems.

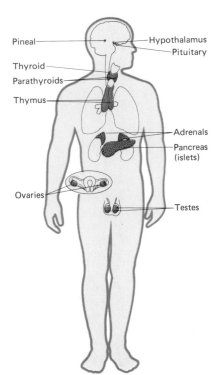

(e) The endocrine system consists of the glands and tissues that release chemical messengers called hormones. The endocrine system works with the nervous system in regulating metabolic activities.

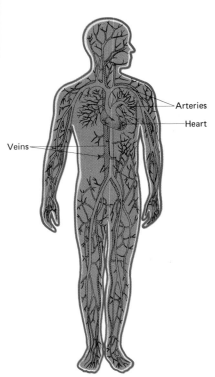

(f) The circulatory system serves as the transportation system of the body. The heart and blood vessels are part of this system.

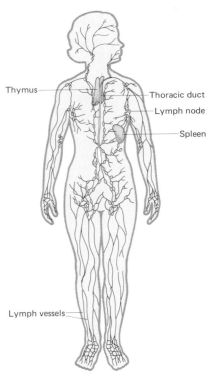

(g) The lymphatic system is a subsystem of the circulatory system. This system defends the body against disease.

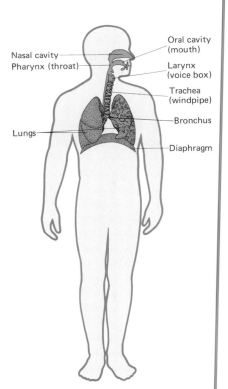

(h) The respiratory system consists of the lungs and air passageways. This system supplies oxygen to the blood and rids the body of carbon dioxide.

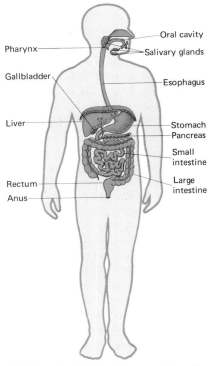

(i) The digestive system consists of the digestive tract and glands that secrete digestive juices into the digestive tract. This system breaks down food and eliminates wastes.

FIGURE 17-4 *Continued*

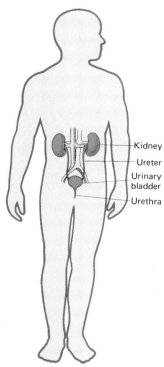

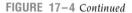

(j) The urinary system is the main excretory system. The kidneys remove wastes and excess materials from the blood and produce urine. This system helps to regulate blood chemistry

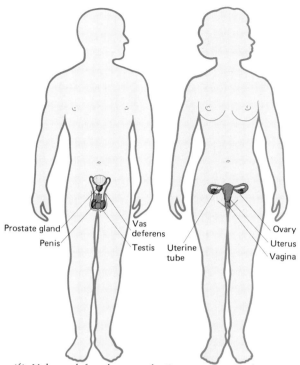

(k) Male and female reproductive systems. Each reproductive system consists of gonads and associated structures. The male reproductive system produces and delivers sperm. The female reproductive system produces ova (eggs) and incubates the developing offspring. The reproductive system maintains sexual characteristics and reproduces the species.

FIGURE 17-4 *Continued*

TABLE 17-1 BODY SYSTEMS, BODY PARTS, AND THEIR FUNCTION

Body System	Body Parts	Function
Integumentary	Skin, hair, nails, and sweat glands	Protects the body from microorganisms
Nervous	Nerves, brain, sensory organs, and spinal cord	Receives and interprets stimuli; conducts impulses
Respiratory	Lungs, bronchi, and other air passageways	Delivers oxygen to and expels carbon dioxide from body cells
Circulatory	Heart, blood, blood vessels, and lymph glands	Transports blood and other substances; defends against disease
Skeletal	Bones, cartilage, and ligaments	Supports the body; protects major organs
Muscular	Cardiac muscle	Pumps blood
	Skeletal muscle	Moves parts of the skeleton
	Smooth muscle	Helps push food through the digestive system
Digestive	Mouth, esophagus, stomach, intestines, liver, pancreas, and gallbladder	Takes in and breaks down food; excretes body waste materials
Urinary	Kidney, ureter, bladder, and urethra	Removes unneeded substances from blood; excretes fluid waste
Reproductive	Ovaries, uterus, and vagina in females; testes, penis, and prostate gland in males	Reproduces the human species; secretes certain hormones
Endocrine	Pituitary, adrenal, thyroid, and other glands	Regulates body chemistry and many body functions
Lymphatic	Thymus, spleen, and lymphatic nodes and vessels	Helps regulate fluids in the blood; defends the body against disease

INTESTINE

the tube that extends from the stomach to the anus

BLADDER

the elastic muscular sac that collects urine before it leaves the body

OVARIES

egg-shaped organs located on each side of the uterus in females; produce the ovum (egg) and hormones

UTERUS

the womb; pear-shaped organ located above the cervix in the pelvic region of females

PERITONEUM

the membrane that lines the abdominal and pelvic cavities

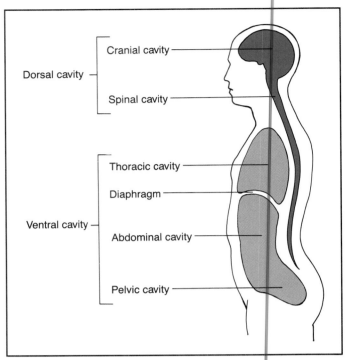

FIGURE 17-5
Major body cavities.

KIDNEY
one of two organs that filter waste products out of the blood to be eliminated from the body
PELVIC
pertaining to the pelvis (the area between the hip bones and the lower spine)

a special membrane called the peritoneum. The **peritoneum** is the membrane that lines the abdominal cavity and another cavity called the pelvic cavity. The **kidneys** are located outside the peritoneum at the back of the abdominal cavity. The **pelvic** cavity is part of the abdominal cavity and is located at the lowest part of the abdomen.

BODY AREAS

ANATOMIC POSITION
the human body standing erect with palms and toes facing forward
SUPERIOR
upward, toward the head; a structure occupying a higher position
INFERIOR
downward, toward the feet; the lower of two structures
ANTERIOR
located toward the front
POSTERIOR
located toward the back
MEDIAL
located in the middle
GROIN
the area from the lower abdomen to the inner part of the thighs
LATERAL
toward the side; away from the middle of a body part

Anatomic position is the term used to describe the human body standing erect with the palms and toes facing forward. The following directional terms will help you locate various body structures (Figure 17-6).

- **Superior**—Upward, toward the head; a structure occupying a higher position. The heart is superior to the kidneys because it occupies a higher position than the kidneys.
- **Inferior**—Downward, toward the feet; the lower of two structures. The toes are inferior to the knees because they are lower than the knees.
- **Anterior**—In the front. The heart is anterior to the spine because it is located in front of the spine.
- **Posterior**—In the back. The spine is posterior to the heart because it is located behind the heart.
- **Medial**—Toward the middle of an imaginary line that goes through the center of the body from the head to the **groin.** The breastbone is medial to the shoulder because it is located where the imaginary lines goes through the center of the body.
- **Lateral**—Toward the side; away from the middle of a body part. The arm is lateral to the trunk of the body because it is located toward the side of and away from the trunk.

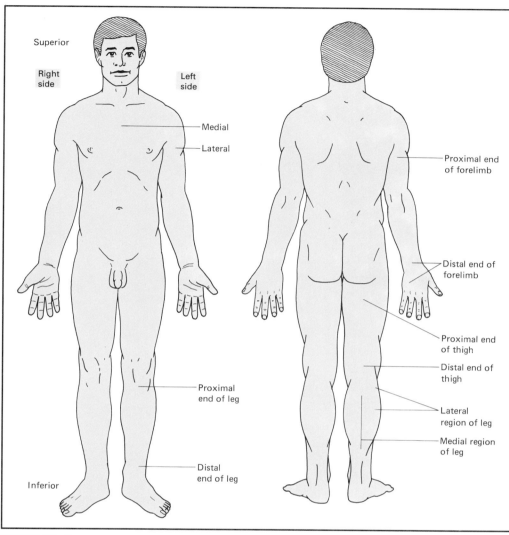

FIGURE 17–6

The human body in anatomic position and some directional terms. (From Solomon EP: Introduction to Human Anatomy and Physiology. Philadelphia, W. B. Saunders Company, 1992.)

- **Proximal**—The nearest point of reference. The knee is the proximal point of the leg because it is nearer than the foot.
- **Distal**—The farthest point of reference. The foot is the distal point of the leg because it is the farthest point of reference on the leg.
- **Superficial**—Near the surface. The wrist bones are superficial because they are located near the surface of the body.
- **Deep**—Located below or away from the surface. The appendix is deep because it is located away from the surface of the body.

PROXIMAL
the nearest point of reference
DISTAL
the farthest point of reference
SUPERFICIAL
near the surface
DEEP
below or away from the surface

CARING COMMENT

Stand up straight in front of a full-length mirror. Turn your palms forward and point your toes straight ahead. This is good body alignment. Patients in bed are in good body alignment when they are lying straight, with palms up and toes pointing upward.

CHAPTER WRAP-UP

- Anatomy is the science of body structure; physiology is the study of body function.
- The cell is the basic unit of any living organism.
- Tissue is a group or layer of cells that all perform the same task. The four main types of tissue are
  - Connective
  - Epithelial
  - Muscle
  - Nervous
- Groups of tissues combine to form organs.
- A body system consists of a group of organs that work together to perform specific body functions. The body systems are as follows:
  - Integumentary
  - Nervous
  - Respiratory
  - Circulatory
  - Skeletal
  - Muscular
  - Digestive
  - Urinary
  - Reproductive
  - Endocrine
  - Lymphatic
- The body contains two major cavities: the dorsal and ventral cavities.
- A variety of directional terms are used to describe the locations of various body structures.
- Anatomic position is the human body standing erect with the palms and toes facing forward.

REVIEW QUESTIONS

1. Define *anatomy* and *physiology*.
2. Name the three things a cell needs for growth and survival.
3. Use directional terms to locate the ankles, the elbow, and the nose.

ACTIVITY CORNER

This chapter lists 11 body systems. Try naming them all. Rate yourself on the scale below.

_____

_____

_____

_____

_____

_____

_____

_____

_____

_____

_____

Number correct: 10–11   Expert
                  7–9   Above average
                  4–6   Average
                  3 or below Check your work

18 Learning About the Senses

Objectives

AFTER YOU COMPLETE THIS CHAPTER, YOU WILL BE ABLE TO:

Describe the structure and function of the five senses.

Identify normal observations of the five senses.

Identify common disruptions in sensory function.

Identify unusual observations of sensory function.

Describe sensory deficit and sensory overload.

Care for patients with disruptions in sensory function.

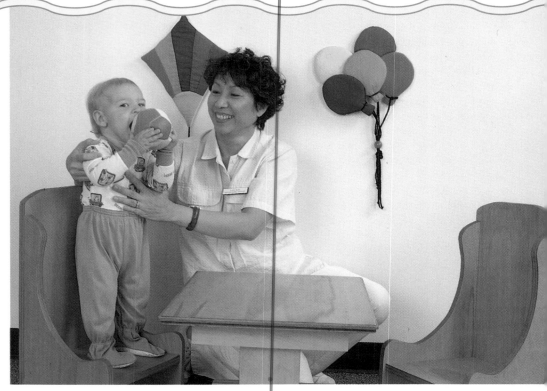

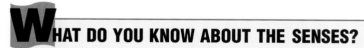

Overview   Some patients under your care will have a problem with the functioning of their eyes, ears, nose, taste buds, or nerve endings in the skin. This affects their senses—their seeing, hearing, smelling, tasting, or feeling. By knowing how to help these patients make adjustments in the way they do things, you can enable them to continue to enjoy the world around them and remain safe.

WHAT DO YOU KNOW ABOUT THE SENSES?

Here are eight statements about the senses of the body. Consider them to test your current ideas about the senses. If you think the statement is true, circle the T; if you think the statement is false, circle the F. Change the false statements to make them true.

1. T F   The sensory organs include the eyes, ears, nose, and taste buds only.

2. T F   The brain receives information from the sensory organs of the body.

3. T F   The gustatory sense is the sense of hearing.

4. T F   The rupture (breaking) of small blood vessels in the nose can result in a nosebleed.

5. T F   Bright light causes the pupil of the eye to constrict (become smaller).

6. T F   Eyelashes are a decorative feature of the body.

7. T F   The odor of food adds to the pleasure of eating.

8. T F   The sense of touch can act as a protective mechanism in the body.

ANSWERS

1. **False.** One other sensory organ is the sensitive nerve endings that are present in the skin and provide the sense of touch.

2. **True.** The brain is the center for processing and interpreting information sent to it by the sensory organs.

3. **False.** The gustatory sense is the sense of taste; the auditory sense is the sense of hearing.

4. **True.** When a blood vessel is ruptured, it bleeds.

5. **True.** The pupil responds to bright light by becoming smaller. This helps regulate the amount of light the eye needs.

6. **False.** Eyelashes protect the eye from dust and debris in the environment that could injure it.

7. **True.** The odor of food helps a person to anticipate and enjoy eating.

8. **True.** The sense of touch may be the first line of defense in a threatening situation.

THE SENSES

SENSES
the ways we receive and interpret stimuli; sight, sound, touch, taste, and smell

STIMULI
Those things that cause an activity to start

SENSORY ORGANS
eyes, ears, nerve endings in the skin, taste buds, nose; the organs that control or regulate vision, hearing, touch, taste, and smell

The **senses** are the way we receive and interpret **stimuli;** the five senses are sight, sound, touch, taste, and smell. The **sensory organs** control our senses. They are the eyes, ears, nose, taste buds, and nerve endings in the skin. The stimuli that we take in through our sensory organs are transmitted to the brain, which interprets them. If the incoming information cannot reach the brain for an explanation, the sensory organs cannot function.

Other terms used to describe sensory function include:

Visual
Auditory
Olfactory
Gustatory
Tactile

OBSERVING FOR SENSORY DEFICITS

SENSORY DEFICIT
a condition in which a person is unable to respond to stimulation

Sensory deficit is the loss of or a reduction in sensory stimulation. When the sensory organs do not receive or interpret outside stimulation, a person has a sensory deficit. Hereditary problems, disease, and accidents can cause deficits in one or more of the five senses. Patients with a sensory deficit need extra care to prevent accidental injury and to help them function (see Looking for Sensory Deficits chart).

VISUAL
pertaining to ability to see

LOOKING FOR SENSORY DEFICITS

Visual Deficit

Subjective Observations

- Ask patients whether they have any problems seeing.
- Do patients tell you when they have double or blurred vision?
- How well do patients see in a darkened room?
- Does bright light irritate the eyes?

Objective Observations

- Do patients own prescription glasses or contact lenses and wear them when they should?
- Observe patients when they read to see how far they hold the reading material from their eyes.
- Do patients squint while trying to recognize something or someone or while trying to read?

Auditory Deficit

Subjective Observations

- Do patients tell you they have a ringing or humming sound in their ears?

Objective Observations

- If a hearing aid has been prescribed, is it used accordingly?
- When patients attempt to communicate, do they speak loudly?
- Do you often have to repeat things to patients?
- Are the television and radio played at louder than usual settings?
- Is there a puzzled expression on patients' face when you communicate?

Olfactory Deficit

Subjective Observations

- Do patients tell you they can smell the flowers in the room, a visitor's perfume, the food in the cart in the hall, or other hospital smells?

Gustatory Deficit

Subjective Observations

- Ask patients about their use of extra seasonings such as salt and pepper.
- Do patients tell you food tastes good?
- Can patients tell whether they are tasting food that is spicy, sweet, or sour?
- Have patients mentioned a taste in their mouth that could not be explained?

Tactile Deficit

Subjective Observations

- Can patients tell you whether an object is hot or cold, sharp or dull, and light or firm when you touch them with the object?

AUDITORY
relating to the sense of hearing

OLFACTORY
associated with the sense of smell

GUSTATORY
associated with the sense of taste

TACTILE
pertaining to touch

THE EYE

The eyes are our windows to the world. Through them we see images and colors. The images that we see in our field of vision stimulate the sensory center in the brain. The sensory center interprets the stimuli so that we can identify the objects in the world around us. The **eye** is a sphere about an inch in diameter. The bones of the skull form the socket in which the eye sits and protect the eye from injury. Muscles control the eye's movements. Special muscles control the pupil. When a person is exposed to bright light, the pupil constricts (becomes smaller) to prevent too much light from entering the eye. Other special muscles enable the pupil to dilate (enlarge) when the light is dim, so that as much light as possible is allowed in. The area that can be seen by the two eyes is called the field of vision. We can see length and width with

EYE
organ of vision

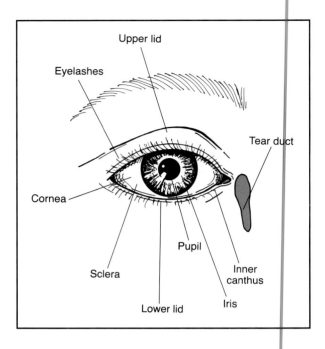

FIGURE 18-1
The external structures of the eye.

one eye, but need both eyes to see depth. Cover one of your eyes with your hand and look at an object. You will be able to see its length and width. Keep the eye covered and reach for the object. You will find that it is easy to mistake the position of the object when you reach for it, because both eyes are needed to see depth.

EXTERNAL STRUCTURES OF THE EYE

The main external structures of the eye are shown in Figure 18-1. They are the

- eyelids
- eyelashes
- sclera and cornea

The eyelids are the moveable folds of skin above and below the eye. They protect the anterior (front) surface of the eye. A delicate membrane called the conjunctiva lines the eyelid and the eyeball. The eyelashes are the hairs that grow along the edge of the eyelids. They protect the eyes from dust and debris in the environment. The **sclera** is the tough, white outer covering of the eyeball. The sclera becomes transparent over the pupil and iris. The clear, transparent part of the sclera over the pupil and iris is called the cornea.

INTERNAL STRUCTURES OF THE EYE

The main internal structures of the eye are shown in Figure 18-2. They are the

- iris
- pupil
- lens
- anterior (front) and posterior (back) chambers
- retina (Figure 18-2)

The **iris** is the circular, colored membrane located behind the cornea. The iris may be blue, green, hazel, brown, or black. The **pupil** is the opening in the

SCLERA
the tough, white outer covering of the eyeball

IRIS
the circular, pigmented (colored) membrane of the eye

PUPIL
the opening in the center of the iris that helps control the amount of light entering the eye

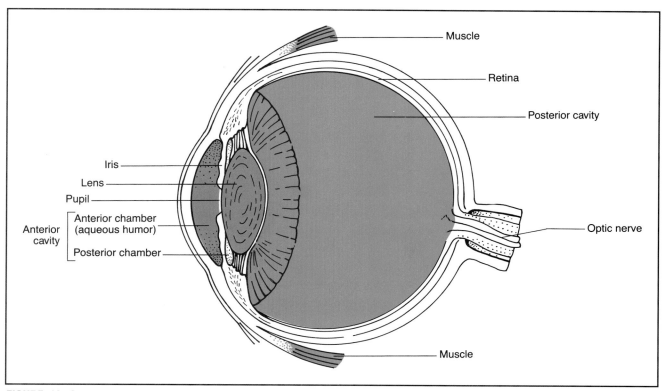

FIGURE 18–2
The internal structures of the eye.

center of the iris that helps control the amount of light that enters the eye. The **lens** is located behind the iris and the pupil. It is a crystal-like material that bends or scatters light rays.

The anterior cavity consists of two **chambers**, the anterior (between the cornea and the iris) chamber and the posterior (between the iris and the lens) chamber. A watery fluid called **aqueous humor** fills the anterior and posterior chambers. The posterior cavity of the eye is filled with **vitreous humor**, a jelly-like, transparent material. The aqueous humor and the vitreous humor help the eye keep its rounded shape.

The **retina** is the light-sensitive inner layer of the eye. When the retina is hit by light rays, it forms images.

OBSERVATIONS OF THE EYE

Your eyes are usually the first thing you notice when you look in the mirror in the morning. If you did not sleep the number of hours your body requires, your eyes may have puffy bags under them. If you were up late studying the night before, your eyes may be reddened or teary. After a night's rest, the eyes should be clear.

The blink **reflex** washes the surface of the eyeball and keeps it moistened and clean. The color of the sclera is normally white. Put your finger just below the lower eyelid and gently pull in a downward direction. The area that is exposed is called the **conjunctiva.** It should be deep pink or red.

Notice that when you open and close your eyes the pupils change in size to control the amount of light that enters (Figure 18–3). Both pupils should be

LENS
glass or other transparent material that bends or scatters light rays

CHAMBER
an enclosed space

AQUEOUS HUMOR
watery fluid that fills the anterior and posterior chambers of the eye

VITREOUS HUMOR
the transparent substance that fills the part of the eyeball between the lens and the retina

REFLEX
an automatic response to a stimulus

CONJUNCTIVA
the delicate membrane that covers the inner eyelids and the eyeball

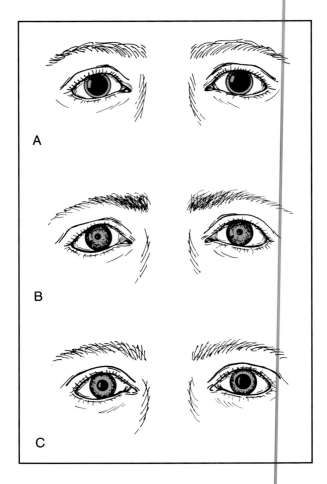

FIGURE 18–3
Pupil sizes. A, Dilated. B, Pinpoint. C, Unequal.

the same diameter (of equal size). The pupils dilate when you are in a dim light. They constrict when the light is bright.

Many people wear glasses to correct vision problems. Some people wear contact lenses. You might need to ask your supervisor or the nurse how to give eye care to patients who wear contact lenses or an artificial eye. Patients often tell you what kind of vision problem they have. They may tell you how far they can see with or without their glasses (Figure 18–4).

UNUSUAL OBSERVATIONS OF THE EYE

Observe both eyes to determine whether any changes have occurred in them. Report to the supervisor or nurse if patients tell you that their eyes hurt or are

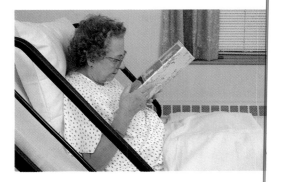

FIGURE 18–4
When you observe patients reading, look to see how far or close they are holding their reading material.

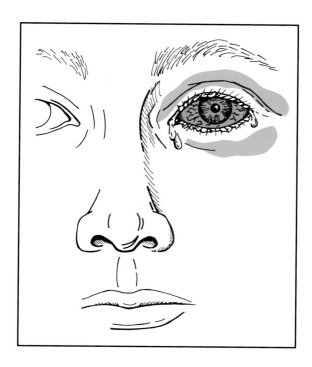

FIGURE 18–5
Unusual observations of the eye.

itchy. Other unusual observations to report include redness or **jaundice** of the sclera. Any discharge should be reported, whether it is clear and watery or yellow or green and thick (Figure 18–5). Observe and report any **periorbital edema.** Always check that the pupils are equal in size. When you notice unequal pupils, report this change to the supervisor or nurse.

CARE OF THE PATIENT WITH COMMON DISRUPTIONS IN VISION

MYOPIA

The most common disruptions in vision are corrected by prescription glasses. **Myopia,** also called **nearsightedness** or shortsightedness, is the ability to see near objects more clearly than distant objects. It is caused by the shape of the eyeball changing from round to too long from front to back. Myopia can occur in children as well as adults. Although there is no cure, myopia can be corrected by prescription glasses. Glasses enable the person to see distant objects more clearly.

HYPEROPIA

In another condition, a person may see distant objects clearly, but near objects are blurred. This is called **hyperopia,** or **farsightedness.** Hyperopia can also be corrected by prescription glasses. The prescription glasses for hyperopia bend the light rays so that near objects are in focus.

PRESCRIPTION GLASSES

When patients are not wearing their glasses, the glasses should be kept in a safe, smooth holder designed for them. Whenever you notice glasses lying on

JAUNDICE
yellowness of the skin, sclerae, mucous membranes, and body excretions caused by an accumulation of bile pigments in the blood

PERIORBITAL EDEMA
swelling surrounding the eye

MYOPIA
nearsightedness; shortsightedness

HYPEROPIA
farsightedness

the bed, ask patients if you can place them on the night stand or in a drawer of the night stand.

When patients' glasses are made of plastic, clean them with soft cotton. *Never* use paper to clean or shine lenses because paper scratches the lenses.

Never lay a pair of glasses directly on the lenses. This could accidentally scratch the lenses.

Clean patients' glasses for them and hand them to the patients when they prefer to put their glasses on themselves. When handing patients their glasses, offer them by the temples so that patients can easily put them on without smearing the glass. When you put glasses on a patient, make certain you place them on the bridge of the nose and over the patient's ears correctly. To prevent loss of prescription glasses, assist patients in putting their name on the frame of the glasses. Your actions are important in helping patients take care of their glasses.

PROCEDURE

PRESCRIPTION
an order for a procedure, medication, diet, or other service written by a physician

Caring for Prescription Glasses

Clean patients' glasses to provide a clear field of vision for them. Clean patients' glasses once a day, preferably at bath time, and any time they are soiled. The procedure is usually performed at the patient's sink.

GATHER EQUIPMENT

Running water
Lint-free cotton cloth

Commercial cleaning spray (optional) (Figure 18−6)

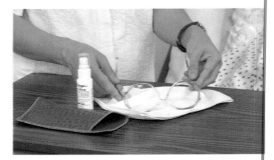

FIGURE 18−6

A commercial spray for cleaning glasses can be used at the bedside.

ACTION	RATIONALE
Procedural Steps	
1. Hold the glasses by the temples.	Glasses held in this manner are secure.
2. Turn on the tap and adjust for a slow flow of cool water.	Hot water can damage the shape of plastic frames.
3. Place glasses under the running water.	Loosens dirt and debris.

4. Hold glasses under the running water long enough for all debris to loosen.

All soil should be removed before the glasses are dried.

5. Turn off the water when the glasses are clean.

Allows the glasses to begin air drying.

6. Dry and polish the glasses with a soft, clean, cotton cloth (Figure 18–7).

Cotton does not scratch the glass; other materials can.

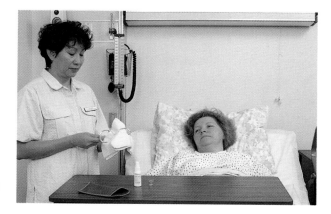

FIGURE 18–7

Polish lenses until they are clean and clear, with no streaks.

7. Store cloth for reuse.

Cloth will be available for the next time the glasses need to be cleaned.

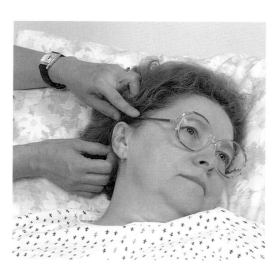

FIGURE 18–8

When you position glasses on a patient, make sure you check that the temples fit comfortably over the ears.

8. Ask patients if they would like to put their glasses on themselves or would like you to apply them (Figure 18–8).

CONTACT LENSES

Contact lenses are an item of choice for many patients. They are not as noticeable as glasses. "Contacts" are manufactured in different forms. Hard contacts are firm lenses that must be removed each time a person plans to sleep. Soft contacts are available as daily or extended wear lenses. Extended wear contacts may be worn for more than one day. Contacts also come in a range of colors.

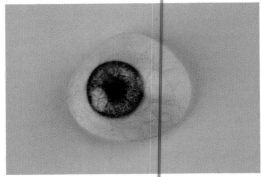

FIGURE 18-9
The modern artificial eye is lightweight and life-like.

The most important feature of contact lens care is to maintain cleanliness. Remind patients to wash their hands before they insert and remove their contact lenses. When contacts are removed for the night, place them in a secure area. A special storage holder can be purchased in stores. Special cleaners are used to keep the contact lenses as clean as possible to prevent eye infections.

Most patients who wear contact lenses prefer to perform their own eye care. Usually they choose to insert and remove their own contact lenses as well. Whenever a problem arises with a patient's contact lenses, notify the supervisor or nurse.

ARTIFICIAL EYES

HYGIENE
the practice of cleanliness to promote health

Patients who have lost an eye to disease or injury may choose to wear an artificial eye in the remaining eye socket. Artificial eyes, once made of glass, are now made of a plastic material (Figure 18-9). They come in various sizes so that the fit is as comfortable as possible. Artificial eyes come in a variety of colors to match the wearer's real eye. An artificial eye is preferred for cosmetic and psychological reasons. Daily **hygiene** care is needed to prevent infection and the accumulation of dried mucous secretions in the eye socket. You may be asked to care for the eye socket and the artificial eye when patients are unable to do so themselves.

PROCEDURE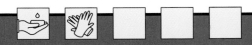

Caring for an Eye Socket and Artificial Eye
Clean the eye socket and artificial eye to remove mucus and prevent the growth of harmful microorganisms.

GATHER EQUIPMENT
Eyecup (or a clean denture cup) with patient's name and room number on it
Bath thermometer
Two pieces of 4 × 4 gauze

Small plastic bag
Special cleansing solution if ordered by the physician (two kinds of solutions may be used for care of the eye

Four or more cotton balls
Clean disposable gloves
Clean emesis (kidney-shaped) basin with
lukewarm (100° F) water

socket—one for irrigation and one for
lubrication)

ACTION	RATIONALE
Preparation	
1. Wash hands.	Prevents the spread of microorganisms.
2. Identify yourself and the patient.	Maintains patients' rights.
3. Provide privacy.	Maintains patients' rights.
4. Explain the procedure.	Informs patients what is happening.
Procedural Steps	
5. Cuff the edges of the plastic bag and place it within your reach.	
6. Put on the clean gloves.	Prevents you from coming in contact with body secretions.
7. Place patients in as low a position as they can tolerate.	Prevents dropping the artificial eye on a hard surface.
8. Ask patients to close their eyes. Moisten a cotton ball in the lukewarm water in the emesis basin.	
9. Wipe the upper lid from the inner corner of the eye to the outer edge. Use a newly moistened cotton ball each time you wipe. Discard soiled cotton balls into the plastic bag.	The inner part of the eye is considered to be cleaner than the outer edge of the eye. (Always cleanse from clean to soiled areas.)
10. Place a 4 × 4 gauze in the bottom of the eyecup.	Pads the bottom to prevent damage if the eyecup is dropped.
11. Remove the artificial eye. Use your thumb to gently pull down the lower eyelid. Use your forefinger to open the upper lid.	Releases the artificial eye from the eye socket.
12. Grasp the artificial eye as it leaves the eye socket and place it on the gauze in the eyecup.	Prevents dropping the artificial eye.
13. Use new cotton balls moistened with water (or an irrigating solution, if ordered) to remove any accumulation from the now empty eye socket. Dry the eye socket gently, using a clean, dry cotton ball for each wipe.	Prevents spread of harmful microorganisms.
14. Carry the eyecup to the bathroom.	The cleaning of the artificial eye can take place in the patient's bathroom under running water.
15. Plug the drain in the sink. Fill the sink about one-third full of lukewarm water (100° F, or as suggested by your institution).	Prevents loss or damage if eye is dropped. Hot water may change the shape of the eye.
16. Hold the eye securely and wash it under running lukewarm water. Use the gauze to loosen accumulation from the eye.	Use only water or the special solution ordered by the physician. *Any other solution may dissolve or damage the artificial eye.*
17. Rinse the eye. Rinse the eyecup, discard the water, and place the eye, still wet, on a dry 4 × 4 gauze.	A moist eye is easier to insert into the eye socket. If the eye is to be stored, fill the eyecup half full of water, place the eye

Continued on following page

PROCEDURE

Caring for an Eye Socket and Artificial Eye
Continued

in it, and store it in the drawer of the bedside stand.

18. Remove gloves.
19. Wash your hands and carry the eye to patients' bedside.
20. Explain to patients what you are going to do.

Informs patients what is happening.

21. Insert the artificial eye into the eye socket. Position the notched edge toward patients' nose. Lift the upper lid with the forefinger of one hand. Insert the eye in the eye socket with the other hand. The eye will slip into place. Press down slightly on the lower eye lid so it slips over the eye.

If patients are able to insert eye, provide the equipment for them to wash their hands first.

22. Assist patients to a position of comfort.
23. Open the privacy curtains and place the call signal within patients' reach.

Leaves patients with a means to communicate.

Follow-Through

24. Wash hands.

Prevents the spread of infection.

25. Report to the nurse that the artificial eye was cleaned and reinserted. Report any unusual observations and how the patient tolerated the procedure.

The nurse has responsibility for a decision in the case of unusual observations made during a procedure.

CARE OF THE BLIND PATIENT

BLINDNESS
inability to see

A blind person is someone who has lost the sense of sight. There are various degrees of blindness. Some of your patients will be totally blind, and others may be able to see shadows. Two diseases that can cause **blindness** are cataracts and glaucoma. Injury and infection can also cause blindness, as can damage caused by certain brain tumors. Many assistive devices are available to help blind patients function in a "sighted" world:

- Specially trained seeing-eye dogs help their master at home and outside.
- A red-tipped white cane helps the blind person probe what is in the environment.

BRAILLE
a system of writing/reading used by persons who are blind

- **Braille** enables blind persons to read. In Braille, letters take the form of raised dots on special paper. By running their fingertips over the raised dots, blind persons can read.
- Talking clocks help the blind person in the home. The person presses a button to activate a voice message that announces the time.
- A clock-based directional system makes it easier for blind persons to eat by telling them where certain foods are located on the plate. For example, you may tell a patient that the meat is located at 12 o'clock and the vegetable is located at 5 o'clock.

The only sense a blind person has lost is the sense of sight. Unless you are informed of a change in hearing, remember to speak in a normal tone of voice.

Furniture placement in the home as well as in the health care institution is important. Always inform the patient when furniture has been moved. A blind person would not notice the changed position of the furniture and could be at risk for an accident and injury.

DISRUPTIONS IN VISUAL FUNCTION

CATARACT

A **cataract** is an opacity on the lens of the eye. You can observe the cataract by looking for a milky, cloudy spot on the eye (Figure 18–10). If **opacity** is present, light rays cannot penetrate the lens, which is normally transparent. Cataracts may be hereditary (a baby can be born with cataracts) or may be caused by injury to the eye, great heat, or radiation. In addition, cataracts occur as a result of the aging process. Patients may tell you that their vision is dim or blurred. They may use a brighter light when reading or hold printed material closer to their eyes than usual. Patients who have a cataract may experience double vision or have the prescription for their eyeglasses changed frequently.

The person who is blinded by cataracts needs safe nursing care and protection from injury. Cataracts cause varying degrees of blindness—ask patients how much they are able to see. They may be able to see large printed letters or vivid colors. Plan your care around how much the patient can see. The measures that help in the care of the blind patient also help the patient who has cataracts. The only treatment for a cataract is surgery. After surgery, special prescription lenses help the patient see again.

CATARACT
a milky, cloudy spot (an opacity) on the lens or the capsule of the eye
OPACITY
a condition in which light rays cannot penetrate a normally transparent object

GLAUCOMA

Glaucoma is a group of eye diseases that result in increased **intraocular pressure.** The pressure can damage the retina and **optic nerve** and lead to blindness when not treated. Remember that the eye is normally filled with aqueous humor. In a person who has glaucoma, more fluid than is needed is formed and it does not escape by the usual routes. This buildup of fluid causes the pressure inside the eye. Certain medications are used to treat glaucoma

GLAUCOMA
a group of eye diseases that result in intraocular pressure
INTRAOCULAR PRESSURE
increased pressure inside the eyeball
OPTIC NERVE
the nerve in the eye that carries impulses for the sense of light

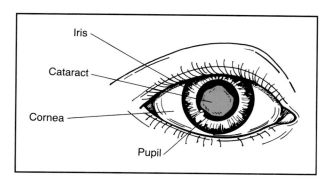

FIGURE 18–10
A cataract.

and must be used each day to prevent permanent damage. If left untreated, glaucoma causes damage to the retina and optic nerve that cannot be repaired.

Patients may tell you that they are losing their side vision or that they see halos or rings around lights. If glaucoma occurs quickly, acute pain may be present. The care of the patient with untreated or unsuccessfully treated glaucoma is comparable to care of the blind person.

THE EAR

EAR
organ of hearing and balance

The **ear** catches stimuli made up of sound waves. The ears receive the sound waves and transmit them to the auditory center of the brain for interpretation. In addition, certain parts of the inner ear send impulses to the brain to help the body maintain balance when the head or other body parts move.

A person learns to recognize a great variety of sounds: music, laughter, words, and other sounds. The fetus in the womb can hear the beat of its mother's heart as well as outside sounds.

CARING COMMENT

Remember that even the person who is not conscious is able to hear, because the sense of hearing remains active. If you discuss anything while you care for an unconscious patient, the patient may recall your discussion upon awakening.

PINNA
the part of the ear that projects outside the head; also known as the auricle

AUDITORY CANAL
the tube in the ear through which sound waves travel

TYMPANIC MEMBRANE
the thin membrane that stretches across the ear canal, separating the middle ear from the outer ear; eardrum

EUSTACHIAN TUBE
the auditory tube; the narrow channel between the tympanum and the nasopharynx

NASOPHARYNX
the part of the pharynx located above the soft palate

OSSICLE
a small bone, especially of the middle ear

MALLEUS
the largest of the three ossicles; also called the hammer

INCUS
the middle ossicle of the ear; also called the anvil

STAPES
the innermost ossicle of the ear; also called stirrup

PARTS OF THE EAR

The ear is divided into three parts (Figure 18–11):

- outer (or external) ear
- middle ear
- inner ear

The outer ear is made up of the **pinna** and a canal called the **auditory canal** that directs sound waves to the tympanic membrane. The **tympanic membrane** is also known as the eardrum; it separates the middle ear from the outer ear.

The middle ear consists of the

- eustachian tube
- ossicles

The **eustachian tube** extends from the tympanic membrane into the **nasopharynx** and helps make the pressure in the middle ear equal to the pressure in the air outside. When you fly in a plane, you can feel the changes in pressure as the plane takes off and lands. Sometimes simply driving down a steep hill at a high rate of speed can produce changes in pressure and cause a similar feeling of discomfort inside the ear.

The **ossicles** are the three tiny bones in the middle ear known as the

- hammer (**malleus**)
- anvil (**incus**)
- stirrup (**stapes**)

These special bones transmit the sound waves from the eardrum to the inner ear.

The structures in the inner ear include the

- cochlea
- semicircular canal

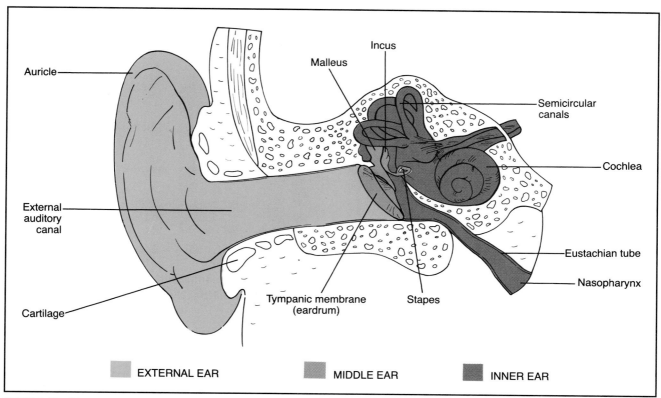

FIGURE 18–11
Structures of the ear.

The **cochlea** is shaped like a snail and contains fluid that vibrates when sound waves are sent through it by the stapes. The **semicircular canal** contains a special liquid and tiny "hairs" that bend when the liquid moves. The liquid moves when the head and body move. This creates impulses that the brain uses to help the body maintain a sense of balance.

The fluid in the semicircular canals works like the fluid in a carpenter's level. When a board or a wall is straight, place a carpenter's level against it and the bubble in the fluid is in the center. It tells the carpenter the board or wall is level. The fluid in the semicircular canals works in a similar way to tell the brain whether the body is balanced or imbalanced.

COCHLEA

the essential organ for hearing; a snail-shaped tube that forms part of the inner ear

SEMICIRCULAR CANAL

the passage shaped like a half-circle in the inner ear that controls the sense of balance

OBSERVATIONS OF THE SENSE OF HEARING AND BALANCE

The following are some hearing- and balance-related observations to make of your patients.

- When speaking to patients, notice whether they can hear you when you use a normal tone of voice.
- Is the radio or television volume kept on so loud it disturbs conversation?
- Do patients hear better in one ear?
- You may notice **cerumen** in a patient's ear. You should check the ears of your elderly patients daily for any accumulation of wax. Wax inside the ear can impair hearing.
- Check whether patients are wearing a **hearing aid** in one or both ears.
- Note whether patients walk erectly and straight or weave.

CERUMEN

earwax

HEARING AID

a device that makes sounds louder for persons who are hard of hearing

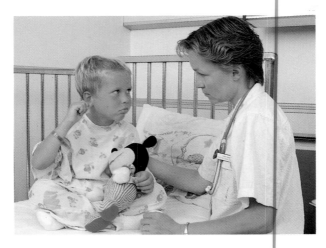

FIGURE 18-12

Children may pull their ear in response to pain from an ear infection.

Unusual Observations

Patients may report that they are hard of hearing and wear a hearing aid. They may tell you there is pain in their ear(s). Often, the pain causes the person to pull or tug at the ears. In children who have not learned to talk, this may be an indication of an ear infection (Figure 18-12).

A patient may also mention a ringing sound **(tinnitus)** in the ears. Ears can also itch, so you may notice patients scratching their ears. Patients may scratch their ears in response to pain or discomfort, which may be caused by an infection.

You may notice a discharge from the ears. Report the consistency (thin or thick) of the discharge. Describe the color of the discharge; it may be clear, yellow, or greenish. Note if the discharge has an odor.

When an infection is suspected, you may be asked to measure the patient's temperature. Remember to observe the patient's sense of balance. Report any changes in hearing or balance to the supervisor or the nurse.

TINNITUS

noise (ringing, buzzing, or roaring) in the ears

CARE OF PATIENTS WITH COMMON DISRUPTIONS IN HEARING

DEAFNESS

Deafness is the complete or partial lack or loss of the sense of hearing. A person who is deaf or has some degree of deafness may be regarded as hearing impaired. Complete or partial lack or loss of hearing may be caused by:

- inheritance
- disease
- trauma to the ear

In certain kinds of damage to the hearing organs, the sense of hearing cannot be restored, and the person must wear a device called a hearing aid that improves the ability to hear. Dogs can also be trained to assist hearing-impaired persons.

CARING COMMENT

A hearing aid is an instrument that amplifies sounds. Because it amplifies all sounds in the environment, the person who uses one needs to be trained to filter out the background noises and concentrate on the desired sound.

Sound is conducted to the inner ear for translation in the brain in two ways:

Air

Bone

A hearing aid inserted into the external ear catches sound waves and conducts them to the inner ear through air. Another type of hearing aid can be worn behind the ear or hidden in the temple of a pair of eyeglasses. This type of hearing aid works by conducting sound waves through the bone.

THE HEARING AID

You must be able to recognize the main parts of a hearing aid:

- earmold
- cord
- microphone
- control switch (on/off)
- battery compartment

Types of Hearing Aids

Hearing aids are made in a variety of styles. Each of the following styles has the same basic working parts:

- **body pack hearing aid**—The earmold is placed in the ear and is connected by a cord to a case that contains the working parts; the case is carried in a shirt or blouse pocket (Figure 18–13).
- **in-the-ear hearing aid**—All working parts are contained in an earmold that is placed in the ear (Figure 18–14).
- **behind-the-ear hearing aid**—The earmold is connected to a small case (containing the working parts) that fits over the ear; the hearing case is shaped to fit behind the ear (Figure 18–15).

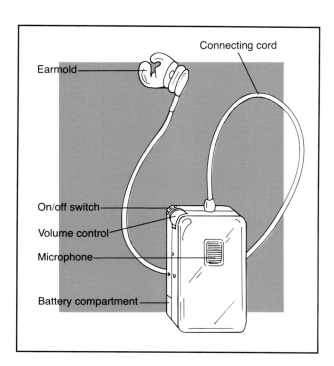

FIGURE 18–13

The parts of a hearing aid.

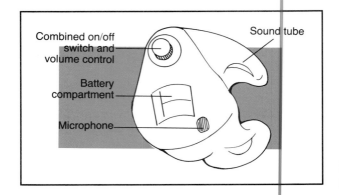

FIGURE 18–14
In-the-ear hearing aid.

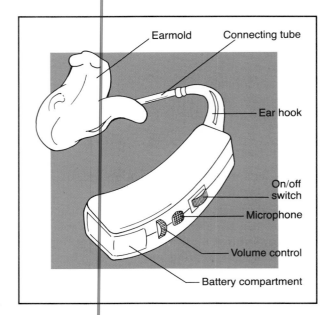

FIGURE 18–15
Behind-the-ear hearing aid.

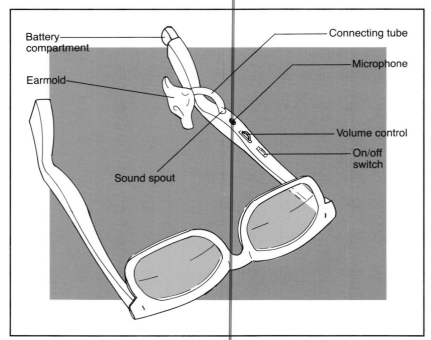

FIGURE 18–16
Eyeglass hearing aid.

- **eyeglass hearing aid**—An earmold is connected to the temple of the eyeglasses (Fig. 18–16). The controls are in the temple.

Placement of a Hearing Aid

Patients may wish to insert their hearing aid themselves, or they may ask you to do it for them. If you are asked to do it, check the batteries before you insert the hearing aid into the patient's ear. Check also that the batteries are the correct ones for that particular hearing aid. To check for battery function,

1. Turn the control switch to the on position.
2. Turn up the volume control and listen for a whistling sound by holding the hearing aid close to your ear.
3. If there is no whistling sound, change the batteries.
4. After you have changed the batteries, the case should close easily; if not, reposition the batteries.

CARING COMMENT

Never wash a hearing aid. Instead, the supervisor, nurse, a friend, or family member should arrange to return it to the dealer for proper cleaning.

Never let a hearing aid be exposed to heat or moisture, even from shower steam or an aerosol can.

Be careful not to drop the hearing aid, because the case can crack easily.

When the hearing aid is not in use, store it in a container labeled with the patient's name and room number.

The hearing aid is removed at bedtime. Remove the batteries before you store the hearing aid for the night.

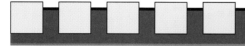

PROCEDURE

Placing a Hearing Aid

Prepare the hearing aid by testing the battery for proper function. Check the hearing aid to make sure the connections are secure. Check the ear to make sure it is free of wax, cotton, or other debris.

GATHER EQUIPMENT

Hearing aid   Battery

ACTION	RATIONALE
1. Open the hearing aid to make sure battery is working properly (Figure 18–17).	
2. Turn the control switch to the on position. Turn up the volume control, hold the hearing aid close to your ear, and listen for a whistling sound.	If you do not hear whistling, batteries need to be changed.
3. Turn down the volume.	
4. Line up the hearing aid with the patient's ear (Figure 18–18).	

Continued on following page

PROCEDURE

Placing a Hearing Aid *Continued*

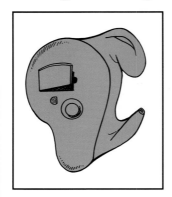

FIGURE 18–17

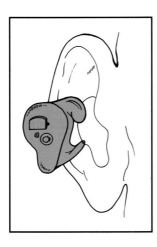

FIGURE 18–18

5. Rotate hearing aid (ear mold part) slightly and begin to insert it into the ear (Figure 18–19).

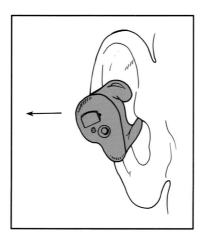

FIGURE 18–19

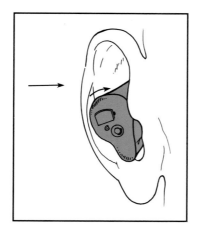

FIGURE 18-20

6. Press the hearing aid in while rotating it backwards (Figure 18-20).

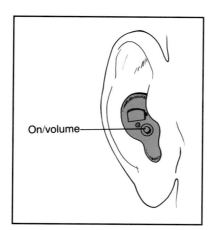

On/volume

FIGURE 18-21

7. Adjust the volume so that it is comfortable for the patient (Figure 18-21).

CARING COMMENTS

If patients tell you they hear an unpleasant whistling or squealing sound, reposition the hearing aid in their ear.

The hearing-impaired patient may enjoy listening to music or special tapes through earphones (Figure 18-22).

COMMUNICATION TOOLS

When we communicate we depend on sound: hearing it and delivering it. Persons who have a hearing impairment can develop tools that help them

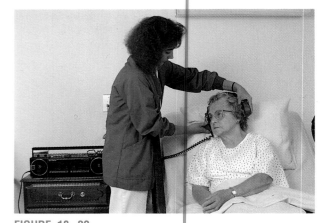

FIGURE 18–22
Position earphones so they fit snugly over the patient's ears.

COMMUNICATION
an exchange of information
SIGN LANGUAGE
a formal language that uses hand and matching mouth gestures to communicate words and meanings to people who cannot hear

communicate. Lip reading is one tool that assists **communication.** A person can be taught to read lips. **Sign language** is another tool that can be taught. People who do not have a problem with hearing can learn to read lips and use sign language to communicate with hearing-impaired persons.

Many television programs are broadcast with captions that can be read by hearing-impaired persons. A special device is needed for the captions to be seen on the television screen. People who have some degree of hearing may be able to use the telephone with the help of a special volume adaptor.

You must be acutely aware of the needs of any hearing-impaired patient in your care. You should

- Always position yourself in front of hearing-impaired persons when speaking to them.
- Speak slowly and allow patients to see you so that they can read your lips and interpret your body language.

CARING COMMENT

Remember that hearing-impaired patients may not hear normal danger signals, such as a fire alarm or siren. During an emergency, you must take special care to help communicate danger to hearing-impaired patients. Try not to speak too quickly for the patient to understand your directions correctly.

CERUMEN

Hearing impairment can be caused by cerumen. Cerumen is an accumulation of a waxy substance secreted by glands in the auditory canal. The cerumen cleans the external ear canal as it moves outward. Dead cells and foreign particles are removed from the ear canal in this way. The cerumen sometimes becomes hard and remains in the ear canal, where it can form into a waxy ball the size of a pea or larger. Cerumen can impair hearing by blocking sound waves so they cannot be interpreted correctly.

When you notice that patients ask you to repeat questions or do not respond to their name as usual, report this observation to the supervisor or nurse.

The physician can order special ear drops to loosen the wax so it can drain to the outside naturally. Sometimes the registered nurse must perform an ear irrigation. A water solution is directed into the ear and flushes the cerumen out.

CARING COMMENT

Never attempt to clean the ear canal with cotton swab sticks; the tympanic membrane (eardrum) may be punctured.

OTITIS MEDIA

Otitis media is an inflammation of the middle ear. It occurs most often in children. It is seen often in infants who are bottle fed, because the formula sometimes enters the eustachian tubes. Breastfed babies are held at a higher angle by the mother during feeding, so there is less chance of milk entering the eustachian tubes. Otitis media also often occurs after a respiratory infection.

A child with pain in the ear may be seen pulling or tugging at the affected ear. The pain is constant and can occur in one or both ears. The child may be irritable and difficult to comfort. A fever of about 102° F can develop. When examining the ear with a special instrument called an **otoscope**, the physician will see changes in the tympanic membrane and order an antibiotic to clear up the infection. A series of otitis media infections can result in hearing loss.

OTITIS MEDIA
inflammation of the middle ear; occurs most often in infants and children

OTOSCOPE
an instrument used to inspect the ear

CARE OF THE PATIENT WITH A DISRUPTION IN BALANCE

VERTIGO

Vertigo is the sensation that one's body or one's surroundings are moving. It is more commonly called dizziness. The dizziness can range from a mild transient (passing) dizziness to a dizziness that causes persons to lose their balance and fall. Although vertigo can be caused by diseases of the brain, it is often a result of a disturbance in parts of the inner ear. The physician treats the cause when it can be identified. Your responsibilities in caring for patients with vertigo are as follows:

VERTIGO
dizziness; a feeling that one's body or one's surroundings are moving

- Keep patients safe from falls.
- Assist patients when they walk. Patients can use handrails for support on one side while you support their other side.
- Always place patients' call signal within reach so that they can summon assistance quickly.
- Try to anticipate patients' needs and allow them as much independence as possible.

In some cases, patients with vertigo may use a wheelchair to move around on their own. Walks can be planned when you have enough help to ensure safety.

THE NOSE

The **nose** is the organ of smell as well as the entryway for oxygen that is carried to the lungs. When air enters the openings in the nose, tiny particles are

NOSE
the organ of smell and the means of bringing air into the lungs

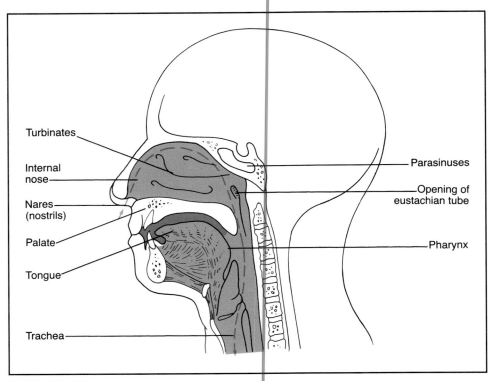

FIGURE 18-23
The structures of the nose.

filtered out before the air continues to the lungs. Pollen and dust are filtered out because they stimulate the nerve endings in the nose. This stimulation triggers a sneeze, which forcibly ejects the unwanted material from the breathing passages. Another function of the nose is to permit the drainage of fluids from the sinuses.

STRUCTURES OF THE NOSE

BONE
the hard, rigid connective tissue that makes up most of the skeleton

CARTILAGE
fibrous, semi-rigid tissue found in adults

NOSTRILS
the two external openings of the nasal cavity

The outside of the nose is made of **bone** and **cartilage** covered with skin (Figure 18–23). Two nasal openings, called **nostrils,** allow the entrance and exit of air. The nostrils lead into the inner part of the nose, which is lined with a mucous membrane that contains cilia (short hairs). The cilia trap and filter out incoming particles. Small blood vessels in the mucous membrane warm the air before it enters the lungs. The nostrils continue to the upper part of the nasal cavity, where nerve endings in the mucous membrane provide the sense of smell. The nose can tell the difference between many odors.

Special bony ridges called **turbinates** divide the nasal cavity into passages for air. These passages at the back of the nose lead to the pharynx. The same passages allow fluids to drain into a special cavity (the parasinuses). Another opening leads to the eustachian tubes, which air enters so that pressure on both sides of the eardrum is equal.

TURBINATES
thin membranes over bony cartilage that support the walls of the nasal chambers

OBSERVATIONS OF NASAL FUNCTION

Normal Observations

The nostrils should be clear to allow for the passage of air into the lungs. Patients' sense of smell may be noted when they tell you about odors they are able to identify. The easiest odors to identify are pungent (sharp) odors like vanilla or rubbing alcohol.

Unusual Observations

The lining of the nose reacts to irritation by producing a discharge from the mucous membranes. You need to observe the color of the discharge. It may be clear and watery, or it may be thick with a white, yellow, or greenish tint. A red or rusty tint can indicate the presence of blood in the discharge. You should also note the amount of drainage and whether drainage is constant. Observe whether patients breathe through their nose or through their mouth. Report anything patients tell you about a decreased ability to smell to your supervisor or the nurse.

CARE OF PATIENTS WITH DISRUPTIONS IN NASAL FUNCTION

NASAL DISCHARGE

Nasal discharge occurs when the mucous membranes inside the nose become irritated and inflamed. The body responds by producing the discharge, which contains dead cells and debris, and allowing it to escape. The discharge may contain harmful microorganisms that can infect others who contact it. Provide the patient with the following:

- a box of tissues and a waste container for used tissues (Figure 18–24)
- extra fluids, when allowed, to help liquefy thick secretions (Figure 18–25)
- fresh water or other fluids, as desired (milk is not advised because it thickens secretions)
- **humidity**, when ordered, to help the patient breathe easier and break up

HUMIDITY
moisture

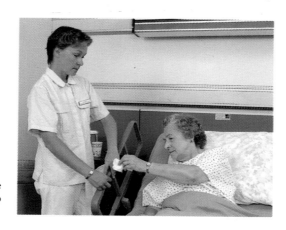

FIGURE 18–24
A bag can be taped to the side rails of the bed for the patient with nasal drainage to dispose of tissues.

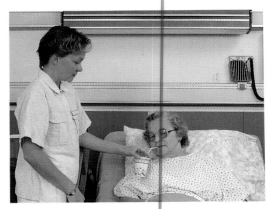

FIGURE 18–25
Offer fluids to patients at least every 2 hours.

HUMIDIFIER
a device that produces a fine mist of water particles

thick mucous secretions (check frequently to make sure the **humidifier** contains water and is producing a mist)

EPISTAXIS

EPISTAXIS
nosebleed; rupture of small blood vessels in the nose

A nosebleed is a frightening occurrence for any person. The medical term for a nosebleed is **epistaxis.** Epistaxis can occur spontaneously or as a result of injury to the nose. In most cases, quick action on your part can help stem the flow of blood (Figure 18–26):

1. Raise the bed to the high Fowler's position.
2. Apply firm, persistent pressure over the bridge of the nose for about 2 minutes or until the bleeding stops.
3. Call your supervisor or nurse, who will assess the patient and decide on the course of action.

TASTE BUD
organ of taste; located on the tongue
TONGUE
organ of taste; also aids in chewing, swallowing, and speaking

SENSE OF TASTE

The sensory organs of taste are the **taste buds** that are located on the surface of the **tongue** (Figure 18–27). The nerve endings in the taste buds send a

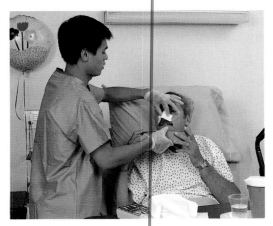

FIGURE 18–26
Note that disposable gloves are worn when caring for the patient with a nosebleed.

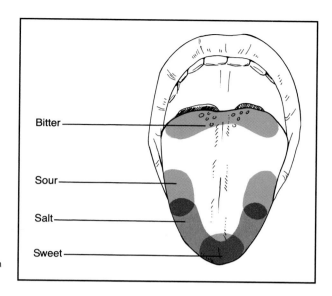

FIGURE 18-27
Locations of the taste buds on the tongue.

Bitter

Sour

Salt

Sweet

message to the brain. The brain interprets whether the message is sweetness, sourness, bitterness, tanginess, or saltiness.

CARING COMMENT

The sense of taste helps a person to enjoy food. The sense of smell is important in this process. When patients tell you food does not taste very good anymore, they may have a problem with their sense of smell. Smell has a lot to do with the way food tastes.

IMPAIRMENT OF TASTE

Impairment of taste can occur as a result of illness, the aging process, and certain medications. Be aware that some illnesses eliminate the sense of taste and the patient is not tempted to eat even though you offer a favorite food or beverage. The aging process affects the taste buds; they become more ineffi-cient as we age. When this occurs, foods no longer taste the same and the patient loses the enjoyment associated with eating. Certain medications can affect the sense of taste by interfering with the message sent to the brain. When persons cannot distinguish what they are tasting, they may lose interest in eating.

CARE OF THE PATIENT WITH AN IMPAIRED SENSE OF TASTE

A balanced diet and plenty of foods help maintain and restore health for all persons. You can help patients by learning what they like and dislike in food. Because strong flavors can stimulate the sense of taste more than weak flavors, you may observe your patients using more salt and pepper on their food. In addition, different textures (for example, soft or lumpy) of food help stimulate the taste buds.

The food that is prepared for patients is purposely planned to please the eye. Variety in texture and color can stimulate appetite in the patient with an impaired sense of taste.

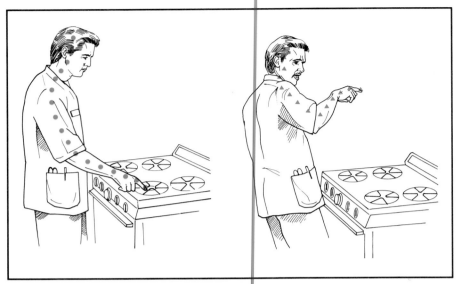

FIGURE 18–28

A, A situation that causes pain, such as touching something hot, sends a message to the brain. B, The brain responds by sending a message to the painful body part to move away from the painful situation.

Report to the supervisor or nurse anytime patients tell you their tastes have changed or you observe that they are using extra salt and pepper to improve the taste of foods. The dietary department will work with patients to provide foods that suit their taste needs.

SENSE OF TOUCH

Nerve endings in the skin receive stimuli and transmit the information to the brain for interpretation (Figure 18–28). Nerve endings for this purpose are located all over the surface of the body. The response to touch may be one of pleasure or discomfort. Many nerve endings are located in the tips of the fingers. The nerve endings are sensitive to a variety of sensations. For example, through the sense of touch, a person can distinguish between hot and cold and sharp and dull and can feel and identify shapes of objects.

CARE OF THE PATIENT WITH AN IMPAIRED SENSE OF TOUCH

You are responsible for providing a safe environment for the patient with an impaired sense of touch. The fingers and toes are supplied with a rich sense of touch. They may be used to test the temperature of objects as well as to determine the sharpness of objects. Patients whose sense of touch is impaired can be injured unknowingly. They may burn or cut themselves and be unaware of the injury because their brain does not interpret the touch sensation as expected. Take the following precautions with patients who have an impaired sense of touch:

- Determine the temperature of the bath water before you allow the patient to bathe.
- Allow time for hot beverages to cool before you serve them, or tell the patient they are hot.
- Keep all sharp objects safely out of reach. Use extra care in the transfer

of touch-impaired patients; they might not react to pain in the normal way.

- Check the affected extremities carefully and promptly report any redness or break in the skin.

SENSORY DEPRIVATION AND SENSORY OVERLOAD

SENSORY DEPRIVATION

Sensory deprivation is the condition of inadequate stimulation, in terms of both quality (type of stimulation) and quantity (amount of stimulation). Sensory deprivation can be caused by an environmental situation such as a room with colorless walls; dim lights; and no windows, pictures, calendars, or books. Life becomes dull without the stimulation of all the senses.

Sensory deprivation can also be caused by the patient's condition. Patients who are in an isolation room because of infection or who cannot move because of a cast may be deprived of the sensory stimulation they normally enjoy. Deprivation can also be caused by a deficit of one of the five senses. In this case, because patients cannot receive stimuli, they are deprived of normal, healthy stimulation of the senses.

Another reason sensory deprivation may occur is that a patient is not able to process (use) stimuli. This means that although sensory organs receive stimulation, they are not able to understand or interpret the stimuli in the usual way. Diseases that affect the brain (for example, stroke and cancer) can interfere with the ability to process stimuli. In diseases that cause necrosis (death of tissue) in the brain, the affected part of the brain can no longer receive and interpret sensory information.

Drugs that depress brain function, such as alcohol and narcotics, can also interfere with the person's ability to process incoming stimuli. When alcohol is present in the body, it decreases the function of the brain. It does not send messages to the body as quickly as usual.

Finally, sensory deprivation can result if there is a language barrier. The patient may not be able to understand information without the help of an interpreter. They can hear when spoken to, but do not understand what is said because of a lack of knowledge of that specific language.

SENSORY DEPRIVATION
a condition in which a person receives less than normal sensory input; there is inadequate quality or quantity of stimuli

Observations of the Patient with Sensory Deprivation

The patient who experiences sensory deprivation may exhibit a variety of behaviors. It may be difficult to communicate with this patient. Ask simple questions about usual events in the patient's life. Observe for fatigue, boredom, and decreased interest in surroundings. The deprivation may cause the patient to have a poor appetite or sleeping problems such as **insomnia** or restlessness. Patients may tell you they have physical discomforts (for example, headache or stomachache) that are unexplained. Sensory deprivation is most notable in patients who are in the intensive care unit. Think about the dull, sterile environment of the special care units found in the hospital.

INSOMNIA
the inability to fall asleep easily or remain asleep throughout the night

Care of the Patient with Sensory Deprivation

You need to provide patients who have sensory deprivation with the sensory stimulation that is missing. For example, to give the patient a sense of the time of day, you can

- Use less lighting during the night.
- Put day clothing on the patient during the day and night clothes on at night whenever possible.

- Keep a calendar or clock in the room to help orient the patient to time.
- While you are giving care, mention the time of the day, week, or month to the patient.
- Mention any changes in the seasons.

To provide other sensory stimulation, you can

- Sit the patient in a chair by the window for visual stimulation.
- Use color and activity to stimulate the patient's senses.
- Provide music during the day for auditory stimulation. You should ask a family member about the patient's preference in music.
- Encourage visitors to add stimulation to the environment by their presence and efforts to talk with the patient.

SEIZURE DISORDER, A DISRUPTION IN SENSORY FUNCTION

SEIZURE

a change in body function caused by abnormal electrical activity in the brain; convulsion

A **seizure** is a change in body function caused by abnormal electrical activity in the brain. A seizure is also known as a convulsion. There are many different types of seizures. A person who experiences any type of seizure is said to have a seizure disorder. If your patient has a history of seizure disorder, you will be notified of this when you receive a report from the nurse or your supervisor before you give care.

You should observe for the following:

AURA

an odd feeling, such as numbness or dizziness, just before a seizure or migraine headache starts

- patient reports of an **aura**
- sudden stiffening of the limbs
- jerking movements of the limbs
- changes in consciousness, such as appearing to daydream or the inability to respond to commands
- eye changes such as
    Turning of the eye and head to one side or the other
    Changes in the size of pupils
- other changes may include
    An increase in saliva
    Tongue or lip biting
    Incontinence of bowel or bladder
    Changes in the breathing pattern, such as appearing to stop breathing

Each person responds to a seizure disorder differently. You will not observe all of the changes listed above in all patients with seizure disorders. This list just gives the changes most commonly observed. Many other changes might occur, depending on the part of the brain that is affected. Observe for anything different from the usual.

A person is a high risk for injury during a seizure. As a nursing assistant, you should be familiar with the seizure precaution policy in your health care institution. If a seizure occurs, you should:

- Note the time the seizure began.
- Turn patients on their side, if possible.
- Support the head with a pillow.
- Call for help by turning on the call signal:
    The nurse may need to use suction equipment if saliva closes off air supply to the lungs.
    The nurse may decide to give oxygen.
- Stay with the patient and observe for any changes.
- Note the time the seizure ends.

After the seizure is over, the patient may

- Be difficult to wake up.

- Be unaware that a seizure occurred.
- Feel sleepy and sleep for several hours.

You should make the patient comfortable and make the room quiet and comfortable for sleep. After the seizure is over, report and record your observations.

In recent years, the focus of caring for the patient with seizure disorder has changed. The focus now is on keeping the patient safe. Follow these guidelines to keep patients safe during a seizure.

- *Never* place a padded tongue blade between the teeth. During a seizure, the jaws tighten. Forcing a tongue blade between the teeth can chip the enamel and place the patient at risk for breathing the pieces into the lungs.
- Padded side rails are not encouraged because of the embarrassment they may cause the patient and family.
- If patients are doing something active when the seizure occurs, you may need to help them lie down in a safe place.

SENSORY OVERLOAD

Sensory overload occurs when a person receives an excessive amount of sensory stimulation. It is generally more stimulation than can be tolerated by the individual within a given time period. The brain reacts to the sensory overload by not responding appropriately. You are responsible for observing the behavior of a patient who may have sensory overload. The response to sensory stimulation is very individualized.

SENSORY OVERLOAD
a condition in which a person receives too many stimuli to the senses

Observation of the Patient with Sensory Overload

The patient with sensory overload may display nervous or anxious behaviors (for example, irritability or crying). You may notice that the patient who tires easily may have disturbed sleep. Too much stimulation for the brain to interpret may cause a change in appetite. The patient may have no desire to eat and may just move the food around until it is taken away. In sensory overload, the brain cannot concentrate and you will observe a short attention span.

Care of the Patient with Sensory Overload

Whenever there is an overabundance (too much) of stimulation, you need to change the environment to block the incoming stimulation. The following are some measures you can take to help decrease stimuli in the patient's environment.

- Reduce bright lights and eliminate extra movement in the surroundings.
- Place a folded washcloth over patients' eyes to lessen visual overstimulation.
- Decrease offensive noises in the environment.
- Encourage the patient to listen to soft music through a set of earphones.
- Remember that patients with sensory overload may need help interpreting information and understanding it.
- Explain to patients what you are doing and what is happening around them.
- Use simple words and short sentences.
- Ask patients to take deep breaths and imagine themselves in a quiet place.
- Whenever possible, reduce any stimulation that is more than patients can handle.

CHAPTER WRAP-UP

- The five senses are seeing, hearing, smelling, tasting, and touching.
- The sensory organs have nerve endings that receive stimuli and transmit them to the brain for interpretation. The body responds to the brain's message and initiates the appropriate sensory response.
- The sensory organs are the eyes, ears, nose, taste buds on the tongue, and finger tips and other areas of the skin with nerve endings.
- When one or more of these sensory organs are impaired or damaged permanently, the brain either does not respond to stimuli or responds incorrectly.
- Your observations of your patients should include each of the sensory organs and their function every day.
- Care of patients with impairment of the senses consists of helping them stay safe and perform their activities of daily living.
- Sensory deficit is the lack of receiving incoming sensory stimulation.
- Sensory deprivation is inadequate quality and quantity of stimulation in the environment.
- A seizure is abnormal electrical activity in the brain.
- Sensory overload is excessive sensory stimulation.

REVIEW QUESTIONS

1. Name the sensory organs.
2. Give an example of how the sensory organs work together.
3. Identify common disruptions in seeing, hearing, and the senses of smell, taste, and touch.
4. What is sensory deficit? Sensory overload?
5. Explain the care of patients who have an impairment of one or more of the five senses.
6. List the observations of the patient having a seizure.

ACTIVITY CORNER

Prepare yourself for an evening of television and snacks in the following manner:

Place a bowl of snacks within reach.
Put on a pair of glasses that have cream or lotion smeared on the lenses.
Put a cotton ball in each ear.
Put on a pair of disposable gloves.
Turn on your television set.
Sit down and relax while you "watch" a favorite program.
When you eat some of the snacks, pinch your nose shut while you place the food in your mouth and chew and swallow.

Watch an entire program while your senses are blocked in these ways. Describe how it felt to

See through clouded lenses _____

_____

Hear with cotton balls in your ears _____

_____

Touch things with gloves on _____

_____

Smell when your nose was pinched shut _____

_____

Taste food when you could not smell it _____

_____

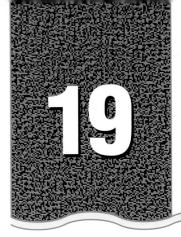

19 Learning About Foods and Fluids

Objectives

AFTER YOU COMPLETE THIS CHAPTER, YOU WILL BE ABLE TO:

Describe the structure and function of the upper gastrointestinal system.

Define the terms *nutrition* and *metabolism*.

Name foods that contain carbohydrates, proteins, fats, vitamins, and minerals.

List the five food groups.

Name the different types of special diets.

Record the amount of food and fluids patients take in.

Identify the reasons why the body needs fluid.

Measure weight and height of the patient.

Describe common disruptions in nutrition and metabolism.

Care for patients with common disruptions in nutrition and metabolism.

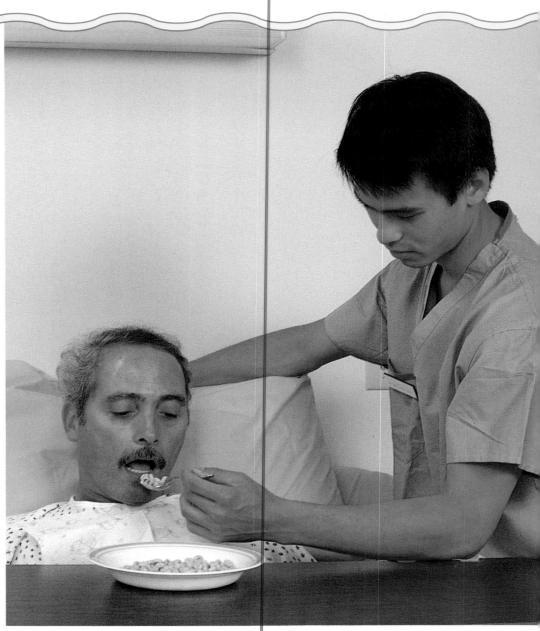

Overview Food and fluids are the fuel that provides the body energy. All tissues of the body need energy to perform their work. The foods from the five food groups are eaten and broken down for use by body tissues. Proper nutrition is necessary in building a sound body that can heal when illness strikes.

WHAT DO YOU KNOW ABOUT NUTRITION AND METABOLISM?

Here are nine statements about nutrition and metabolism. Consider them to test your current ideas about the food you eat. If you think the statement is true, circle the T; if you think the statement is false, circle the F. Change the false statements to make them true.

1. T F   Digestion begins in the stomach.
2. T F   Carbohydrates are found in grains and cereals.
3. T F   Fats are the body's biggest source of energy.
4. T F   Most vitamins are provided by protein in the diet.
5. T F   Vitamin K helps the blood clot.
6. T F   Iron is needed to carry oxygen to the cells of the body.
7. T F   Eggs can be used as a meat substitute.
8. T F   The adolescent needs a high-calorie diet.
9. T F   A clear liquid diet includes creamed soups.

ANSWERS

1. **False.** Digestion begins when food mixes with saliva in the mouth.
2. **True.** Grains and cereals provide carbohydrates needed by the body.
3. **True.** The body gets more energy per gram from fat than from carbohydrates or proteins.
4. **False.** Vitamins are provided by a diet that includes foods from all five food groups.
5. **True.** Vitamin K is important to the blood-clotting process.
6. **True.** The only way oxygen can reach the cell is to be carried there by the iron in red blood cells.
7. **False.** Meat substitutes include nuts, peanut butter, and dry beans.
8. **True.** Because adolescence is a time of rapid growth, a high-calorie diet is important.
9. **False.** Only food or fluid that can be seen through can be eaten in a clear liquid diet.

STRUCTURE AND FUNCTION OF THE UPPER GASTROINTESTINAL SYSTEM

STRUCTURE

The upper gastrointestinal system is made up of the following structures (Figure 19–1).

- **Oral cavity**—consists of the mouth, salivary glands, tongue, and teeth. It is covered by a skin called a **mucous membrane.** The **tongue** is a muscle and is very flexible. The teeth are made of a long-lasting enamel. They have roots reaching into the gums to secure them in the jaw.
- **Pharynx**—a muscular tube located at the top of the esophagus. It is covered with a mucous membrane.
- **Esophagus**—a muscular tube from the pharynx to the top of the stomach. Food enters the esophagus from the pharynx.
- **Stomach**—a pouch-like organ located on the left side of the body at the end of the esophagus. It is lined with a special lining that is not affected by the acid produced in the stomach.

Other organs that assist in the **digestion** of food are the following (see Figure 19–1B):

- **Liver**—the largest organ in the body. It is located in the upper right abdomen. It secretes bile and plays a role in fat breakdown. It has special ducts (small tubes) that are connected to the gallbladder.

ORAL CAVITY
the opening in the body that consists of the mouth, salivary glands, tongue, and teeth

MUCOUS MEMBRANE
the covering of skin that lines the organs of the gastrointestinal tract (from lips to anus)

TONGUE
organ of taste; also aids in chewing, swallowing, and speaking

PHARYNX
the throat; the muscular tube located at the top of the esophagus

ESOPHAGUS
a muscular tube from the pharynx to the top of the stomach

STOMACH
pouch-like organ located on the left side of the abdomen; the widest part of the gastrointestinal system

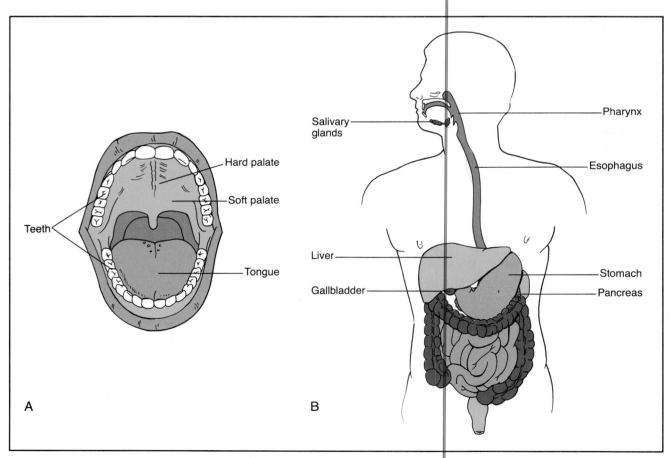

FIGURE 19–1
A, The oral cavity. B, The upper gastrointestinal system.

- **Gallbladder**—a small, pear-shaped sac located under the liver. It serves as a storage place for bile.
- **Pancreas**—a gland located below and behind the stomach and the liver. It secretes a juice that helps in breakdown of fats, proteins, and carbohydrates. Special cells secrete insulin.

FUNCTION

The upper gastrointestinal system begins the work of changing food into a form that can be used by the body (see Figure 19–1B). The body needs food and fluid to be changed into a form it can use in order to maintain health.

The oral cavity provides a place for food and fluid to enter the body. The mouth is the entrance to the gastrointestinal system. When food enters the oral cavity, the salivary glands secrete **saliva.** By mixing in with food, saliva begins the breakdown of food. The teeth are used to help mix food with the saliva and to chew food into a softer **consistency.** The tongue is a sensory organ that contains taste buds and also pushes food into the pharynx. **Taste buds** are special cells on the tongue that help a person tell the difference between sweet, sour, salty, and bitter tastes.

The pharynx allows the passage of food from the mouth into the esophagus. The pharynx and esophagus are made of muscle that contracts to move food into the stomach. The stomach is a temporary storage place for food. **Gastric** secretions in the stomach continue the breakdown of food that started in the oral cavity. Food cannot be used by the body until it is broken down for digestion. After the food is broken down, it passes into the lower gastrointestinal system.

The liver, gallbladder, and pancreas are the accessory organs of digestion. The liver has several important functions:

- Stores red blood cells.
- Turns fats and proteins into glucose (sugar).
- Produces **bile** that helps break down fat.
- Assists in storing glucose for later use by the body.

The gallbladder is the storage place for the bile that the liver makes. The gallbladder concentrates (reduces the liquid amount of) the bile and stores it until the body uses it to break down **fat.** When a person eats a fatty meal, bile is released when the food reaches the duodenum (the first part of the small intestine). The pancreas helps break down **protein** and **carbohydrates.** Two important hormones secreted by the pancreas are

Insulin

Glucagon

Insulin regulates how the body converts sugar into energy. Glucagon helps increase the concentration of sugar in the blood.

NUTRITION

Nutrition is the study of food as it relates to the health of the body. Nutrition includes study of the

- body's needs for food and fluid
- ways the foods and fluids are provided for the body
- effects of poor food intake on the body

Food and fluids contain **nutrients** that the body needs. Certain body processes change the nutrients into a chemical form that the body can use. The body processes involved are

- **Ingestion**—the act of taking in food and fluid by mouth
- **Digestion**—the act of breaking down food

DIGESTION
the mechanical and chemical breakdown of food into forms the body can use

LIVER
the largest organ in the body; stores red blood cells and secretes bile

GALLBLADDER
small pear-shaped sac under the liver that concentrates and stores bile

PANCREAS
organ behind the stomach that secretes insulin

SALIVA
watery substance secreted from the salivary glands; moistens food and makes it easier to swallow

CONSISTENCY
the degree of thickness of a substance

TASTE BUDS
cells on the tongue that distinguish salty, sweet, sour, and bitter tastes

GASTRIC
pertaining to the stomach

BILE
substance secreted by the liver that breaks down fat in the duodenum

FAT
source of energy in the body; adipose tissue

PROTEIN
a material needed for cells to grow

CARBOHYDRATE
a source of energy in the body; found in sugar and starches

NUTRITION
the study of food's relationship to health; the act of providing food to nourish the body

NUTRIENT
a chemical substance that helps the body break down, absorb, and use foods and fluids

INGESTION
taking in food and fluid by mouth

ABSORPTION
the way the body makes use of the end products of digestion (nutrients); the passage of fluids and other substances into the bloodstream

ELIMINATION
the way the body rids itself of unusable food and fluid; the discharge of the waste products created by the body's metabolism

- **Absorption**—the passage of nutrients into the bloodstream
- **Elimination**—the way the body rids itself of unusable food and fluid; the discharge of the waste products of the body's metabolism

These body processes make nutrients available to the tissues of the body.

THE NUTRIENTS

Nutrients are chemical substances that help the body break down, absorb, and use the foods and fluids that are eaten. The body needs nutrients to perform the following functions:

- To provide heat or energy.
- To make and repair tissue.

TABLE 19–1 NUTRIENTS AND THEIR FUNCTIONS

Nutrient	Functions
Carbohydrates	Break down into sugars during digestion. (Sugar provides energy for the body. Unused sugar is stored in the liver. Excess sugar is changed into body fat when there is no storage space left in the liver.)
	1 gram of carbohydrate gives the body 4 calories.
	Are found in breads and cereals, fruits, vegetables, and sugar.
	Are usually inexpensive and readily available.
	Make up about 50% of the average person's diet.
	Provide quick energy (for example, orange juice).
	Provide energy over time (for example, cereals and grains).
	Contribute **fiber** to the diet.
Proteins	Are needed for growth and repair of body tissues.
	1 gram of protein gives the body 4 calories.
	Are basic to the structure of all living cells.
	Are found in all body **fluids.**
	Are found in meats, fish, poultry, eggs, milk, and dairy products (animal sources).
	Are found in peas, beans, corn, and wheat (plant sources).
	Are expensive.
	Should contribute to about 15% of daily food intake.
	Are needed for growth; requirements vary with age and also increase if stress, surgery, burn, or fever is present.
Fats	Are body's most concentrated source of energy.
	1 gram of fat gives the body 9 calories.
	Carry the fat-soluble vitamins in the body (A, D, E, and K) so the body can use them.
	Give a feeling of fullness after eating.
	Help foods taste better.
	Should make up 30% or less of daily calories; the average American's diet is 50%.
	Are found in meats, dairy products, cooking oils, egg yolks, and nuts.
	Excess fat is stored as body fat (adipose tissue).
	Stored fat is a reserve source of energy.
	Include cholesterol, found only in foods from animal sources (large amounts are found in egg yolks, liver, and organ meats such as kidney and brain; smaller amounts are found in dairy products and the fat in nonorgan meat).
Vitamins	Maintain life and promote growth.
	Contain no calories.
	Are provided by a diet that includes food from the five food groups.
	Help release energy from carbohydrates, proteins, and fats.
	Are fat-soluble (A, D, E, and K) or water-soluble (B and C).
	Water-soluble vitamins (B and C) must be replaced every day because the body eliminates any amount of them that is not used.
	Because fat can be stored in the body, the fat-soluble vitamins are stored.
Minerals	Are needed daily for important body functions.
	Are needed for good bones and teeth.
	Help with nerve and muscle function.
	Help the body regulate its water balance.
	Are found in almost all foods except table sugar and oil.

FIBER
the portion of food that passes through the intestine and colon undigested; increases the bulk of the stool and makes it softer

FLUIDS
liquids

- To control body processes such as fluid balance, growth, hormone production, etc.

The essential nutrients needed for a healthy body have been identified by scientists (Table 19–1). The nutrients are divided into the following groups.

CARBOHYDRATES Carbohydrates are a source of energy in the body and are found in sugar and starches. Carbohydrates that are not used are stored in the liver. When a person takes in too many carbohydrates, the excess sugar is changed into body fat and stored in the tissue. Simple carbohydrates, such as donuts or other bakery sweets, are those that the body uses quickly. A person may feel hungry soon after eating simple carbohydrates. Complex carbohydrates take longer for the body to break down and use. A person does not feel hunger as quickly when eating complex carbohydrates, such as cereals and grains. Cereals and grains include wheat, rice, oats, and bran. Fruits and vegetables are also sources of complex carbohydrates.

PROTEIN Protein is the material cells need to grow and to repair themselves. Protein is found in all body cells and all body fluids. In the diet, protein comes from meats, fish, poultry, eggs, milk, and dairy products.

FAT Fat is another source of energy in the body. Another name for fat is adipose tissue. Fat is a concentrated form of energy that is stored in the body. Fats are important because they carry the fat-soluble vitamins (vitamins A, D, E, and K). Meats, dairy products such as milk and cheese, cooking oils, egg yolks, and nuts are rich sources of fat in the diet. Fat also includes cholesterol. **Cholesterol** is a fatty substance that attaches to the lining of arteries and makes them narrow. Too much cholesterol in your body can cause serious health problems.

CHOLESTEROL
fatty substance that attaches to the lining of arteries; comes from animal fats and oils

VITAMINS **Vitamins** are essential elements needed in small amounts for a healthy body. Vitamins may be **fat-soluble** or **water-soluble.** The fat-soluble vitamins (A, D, E, and K) can be stored in the body's fat cells. Water-soluble vitamins cannot be stored and must be taken in by the body every day. Vitamin C and the B vitamins are water-soluble (Table 19–2).

VITAMIN
an organic substance that is essential in small amounts to the body's health

FAT-SOLUBLE
able to dissolve in fat

WATER-SOLUBLE
able to dissolve in water

MINERALS **Minerals** are substances that work to help the body maintain good function. Minerals such as chloride, copper, phosphorus, fluoride, and many others are needed in various amounts. Minerals must be taken in by the body daily. They are important for good bones and teeth and help with nerve function. A varied diet that includes foods from the five food groups provides the amounts of vitamins and minerals needed for a healthy body. Minerals are found in almost all foods, except table sugar and oils (Table 19–3).

MINERAL
an inorganic (neither animal nor vegetable) substance needed for health

WATER **Water** is a clear, odorless, tasteless fluid. Water carries important substances to the cell and takes away the waste products produced by the cell. Our bodies cannot survive for very long without water.

WATER
clear, odorless, tasteless fluid

METABOLISM

Metabolism is the process that produces energy in the body and gives cells energy to grow and repair. Metabolism is the result of physical and chemical processes that take place in the body. Food is metabolized after it is eaten and digested. The body digests and metabolizes carbohydrates, fats, and proteins to produce the energy the body needs.

METABOLISM
the process that produces energy in the body, allowing cells to grow and repair

CALORIES

A **calorie** is a measure of the energy produced by the breakdown of food in the body. Calories are measured in **grams.** One gram of carbohydrate or protein

CALORIE
a measure of the energy produced by the breakdown of food in the body

GRAM
a unit of weight used in the metric system

TABLE 19-2   **VITAMINS, THEIR FUNCTIONS, AND THEIR SOURCES**

Vitamin	Chief Functions	Sources
Fat-soluble vitamins		
Vitamin A	Prevents night blindness Promotes bone and skeletal growth in children Helps keep skin from drying	Animal sources: liver, egg yolk Fruits and vegetables: yellow fruits and vegetables, such as carrots, squash, and apricots; green vegetables such as spinach Milk may be fortified with vitamin A
Vitamin D	Helps teeth and bones develop Helps the body use certain minerals	Few food sources (one is Vitamin-D-enriched milk) Exposure to sunlight helps the body make vitamin D
Vitamin E	Protects red blood cells from breaking down	Vegetable oils; green, leafy vegetables; cereals; meats; fish; eggs; and milk
Vitamin K	Helps the blood clot	Bacteria in the intestines Liver; egg yolk; and green, leafy vegetables
Water-soluble vitamins		
Thiamine (B$_1$)	Helps appetite and muscle tone Helps form energy from fats and carbohydrates Helps with nerve function	Yeast, pork, liver, grains, and enriched cereal and bread
Riboflavin (B$_2$)	Helps vision Enhances skin tone Needed for cell function	Best source: milk Also in eggs, meat, and green vegetables
Niacin (B$_3$)	Needed for body energy, growth, and healthy skin Helps nervous and gastrointestinal systems function	Meat, poultry, fish, grains, cereals, green vegetables, nuts, and bran
Vitamin B$_6$	Helps the body use nutrients	Same as other B vitamins
Vitamin B$_{12}$	Needed for red blood cell formation Helps function of the nervous and gastrointestinal systems Helps the body use fats, carbohydrates, and proteins	Animal sources such as meats
Vitamin C	Helps the body absorb and use iron Needed for healthy blood vessels Helps protect the body against infection	Citrus fruits, melons, strawberries, tomatoes, potatoes, cabbage, and green pepper

TABLE 19-3   **MINERALS, THEIR FUNCTIONS, AND THEIR SOURCES**

Minerals	Chief Functions	Sources
Calcium	Helps blood clot Helps nerves carry sensations Helps muscle fibers contract Helps teeth and bones develop	Milk, cheese, other dairy products (except butter)
Sodium	Maintains body's fluid balance Helps with nerve function Works with potassium to relax muscles Helps the body absorb nutrients	Almost all food; a heavy concentration in processed foods like luncheon meats and ham
Potassium	Helps in release of energy in the body Needed for good heart and nerve function	Fruits, vegetables, meats, cereals
Iron	Needed to carry oxygen to the cells Prevents **anemia**	Liver and other organ meats, dried fruits, nuts, whole grains, enriched cereals
Iodine	Needed for thyroid gland function and metabolism	Seafood, iodized table salt

ANEMIA
reduced number of red blood cells

produces 4 calories of energy. One gram of fat produces 9 calories of energy.

Individuals should eat enough calories to produce the energy their body needs for tissue growth and repair and to get through the day. Complex carbohydrates (grain, cereal, fruit, and vegetables) provide the best energy bargain for the body. They give a person energy over a longer period of time because they take longer to digest and metabolize. Simple carbohydrates (donuts, potato chips, etc.) metabolize quickly and are easily stored as fat in the body. Protein (meat, dairy products) that is not used by the body may also be stored as fat. Fats (butter and oils) give the body energy when they are digested and metabolized, but they do not have much nutrient value. Any fat not used by the body is stored for reserve energy.

EXAMPLE

If you eat 3 grams of carbohydrate, 4 grams of protein, and 2 grams of fat, which will give you the most calories?

3 grams carbohydrate = 12 calories

4 grams protein = 16 calories

2 grams fat = 18 calories

You might eat less fat, but it is high in calories.

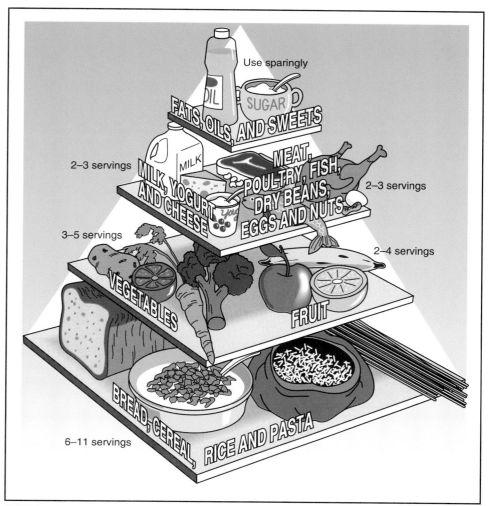

FIGURE 19-2

Meals are planned using the five food groups.

THE FIVE FOOD GROUPS

The U.S. Department of Agriculture has divided foods into five categories called food groups (Figure 19–2). The five food groups can be used to plan balanced meals. The five food groups are

- Fats, oils, and sweets
- Milk, yogurt, and cheese
- Meat, poultry, fish, dry beans, eggs, and nuts
- Vegetables and fruit
- Bread, cereal, rice, and pasta

The number of servings from each of the five food groups that a person's daily food intake should include is shown in Figure 19–2. Table 19–4 lists examples of food in each food group and the nutritional benefit of each. You need to know which foods are high in calories as well as which foods contain fiber, because the five-food-group categorization does not identify them.

High-calorie foods are generally recommended for persons who have experienced weight loss. They are important during the healing process because they provide the body with the energy needed to heal. The following are examples of high-calorie foods:

- Ice cream
- Custard or pudding
- Milk shake
- Chocolate candy

TABLE 19–4   THE FIVE FOOD GROUPS

Food Group	Examples	Benefits	Uses in the Body
Fats, oils, and sweets group	Cooking oils, lard, cake, candy bars	Fat	Helps body use fat-soluble vitamins
Milk, yogurt, and cheese group	Milk, cheese, ice cream, yogurt	Calcium Protein Vitamins	Tooth and bone growth Muscle function Muscle function Builds and repairs tissues Growth and health
Meat, fish, poultry, dry beans, eggs, and nuts group	Red meat (beef, pork), poultry (chicken, turkey)	Protein Vitamins Iron	Muscle function Builds and repairs tissue Growth and health Carries oxygen in the blood
Meat substitutes	Nuts, peanut butter, dry beans	Same as above	Same as above
Vegetable and fruit group	Green, leafy vegetables (lettuce, kale, and spinach); tomatoes; green beans; peas; corn; other vegetables; fruits such as apples, oranges, peaches, berries	Vitamins (mainly A and C)	Growth and health
Bread, cereal, rice, and pasta group	Breads: white, rye, wheat; cereals: bran, wheat, oat; pasta: macaroni, spaghetti, noodles	Vitamins Protein Iron	Growth and health Muscle function Carries oxygen in the blood

Fiber is the portion of food that passes through the intestine and colon undigested; it increases the bulk of the stool and makes it softer. Therefore, it helps prevent and treat constipation. It also helps the stool move quickly through the intestines so that waste products are carried out of the body faster. Fiber has been linked to decreased risk of colon cancer. Foods that contain fiber are plant foods such as

- Vegetables
- Fruits
- Whole grain breads and cereals
- Nuts
- Legumes (dried beans)

FLUIDS

Water is almost as important to life as oxygen. Human beings cannot live more than a few days without water. About two-thirds of the body's weight comes from water. All chemical changes that take place in the body need the presence of water. These changes also produce water in the body. Water carries nutrients to cells and wastes out of them. Body fluids are water based:

- blood
- saliva
- digestive juices
- perspiration

The body receives water from beverages in the diet and fruits and vegetables that contain a lot of water (e.g., watermelon). Most foods we eat contain water. A person needs about 2–2½ quarts of water each day or 1,500–2,000 ml per 24 hours. The need for water increases during hot weather and certain **disruptions** in health, such as

DISRUPTION
an interruption of normal function or activity

- Vomiting
- Diarrhea
- Fever
- **Excessive** sweating
- Burns

EXCESSIVE
too much

THE IMPORTANCE OF FLUIDS

Fluids are needed to sustain life. Fluids are inside and outside each cell in the body and are needed to maintain each bodily function. The body has special controls to keep the water in the proper balance. Fluid balance is the balance between the fluids inside and outside the cells. Any changes in an infant's or young child's fluid balance can be serious. When the body retains (keeps) too much fluid or loses too much fluid, body functions are affected.

ENCOURAGING PATIENTS TO DRINK FLUIDS

Illness can change the way a person takes in fluids. Persons who are ill may

- Be too weak to hold a cup or glass.
- Be unable to get to a refrigerator or sink.
- Lose their appetite because of their illness or their medication.
- Need to get into the habit of drinking a certain amount of fluids each day.
- Desire a fluid that they are not permitted to drink.

ILLNESS
sickness; a condition different from the normal health state; any change, temporary or long-lasting, in a person's physical, emotional, or spiritual health and well-being

An important part of the care you give as a nursing assistant is to encourage patients to drink fluids. You should

- Hold a glass or cup against patients' lips if they cannot do so.
- Offer a straw to patients strong enough to use one.
- Bring patients fresh water or other fluids they desire (if there are no restrictions).
- Find out what fluids patients like and try to get these fluids from the dietary department or a family member.
- Make sure that the fluid is an appropriate temperature. Ask patients whether they prefer ice water or cold tap water.
- Offer frequent sips of fluids (15 ml = ½ ounce; 30 ml = 1 ounce).
- Follow the nurse's instructions after she or he has taught the patient about the need for drinking fluids.
- Remember to document all fluids (large and small amounts) on the intake and output (I&O) record.

CARING COMMENT

Some older adults believe that if they drink less water, they will urinate less often. This is not true. Encourage older adults to drink fluids unless their physician has restricted their fluid intake.

SERVING FLUIDS AND BETWEEN-MEAL NOURISHMENT

In health care institutions, fresh ice water is placed in a pitcher within the patient's reach. Other fluids patients desire can be ordered for them unless there are fluid restrictions.

NOURISHMENT
a food or fluid that adds carbohydrates, proteins, and/or fats to the diet

Between-meal **nourishment** (also called nutritional supplement) is provided to patients to supplement the three meals a day served in the health care institution. Between-meal nourishment provides extra calories to the patient. When patients are hungry and are under no dietary restrictions, you can serve them food or fluid as requested. Examples of nourishment include servings of gelatin (Jello); pudding; ice cream; juice; soda; milkshakes; and commercially prepared high-calorie, high-protein, or high-carbohydrate drinks, crackers, and cookies.

PROCEDURE

Serving Fluids and Between-Meal Nourishment

When ordered, nourishments are usually provided midmorning, midafternoon, and at the hour of sleep.

GATHER EQUIPMENT

Serving container such as a pitcher and glass
Ice
Straw for fluids

Nourishment
Eating utensils such as a spoon and fork
Small tray if available
Paper napkin

ACTION	RATIONALE

Preparation

1. Ask the nurse or check the patient's care plan for fluid and dietary restrictions.

Helps the patient keep intake within the restrictions.

2. Wash hands.

Prevents the spread of microorganisms.

Procedural Steps

3. *For ice water:*
   Follow your institution's procedure for getting ice and take a pitcher with ice into the patient's room. Pour tap water into the pitcher. Pour water and ice into the glass, place a straw in the glass, and place the glass within the patient's reach. Assist persons who are unable to hold a glass themselves.

Procedures are written to prevent contamination of ice through improper handling.

   For other fluids:
   Check in the refrigerator for fluids marked with the patient's name and room number. Place ice in a glass and pour in fluid.

Prevents you from using fluids or foods that are designated for others. Special nourishments are provided by the dietary department and are marked with the patient's name and room number and the time they should be served.

   For milkshakes and commercially prepared drinks:
   Do not add ice unless indicated on the label. Take the drink to the patient's room and pour the fluid into the glass, place a straw in the glass, and place the glass within the patient's reach.

   For between-meal nourishment:
   Check the refrigerator or other designated place for the nourishment that is marked with the patient name and room number. Take the food and correct eating utensil to the room and place them within the patient's reach. Assist in opening packages if the patient is not able to open them.
   Note: Between-meal nourishment may be food or fluid.

4. Place a paper napkin within the patient's reach. If necessary, place the napkin across the patient's chest.

5. Encourage the patient to eat and/or drink. If necessary, feed the patient or hold the glass and straw for the patient.

6. After the patient is finished, dispose of soiled containers, utensils, and napkins properly.

Follow-Through

7. Record the amount taken in by the patient if he or she is on an I&O order. Report and record intake on any other required forms.

NUTRITIONAL NEEDS ACROSS THE LIFE SPAN

Nutritional needs vary across the life span. More nutrition is needed during periods of rapid cell growth: infancy, adolescence, pregnancy, and illness.

INFANT

The first year of life is a time of very rapid growth in humans. The nutritional needs are very high. After the first few months of life, cereal, fruits, vegetables, meats, and eggs provide calories and variety in the diet. For the first few months, all the **infant** takes in is milk. Milk is available in the form of breast milk or prepared infant formula.

Breast Milk

The mother's breast milk is a readily available and money-saving way to feed the infant (Figure 19–3). It contains all the necessary nutrients for growth. Breast milk also contains substances that protect the infant in the early months of life from certain diseases.

The mother who is breastfeeding her infant has special fluid and dietary needs. She should drink four to six 8-ounce glasses (a total of 32–48 ounces) of milk each day. She also needs to take in more calories because her system uses about 1,000 calories more per day to produce milk. Table 19–5 indicates the amount of food from each food group that should be included in the diet of the woman who is breastfeeding.

The mother who is breastfeeding can eat any food that does not cause her a problem (such as **constipation** or gas). She should limit food or beverages that contain **caffeine** because the caffeine may harm the infant. This includes

INFANT

the person at the beginning of life (from birth to 1½ years), for whom all needs are met by others

CONSTIPATION

inability to have or difficulty in having a bowel movement

CAFFEINE

a substance in coffee, tea, colas, and chocolate that acts as a stimulant and diuretic

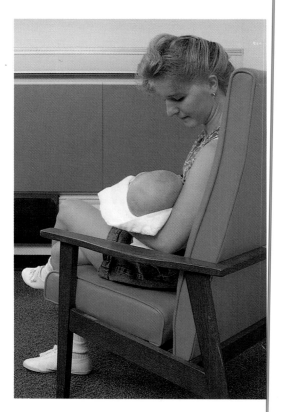

FIGURE 19–3
This young mother is feeding her infant breast milk, the ideal food for infants.

TABLE 19–5   AMOUNT OF FOOD FROM EACH
FOOD GROUP REQUIRED FOR A
BREASTFEEDING WOMAN DAILY

Food Group	Daily Amount
Milk	Four to six 8-ounce glasses
Meat	Three to four servings
Eggs	One
Vegetable	
Green or yellow	One
Other	Two or three servings
Fruit	
Citrus	At least two servings
Other	Two servings
Bread and cereal	Four servings

chocolate, coffee, tea, and colas. The nursing mother should take medications only under the supervision of her physician because the medication may appear in the breast milk and affect the infant.

Prepared Infant Formula

Prepared infant **formula** is a milk mixture used to feed babies. It is designed to provide the nutrients necessary for growth. Formula is available in liquid and powder forms. The formula may be fortified with iron. Special formulas are also available, such as a soy-based formula for the infant who cannot digest the **lactose** in milk.

FORMULA

milk mixture that is fed to babies

LACTOSE

a sugar present in milk; many persons lack the enzyme that breaks down lactose for use by the body

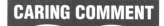

CARING COMMENT

Be sure to read the directions on the bottle of infant formula. Do not add water unless directed to do so by the label.

Feeding Schedule

The infant is often fed on a schedule. The feeding schedule may be determined by the parents or the health care provider. In some cases, infants may be permitted to feed on demand. If this is the case, feeding time occurs whenever the infant is hungry.

TODDLER

During the **toddler** years, growth begins to slow. Muscle and bone development is very important, because toddlers are beginning to walk. Thus they need protein to help their muscles grow and function and **calcium** to make their bones grow and become strong. By the end of toddlerhood, children are feeding themselves most table foods.

TODDLER

the child from 1½ to 3 years of age

CALCIUM

the chemical element that is important to bone and tooth formation

PRESCHOOLER

The preschooler does well with three meals a day plus nourishing snacks (Figure 19–4). Growth continues, so protein continues to be needed in the

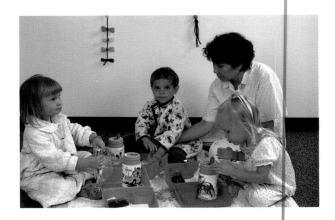

FIGURE 19–4
During the preschool age, play and physical activity result in high energy needs. Nourishing snacks such as carrot sticks, muffins, and fruit help meet these needs.

PRESCHOOL AGE
the child from 3–6 years of age

diet. A child of **preschool age** should drink two to three 8-ounce glasses of milk each day.

SCHOOL-AGE CHILD

SCHOOL AGE
the child from 6 to 12 years of age (the years before adolescence)

PUBERTY
the developmental and physical changes that result in adult sexual characteristics and the ability to reproduce

GROWTH SPURT
when a child gains weight and adds inches in a short period of time

ADOLESCENCE
13–18 years of age; a time of transition from childhood to adulthood

MENSTRUATION
the discharge through the vagina of blood and tissue from the uterus of the nonpregnant female; also called monthly flow, menses, and period

Body growth continues but slows down during the **school-age** years. The body begins to get ready for the rapid growth of **puberty.** Food intake is influenced by individual appetite patterns, **growth spurts,** and type and amount of activity.

ADOLESCENT

Growth spurts continue to occur in **adolescence.** A high-calorie diet is important. The amount of food needed increases with the demands of a growing and changing body. Because muscle and bone are still developing, adequate amounts of protein and calcium are still needed. Once **menstruation** begins in girls, their need for iron increases (see Table 19–3 for good sources of iron).

ADULT

Nutritional requirements vary for adults. They may increase during the reproductive (childbearing) years. The amount of food eaten may decrease depending on the activity level and the type of food eaten by the individual. Enough food should be ingested to meet the needs for healthy body function.

THE ELDERLY

Many body functions that are associated with eating change with age. These changes include

- slowing of digestion
- decrease in saliva production
- loss of teeth
- possible loss of appetite
- decrease in the senses of taste and smell
- decreased need for calories

Elderly persons should eat enough food to maintain the proper weight for their height, maintain activities of daily living, and enjoy the benefits of socializing. See Chapter 31 for further information about changes in the elderly person's nutrition and metabolism.

DIETARY GUIDELINES

Dietary guidelines issued by the U. S. Department of Agriculture help individuals meet their needs for nutrition. These guidelines suggest that individuals

- Eat a variety of foods.
- Maintain a desirable weight.
- Avoid too much fat and cholesterol.
- Eat food that has adequate starch and fiber.
- Avoid too much sugar.
- Avoid too much sodium (salt).
- Drink alcoholic beverages in moderation, if they are permitted.

SPECIAL PATIENT DIETS

The physician may order a special **diet** to help meet a patient's particular nutritional need. A special diet may also be called a **therapeutic diet** or a modified diet. Special diets may be needed during a disruption in one or more body functions. Special diets may be needed to

- Provide nutrients in the correct amounts.
- Provide a consistency that the patient can eat.
- Assist the individual in maintaining or regaining health.

The nutrition specialist (may be the dietician) consults with patients to discover their likes and dislikes in foods and beverages. When patients' preferences are included in their special diet, they are more likely to follow the diet. Some special diets commonly used are

Clear liquid
Full liquid
Soft
Puree
Regular
Diabetic

DIET
the total amount of food eaten by an individual

THERAPEUTIC DIET
diet that helps meet a patient's particular nutritional need; also called special, modified, or restricted diet

PUREE
strained food

CLEAR LIQUID DIET (Figure 19–5)

- A clear liquid diet is ordered for patients who have had surgery, acutely ill patients, to relieve thirst, or to provide fluids for persons with a temporary food intolerance (such as vomiting or diarrhea).

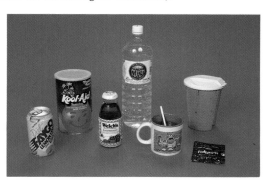

FIGURE 19–5
The patient can drink water and any clear fluid on a clear-liquid diet.

- All fluids are clear enough to see through, including
     soup broth and bouillon
     juices
     ginger ale
     coffee
     tea
     plain gelatin
- This diet is used only for a short time because it does not provide enough nutrients for good health.
- Clear liquids do not stimulate the digestive system or cause gas to form.

FULL LIQUID DIET

- A full liquid diet is ordered for patients who have had surgery, patients with stomach disruptions, patients with an elevated body temperature, and patients who have an intolerance for solid foods.
- It includes all liquids used in the clear liquid diet, plus strained soups; milk and milk products like ice cream, eggnog, and custard; fruit and vegetable juices; and thinned, cooked cereal.
- In order for the diet to provide enough nutrients, meal planning is required.
- This diet is used as a transition from clear liquid to a soft diet.

SOFT DIET

- A soft diet is ordered for patients with chewing or gastrointestinal problems and as a stepping stone to a regular diet.
- A soft diet includes all liquids, pureed fruits and vegetables, strained cereals, ground-up meat, and pudding. Eggs and toast may be included when permitted.
- Foods in this diet require no chewing and are easy to digest.

PUREED DIET

- A pureed diet is ordered for patients who cannot chew solid foods or have difficulty swallowing.
- All food is ground up into a soft consistency, with no lumps.

CARING COMMENT

A soft or pureed diet may look unappetizing to the patient. You can help by making sure that foods are the correct temperature. When you feed patients, offer only one food at a time so that they can taste each food.

REGULAR DIET

- A regular diet is used for all patients who do not require a special diet.
- A regular diet includes all the foods from the five food groups in their regular consistency (not pureed or ground up).

DIABETIC DIET

- A diabetic diet is ordered for the individual with diabetes.
- Food is balanced to provide an appropriate amount of nutrients to help keep the glucose in the blood at an acceptable level.
- A prescribed number of calories and certain proportions of fats, carbohydrates, and proteins form the basis of the diet.
- There are six exchange food groups from which the person can plan a diabetic diet. Items in each food group can be exchanged for each other in specified amounts.
- Individuals choose a certain amount of food from these groups to meet the dietary requirements specified by their health care provider.
- The six exchange food groups are
    Milk
    Vegetable
    Fruit
    Bread
    Meat
    Fat
- It is important for the patient who is diabetic to eat meals at scheduled times and stay on the planned diet.

CARING COMMENT

When patients do not eat the food they have been given, find out if there is another food they might like to eat instead. If they specify a preference, tell the nurse or supervisor so that it can be added, if possible, to the ordered diet.

OTHER SPECIAL DIETS

Bland Diet

- A bland diet is ordered if the organs of the digestive system (intestines, stomach, or esophagus) are irritated.
- This includes mild foods.
- Spicy foods are excluded.
- The food is easily digested.

Low-Fat Diet

- A low-fat diet is ordered for patients who have difficulty digesting fats.
- Restricted foods are dairy products, fried foods, and fatty meats.

Low-Residue Diet

- A low-residue diet may be used for patients who have an irritation or disease of the intestines.
- Foods high in fiber (vegetables, fruits, etc.) are restricted.
- Low-fiber food (milk, white bread, lettuce, etc.) is easier on digestion.

High-Protein Diet

- A high-protein diet is ordered to help a person gain weight.

- Foods from the dairy, meat, fish, poultry, and bean food groups are included.
- Protein is needed for tissue healing.

High-Calorie Diet

- A high-calorie diet is ordered for the patient who has lost weight or is losing weight.
- A **calorie count** may be ordered. Write down the type and amount of food the patient has eaten at each meal; a member of the dietary staff will collect the information and calculate the number of calories the patient has eaten in a 24-hour period.
- Foods that are high in calories are ordered, such as dairy products (milk shakes, etc.).
- Special supplements such as fortified milk shakes and Ensure (a commercial preparation high in calories) are also given.
- Daily weight measurements may be ordered to track the patient's weight gain.

CALORIE COUNT
a record of the amount of calories eaten

Low-Calorie Diet

- A low-calorie diet is ordered for the patient who needs to lose weight.
- Foods high in calories (sweets, dairy products, etc.) are restricted.
- Daily weight measurements may be ordered to track the patient's weight loss.

Low-Sodium (Salt) Diet

- A low-sodium diet is ordered for the person with heart and/or kidney problems.
- Foods that contain sodium, such as processed meats (ham and luncheon meats) are restricted.
- The use of the table salt is restricted; no salt is placed on the patient's tray.
- Foods are not salted during preparation and cooking.
- A sodium-free diet is completely sodium free.

CARING COMMENT

A salt substitute may contain potassium. Check with the nurse to be sure the patient is allowed to use such a salt substitute.

METHODS USED TO SUPPLY NUTRITION TO PATIENTS WHO CANNOT EAT

If the patient is not able or is not allowed to take food in through the mouth, nutrition is provided through tube feeding or hyperalimentation.

TUBE FEEDINGS

TUBE FEEDING
giving fluids or nutritional supplements through a tube inserted into the stomach

Tube feedings are done after a tube is placed directly into the patient's stomach by a registered nurse or a physician. The tube is inserted through a nostril and pushed down the throat into the stomach. If tube feeding is to continue for a long time, a gastrostomy tube is inserted by a surgeon directly into the stomach.

The patient receives liquids through the feeding tube. The liquids are special formulas that are rich in calories and nutrients. The nurse or supervisor is completely responsible for tube feedings.

HYPERALIMENTATION

In **hyperalimentation** (also known as total parenteral nutrition, TPN, or hyperal), the patient is given needed proteins, carbohydrates, vitamins, and minerals by direct injection of a solution into a large vein. The solution can be specially made up for the individual patient. Hyperalimentation is prescribed for patients who have a problem digesting food. It gives the bowel an opportunity to rest and heal. The nurse or supervisor is responsible for monitoring the hyperalimentation feeding of the patient.

HYPERALIMENTATION
delivery of proteins, carbohydrates, vitamins, and minerals through a large vein

INTRAVENOUS FLUIDS

An **intravenous** line is another way of replacing and maintaining fluids in the body, but it does not provide enough calories and other nutrients to maintain life. A 1000-ml bag of intravenous solution usually has about 170–200 calories. The normal adult needs 1200–2000 calories a day for energy, tissue growth, and repair.

INTRAVENOUS
through the vein

FLUIDS

PROBLEMS WITH FLUID BALANCE

Fluid Excess

When the body retains fluids, it is in a state of **fluid excess.** The heart and blood vessels, lungs, and kidneys can no longer do an efficient job of getting rid of fluid. Fluid excess can take the form of either

- **Edema**—an abnormal accumulation of fluids in the cells
- **Hypervolemia**—an abnormal accumulation of fluid in the blood

FLUID EXCESS
condition in which the body's tissues hold extra fluid
EDEMA
an abnormal accumulation of fluid between cells
HYPERVOLEMIA
an increase in the volume of fluid circulating in the body

OBSERVATIONS

- Increased weight—Fluid trapped in the cells or the circulation results in a weight increase when daily weight figures are compared.
- Edema—Because trapped fluid has nowhere else to go, it causes swelling until heart and/or kidney function is restored or the excess fluid is removed. For example, a special medication (a diuretic) increases fluid output through the urine.
- Decreased fluid output—When fluid output is compared to what the patient takes in, it becomes obvious that the extra fluid is somewhere in the body. For example, for a person whose intake is 2,000 ml and output is 800 ml in a 24-hour period, the body is holding the "missing" 1,200 ml of fluid (2,000 − 800 = 1,200).
- A cough—Fluid may irritate the lining of the lungs, causing the patient to cough.
- Congested breathing—Fluid trapped in the cells of the lungs forces the air to travel through the extra fluid.

CARE OF THE PATIENT WITH EXCESS FLUIDS

Care of the patient with excess fluids in the body is important for two reasons:

- Because the heart, lungs, and kidneys work harder as they try to rid the body of the excess fluids, the patient may tire very easily. The body uses all its energy in trying to restore water balance.

- The skin of the extremities (limbs) and other parts of the body where edema forms may break down because the pressure from the edema interferes with the proper function of the skin.

In caring for patients with excess fluids, you should

- Handle the edematous (swollen) extremities gently, because the skin is fragile and may break open.
- Offer a special diet as directed by the nurse or supervisor who has read the physician's order.
- Elevate the edematous extremities (as indicated by the nurse) above the level of the heart (about 18 inches) to help the circulation work more efficiently. This also decreases the work of the heart.
- Measure, record, and report vital signs, because changes may mean that the body organs are working too hard or are not able to keep up with the job of getting rid of the excess fluid.
- Weigh the patient every day at the same time and record and report the information, because an increase in weight may mean that the body is not clearing the extra fluids from the cells or the circulation.

Fluid Deficit

FLUID DEFICIT
condition in which the body loses fluid and fluid is not replaced in the amount needed by the body

DEHYDRATION
removal of water from the body or a tissue; or the condition that results from undue loss of water

Fluid deficit occurs when the body loses fluid and the fluids are not replaced with the amount needed for proper body function. When the patient has fluid deficit, the body becomes **dehydrated.** Dehydration occurs when a large amount of fluid is lost through vomiting, diarrhea, or blood loss and is not replaced. Fluids in the body are replaced by

- Oral fluids
- Intravenous fluids

OBSERVATIONS

- Weight loss—Because fluid is lost from cells or the circulation, body weight is also lost.
- Dry mucous membranes and skin—Cells need fluid to survive and function; the loss of fluid has a drying effect on the body's tissues.
- Thirst—Patients tell you they are thirsty, because the cells are sending the message to the brain that they need fluids.

CARING COMMENT

The infant who is dehydrated is not able to say, "I'm thirsty." It is important to observe for the following in infants and report any observations to the nurse.
- sunken eyes and sunken fontanelles (soft spots) on the head
- decrease in tears or lack of tears when crying
- listlessness
- decreased urine output

CARE OF THE PATIENT WITH FLUID DEFICIT

Care of the patient with fluid deficit is important for the following reasons:
- The cells of the body cannot survive without enough water.
- Cells use water in all the chemical processes of the body. For example, metabolism is a chemical process.
- Enough fluid must be in the circulation so the blood can deliver the oxygen cells needed and take carbon dioxide away from cells.

In caring for patients with a fluid deficit, you should

- Check fluid intake. The nurse or supervisor will tell you when fluid intake needs to be recorded. Keeping an I&O record makes it easy to monitor the water balance in the body.
- Weigh the patient daily. An increase in weight may mean that the body is retaining the fluids it needs to function properly.
- Offer fluids. Patients should be encouraged to take in fluids by mouth when permitted to do so. You can help by offering fluids they like.
- Observe intravenous fluids. IV fluids may be ordered to help the body maintain a fluid balance. The nurse is responsible for the patient's intravenous fluid therapy. The nursing assistant should report any problems (fluid not dripping into tubing, patient's statements of pain at the site of the IV, bag almost empty of solution, etc.) to the nurse.

MEASURING FLUIDS

Fluids that are taken in by the patient are measured, recorded, and reported in milliliters (Figure 19–6). It is important to remember that

5 ml = 1 teaspoon

30 ml = 1 ounce

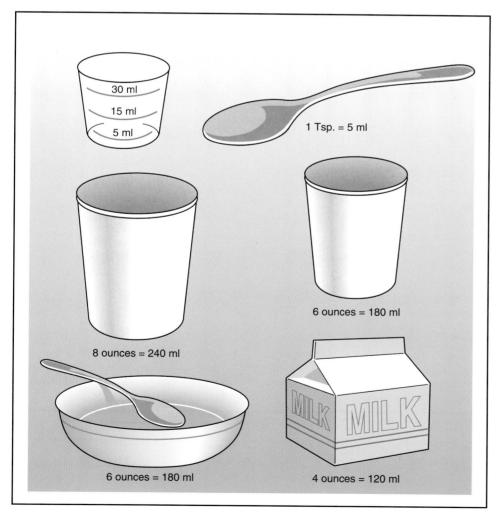

30 ml
15 ml
5 ml

1 Tsp. = 5 ml

6 ounces = 180 ml

8 ounces = 240 ml

6 ounces = 180 ml

4 ounces = 120 ml

MILK   MILK

FIGURE 19–6

The number of milliliters (ml) in a variety of common containers. Tsp., teaspoon.

EXAMPLE

For example, if the patient drinks 8 ounces of fluid this is recorded as 240 ml:

8 ounces × 30 ml per ounce = 240 ml

If the patient takes in 3 teaspoons of fluid, you record 15 ml on the I&O record:

3 teaspoons × 5 ml per teaspoon = 15 ml

The I&O record is used to keep track of the patient's water balance. The total amount of fluid taken in and the amount of output should match. If the fluid intake is greater than the fluid output, the patient may be keeping fluids in the body. Edema may result. If the fluid output is greater than the fluid intake, the patient may be losing too much fluid and may become dehydrated.

PROCEDURE

Measuring and Recording Intake

The measuring and recording of fluid intake is an important responsibility of the nursing assistant. Each time the patient takes in fluids, the amount should be recorded in the correct time slot on the I&O record.

GATHER EQUIPMENT

Blank I&O record with the patient's name stamped on it
Pen

Fluid for patient to drink
Container to measure the amount of fluid patient drinks

ACTION	RATIONALE
Preparation	
1. Explain to patients the need to measure the fluids they take in.	Patients often want to help keep track of the amount of fluids they take in. This is good because it involves them in their own care.
Procedural Steps	
2. Check patients' care plan.	Specifies the amount of fluid intake required. The most common amount is 240 ml per waking hour.
3. Provide and encourage fluids every hour. Place the fluids within reach. Ask patients what fluids they prefer and provide them if there are no restrictions.	Placing fluids within patients' reach on the over-bed table or the bedside stand helps patients.
4. Measure the amount of fluid patients drink.	
Follow-Through	
5. Record the amount of fluid taken in on the I&O record (Figure 19–7). Be sure to write the amount in the correct time slot.	An I&O record is usually kept for 24 hours. At the end of the 24-hour period, the information is documented in the patient's chart.

FIGURE 19–7

Sample Intake and Output Record. (Courtesy of Woman's Christian Association Hospital, Jamestown, NY.)

Time	IV Type and Amt.	Amt. Left	Amt. Absorb.	Partial Fill IV Meds	Oral	Urine		Urinary Irrigation		Emesis	NG / IRR	
											INTAKE / OUTPUT	
2400												
0100												
0200												
0300												
0400												
0500												
0600					240	350						350
11-7 Shift Summary					240	350					+ −	350
0800					240							
0900						250				100		350
1000					120							
1100												
1200					420							
1300												
1400						325						325
7-3 Shift Summary					780	575				100	+ −	675
1600					100							
1700						375						375
1800					360					50		50
1900												
2000					240							
2100						300						300
2200												
3-11 Shift Summary					700	675				50	+ −	725
		IV		Partial Fill IV Meds	Oral	Urine		Urinary Irrigation		Emesis	NG / IRR	
24 HOUR TOTALS					1720	1600				150		1750

DATE: Oct 1, 1992

WCA HOSPITAL INTAKE AND OUTPUT 24 HOUR SUMMARY

ML AMOUNTS FOR COMMON CONTAINERS

Container	ml
Small juice (4 oz.)	120
Large juice (6 oz.)	180
Styrofoam cup (8 oz.)	240
Coffee mug (8 oz.)	240
Plastic glass (6 oz.)	180
Can of soda (pop) (12 oz.)	360
Milk carton (4 oz.)	120
Soup or cereal bowl	180
Jello or ice cream (4 oz.)	120

FIGURE 19-7 *See legend on opposite page*

CARING COMMENT

The nurse tells you if the patient needs to be weighed every day. You may hear the term "daily weights" used to refer to the order that the patient be weighed every day. If the patient is to be weighed daily, take the measurement at the same time every day and use the same scale. The patient should be dressed in similar clothes for each measurement. Ask the patient to void before the measurement is taken.

COMMON DISRUPTIONS IN NUTRITION

OBESITY

OBESITY
overweight; the presence of too much fat in the body

One of the most common disruptions in nutrition is **obesity.** The person who is obese carries an accumulation of fat in the body. Obesity is an increase in weight above what is recommended for the individual's height and body build. The percentage of increase above normal determines whether a person is overweight, obese, or grossly obese.

- **Overweight**—10% above recommended weight
- **Obese**—15% above recommended weight
- **Grossly obese**—20% or more above recommended weight

Causes of Obesity

EXCESSIVE INTAKE   The amount of food or fluids taken in is more than the body needs to function. Often the intake consists of high-calorie and high-fat foods and fluids.

LACK OF EXERCISE   The body needs exercise to burn off calories. The best exercise is walking. To be effective, exercise must be done three or four times a week for 20–30 minutes.

DISEASE THAT AFFECTS METABOLISM   In certain diseases such as hypothyroidism, obesity may occur despite a proper diet and adequate exercise.

Disruptions of Body Functioning Caused by Obesity

The person who is obese may experience the following disruptions in body functioning:

- Stress on the heart and lungs; these organs must worker harder to circulate body fluids to the added cells
- **Hypertension**
- Inability to tolerate activity due to shortness of breath
- Stress on the pancreas, which produces insulin (in some people, this results in diabetes mellitus)

HYPERTENSION
persistent high blood pressure

Care of the Obese Patient

The person who is overweight should be under the care and supervision of a health care professional. The health care professional recommends diet and exercises for the individual. You can help by providing support and encouragement to the patient.

ANOREXIA

Causes

Another disruption in nutrition is **anorexia.** Anorexia can be caused by diseases (such as cancer), certain medications that affect gastrointestinal functioning, or psychological factors. Because a daily intake of foods and fluids is needed to maintain a healthy body, the physician tries to discover cause of the anorexia.

ANOREXIA

loss of appetite

Recording the Anorexic Patient's Intake

You may be asked to record the amount of food taken in by the anorexic patient using terms such as *good*, *fair*, or *poor*. Check your institution's guidelines when asked to use these words to describe intake. A scale such as the following may be used:

- Good—The patient ate 75% or more of the meal.
- Fair—The patient ate 50% of the meal.
- Poor—The patient ate less than 50% of the meal.

You may also want to record the specific amounts of food and fluids the anorexic patient has eaten. For example,

Half of a tuna salad sandwich
Half of a bowl of chicken soup
Two cups of black coffee
One cup of pudding
Half of a cup of pureed carrots

Care of the Anorexic Patient

The anorexic patient may be fatigued (tired) and uninterested in food or fluid. You have the following responsibilities in the care of the anorexic patient:

- Make mealtime pleasant. Place the patient in a sitting position if allowed. Help the patient with toileting before mealtime. Do not hurry when you take the meal into the room.
- Check the environment. Make sure no noxious (foul) odors are present when the meal is served.
- Provide support. Eating is a social activity, so your presence may encourage a patient to eat more.
- Provide the prescribed diet. The nurse tells you the diet that has been ordered for the patient. Match the diet slip with the patient's identification bracelet to be certain you are giving the correct diet to the patient.
- Provide small amounts of food or fluid frequently. A patient may be able to tolerate small amounts offered often better than large amounts of food offered infrequently.
- Weigh the patient daily. A record of daily weight measurements shows when the patient gains weight.

Alternate routes for feeding: The patient may require tube feedings through a tube inserted into the stomach or through a special tube inserted into a vein (hyperalimentation). The nurse is responsible for these alternate feedings.

INABILITY TO FEED SELF

Patients may have a disruption of nutrition because they cannot feed themselves. For example, patients who have a broken arm, are unable to move, or are weak often need help with meals. You may be responsible for feeding patients who are unable to feed themselves.

CARING COMMENT

Patients may be able to feed themselves if you open the packages that are on the tray (milk carton, salt and pepper packets, etc.). Patients who can can feed themselves should do so. Always be sure to check back with patients who feed themselves to see if they need any help.

PROCEDURE

Serving Food

Check patients' care plan or your notes from the shift report for the type of diet that has been ordered. Meals are ready to be served when the dietary cart arrives on the unit.

GATHER EQUIPMENT

Meal tray
Menu

ACTION	RATIONALE
Preparation	
1. Wash hands.	Prevents the spread of microorganisms.
2. Identify yourself and the patient.	Maintains patients' rights.
3. Provide privacy.	Maintains patients' rights.
4. Explain the procedure.	Informs patients what is happening.
Procedural Steps	
5. Offer the bedpan or assist patients to the bathroom before the meal.	Makes patients comfortable and able to enjoy eating.
6. Offer a damp, warm washcloth so patients can wash their hands before meals.	
7. Assist patients into a sitting position for the meal. Place the bed in a high Fowler's position or assist patients to a chair, if this is permitted.	
8. Place the over-bed table at a height comfortable for patients.	
9. Remove patients' tray from the dietary cart. Check the menu for patients' name and type of diet ordered.	
10. Close the dietary cart after you take out the tray.	Keeps foods warm and free from contamination.
11. Check your notes to be certain that the correct diet is on the tray.	Ensures that patients are receiving the correct diet.
12. Take the tray into patients' room and place it on the over-bed stand.	
13. Place the stand within patients' reach.	
14. Open packages, cartons, and other containers if necessary.	Helps patients who are weak or unable to use their hands.

15. Ask patients if they need to have the food cut or liquids poured.

16. Ask patients if they desire anything else. Make certain that all food ordered is present by checking the menu against the food that is on the tray.

Gives patients the opportunity to express their needs.

17. If extra (not ordered) food is on the tray, check with the nurse or supervisor to make sure patients can have the food.

Prevents giving patients food that they are not permitted to have.

Follow-Through

18. If patients are on I&O, calculate and record the amount of fluids taken in during the meal.

19. If patients are on a calorie count, record the type and amount of food eaten.

The dietician does a calorie count from this information and monitors calorie intake every 24 hours.

20. When patients have finished eating, place the tray back on the cart to be returned to the dietary department.

21. Assist patients to a position of comfort after the meal.

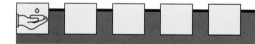

PROCEDURE

Feeding Patients

Patients need to be fed when they are not able to feed themselves. Patients who are very weak, are unable to move, or have experienced injury to the hands or arms may need you to feed them.

GATHER EQUIPMENT

Patients' food tray
Eating utensils

Over-bed stand
Towel

ACTION

RATIONALE

Preparation

1. Wash hands.

Prevents the spread of microorganisms.

2. Identify yourself and the patient.

Maintains patients' rights.

3. Provide privacy.

Maintains patients' rights.

4. Explain the procedure.

Informs patients what is happening.

Procedural Steps

5. Check the care plan or ask the nurse for the prescribed patient diet.

Ensures that patients receive the correct diet.

6. Place patients in the semi- or high Fowler's position (Figure 19–8). Place a protective towel across patients' chest.

Helps prevent choking.
Protects clothing.
Preserves patient's dignity.

7. Tell patients what food is on the tray.

Informs patients what foods they will be receiving.

Continued on following page

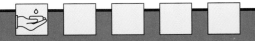

PROCEDURE

Feeding Patients *Continued*

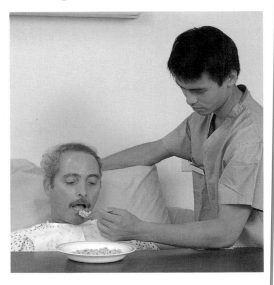

FIGURE 19–8

A sitting position helps food go down the esophagus by gravity.

Step	Rationale
8. Check the temperature of the food and fluids. Add an ice cube or two to foods that are steaming hot.	Prevents burns from hot foods or fluids.
9. If the meal is a regular diet, cut the food into bite-sized pieces.	
10. Prepare patients' beverages. Add cream or sugar if preferred.	
11. Place a spoonful of food in patients' mouth. Tell patients which food is on the spoon.	Part of the enjoyment of eating is seeing or hearing about the food one eats.
12. Vary the food served from teaspoon to teaspoon.	Varies the texture of foods; adds to enjoyment.
13. Give patients time to chew or swallow.	Prevents choking.
14. Offer sips of fluids between the spoonfuls of food.	Provides a break in eating solids. Also helps wash the food down into the stomach.
15. Make mealtime a social time. Talk with patients.	Encourages an increase in dietary intake and increases patients' awareness of their environment.
16. Use a napkin to keep patients' face clean.	Preserves patients' dignity.
17. Give positive feedback while feeding patients.	Lets patients know how well they are eating. Encourages patients to continue eating.

Follow-Through

Step	Rationale
18. After the patient has been fed, wash patients' face and hands.	Refreshes patients' skin.
19. Wash hands.	Prevents the spread of microorganisms.
20. Record, if required, the amount of food and fluids taken in.	

You may be asked to help patients fill out a menu. Read the foods listed on the menu to patients and let them make selections. Mark patients' choices on the menu when they cannot do so.

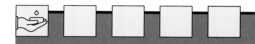

PROCEDURE

Feeding Patients with a Syringe

Patients may be fed by placing a syringe filled with food or fluid into their mouth. A patient needs to be able to swallow to receive a syringe feeding. Many health care institutions require a physician's order for a syringe feeding. The nurse tells you when to use a syringe to feed a patient.

GATHER EQUIPMENT

Fluid or pureed food tray
60-ml bulb **syringe** (or a piston syringe)

Protective towel or other item to cover patients' clothing

SYRINGE
instrument used to inject fluids into or remove fluids from the body

ACTION	RATIONALE
Preparation	
1. Wash hands.	Prevents the spread of microorganisms.
2. Identify yourself and the patient.	Maintains patients' rights.
3. Provide privacy.	Maintains patients' rights.
4. Explain the procedure.	Informs patients what is happening.
Procedural Steps	
5. Check the care plan for the correct diet for the patient.	Ensures that patients receive the correct diet.
6. Place patients in the semi- or high Fowler's position.	Allows ease in swallowing.
7. Place the protective towel across patients' chest.	Protects clothing. Preserves patient's dignity.
8. Tell patients what food is on the tray.	Maintains patients' right to courtesy. Informs patients what kind of food is coming.
9. Check the food's temperature.	Prevents burning or scalding the tissues of the mouth.
10. Fill the syringe with 10 ml of food. 10 ml is equal to about 2 teaspoons.	A small amount of food is easier for the patient to swallow.
11. Ask patients to open their mouth and place the tip of the syringe in either the right or left inner cheek area (Figure 19–9).	
12. Tell patients they will feel the food coming into their mouth.	Lets patients get ready to swallow.
13. Encourage patients to swallow.	
14. Alternate foods and fluids; tell patients what is being placed in their mouth each time.	Increases the pleasure of mealtime.
15. Talk to patients while feeding them and provide verbal feedback about the progress of the meal.	Provides an opportunity for socialization. Motivates patients to eat.

Continued on following page

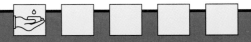

PROCEDURE

Feeding Patients with a Syringe *Continued*

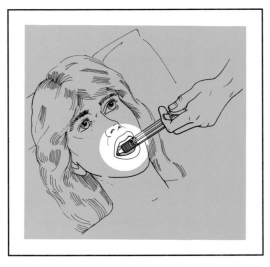

FIGURE 19-9

Place the filled syringe in the inner cheek area and push the plunger in slowly. Check that the patient swallows the food.

Follow-Through

16. When finished, wash patients' face and hands.	Refreshes patients' skin.
17. Rinse, dry, and store equipment for the next use.	Readies equipment for the next meal.
18. Wash hands.	Prevents spread of microorganisms.
19. Record in the appropriate place the amount of food and fluid taken in.	Intake records are kept for patients who are not able to feed themselves.

CARING COMMENTS

Towels or special cloths may be placed around patients' neck or on their chest to keep clothing clean during meals. Refer to these towels or cloths as napkins. Do not refer to them as bibs, because the patient or family may think you view the patient as a baby.

Many health care institutions require that feeding syringes be marked with the patient's name and the date it was first used. Syringes are usually replaced every 24–48 hours.

MEASURING HEIGHT AND WEIGHT

Weight and height measurement are part of patients' admission process. The weight measurement provides a baseline for comparison in case patients' weight changes while they are in the health care institution. It is important to monitor patients' weight to see if a change in diet (type of diet or amount of food) is necessary.

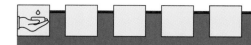

Measuring Patients' Height and Weight with a Standing Scale

GATHER EQUIPMENT

Scale   Pencil
Piece of paper

ACTION	RATIONALE
Preparation	
1. Wash hands.	Prevents the spread of microorganisms.
2. Identify yourself and the patient.	Maintains patients' rights.
3. Provide privacy.	Maintains patients' rights.
4. Explain the procedure.	Informs patients what is happening.
Procedural Steps	
5. Balance the scale before weighing patients. The pointer at the end of the scale should balance itself in the middle (Figure 19–10). If it does not, turn the balance screw until the pointer is in the middle.	Ensures accuracy.

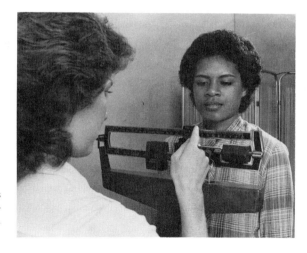

FIGURE 19–10
(From Bonewit K: Clinical Procedures for Medical Assistants, 3rd ed. Philadelphia, W. B. Saunders Company, 1990.)

ACTION	RATIONALE
6. Assist patients in removing their robe if necessary.	Extra clothing increases the weight measurement.
7. Assist patients to stand with both feet securely on the scale. Place a paper towel or other protector on the scale for patients to stand on.	Ensures accuracy.
8. Move the bottom weight (marked in 50-pound sections) to begin. Slide the weight to the closest approximation (idea) of patients' weight.	Helps save time.
9. Move the top balance weight to get	

Continued on following page

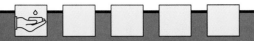

PROCEDURE

Measuring Patients' Height and Weight with a Standing Scale *Continued*

the balance pointer to steady itself in the middle.

10. Add the top and bottom numbers together (Figure 19–11).

Determines patients' total weight.

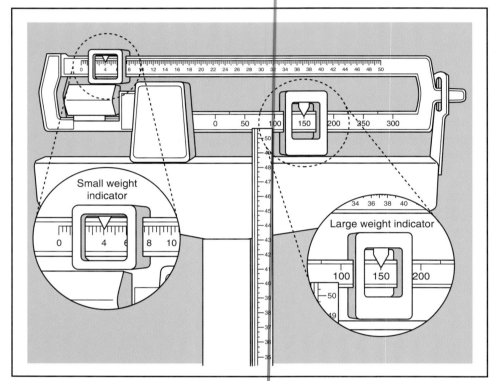

Small weight indicator

Large weight indicator

FIGURE 19–11
Add the top figure (4) to the bottom figure (154) to get the total weight. The scale shows that this patient weighs 154 pounds.

11. Write down the weight.	Comes in handy when recording patients' weight on their chart.
12. Ask patients to turn around with their back to the scale. Their heels should touch the edge of the measuring bar.	Places patients in correct position for measuring height.
13. Ask patients to stand up straight.	Ensures accurate measurement.
14. Pull up the measuring bar until it is above patients' head.	Prevents injury to patients.
15. Flip up the end of the measuring bar.	
16. Slide the measuring bar so that its end is on the top of patients' head (Figure 19–12).	
17. Read the height.	
18. Write down the number.	

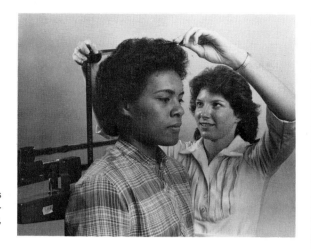

FIGURE 19–12
(From Bonewit, K: Clinical Procedures for Medical Assistants, 3rd ed. Philadelphia, W. B. Saunders Company, 1990.)

19. Slide the measuring bar up out of patients' way and flip the end of the bar down. Then push down the end of the measuring bar.

Prevents injury when patients step off the scale.

Follow-Through

20. Assist patients to step off the scale.

Prevents injury from falling.

21. Record measurement in the appropriate place on the chart.

Your health care institution may require that patients' weight be documented in kilograms. The chart below shows how to convert pounds to **kilograms.**

KILOGRAM
a unit of weight used in the metric system

WEIGHT CONVERSION

To change pounds to kilograms, divide the number of pounds by 2.2.
   Example: 44 pounds divided by 2.2 = 20 kilograms
To change kilograms to pounds, multiply the number of kilograms by 2.2.
   Example: 100 kilograms $\times$ 2.2 = 220 pounds

The standing scale is the most convenient scale for measuring patients' weight. If the patient is unable to stand on the standing scale, there are a variety of other scales that can be used. These include a bed scale, a mechanical lift scale, and a wheelchair scale. If you use a mechanical lift scale to measure a patient's weight, be sure to do the following:

- Keep the batteries charged.
- Adjust the scale to zero with the canvas sling in place before you place the patient in the sling for weighing.
- The canvas sling should be high enough to prevent the patient's feet from touching the bed.
- Talk with the patient to decrease anxiety during the weighing procedure.

When using a wheelchair scale, place the wheelchair (or the geri-chair) on the scale and weigh it. Mark its weight on a piece of tape on the back of the chair. Be sure to use the same chair with same equipment each time you weigh the patient to ensure accuracy.

DISRUPTIONS IN METABOLISM

DIABETES MELLITUS

DIABETES MELLITUS
a disorder that affects the body's ability to use glucose (sugar) because the body cannot use or produce insulin

GLUCOSE
sugar

INSULIN
a hormone produced by cells in the pancreas that helps the body use sugar for energy

Diabetes mellitus is a disorder that affects the body's ability to use **glucose.** The cells in the pancreas that secrete insulin do not secrete enough insulin for the body's needs. The cells are located in the islets of Langerhans in the pancreas.

Insulin is important because it carries sugar into the cell so that the cell can use it for energy. There are two types of diabetes mellitus:

- **Insulin-dependent diabetes mellitus (IDDM)**—IDDM is also known as Type I or juvenile-onset diabetes mellitus. This type requires insulin injections.
- **Non–insulin-dependent diabetes mellitus (NIDDM)**—NIDDM is also known as Type II or adult-onset diabetes mellitus. This type does not require insulin injections.

Insulin can be made artificially in a laboratory. When the patient's cells can secrete some insulin, an oral medication may be ordered by the physician. Children who develop diabetes mellitus always require insulin injections. Diabetes mellitus is treated by a combination of

- diet
- exercise
- medication as needed

Observations of Diabetes Mellitus

The classic signs of diabetes mellitus are known as the "three polys":

- **Polyuria**—increased urine production and output
- **Polydipsia**—excessive thirst
- **Polyphagia**—excessive food intake

Other observations may be

VAGINA
the canal from the cervix to the vaginal opening that stretches during intercourse and childbirth in females

- Fatigue and muscle weakness
- A longer time than usual for sores to heal
- Vaginitis (inflammation of the **vagina**) in females
- Poor vision
- Decreased sensation in the extremities

Upon examination, an excess of glucose is found in the blood.

Understanding Diabetes Mellitus

People who have diabetes mellitus are known as diabetics. Diabetics are at risk for a variety of disruptions in functioning, such as

INFECTION
the body's response to invasion by harmful microorganisms and their multiplication in the body

- **Infection**
- Slow healing
- Circulation problems
- Vision problems
- Nervous system problems

Diabetics can reduce their risk for disruptions by following the diet and exercise plan recommended by their physician and taking the medications that have been prescribed for them.

The following are aspects of diabetes mellitus you should know about.

HYPERGLYCEMIA   Hyperglycemia is an abnormally high amount of sugar in the blood.

HYPOGLYCEMIA   Hypoglycemia is an abnormally low amount of sugar in the blood.

DIABETIC COMA   A diabetic coma (unconscious state) results when the diabetic patient lacks insulin. It occurs when the patient does not receive enough insulin, for example, when the body has an increased need for insulin (such as during infection or other body stress). Diabetic coma usually has a gradual onset.

INSULIN SHOCK   Insulin shock results when the diabetic receives too much insulin; this results in low blood sugar. Insulin shock has a sudden onset.

BLOOD GLUCOSE   This refers to the level of sugar present in the circulating blood. A blood test is the most accurate test of the glucose level in the blood. A quick blood test (finger stick) performed by the nurse at the bedside indicates the amount of glucose circulating in the bloodstream.

FINGER STICK   A drop of blood is produced by piercing the finger with a special instrument (lancet). The drop is immediately placed on a specially treated strip of plastic. The results are read by one of two methods: Either the change in color on the strip is compared against a color chart on the container in which the strips are stored, or the strip is inserted into a battery-operated glucose monitoring machine. The machine reads the reaction on the strip and prints out the results. These machines are often used by diabetic patients to monitor their blood glucose levels at home.

URINE GLUCOSE   Urine glucose is a test of the urine, using special dipsticks (see Chapter 21), to determine whether glucose is present. The urine glucose test is not accurate because it does not reveal the specific amount of glucose that is present in the blood. Nursing assistants can perform this test. In addition to glucose, you test for two other elements to the urine:

- **Acetone**—a chemical found in the blood and urine of diabetic people
- **Ketones**—substances produced when the body is burning fat reserves

Observations of Diabetic Coma or Insulin Shock

You may be asked to observe the diabetic patient for signs and symptoms of diabetic coma or insulin shock. Signs of diabetic coma include

- dry, flushed skin
- increased thirst
- sweet or fruity odor of the breath
- increased respirations with signs of air hunger and difficulty breathing (patients with air hunger look like they cannot get enough air)
- loss of consciousness
- general weakness
- nausea or vomiting, loss of appetite
- possible abdominal pain

Signs of insulin shock include

- headache, dizziness
- general weakness

- problems with vision (blurring or difficulty seeing)
- numbness of lips and tongue
- sweating or cool, clammy skin
- hunger
- irritability

Caring for Patients with Diabetes Mellitus

GENERAL CARE

Your responsibility in the care of diabetics is to help them reduce their risk for disruption of body functioning by helping them adhere to the diet and exercise ordered by their physician. You are also responsible for

- observing for any changes in the skin
- using caution when moving or transferring patients, to prevent any skin injury
- assisting in monitoring patients' food and fluid intake
- assisting in monitoring patients' urine glucose level by performing urine testing when asked

SPECIAL NEEDS

Diabetic patients have special skin needs. They are taught to prevent skin irritation. Diabetic persons often experience circulation problems that result in a decreased blood supply to the tissues of the extremities, especially the legs and feet. This lack of blood supply interferes with healing of the body's tissues.

The nervous system is also affected by diabetes mellitus. There is a loss of sensation in the feet due to a condition called peripheral neuropathy. Because persons with peripheral neuropathy cannot feel anything with their feet, they are not aware of injuries to their feet.

GANGRENE
death of body tissue caused by lack of blood supply
AMPUTATION
removal, either surgical or accidental

The diabetic patient is also at risk for **gangrene** of the foot or toe because of a lack of blood supply to these extremities. The lack of blood supply causes the toes or foot to turn black. Gangrene often results in **amputation** of the extremity.

Diabetic patients also have psychologic needs. They need to make changes in their life-style that can include

- eating a special diet that they may consider restrictive
- exercising to help their body use insulin
- taking a medication or injecting themselves with insulin daily
- realizing that there is no cure for diabetes and the disease is life-long
- examining their body daily for signs of skin irritation

Take time to listen to patients' concerns. Report any problems to the nurse. Patients may be referred by the nurse or physician to a diabetic support group, where they and their family can find information that helps in living with diabetes.

Because diabetic patients have difficulty healing from injury, they are taught precautions they must incorporate into their life, and you should help them continue these practices in the health care institution or at home. Diabetic persons are taught to

- Bathe or shower daily and pay special attention to washing and drying the feet. Apply lotion to keep the skin soft.
- Examine the feet under a good light at least once a day. Look for

bruising, red spots, or any breaks in the skin. Any signs of skin irritation should be reported to the nurse or supervisor.

- Wear sturdy, protective shoes to protect the feet from injury. Never walk barefoot, indoors or outside.
- Wear shoes that fit without rubbing to prevent a skin irritation that would be difficult to heal.
- Avoid wearing garters or stockings with tight elastic because these interfere with circulation. Do not use rubber bands to hold up stockings.
- Avoid crossing the knees (while sitting or lying down) because this interferes with circulation.
- Never use the toes to test bath or shower water. A burn could result because of the impairment in feeling due to neuropathy.
- Cut toe nails straight across or as directed by the physician. Go to a podiatrist for care of the feet. Improper cutting may result in ingrown toe nails that can become infected. If you are asked by the patient to cut his or her toe nails, check the health care institution's policy, and check with the nurse before you proceed.
- Wear an identification bracelet. Identification bracelets may be purchased in a pharmacy.
- Follow the prescribed treatment of diet, exercise, and medication (when indicated).

FACTORS THAT AFFECT A PERSON'S NUTRITIONAL INTAKE

Eating is an event that is often shared; most people enjoy food and relax when eating in the company of others. Patients may eat and drink more when you stay in their room and sit near them during mealtime. Infants learn to trust other people when their basic nutritional needs are met.

FINANCES

Finances are an important influence on a person's nutritional intake. When money is needed to pay bills, the food budget may be cut and not enough food is available for the person to maintain a healthy body. Money may also be spent unwisely on food that is inexpensive but has empty calories, such as potato chips, soda, and candy bars. Federal programs such as the food stamp program and private agencies such as food banks and churches often assist people who do not have enough to eat.

CULTURE AND RELIGIOUS BELIEFS

A person's culture can determine what is acceptable in the diet. For example, the Italian people are associated with a love for pasta. People of Hispanic origin are known for spicy foods like burritos and chili. Common food traditions of different cultural groups are listed in Table 19–6.

Religious beliefs may also determine acceptable foods in the diet. For example, the Jewish religion teaches followers to refrain from eating dairy and meat products at the same meal. Many Christians fast (go without food) for a certain amount of time before some holidays. In some religions, for example, the Jewish religion, followers must prepare food in a special way. You should

TABLE 19–6 **COMMON FOOD TRADITIONS OF DIFFERENT CULTURAL GROUPS**

African American

Food choices are not significantly different from others in the same geographic area. Southern black and white cooking tradition includes greens (collard, turnip, etc.), okra, pork products, corn bread, and hominy grits.

Native American

Traditional foods vary among tribes. Corn, beans, squashes, and chili peppers are common.

Mexican American

Characteristic foods are tortillas, tamales, tacos, and enchiladas. Beans, rice, tomatoes, carrots, onions, and chili peppers are used in traditional cooking. Milk drinking is low, but cheese is used.

Puerto Rican and Cuban

In Caribbean areas, a wide range of fruits and vegetables are used—plantain, sweet potato, green bananas, okra, mango, avocado, and citrus fruits. In mainland cities, diets may suffer because these fruits and vegetables are not available or are too expensive.

Chinese

Food is cut into very small pieces and cooked quickly. Rice is a staple in some regions; wheat-flour noodles or dumplings are a staple in other regions. Soybean products such as bean curd (also called tofu), oil, and sauce are used. Cooked vegetables include bean sprouts, bamboo shoots, greens, mushrooms, and snow peas.

Middle Eastern

The countries around the eastern end of the Mediterranean (Greece, Turkey, Lebanon, Syria, Iraq, Iran, Israel, Jordan, and Egypt) sea share certain food traditions. The religious dietary differences between Moslems, Jews, and Christians are important. Lamb and goat are staple meats. Bread, rice, beans, lentils, chick peas, olives, and eggplant are staples. Moslems and Jews avoid pork products and animal shortenings. Observant Jews do not mix meat and dairy products. Milk is used little in some groups; yogurt is popular in most.

Adapted from Foster RFR, Hunsberger MM, Anderson JJT: Family-Centered Nursing Care of Children. Philadelphia, W. B. Saunders Company, 1989.

be aware of religious considerations and ask patients if they have any problems with eating the food and fluids that are served in the health care institution. Report such a situation to the nurse, who should secure an appropriate diet for the patient.

ALLERGIES

ALLERGY

an abnormal response caused by exposure to an allergen (for example, dust or food)

An **allergy** is an abnormal response caused by exposure to an allergen such as dust, drugs, or food. Allergies to certain food or fluids limit the kinds of food a person may be able to eat. Foods that commonly cause allergies are

- milk and dairy products
- eggs and products made with eggs
- wheat
- fruits or vegetables
- chocolate

Be sure to check patients' care plan for information about allergies.

PERSONAL PREFERENCES

People have a personal preference in their dietary choices. For example, a vegetarian diet excludes all meat. There are several different kinds of vegetarian diets. Most consist of a diet made up of fruits, vegetables, and grains. Some vegetarians also consume milk and dairy products.

CHAPTER WRAP-UP

- The organs of the gastrointestinal system include the
    Oral cavity
    Pharynx
    Esophagus
    Stomach
- The upper gastrointestinal system begins the work of changing food into a form that the body can use.
- Nutrition is the study of food's relationship to health.
- The body breaks down food through the following processes:
    Ingestion
    Digestion
    Absorption
- Food is broken down into nutrients. The nutrients the body needs are
    Carbohydrates
    Proteins
    Fats
    Vitamins
    Minerals
    Water
- The daily diet should include foods from the five food groups:
    Fats, oils, and sweets group
    Milk, yogurt, and cheese group
    Meat, poultry, fish, dry beans, eggs, and nuts group
    Vegetable and fruit group
    Bread, cereal, rice, and pasta group
- Nutritional needs change across the life span. They increase during periods of rapid growth, such as infancy and late adulthood, and during periods of stress and illness.
- A special diet is ordered to help a patient maintain a good nutritional state. Examples of common special diets are
    Clear liquid
    Full liquid
    Soft
    Diabetic
- Fluids are needed to sustain life. Too much fluid in the body results in fluid excess. Fluid excess can cause edema and/or high blood pressure. When you care for patients with fluid excess, you
    Elevate the extremities above heart level.
    Handle extremities gently.
    Weigh patients every day.
    Monitor vital signs as directed.
    Offer food or fluids as directed.
- When the body loses fluid, a condition known as fluid deficit occurs. The body becomes dehydrated because not enough fluid is taken in by the patient. When you care for patients who are dehydrated, you
    Monitor fluid intake.
    Weigh patients every day.
    Offer fluids as directed.
- When patients cannot feed themselves you may be asked to
    Feed patients with a spoon or fork.
    Use a syringe to feed patients.
- Common disruptions in nutrition include
    Obesity

Anorexia
Diabetes mellitus

REVIEW QUESTIONS

1. List the nutrients that help the body function.
2. How does the body turn food into a nutrient that the body can use?
3. Give examples of foods that contain carbohydrates, proteins, and fats.
4. List the fat-soluble vitamins.
5. How do vitamins and minerals help the body?
6. Give examples of foods in each of the five food groups.
7. What foods are included in the following diets? Clear liquid, full liquid, soft, and regular.
8. Describe the special needs of patients with
   - Diabetes mellitus
   - Fluid excess
   - Fluid deficit
   - Obesity
   - Anorexia
   - An inability to feed themselves

ACTIVITY CORNER

Use a measuring cup to measure the amount of fluid (in ounces) your favorite cup or glass holds.

_____ Ounces

Keep track of how many cups or glasses of fluid you drink during the next two meals.

_____ Cups or glasses

Write down how many ounces of fluid you drank.

_____ Ounces from first meal

_____ Ounces from second meal

_____ Total ounces of two meals

Convert the ounces to milliliters (ml):

_____ ounces $\times$ 30 ml per ounce = _____ ml

Are you drinking enough fluids every day? Yes _____ No _____ If no, how can you increase your fluid intake?

Write down the foods and fluids you ate for Sunday dinner in the first column. Write down the name of the food group in which it belongs in the second column.

Name of Food or Fluid	Name of Food Group

Were all food groups represented in your meal?

Yes _____ No _____ If no, what foods do you need to add to make your meal well balanced?

_____

_____

_____

20 Learning About Bowel Elimination

Objectives

AFTER YOU COMPLETE THIS CHAPTER, YOU WILL BE ABLE TO:

Describe the structure and function of the lower gastrointestinal tract.

Describe normal observations associated with bowel elimination.

Explain how a stool specimen is collected.

Explain how a stool specimen is tested.

Identify common disruptions in bowel elimination.

List artificial devices that help eliminate a bowel movement from the body.

Give an enema.

Insert a suppository.

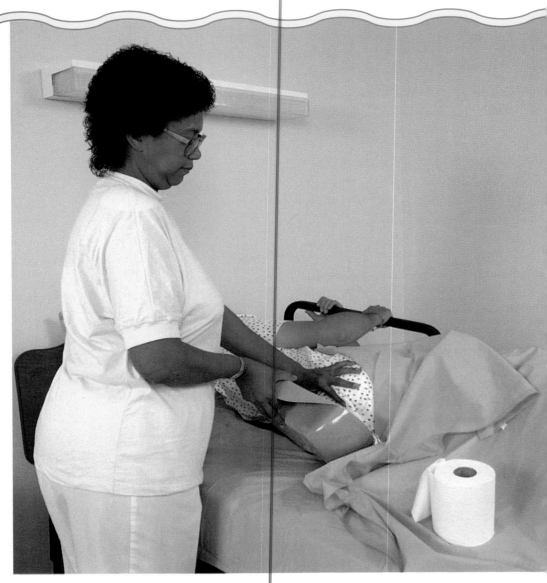

Overview The elimination of solid waste is performed by the gastrointestinal system. This body function is commonly known as bowel elimination. An ill person may need your assistance when the need for elimination occurs.

WHAT DO YOU KNOW ABOUT BOWEL ELIMINATION?

Here are five statements about bowel elimination. Consider them to test your current knowledge. If you think the statement is true, circle the T; if you think the statement is false, circle the F. Change the false statements to make them true.

1. T   F   A person should have at least one bowel movement per day.
2. T   F   Another term for *bowel movement* is *stool*.
3. T   F   The purpose of incontinence pants is to keep the bed linens dry.
4. T   F   Disposable gloves should be worn whenever contact with body waste is possible.
5. T   F   The person who is constipated has loose, watery stools.

ANSWERS

1. **False.** There is no definite number of bowel movements a person should have every day. The number of daily bowel movements is very specific to the individual.
2. **True.** *Stool* and *feces* are other terms used in place of *bowel movement*.
3. **False.** The purpose of incontinence pants is to contain the urine or stool that leaves the body involuntarily. Incontinence pants also protect the patient's dignity.
4. **True.** Disposable gloves are worn whenever contact with body waste products is possible.
5. **False.** The person who is constipated has dry, hard stools. The person with diarrhea has loose, watery stools.

ELIMINATION
the way the body rids itself of unusable food and fluid; the discharge of waste products created by the body's metabolism

METABOLISM
the process that produces energy in the body, allowing cells to grow and repair

BOWEL
the intestine

GASTROINTESTINAL TRACT
the large and small intestines

INTESTINE
the tube from the stomach to the anus

DUODENUM
the first part of the small intestine; where bile breaks down fat in the body

JEJUNUM
the part of the small intestine between the duodenum and the ileum

ILEUM
the last part of the small intestine

DIGEST
to break down chemically and mechanically

NUTRIENT
a chemical substance that helps the body break down, absorb, and use foods and fluids

COLON
the large intestine; extends from the end of the small intestine to the rectum

RECTUM
last part of the large intestine that ends at the anal canal

Elimination is the way the body rids itself of unusable food and fluids; it is also the discharge of the waste products of the body's **metabolism.** Normal body waste is produced in two forms:

- the solid (soft to hard) form eliminated by the **bowel**
- the liquid form eliminated by the bladder (see Chapter 21)

The eliminated waste is composed of the materials the body does not need to survive (unusable food and fluid) or that may be harmful to the body.

STRUCTURE AND FUNCTION OF THE LOWER GASTROINTESTINAL TRACT

The organs of the lower **gastrointestinal tract** are the small and large **intestines** (Figure 20–1). The small intestine is divided into three parts:

Duodenum
Jejunum
Ileum

If stretched out, the small intestine is about 18 feet in length. It functions to absorb **digested nutrients** from food into the bloodstream.

The large intestine is divided into the

Colon
Rectum
Anal canal

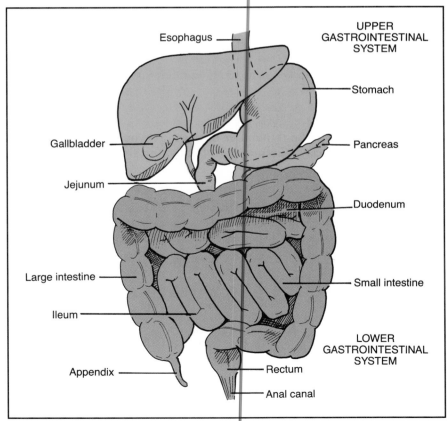

FIGURE 20–1
The major organs of the lower intestinal tract are the large and small intestines.

The functions of the large intestine are to
- Remove water from the digested material and send it back to the circulation.
- Expel solid waste.

The organs of bowel elimination move in a special way called **peristalsis.** Peristalsis pushes the waste material toward the anal canal. When the waste material reaches the anal canal, it is ready to be expelled by the body. When the rectum fills with waste material ready to be expelled, it sends a message to the brain. The person is alerted that the bowel needs to be emptied. The material expelled from the body is known as the bowel movement.

PERISTALSIS
a wave-like action caused by the contraction and relaxation of the muscles of the intestines

OBSERVATIONS OF BOWEL MOVEMENTS

The **bowel movement** is the waste material that is formed as the food moves from the digestive tract through the intestinal tract. Other words for bowel movement are *feces* and *stool*.

BOWEL MOVEMENT
the waste material that forms as food moves from the digestive tract through the intestinal tract; also called feces and stool

SUBJECTIVE OBSERVATIONS

Ask patients about their bowel movements. You can use questions such as

"When was your last bowel movement?"
"How often do you move your bowels?"
"Do you have pain when you move your bowels?"

OBJECTIVE OBSERVATIONS

Make the following observations of patients' bowel movements:
- color (usually brown)
- **consistency**
- frequency (how often patients have a bowel movement)
- amount (usually described as small, medium, or large)

CONSISTENCY
the degree of thickness of a substance

UNUSUAL OBSERVATIONS OF BOWEL ELIMINATION

An ill person may have changes in bowel elimination that are important for you to observe. Changes may be caused by
- disease
- foods the person has eaten
- medications
- lack of fluid or fiber in the diet
- lack of daily exercise

The nurse or supervisor may tell you to observe each bowel movement.

In most health care institutions, a record of patients' bowel movements is kept. Learn to make a note of your observations about patients' bowel movements on your small notepad so that you will remember to record the information in the appropriate place, for example, on patients' chart or on the worksheet at the nursing station (Table 20–1).

CHANGES ASSOCIATED WITH AGING

The movement of food through the intestine slows as a person ages. Because food is in the intestine longer, more water is reabsorbed by the body, resulting

TABLE 20–1   UNUSUAL OBSERVATIONS OF BOWEL ELIMINATION

Observation	Description and Cause
Color	White or chalky stool is caused by barium, a chalky, somewhat thick substance that is given in an enema so that an outline of the intestine shows on the x-ray.
	Tan or gray stool is caused when bile is not present in the duodenum (see Figure 20–1). When bile is present in the intestine, it gives the stool a familiar brown color.
	Tarry or black stool can be caused by blood that has traveled through the digestive system. It is often a pasty, sticky type of stool. A person who takes iron supplements may also produce black, tarry stools.
	On occasion, bright red might be noticed when the feces is expelled. When the stool is bright red, it usually means that there is bleeding somewhere near the anus.
	Mucus or fat might be observed. This is caused by specific diseases of the gastrointestinal tract.
Odor	Note any foul or unusual odor that occurs with a bowel movement. Infection caused by a bacteria may cause an odor that is different from usual.
Consistency	Hard stools may occur because a person lacks an appropriate amount of fluid or fiber in the diet.
	Hard stools may also be caused by certain medications.
	Unformed stool is usually associated with changes in diet and fluid intake as well as certain medications.
	Watery stools occur when there is a disruption in bowel function that may be caused by the presence of disease in the gastrointestinal system.
Frequency	Individuals' frequency of stool elimination varies. You need to know each of your patients' daily pattern of bowel elimination. To get this information, make a note when you receive a report from the nurse.
	Less frequent elimination than is normal for the person may indicate that peristalsis has slowed.
	More frequent elimination than is normal for the person may indicate peristalsis has increased.
Amount	Although the amount of stool varies depending on the patient, you can use the following terms to describe the amount of stool in the plastic container that is placed on the toilet to catch the stool while the patient has a bowel movement.
	• *small*—the stool would not cover the bottom of the container if it were spread out
	• *moderate*—the stool covers the bottom of the container and would fill the container to ½–1 inch if it were spread out
	• *large*—the stool would fill the container to over an inch if it were spread out

FIBER

the portion of food that passes through the intestine and colon undigested; increases the bulk of the stool and makes it softer

in a stool that is more solid and difficult to expel. The older person may not eat enough **fiber** or drink enough fluids for the stool to move quickly through the intestine. Lack of exercise also results in less efficient movement of fecal material through the intestinal tract. As a result, an elderly patient may be constipated (see Chapter 31 for discussion of the changes in bowel elimination that occur with age).

ASSISTING WITH ELIMINATION NEEDS

Patients in a health care institution vary in their ability to meet their own toileting needs. You may be asked to assist patients to the bathroom and help them to the toilet (Figure 20–2). Patients may be permitted to use a bedside commode (portable toilet) when assisted by the care giver (Figure 20–3). After patients have emptied their bowels or bladder, you may need to assist them back to their bed or a chair.

When patients are unable to leave the bed, they use a bedpan or a urinal (container into which a person urinates) for toileting (Figure 20–4). This equipment is kept in the lower drawer of each patient's bedside stand and is used only for that particular patient. The standard bedpan is available in an adult

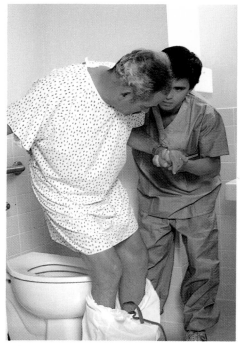
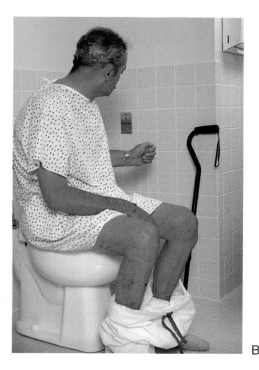

A   B

FIGURE 20-2

A, Help the patient to sit on the toilet. B, Provide privacy when the nurse tells you the patient is able to remain alone while emptying the bowels. Be sure to hand the call signal to the patient for safety.

size and a child size. A **fracture pan** is a bedpan that is used for patients who are unable or not allowed to raise their hips high enough to lift themselves onto a regular adult bedpan. A fracture pan is smaller and easier to slide under a patient than a regular bedpan. A urinal is used for males who need to urinate. A specially designed urinal, rarely used, may be available for female patients.

FRACTURE PAN

a small bedpan that slides easily under the hips, generally used for patients with a hip fracture

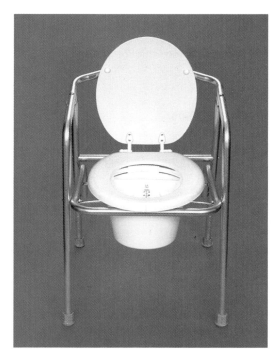

FIGURE 20-3

The bedside commode is used by the patient who is unable to walk as far as the bathroom.

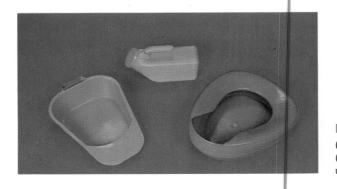

FIGURE 20-4
(Right) A regular-size bedpan.
(Left) A fracture bedpan. (Top) A
urinal.

Nursing assistants are often required to perform the following procedures, so it is very important that you know how to do them correctly.

PROCEDURE

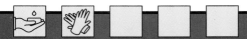

Providing a Bedpan for Patients Who Can Assist

Patients who are on bed rest may ask for a bedpan so they can empty their bowel. Male patients use the bedpan to empty the bowels and a urinal to empty their bladder. Female patients empty both their bladder and bowel into a bedpan. The same procedure used for a regular bedpan is used for a fracture pan.

GATHER EQUIPMENT

Two towels   Disposable gloves
Three disposable or reusable washcloths   Bedpan
Bath blanket   Toilet paper
Bedpan cover

ACTION	RATIONALE
Preparation	
1. Wash hands.	Prevents the spread of microorganisms.
2. Identify yourself and the patient.	Maintains patients' rights.
3. Provide privacy.	Maintains patients' rights.
4. Explain the procedure.	Informs patients what is happening.
Procedural Steps	
5. Unfold the bath blanket and place it over patients. Ask patients to hold the top edge of the bath blanket while you pull the top sheet and blanket down to the bottom of the bed.	Provides warmth and privacy for patients. Helps keep bed linens clean.
6. If using a metal bedpan, rinse it under warm, running water and dry it before use.	A warm bedpan is more comfortable for patients.
7. Raise the bed to the high position and lower the side rail on the side nearest you.	Helps you use good body mechanics.
8. Ask patients to help lift themselves onto the bedpan. If patients are able to do this, slide the bedpan under the buttocks (Figure 20–5A). You can give	Allows patients to assist in their care and provides an opportunity for exercise.

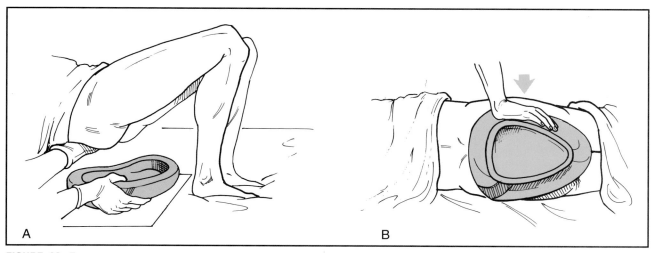

FIGURE 20-5

patients assistance by placing your free arm under their lower back to help them as they lift their buttocks.

9. If patients are not able to help, roll them to their side away from you and place the bedpan against their buttocks. With your hand on patients' hip, roll them toward you onto their back with the bedpan underneath (Figures 20–5A and 20–6).

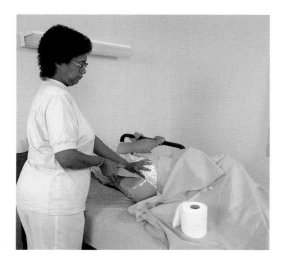

FIGURE 20-6

10. Be sure the bedpan is located correctly so that the waste products will be expelled into it.

Prevents accidental soiling of the bed linens.

11. Raise the head of the bed to Fowler's position.

Places patients in a more natural sitting position for elimination.

Continued on following page

PROCEDURE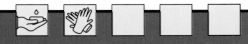

Providing a Bedpan for Patients Who Can Assist
Continued

12. Before leaving patients,
    * Place the toilet paper within their reach (Figure 20–7).
    * Put the bed in the low (horizontal) position.
    * Raise the side rails.
    * Place the call signal within patients' reach.
    * Tell patients to use the call signal when they are ready to get off the bedpan.
    * Close the privacy curtain or door.
13. When you return to remove patients from the bedpan, determine whether patients have been able to use the toilet paper. If patients were unable to wipe, go to step 19.

Provides privacy and allows patients to help with their care

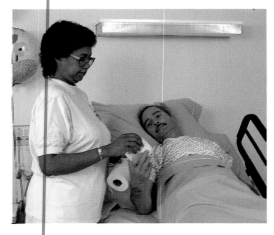

FIGURE 20–7

14. If patients were able to wipe, raise the bed to the high position and lower the side rail nearest you.

Helps you use good body mechanics.

15. Put on a pair of disposable gloves.

Prevents contact with body secretions.

16. Ask patients to help lift themselves by pressing down on the mattress with the feet and arms to help lift up the body so you can remove the bedpan.

Gives patients an opportunity to exercise.

17. Remove the bedpan and place it securely within your reach.

18. Place the bedpan cover on the bedpan.

19. When patients need assistance in cleaning after elimination, do the following before you remove the bedpan:
    • Put on disposable gloves.
    • Wet the disposable washcloths with warm water and take them to the bedside.
    • Assist patients to roll over onto their side.
    • Use enough toilet paper to remove waste materials from the surface of the skin.
    • For female patients, wipe from front to back.
    • Use one washcloth to wash the front part of the **perineal area.**
    • Use the second washcloth to wash the anal area.
    • Discard disposable washcloths into the waste container or place reusable washcloths into the dirty linen hamper.
    • Use the towel to dry the area thoroughly.
    • Discard gloves into the waste container.
    • Assist patients into a comfortable position.

20. Dampen the third washcloth with warm water and ask patients to wash their hands. Offer a different towel to dry hands after washing.

21. Remove the bath blanket and cover patients with the top sheet and blanket.

22. Place the bed in the lowest position and raise the side rails. Adjust the head of the bed according to patients' comfort needs. Place the call signal within patients' reach. Open the privacy curtain or door.

    Ensures patient safety.

23. Take the covered bedpan to patients' bathroom. Close the door and remove the cover.

24. Observe the bowel movement for color, consistency, odor, and amount.

25. If any of your observations are unusual (foul odor or whitish, gray, red, or any other unusual color), save the specimen to show the nurse or supervisor.

    May mean that a disease is present.

26. Gather a stool **specimen** if one is required (see the procedure for collecting a stool specimen).

27. Empty the contents into the toilet and flush.

PERINEAL AREA
the area between the legs, including genitals and anus

Continued on following page

PROCEDURE

Providing a Bedpan for Patients Who Can Assist
Continued

28. To rinse the bedpan, place the flush sprayer in the down position and flush the bedpan with clean water until the waste material is completely removed. Dry the bedpan.

29. Remove gloves and place them in a waste container.

30. Replace the bedpan and toilet paper in the bedside stand.   Equipment is ready for the next use.

31. Place any soiled linen in the linen hamper.

Follow-Through

32. Wash hands.   Prevents spread of microorganisms.

33. Report normal and unusual observations to the nurse or supervisor.

34. Record your observations in the appropriate places:
    • patient chart
    • worksheet on the unit

COLLECTING A STOOL SPECIMEN

PARASITE
one who depends on another for support without giving anything back

SPECIMEN
a sample; a small piece of a body tissue or a secretion used for examination

A stool specimen may be ordered to determine whether foreign bodies, ova and **parasites** (for example, hookworms and pinworms and their eggs), or blood is present in patients' waste material. Patients are asked to provide a stool specimen by eliminating into a special collection container that fits over the toilet under the toilet seat. In some areas, this container is called a "hat" because it resembles one. For patients on bed rest, a specimen is obtained from the bedpan.

The specimen is taken to the laboratory for examination as soon as possible after it is collected. A laboratory order slip needs to accompany the specimen to the laboratory. The laboratory slip indicates the kind of test the physician wants performed on the specimen.

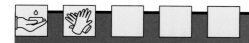
Collecting a Stool Specimen

The nurse or supervisor tells you when a stool specimen needs to be taken. Before beginning the procedure, label a specimen container with the patient's name and room number, the date, and the time.

GATHER EQUIPMENT

Disposable gloves
Specimen container

Paper towel
Wooden tongue blade

ACTION	RATIONALE

Preparation

1. Wash hands.	Prevents the spread of microorganisms.
2. Identify yourself and the patient.	Maintains patients' rights.
3. Provide privacy.	Maintains patients' rights.
4. Explain the procedure.	Informs patients what is happening.

Procedural Steps

5. Go into patients' bathroom and put on the disposable gloves.	
6. Place a clean paper towel on the side of the sink.	Protects the sink from soiling.
7. Open the specimen container and place the lid on the clean paper towel.	
8. Use the wooden tongue blade to pick up a sample of the specimen from the bedpan or other collection container and transfer the sample to the specimen container (Figure 20–8).	Allows you to transfer a specimen without soiling or contaminating yourself.

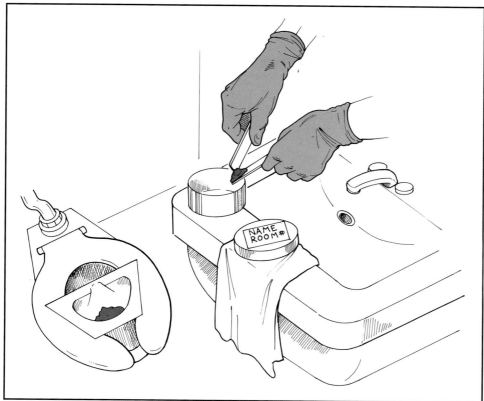

FIGURE 20–8

Continued on following page

PROCEDURE

Collecting a Stool Specimen *Continued*

9. Turn the wooden blade around and pick up another sample from another part of the stool. Repeat once more. Take enough stool to fill at least half the collection container.

Provides a specimen from three different parts of the stool.
Ensures that enough of a specimen is provided that the ordered test can be done.

10. Discard the wooden blade into the waste container.

11. Place the lid on the specimen container.

12. Flush the remaining waste material down the toilet.

13. Remove the disposable gloves and discard them into a waste container.

Follow-Through

14. Wash hands.

Prevents the spread of microorganisms.

15. If the specimen container is made of clear plastic, wrap it in a paper towel before you take if from patients' room.

Provides a more pleasing appearance.

16. Take the specimen or arrange to have it taken to the laboratory for examination immediately.

Certain tests must be done as soon as possible after the specimen is collected.

17. Report and record the time the stool specimen was obtained and that it was taken or sent to the laboratory.

PROCEDURE

Testing a Stool Specimen on the Unit

A stool specimen may be tested for the presence of occult (unseen) blood. The nurse or supervisor tells you how often a patient should have a stool specimen tested.

GATHER EQUIPMENT

Hemoccult test packet or other equipment to test for blood in the stool
Developer

Disposable wooden blade
Disposable gloves

ACTION	RATIONALE

Preparation

1. Wash hands.

Prevents the spread of microorganisms.

2. Identify yourself and the patient.

Maintains patients' rights.

3. Provide privacy.

Maintains patients' rights.

4. Explain the procedure.

Informs patients what is happening.

Procedural Steps

5. Take all equipment into patients' bathroom and place it on a clean paper towel on the sink.

Performing the test in the patient's bathroom prevents contamination of other areas.

6. Put on the disposable gloves.

Prevents contact with body secretions.

7. Open the back of the test packet and notice the two paper squares that are set into the packet (Figure 20–9).

The packet is designed so that you never touch the stool specimen directly.

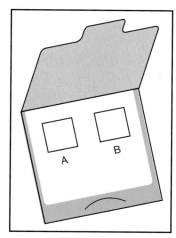

FIGURE 20–9

8. Use the wooden blade to pick up a small amount of the stool specimen and smear it on the thin paper square on side A of the test packet (Figures 20–10 and 20–11).

Only a small amount of stool is needed.

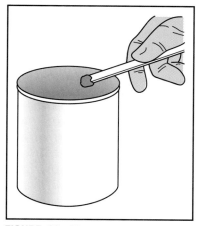

FIGURE 20–10

9. Turn the wooden blade around and pick up another small amount of stool from another part of the specimen. Smear it on the thin paper square on side B of the packet.

Allows more accurate testing.

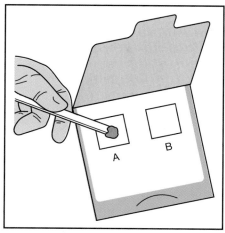

FIGURE 20–11

Continued on following page

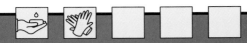

Testing a Stool Specimen on the Unit *Continued*

10. Close the packet (Figure 20–12).

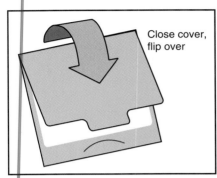

Close cover, flip over

FIGURE 20–12

11. Turn the packet over and open it to expose the thin paper areas with the stool specimen under them. Notice the test area marked positive (+) and negative (−).

12. Open the developer and place 1 drop on the positive and negative parts of the test area. Wait 10 seconds for the reaction to take place (Figure 20–13).

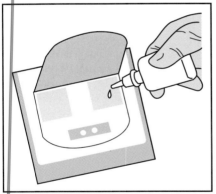

FIGURE 20–13

13. The test area marked positive should turn blue. This indicates the test is working.

14. If the positive area turns blue, place two drops of the developer on each of the thin paper squares. Read reactions within 1 minute (Figure 20–14).

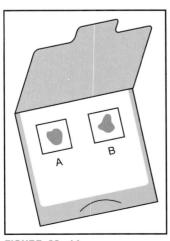

FIGURE 20–14

15. Replace the cap on the developer.

16. If there is no change in color on the paper squares, the test for occult blood is negative. If the color changes to blue, the test for occult blood in the stool is positive.

17. Save the test packet if your nurse or supervisor has asked to check the results.

18. Discard the packet after the results have been checked.   The packet is designed for one use only.

19. Flush any remaining stool specimen down the toilet.

20. Discard the wooden blade in the waste container. Remove the disposable gloves and discard them into the waste container.

21. Return the developer to its storage place.   Readies the developer for the next use.

Follow-Through

22. Wash hands.   Prevents the spread of microorganisms.

23. Report the results to the nurse or supervisor.   Reporting and recording the results of testing a stool specimen on the unit are important responsibilities.

24. Record results as positive or negative in the appropriate places:
    • patient chart
    • worksheet on the unit

COMMON DISRUPTIONS IN BOWEL ELIMINATION

INCONTINENCE

Incontinence is the inability to control the urge to eliminate the waste products (urine or bowel movements) of the body. A person becomes incontinent when **disease** or injury of the nervous system interferes with the ability to control elimination. Incontinence may occur because:

DISEASE

sickness; a condition of the body or one of its parts that causes change in the body's functioning

• The muscle that surrounds the anus or urethra is weak.
• Patients are unable to get to the bathroom by themselves on time.
• The brain cannot send the message to eliminate body wastes as usual.

Incontinence can have a negative effect on patients' self-esteem because they no longer have control over their body functions. You can assist patients by keeping an understanding and nonjudgmental attitude when providing care.

Bowel retraining (often combined with bladder retraining) may help patients relearn how to control the urge to eliminate (see Chapter 21). You are asked to help these patients in their bowel and bladder retraining activities. Patients are placed on the bedpan or assisted to the commode at intervals of about every 2 hours or whenever they request it.

You can best care for patients who are incontinent of the bowel by performing the following activities:

• Keep the skin of the buttocks and anal area clean and dry.
• Assist patients onto a bedpan or to the bathroom.
• Keep patients clean and odor free.

- Realize that there is no correct number of bowel movements for a person to have every week.
- Assist patients with bowel retraining.
- Offer patients emotional support and praise when they are successful in controlling the urge to eliminate.

Another part of your care of incontinent patients consists of placing bed protectors on the bed and putting incontinence pants on patients. Bed protectors are used to help keep the bed linens dry. Incontinence pants are applied to hold the waste contents in one area away from the patient's skin until clean incontinence pants are applied.

CARING COMMENTS

Check patients' incontinence pants every hour so that you can change them as soon as possible after elimination has occurred.

Many health care institutions have determined that a patient should have a bowel movement at least every 3 days. Be sure to know the policy of your health care institution.

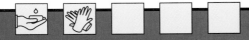

PROCEDURE

Placing a Bed Protector and Draw Sheet on the Bed

A bed protector and draw sheet are used to protect the bed linens from getting soiled by waste products. They are applied whenever the patient is incontinent or is expected to become incontinent (for example, after receiving an anesthetic).

GATHER EQUIPMENT

Draw sheet

Disposable, plastic, or rubber bed protector

Disposable gloves, if needed

ACTION	RATIONALE
Preparation	
1. Wash hands.	Prevents the spread of microorganisms.
2. Identify yourself and the patient.	Maintains patients' rights.
3. Provide privacy.	Maintains patients' rights.
4. Explain the procedure.	Informs patients what is happening.
Procedural Steps	
5. Raise the bed to the high position and lower the side rail nearest you.	Helps you maintain good body mechanics.
6. Ask patients to roll away from you toward the other side rail. If necessary, assist them.	Encourages patient independence in moving.
7. Center the plastic or rubber protector in the middle of the bed and straighten it toward you (Figure 20–15).	

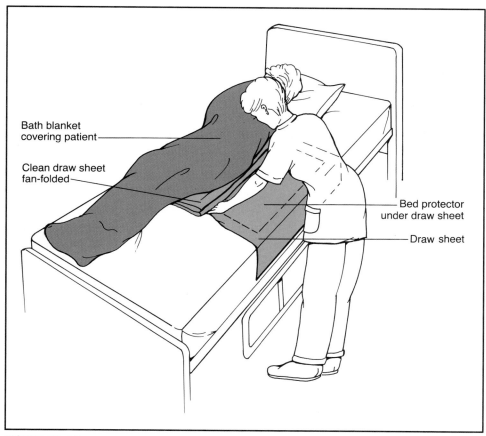

FIGURE 20-15

8. Center the draw sheet in the middle of the bed, with the excess hanging over the side of the bed (see Figure 20–15).

9. Fanfold the excess linen close against the patient's back (see Figure 20–15).

10. Tuck the excess of the draw sheet under the mattress.

11. Assist or ask patients to roll over the bump (created by the fanfolded draw sheet and bed protector) toward you.

12. Raise the side rail and go to the other side of the bed.   Helps keep patients safe.

13. Lower the side rail and pull the bed protector toward you and straighten it out.

14. Pull the draw sheet toward you, tugging to remove any wrinkles.   Wrinkles in the linens can irritate the skin.

15. Tuck the excess linen under the mattress.

16. Assist patients to a comfortable position in the center of the bed and cover them with the top linens.

17. Raise the side rail and place the bed in the low position.   Ensures patient safety.

Continued on following page

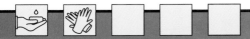

PROCEDURE

Placing a Bed Protector and Draw Sheet on the Bed *Continued*

Follow-Through

ACTION	RATIONALE
18. Place the call signal within patients' reach and open the curtain or door.	Leaves patients with the means to communicate.
19. Wash hands.	Prevents the spread of microorganisms.

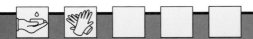

PROCEDURE

Applying Incontinence Pants

Adult incontinence pants are used to contain body wastes in one area away from patient's body. Patients may or may not be able to assist you when you replace their incontinence pants with a new pair. The health care institution may provide incontinence pants made of washable cotton material or disposable plastic pants that are lined with an absorbent material. The disposable incontinence pants are available in small, medium, and large adult sizes. (Most sizes are determined by hip, not waist, measurement.)

GATHER EQUIPMENT

Incontinence pants	Towel
Disposable gloves	Basin of warm water
Bath blanket	Two disposable washcloths

ACTION	RATIONALE
Preparation	
1. Wash hands.	Prevents the spread of microorganisms.
2. Identify yourself and the patient.	Maintains patients' rights.
3. Provide privacy.	Maintains patients' rights.
4. Explain the procedure.	Informs patients what is happening.
Procedural Steps	
5. Raise the bed to the high position and lower the side rail nearest you.	
6. Place the bath blanket over patients and bring the top linens to the foot of the bed.	Provides privacy.
7. Put on the disposable gloves.	Protects you from contamination while handling body wastes.
8. Remove the fasteners from the sides of the incontinence pants and bring the front part of the pants down between patients' thighs.	
9. Remove the incontinence pants: • If patients can assist, ask them to bend their knees and press their feet into the mattress while you remove the incontinence pants from beneath them.	Gives patients the opportunity to participate in their care.

- If patients cannot assist, turn them onto their side. Pull the incontinence pants from between patients' legs toward you while being careful not to spill fecal material or pull patients' skin.

10. Fold the incontinence pants and put them in a secure place.

11. Wash, rinse, and dry the skin of the perineal area and the buttocks. Repeat this action a second time.

    Prevents irritation of the skin.

12. Put a clean pair of incontinence pants on patients:
    - If patients can lift their own buttocks, ask them to do so while you place a clean pair of incontinence pants beneath them.
    - For patients who are on their side, place the clean pair of incontinence pants next to their back (Figure 20–16). Line up the waist of incontinence pants with patients' waist.

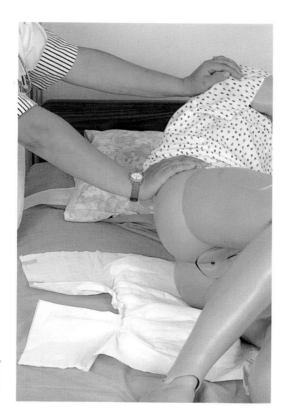

FIGURE 20–16

Place the incontinence pants correctly so that when patients are repositioned on their back the front part of the pants can be brought up between the legs.

13. Bring up the front of the incontinence pants between patients' legs. Be sure to have pants all the way up to patients' crotch.

    Correct positioning of the pants prevents irritation and leakage.

14. At each side, fasten the front of the incontinence pants to the back. Use the attached fastener on the dispos-

Continued on following page

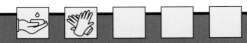

PROCEDURE

Applying Incontinence Pants *Continued*

able pants or pins (or Velcro closures) on the washable cotton pants (Figure 20–17).

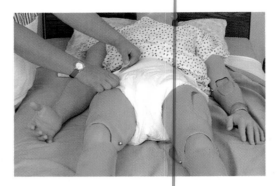

FIGURE 20–17
The incontinence pants should be fastened so they are comfortable and snug. Choose the correct size so that skin does not redden at the edges of the pants.

15. Replace the top linens and remove the bath blanket.

16. Place patients in a position of comfort and place the call signal within their reach.

    Leaves patients with a means to communicate.

17. Raise the side rail and place the bed in the lowest position.

    Ensures patient safety.

18. Observe the contents of the incontinence pants for color, consistency, amount, and odor.

19. Dispose of any fecal material in the incontinence pants in the toilet in patients' room. If a specimen is needed, follow the procedure for obtaining a stool specimen at this time.

    Most agencies require that fecal material be removed from the incontinence pants before the pants are disposed of.

20. Discard disposable incontinence pants into the appropriate waste container. Remove fecal material from washable cotton pants by rinsing the pants in water in the hopper in the soiled utility room. The soiled cotton pants are usually placed in a specially marked linen container.

Follow-Through

21. Remove the disposable gloves and discard them into the waste container.

22. Wash hands.

    Prevents the spread of microorganisms.

23. Record and report your observations.

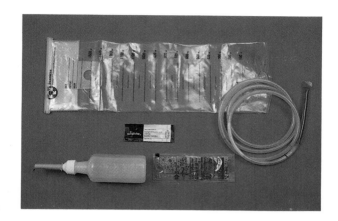

FIGURE 20–18
Enema equipment.

CONSTIPATION

Constipation occurs when the movement of waste material through the intestines slows down. Constipation is difficulty in having or the inability to have a bowel movement. Some of the causes of constipation are

- aging
- disease
- medications
- changes in diet
- lack of exercise
- anesthesia
- decreased fluid intake
- ignoring the urge to have a bowel movement

CONSTIPATION

inability to have or difficulty in having a bowel movement

Treatment for Constipation

ENEMAS An **enema** is a solution that loosens fecal material and stimulates peristalsis of the intestine. An enema is known by the name of the solution that is used. A tap water enema (TWE) is warm water from the faucet that is poured into the enema container. If a soap suds enema (SSE) is ordered, a special liquid soap is mixed with the warm water before it is administered. An oil retention enema is given to lubricate and help remove the fecal material. Another type of enema is a prepackaged enema often referred to by its trademark name, Fleet (Figure 20–18).

ENEMA

a solution that loosens fecal material and stimulates peristalsis of the intestines

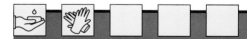

PROCEDURE

Giving a Cleansing Enema

An enema is given to patients who are constipated or are scheduled for a study of the intestines. A study of the intestines provides more accurate results if the bowels are empty.

GATHER EQUIPMENT

Enema kit
Disposable gloves
Washcloth
Towel

Bath blanket
Bedpan if patient must stay in bed
Bedpan cover
Roll of toilet paper

Continued on following page

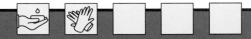

Giving a Cleansing Enema

ACTION	RATIONALE
Preparation	
1. Wash hands.	Prevents the spread of microorganisms.
2. Identify yourself and the patient.	Maintains patients' rights.
3. Provide privacy.	Maintains patients' rights.
4. Explain the procedure.	Informs patients what is happening.
Procedural Steps	
5. Take the enema kit into patients' bathroom and hang the solution container on a hook in the bathroom.	The enema solution is usually prepared in patients' bathroom.
6. Prepare the enema solution according to the enema that has been ordered. The usual amount of water used in the enema solution is 1,000 ml. Always find out from the nurse or supervisor the amount you should use for patients. • For a TWE: Adjust the water until it measures 105° F. Fill the container to the line that indicates 1,000 ml or the amount indicated by the nurse or supervisor. • For an SSE: Do the same as for a TWE but add soap to the water in the container. Seal the container at the top and gently turn it upside down to dilute the soap in the solution.	
7. Open the clamp on the tubing that extends from the container. Allow the enema solution to fill the tubing, expelling the air from the tubing.	Air in the tubing enters patients' rectum and causes discomfort.
8. Hang the container of prepared enema solution next to the bed 18 inches above patients and prepare patients for the procedure.	The higher the container is hung, the faster the solution enters the rectum.
9. Raise the bed to the high position and lower the side rail nearest you.	
10. Cover patients with the bath blanket and fold the top linens toward the foot of the bed.	Offers comfort and privacy to patients.
11. Place patients in the left Sims' position with their right leg bent at the knee and touching the mattress.	Because of the anatomy of the large bowel, allows fluid to flow into the large colon.
12. Put on the disposable gloves and place the bedpan within reach.	Protects you from contamination when handling body wastes.
13. Remove the cap from the tubing and lubricate the tip with a water-soluble lubricant. (In a kit, the tip is usually prelubricated.)	Lubrication helps the tip go through the anal opening without causing trauma to the mucous membrane of the anus.
14. Lift the right buttock so that the anal area is exposed.	

15. Locate the anus and ask patients to take a deep breath while you insert the tip into the anus.

16. Insert the tip as follows (Figure 20–19):
    • Toward patients' navel
    • 3–4 inches in

17. Release the clamp and allow the solution to flow into the rectum.

Helps patients relax and diverts their attention from the enema.

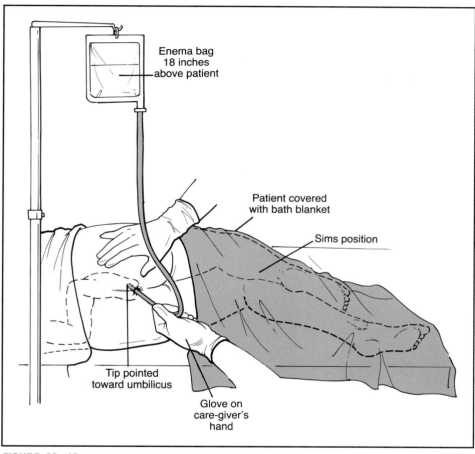

Enema bag 18 inches above patient

Patient covered with bath blanket

Sims position

Tip pointed toward umbilicus

Glove on care-giver's hand

FIGURE 20–19

18. If patients tell you they are having cramps, slow down the rate of solution as it goes in the rectum by adjusting the clamp on the tubing.

19. When the desired amount of solution has flowed into patients' rectum, use the clamp on the tubing to shut off the flow of solution. Remove the tubing from patients and discard the used equipment.

20. Remove and discard the disposable gloves into the appropriate waste container.

21. Ask patients to hold the solution in their rectum as long as they are able. They can lie on their back if they desire.

The longer patients retain the enema solution, the better the results.

Continued on following page

PROCEDURE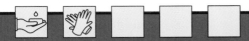

Giving a Cleansing Enema *Continued*

22. If you leave the room do the following:
    - Raise the side rail and place the bed in the lowest position.
    - Place the call signal within patients' reach.

Ensures patient safety. Leaves patients with the means to communicate.

23. When patients indicate they are ready, assist them to the bathroom or place them on the bedpan.

24. If patients use a bedpan, after they have completed the bowel movement, put on a clean pair of disposable gloves and assist them off the bedpan. Cover the bedpan.

25. Clean the rectal area:
    - Position patients on their side.
    - Use toilet paper to clean as much fecal material from the buttocks as possible.
    - Use the washcloth to wash and rinse the area; use the towel to dry the skin thoroughly.

26. Cover patients with top sheet and remove the bath blanket.

27. Place patients in a comfortable position with the call signal within reach.

Leaves patients with the means to communicate.

28. Raise the side rail and place the bed in the low position.

Ensures patient safety.

29. Take the used bedpan to patients' bathroom, remove the cover, and observe the contents.

30. Empty the bedpan into the toilet and flush.

31. Using the flush sprayer, rinse the bedpan. Repeat as needed.

32. Dry the bedpan with paper towels.

33. Remove and discard the disposable gloves. Discard the enema kit if it is disposable. (An enema kit is sometimes used more than once if the patient is receiving several enemas. If this is done in your health care institution, clean and dry the equipment before you store it.)

34. Return the bedpan to the bedside stand.

Equipment is ready for the next use.

Follow-Through

35. Wash hands.

Prevents the spread of microorganisms.

36. Record and report the kind of enema and amount of solution given, the results of the enema, and how patients tolerated the procedure (ask them).

For an SSE, be sure to add soap after the water is in the enema bag and mix gently. If water is added after soap, or if mixing is too vigorous, there may be too many bubbles in the solution.

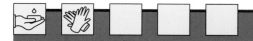

PROCEDURE

Giving a Prepackaged Enema

In the prepackaged enema, the solution is given directly from the bottle in which it is packaged. The tip is prelubricated. The regular enema is quick acting, and the patient can usually retain the solution in the bowel for about 3–5 minutes. The oil retention enema is also prepackaged with a lubricated tip. The oil softens feces.

GATHER EQUIPMENT

Prepackaged (usually Fleet's) enema (regular or oil retention)
Disposable gloves

Bath blanket
Bedpan
Toilet paper
Bedpan cover

ACTION	RATIONALE
Preparation	
1. Wash hands.	Prevents the spread of microorganisms.
2. Identify yourself and the patient.	Maintains patients' rights.
3. Provide privacy.	Maintains patients' rights.
4. Explain the procedure.	Informs patients what is happening.
Procedural Steps	
5. Raise the bed to the high position and lower the side rail nearest you.	Helps you use good body mechanics.
6. Cover patients with the bath blanket and fold the top linens to the foot of the bed.	Provides warmth and privacy.
7. Place patients in the left Sims' position.	Allows the solution to flow more directly into the large colon.
8. Put on the disposable gloves and remove the cover from the prelubricated tip of the enema.	Protects you from contamination when handling body wastes.
9. Lift the right buttock and locate the anal opening.	
10. Ask patients to take a deep breath while you insert the tip into their rectum and squeeze the bottle so that the solution enters the rectum.	Helps patients relax and distracts them from the procedure.
11. Discard the empty solution container.	The prepackaged enema is used only once.
12. Ask patients to keep the solution in the rectum for as long as possible.	The regular solution is very quick acting.
13. Stay in the room and be ready to assist patients to the bathroom or onto the bedpan.	

Continued on following page

PROCEDURE

Giving a Prepackaged Enema *Continued*

14. When patients indicate they are ready, assist them to the bathroom or place them on the bedpan.

15. If patients use a bedpan, after they complete the bowel movement, put on a clean pair of disposable gloves and assist them off the bedpan. Cover the bedpan.

16. Clean the rectal area:
    - Position patients on their side.
    - Use toilet paper to clean as much fecal material from the buttocks as possible.
    - Use the washcloth to wash and rinse the area; use the towel to dry the skin thoroughly.

17. Cover patients with top sheet and remove the bath blanket.

18. Place patients in a comfortable position with the call signal within reach.   Leaves patients with the means to communicate.

19. Raise the side rail and place the bed in the low position.   Ensures patient safety.

20. Take the used bedpan to patients' bathroom, remove the cover, and observe the contents.

21. Empty the bedpan into the toilet and flush.

22. Using the flush sprayer, rinse the bedpan. Repeat as needed.

23. Dry the bedpan with paper towels.

24. Remove and discard the disposable gloves. Discard the empty container.

25. Return the bedpan to the bedside stand.   Equipment is ready for the next use.

Follow-Through

26. Wash hands.   Prevents the spread of microorganisms.

27. Record and report the kind of enema and amount of solution given, the results of the enema, and how patients tolerated the procedure (ask them).

MEDICATIONS   The physician often orders a stool softener or a laxative for the constipated patient. Because this medication is often prescribed on an as-needed basis you need to tell the nurse when patients request the medication to help move their bowels. The nurse is responsible for the administration of medications.

CHANGES IN LIFE-STYLE   The physician or nurse may instruct constipated patients to make changes in their diet, fluid intake, and amount of exercise. These changes often include increasing the amount of fiber and fluids in the diet and increasing exercise by walking a certain distance each day.

SUPPOSITORY A **suppository** is a medication that is administered into a body cavity such as the rectum, vagina, or urethra. A suppository that contains medication to cause a bowel movement may be ordered for constipated patients. If so, you may be asked to insert the suppository. Be sure you are allowed to do this according to the law of your state. Your nursing assistant instructor or the nurse can tell you if state law allows you to perform this procedure.

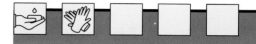

PROCEDURE

Inserting a Suppository

Follow steps 1–3 of the procedure for giving a prepackaged enema. Remember to wash your hands, provide patient privacy, and explain the procedure to the patient.

Check the suppository against the medication administration record by holding it near where the name of the medication is recorded. Read the label on the suppository carefully to make sure you are giving what is recorded. If required by the health care institution, you may take the medication administration record into the patients' room and compare the label on the medication to the record there. You are now prepared to insert the suppository.

Note: Do not hold the suppository in your hand or put it in your pocket because your body heat will cause it to melt, making it difficult to insert. Place the suppository in a small paper cup to carry it into the patient's room.

GATHER EQUIPMENT

Suppository
Lubricant
Disposable gloves
Disposable bed protector

Paper towels
Toilet paper

SUPPOSITORY
a medication administered into a body cavity, such as the rectum, vagina, or urethra

LUBRICANT
a substance that reduces friction

ACTION	RATIONALE
Preparation	
1. Identify patients by matching the name on the medication record to the name on patients' identification bracelet.	Ensures that the correct patient receives the suppository.
2. Place patients in the left side-lying position if they are unable to do so unaided.	Helps the suppository enter the rectum more easily.
3. Place the bed protector next to patients' buttock.	Keeps the linen clean.
4. Open the wrapper and release the suppository. Place it on the bed protector next to patients.	
5. Place a small amount of water-soluble lubricant on the widest part of the suppository.	Helps the suppository enter the rectum without friction.
6. Put on disposable gloves.	Prevents you from contacting body fluids.
7. Use one hand to lift the top buttock. Look for the anal opening.	Allows you to see the anal opening better.
8. Grasp the suppository by the narrow end and slip it into the rectum through the anal canal. Gently, push in. You should feel the suppository slip in beyond the muscle at the entry into the anal canal.	Positions the wider end to go in first.

Continued on following page

PROCEDURE

Inserting a Suppository *Continued*

9. Tell patients they need to hold in the suppository. The nurse will tell you if it needs to be held in for a certain amount of time.

Body heat allows the suppository to melt and be absorbed.

10. Remove your hand from patients' buttock.

Signals the end of the procedure.

11. Use enough toilet paper to remove any lubricant from the anal opening and wrap the toilet paper in the paper towels and discard.

Leaves patients' skin dry.

12. Remove the bed protector and discard it appropriately.

13. Remove gloves and discard them into the waste container.

14. Place patients in a comfortable position with the call signal within reach.

Leaves patients with the means to communicate.

15. Lower the bed.

Ensures patient safety.

Follow-Through

16. Wash hands.

Prevents the spread of microorganisms.

17. Record that the procedure was completed in the appropriate record.

Provides a legal record that the suppository was given.

IMPACTION

IMPACTION
the lodging of hard fecal material in the rectum

CRAMP
the feeling that results from a muscle spasm

Constipation can sometimes result in an **impaction** (Figure 20–20). The patient who is impacted with stool may expel liquid stools. This occurs because the loose stool leaks around the hardened stool and is expelled. Patients with an impaction may experience

• abdominal **cramps** or discomfort

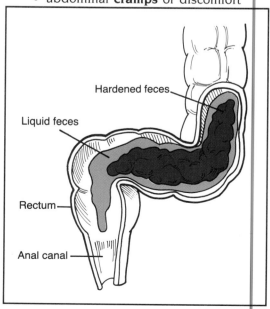

Hardened feces

Liquid feces

Rectum

Anal canal

FIGURE 20–20

Fecal material hardens and stays in the rectum. The patient is unable to expel it. Liquid feces may pass around the hardened stool.

- loss of appetite
- rectal pain caused by straining to have a bowel movement

Two treatments may be ordered for the patient with an impacted stool:

- oil retention enema to soften feces
- digital removal of the stool (using the fingers to remove stool)

CARING COMMENT

Depending on your institution's policy, the nurse may ask you to remove the impaction. Never remove an impaction without instructions from the nurse.

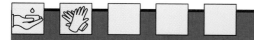

PROCEDURE

Digital Removal of an Impaction

Impacted stool may be removed by inserting the fingers into the patient's rectum and removing it. Allow plenty of time for the procedure, because patients can become very tired as a result of digital removal of stool.

GATHER EQUIPMENT

Bedpan
Toilet paper
Two pairs of disposable gloves
Lubricant
Basin of warm water

Washcloths
Towel
Disposable bed protector
Bath blanket
Room deodorant (optional)

ACTION	RATIONALE
Preparation	
1. Wash hands.	Prevents the spread of microorganisms.
2. Identify yourself and the patient.	Maintains patients' rights.
3. Provide privacy.	Maintains patients' rights.
4. Explain the procedure.	Informs patients what is happening.
Procedural Steps	
5. Raise the bed to the high position and lower the side rail nearest you.	Helps you use good body mechanics.
6. Cover patients with the bath blanket and fold the top linens toward the foot of the bed.	Provides warmth and privacy for the patient.
7. Place patients in the left Sims' position.	
8. Put on the disposable gloves.	Protects you from contamination when handling body wastes.
9. Lift the bath blanket and place the disposable bed protector next to patients, tucking one edge under patients' buttocks. Place the bedpan near patients' buttocks.	
10. Apply lubricant to the first two gloved fingers of your right hand.	Eases the entry of your fingers into the rectum.

Continued on following page

PROCEDURE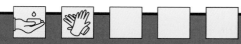

Digital Removal of an Impaction *Continued*

11. Lift the right buttock and locate the anus. The lubricated fingers should be placed at the anus and slipped into the rectum. Ask patients to take a deep breath before you insert your fingers.

    Distracts patients and helps to relax them.

12. Curve your fingers around a small section of stool and bring out the stool.

    Allows your fingers to grasp the stool.

13. Drop the stool into the bedpan and use the toilet paper to remove stool from the patient's buttocks or gloved hands.

14. Repeat steps 12 and 13 until the rectum is empty of stool.

15. Cover the bedpan and put it in a secure place.

16. Remove the gloves and discard them in the appropriate waste container.

17. Put on another pair of disposable gloves and wash, rinse, and dry the rectal area and buttocks.

18. Remove the bath blanket and replace the top sheet.

19. Place patients in a comfortable position with the call signal within reach.

    Leaves patients with the means to communicate.

20. Raise the side rail and lower the bed to the lowest position.

    Ensures patient safety.

21. Discard the soiled linens into the linen hamper.

22. Take the used bedpan to patients' bathroom and empty the contents into the toilet. Use the flush sprayer to rinse and clean the bedpan.

23. Use paper towels to dry the bedpan.

24. Empty the water from the basin and wash and dry it with paper towels.

25. Remove disposable gloves and discard them in the appropriate waste container.

Follow-Through

26. Wash hands.

    Prevents spread of microorganisms.

27. Return the basin, bedpan, and toilet paper to the bedside stand.

    Equipment is ready for the next use.

28. Record and report the following:
    • Amount of stool removed
    • Color, consistency, and odor
    • Time the procedure was done
    • How patients tolerated the procedure (ask them).

Remember that equipment is used for one patient only. Most health care institutions encourage care givers to print patients' name and room number on their particular equipment.

FLATULENCE

Flatulence is the formation of too much gas in the stomach or intestines. A patient may have a distended (enlarged) abdomen and discomfort or pain from the presence of gas. The distention and discomfort can be relieved when the gas is passed out of the body through the anus. **Flatus** is the expulsion of gas from the gastrointestinal tract. If the patient has difficulty in passing gas, the physician may order either of the following:

- insertion of a rectal tube
- administration of a Harris flush enema

FLATULENCE

presence of too much gas in the stomach or intestines

FLATUS

the expulsion of gas from the gastrointestinal tract

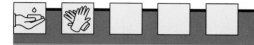

PROCEDURE

Inserting a Rectal Tube

A rectal tube relieves the distention and discomfort that is caused by the presence of gas in the intestine.

GATHER EQUIPMENT

Rectal tube
Water-soluble lubricant
Small plastic cup
Bed protector
Bath blanket

Disposable gloves
Toilet paper
Waxed paper or plastic trash bag
Room deodorant (optional)

ACTION	RATIONALE
Preparation	
1. Wash hands.	Prevents the spread of microorganisms.
2. Identify yourself and the patient.	Maintains patients' rights.
3. Provide privacy.	Maintains patients' rights.
4. Explain the procedure.	Informs patients what is happening.
Procedural Steps	
5. Raise the bed to the high position and lower the side rail on the side nearest you.	Helps you use good body mechanics.
6. Place the bed protector underneath patients.	Protects the bed linens in case of fecal drainage.
7. Place the bath blanket over patients and fanfold the linens down to the foot of the bed.	Keeps patients warm.
8. Position patients on their left side.	Allows for the best release of gas.
9. Put on disposable gloves.	
10. Lubricate the snub-nosed end of the rectal tube.	Prevents injury to anal tissue.
11. Fold back the bath blanket and insert	

Continued on following page

PROCEDURE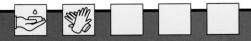

Inserting a Rectal Tube *Continued*

the tube as you would insert the tip of
the tubing for an enema:
- toward patients' navel
- 3–4 inches in

12. Place the open end in the small plastic cup.	Catches drainage that may escape with the gas.
13. Cover patients with the bath blanket and lower the bed. Raise the side rail.	Provides patient comfort and safety.
14. Tell patients to remain in the side-lying position until the tube is removed.	Movement might dislodge the tube.

15. Allow the tube to remain in patients' rectum for the amount of time specified by the nurse or supervisor.

16. After the time is up, remove the tube:
- Put on disposable gloves.
- Lift the bath blanket.
- Pull out the tube, taking care that any drainage does not spill.
- Place the soiled tube and small cup into the waste bag.
- Use toilet paper to remove any lubricant from the rectal area and place the toilet paper in the waste bag. Repeat this step until lubricant is removed.
- Remove the bed protector and place it in the soiled linen hamper (or waste bag if it is disposable).
- Remove the soiled gloves and place them in the waste bag.
- Place patients in a comfortable position.
- Remove the bath blanket and cover patients with the bed linens.
- Discard the soiled items in the soiled utility room.

Follow-Through

17. Wash hands.	Prevents spread of microorganisms.

18. Report and record the following:
- The length of time the rectal tube was in place
- Patients' statements about the release of gas
- Your observation if you heard the gas being expelled
- Any odor

Harris Flush Enema

A Harris flush enema is given to help the patient expel flatus. To administer a Harris flush enema, follow the procedure for giving an enema but make the following changes:

- Allow 100 to 200 ml of the solution to flow into and out of the intestine. Repeat until solution is used up.
- Follow the nurse's or your supervisor's direction for the amount of solution that should be used.

The solution in a Harris flush enema causes peristalsis of the intestine and helps patients expel gas. You should

- Observe for the expulsion of gas.
- Ask patients how they feel after the procedure is completed.
- Report and record that the procedure has been completed, whether flatus has been expelled, and patients' statement about how they feel.

DIARRHEA

Diarrhea is the frequent passage of watery stool. It occurs when fecal material moves too quickly through the bowel for water to be absorbed back into the body. Diarrhea can be caused by

- medication
- food allergy
- disease
- stress
- infection
- food poisoning

The diarrhea stool may be expelled with great force; in some instances, expulsion may occur unexpectedly.

Diarrhea causes loss of fluid from the body. The condition that results is called **dehydration.** The physician may order intravenous fluids to replace lost body fluid. Patients may not be allowed to eat until the diarrhea stops; they will be placed on NPO (nothing allowed by mouth). Ice chips or frequent sips of cool fluids may be permitted by the physician. Loss of fluid may be life threatening for infants and the elderly. A patient with diarrhea may also experience

- abdominal cramping
- nausea and vomiting
- **lethargy**

Care of the Patient with Diarrhea

The patient with diarrhea has many needs that you can meet as a nursing assistant. Table 20–2 shows what you should do for the patient with diarrhea and why.

OSTOMY

The word **ostomy** means artificial opening. The surgeon creates a **colostomy** by creating an artificial opening in the abdominal wall, bringing the colon (or the ureter from one or both kidneys, in which case the term **urostomy** is used) through the new opening, and sewing it to the abdominal wall. The diseased

DIARRHEA
frequent passage of watery stools

DEHYDRATION
loss of body fluid

LETHARGY
abnormal drowsiness and indifference
OSTOMY
an artificial opening
COLOSTOMY
an opening (stoma) made into the abdomen that permits the large intestine to be brought to the surface to provide a route for the evacuation of stool
UROSTOMY
an opening (stoma) made into the abdomen that provides a route for the evacuation of urine from the ureters or bladder

TABLE 20-2   **CARE OF THE PATIENT WITH DIARRHEA**

Action	Rationale
Offer fluids as often as possible when permitted; ask patients what they would like to drink.	Helps replace body fluids that are lost in the watery stools.
Keep the skin clean and dry; wash, rinse, and dry it after each bowel movement.	Helps prevent skin breakdown caused by the frequent watery bowel movements.
Apply incontinence pants when patients are unaware of the bowel movement or are too ill or tired to get to the bathroom as often as needed.	Help contain the stool in one place. May be indicated until the diarrhea stops.
Provide a restful environment because diarrhea is a signal that disease may be occurring in the body.	Helps the body heal.

portion of the colon is removed. The colon that is sewed to the abdominal wall is called a *stoma*. The person who has a colostomy eliminates fecal waste from the body through the colostomy. A colostomy may be done for many reasons:

- disease
- injury
- to rest the bowel

The fecal drainage from a colostomy ranges from liquid to formed stool. The main function of the large intestine is to absorb water from fecal material as it passes through it. The farther fecal material passes through the intestine, the firmer it becomes because it has less fluid in it. The following are general guidelines for fecal consistency found in different types of ostomies:

- If the ostomy is on the right side of the body in the small intestine (*ileostomy*), fecal material in or just leaving the small intestine will be liquid to paste in consistency (Figure 20-21A).
- If the ostomy is on the right side of the body in the large intestine (ascending colon), the fecal material will be a liquid to soft consistency (Figure 20-21B).
- If the ostomy is on the middle of the abdomen (transverse colon), the fecal material will be a soft consistency (Figure 20-21C).
- If the ostomy is on the left abdomen (descending colon) or the lower left abdomen (sigmoid colon), the fecal material will be soft to formed consistency (Figure 20-21D and E).

OBSERVATIONS OF THE PATIENT WITH A COLOSTOMY

When you care for a patient with a colostomy, you need to observe the following:

- Stoma—The normal color should be pink and shiny; no blood should be present.
- Skin around the stoma—The skin should be clean and dry; no excoriation (open areas) should be present.
- Drainage—Check the consistency, odor, and amount of fecal material.

Record your observations in the appropriate place and report pertinent information to the nurse or supervisor. You may also be asked to assist the patient to care for the colostomy.

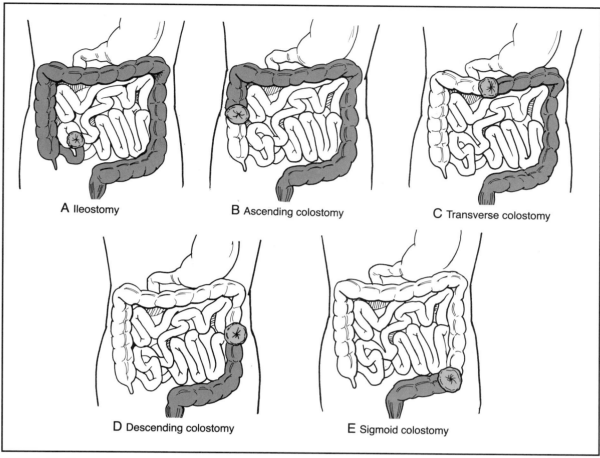

FIGURE 20-21

Ostomy sites and associated problems. A, Ileostomy. The ileostomy drains continuously, and because the fecal material is strong the skin is easily irritated. Odor control may be a problem. B, Ascending colostomy. Leakage around the appliance, skin irritation, and odor control may be problems. C, Transverse colostomy. This colostomy may be temporary. Leakage around the appliance, skin irritation, and odor control may be problems. D, Descending colostomy, and E, sigmoid colostomy. Because the feces is near the end of the intestinal tract, it is more formed. Bowel movement may occur once or twice a day. Leakage around the appliance, skin irritation, and odor control may be problems.

CARE OF A PATIENT WITH A COLOSTOMY

Patients who have received a colostomy may find it very difficult to accept this different way of having a bowel movement. They must wear an appliance to collect the fecal material, and, in most cases, the appliance must be worn at all times. Unless there is a complicating medical condition, most persons with a colostomy can resume their usual activity. They can wear regular clothing, participate in activities such as boating or hiking, and eat foods and fluids that do not cause discomfort. Some foods, such as those that produce gas, may cause discomfort and patients learn to avoid them. Community groups are available in many locations to provide information and support to colostomy patients and families.

CARING COMMENT

You need to be accepting and supportive of the patient with a stoma.

PROCEDURE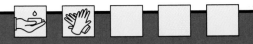

Emptying a Colostomy Appliance

The colostomy appliance (bag) is placed over the stoma so that fecal material can drain into it. The nurse or supervisor will tell you how often to check and change the colostomy bag. In this procedure, the bag is opened at the bottom and the fecal material is allowed to drain out. The bag itself is not removed.

When possible, empty the bag while patients are in the bathroom. They can sit on the toilet, and the fecal contents can drain directly into the toilet. Follow the directions below for opening and closing the bottom of the bag as well as emptying and rinsing it. This procedure addresses emptying the colostomy bag while the patient is in bed.

Note: If your patient has an ileostomy, check the health care institution's procedure.

GATHER EQUIPMENT (when procedure is performed at bedside)

Bed protector (disposable or rubber)   Disposable bulb syringe
Bedpan   Container of water
Toilet paper   Disposable gloves

ACTION	PROCEDURE
Preparation	
1. Wash hands.	Prevents the spread of microorganisms.
2. Identify yourself and the patient.	Maintains patients' rights.
3. Provide privacy.	Maintains patients' rights.
4. Explain the procedure.	Informs patients what is happening.
Procedural Steps	
5. Raise the bed to the high position and lower the side rail nearest you.	Helps you use good body mechanics.
6. Position patients on their side and place the bed protector over the sheet next to them.	Allows gravity to help with drainage.
7. Place the bedpan on the protector next to patients.	
8. Put on the disposable gloves.	Protects you from contamination when handling body wastes.
9. Open the clamp at the bottom of the bag and place the open end into the bedpan (Figure 20–22).	
10. Allow the fecal material to drain into the bedpan. Gently press the bag from top to bottom.	Helps expel the fecal material into the bedpan.
11. When the bag is as empty as possible, fill the bulb syringe with water and put it in the bag through the bottom opening.	
12. Squeeze the bulb and direct the syringe so that any remaining fecal material is dislodged and drained into the bedpan.	
13. Continue filling the syringe with water and rinsing the bag until as much fecal material as possible is removed.	Ensures bag is clean.
14. Wipe the bottom edge of the bag with the toilet paper.	Removes fecal material before reclamping.

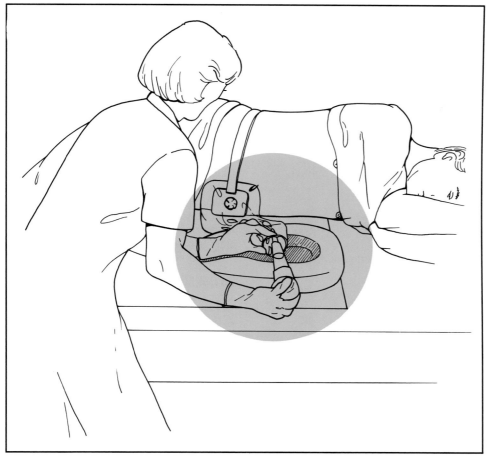

FIGURE 20–22

Emptying and rinsing an ostomy bag.

15. Replace the clamp securely.	Prevents leakage.
16. Remove the bedpan and the bed protector from the bed.	
17. Place patients in a comfortable position with the call signal within reach.	Leaves patients with the means to communicate.
18. Place the bed in the low position and raise the side rail.	Ensures patient safety.
19. Take the bedpan to patients' bathroom and empty the contents into the toilet. Use the flush sprayer to rinse the bedpan until it is clean.	Clean equipment can be stored until needed again.
20. Remove the disposable gloves and dispose of them in the appropriate waste container. Wash your hands.	
21. Dry the bedpan with paper towels until dry.	
22. Put the bedpan and toilet paper in patients' bedside stand.	
23. Discard the bed protector in the appropriate container.	

Follow-Through

24. Wash hands.	Prevents the spread of microorganisms.

PROCEDURE

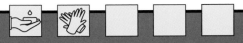

Changing a Colostomy Appliance

The entire colostomy appliance may be changed at regular intervals or according to patients' individual needs. The procedure consists of removing the soiled bag and the sealing ring. Clean and inspect the skin before putting the new equipment in place.

Note: If your patient has an ileostomy, check the health care institution's procedure.

GATHER EQUIPMENT

Bed protector (disposable or rubber)
Bedpan
Basin of warm water
Two washcloths
Towel
Disposable gloves
Clean colostomy bag and bottom clamp

Ring that forms a seal on the skin around the stoma (the nurse will tell you what size ring the patient needs)
Skin powder
Room deodorant
New appliance belt if the one the patient is wearing is soiled

ACTION	RATIONALE
Preparation	
1. Wash hands.	Prevents the spread of microorganisms.
2. Identify yourself and the patient.	Maintains patients' rights.
3. Provide privacy.	Maintains patients' rights.
4. Explain the procedure.	Informs patients what is happening.
Procedural Steps	
5. Raise the bed to the high position and lower the side rail nearest you. Raise the head of the bed to a comfortable position for patients.	Helps you use good body mechanics.
6. Raise patients' gown and fold it across their chest. Cover the exposed area with the bath blanket and fold the top linens toward the foot of the bed.	Prevents soiling of bed linens or night clothes. Provides patient privacy.
7. Place the bed protector next to patients and put the bedpan on it.	
8. Place a basin of warm water, washcloths, and towel on the over-bed stand and arrange the colostomy equipment within your reach.	
9. Put on the disposable gloves.	Protects you from contamination when handling body wastes.
10. Remove the colostomy collection bag and place it in the bedpan. Remove the clamp at the bottom of the bag for reuse.	The clamp can be cleaned with soap and water and saved for the next colostomy change.
11. Peel off the ring that is on the skin around the stoma and discard it into the waste container.	Once the ring is removed, it cannot be used again because it will not stick to patients' skin.
12. Remove the appliance belt if it is soiled. Put a new or clean belt on patients.	The appliance belt is washable and can be reused.
13. Rinse the washcloth in the warm water and cleanse the skin around the stoma (Figure 20–23).	

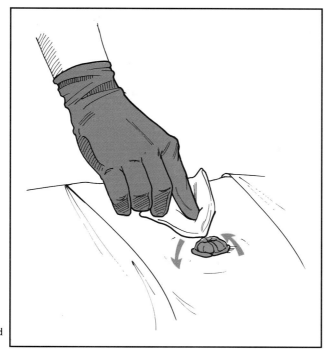

FIGURE 20-23

The skin of the stoma is cleaned by using gentle strokes.

    Note: Change the water and use the second washcloth if a large amount of fecal material is present.

14. Repeat until all fecal material and residue from the ring are removed. Use the towel to pat the skin dry.

15. Inspect the condition of the stoma and the skin that surrounds it.

16. Apply the skin powder to the skin around the stoma where the ring will be attached.

17. Peel off the paper from the ring and

Keeping the skin clean and dry helps to prevent breakdown.

The powder acts as a cement to help seal the ring against the skin.

The ring should fit as closely as possible

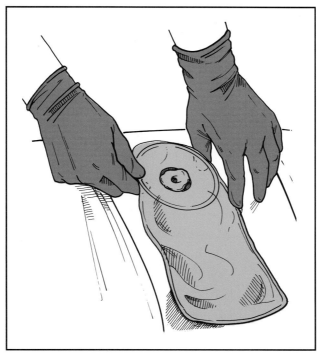

FIGURE 20-24

Place the ring over the stoma. A close fit is needed to provide a good seal and prevent leakage of fecal material onto the skin. Patients will have a supply of colostomy bags with a ring that is the correct size for them.

Continued on following page

Changing a Colostomy Appliance *Continued*

apply the ring to the skin. It should fit closely around the stoma (Figure 20–24.	to the stoma so that the skin is protected from damage by fecal drainage.
18. Connect the appliance belt to the ring.	Secures the appliance in place.
19. Connect the collection bag to the ring and secure the clamp to close off the bottom of the collection bag.	
20. Check to see that all connections are secure.	Leakage can embarrass patients.
21. Place patients in a comfortable position with the call signal within reach.	Leaves patients with the means to communicate.
22. Place the bed in the low position and raise the side rail.	Ensures patient safety.
23. Take the bedpan into patients' bathroom and empty the fecal material from the collection bag into the toilet and flush.	
24. Dispose of the used collection bag and used ring as indicated by your health care institution's policy.	
25. Rinse and dry the bedpan and return it to patients' bedside stand.	Readies equipment for next use.
26. Discard the soiled bed protector into the appropriate container.	
27. Remove and discard the soiled gloves.	

Follow-Through

28. Wash hands.	Prevents the spread of microorganisms.

CARING COMMENT

When you empty or change the colostomy appliance, use a room deodorant to help make the odor in the room pleasant.

CHAPTER WRAP-UP

- Solid waste is eliminated from the body by the lower gastrointestinal system.
- The lower gastrointestinal system includes the small and large intestines.
- The large intestine includes the
  Colon
  Rectum
  Anal canal

- The waste material from the lower gastrointestinal system is known by three names:
    Feces
    Stool
    Bowel movement
- Common disruptions of lower gastrointestinal function are
    Incontinence
    Constipation
    Impaction
    Diarrhea
- An artificial opening brings the bowel out through the wall of the abdomen. The opening is called either a stoma or an ostomy.

REVIEW QUESTIONS

1. Define the terms *constipation, diarrhea, impaction,* and *flatulence.*
2. List the causes of constipation.
3. Describe the normal and unusual observations of a bowel movement.
4. Explain how a stool specimen is collected.

ACTIVITY CORNER

Find a classmate to practice this activity in your classroom or practice area. The classmate should get into a bed. Raise the bed and practice placing a bedpan under the "patient" in two different ways.

The first time, the person should help by lifting his or her body while you position the bedpan under the person and raise the head of the bed. Pour a small amount of water into the bedpan and then try to remove the bedpan without spilling the water.

The second time, roll the person onto his or her side, put the bedpan in place, and roll the person onto the bedpan. Pour a small amount of water into the bedpan. Remove the bedpan without spilling any water.

Reverse roles with your classmate (you become the "patient"), and repeat the two procedures. Talk about how you felt when you were having a bedpan placed under you and how you felt as the person who was placing the bedpan. What feelings did you have? Check any of the following that apply:

_____ Clumsy

_____ Anxious

_____ Ashamed

_____ Embarrassed

_____ Unsure of ability

_____ Other (write in) _____

These are feelings you need to face and talk about before you take care of patients.

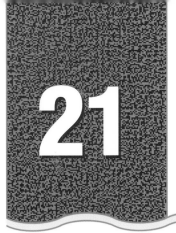

21

Learning About Bladder Elimination

Objectives

AFTER YOU COMPLETE THIS CHAPTER, YOU WILL BE ABLE TO:

Describe the urinary system's structure and function.

Explain why fluid intake is important.

List the normal observations of urinary output.

Describe devices that help drain urine from the body.

Explain how a urine specimen is collected.

Explain how a urine specimen is tested on the nursing unit.

Apply a condom catheter.

Measure and record urine output.

Identify common disruptions in urinary elimination.

Explain how a bowel and bladder retraining program works.

Care for patients with common disruptions in urinary elimination.

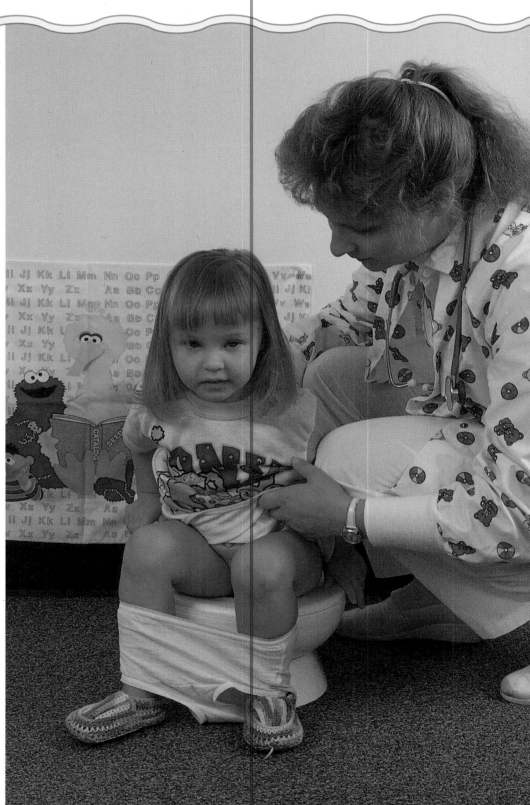

Overview The body eliminates its liquid waste via the urinary system. The kidneys turn waste into urine, and the bladder stores the urine before it is eliminated from the body. As a nursing assistant, you are expected to assist patients in voiding (emptying the bladder) when necessary.

WHAT DO YOU KNOW ABOUT BLADDER ELIMINATION?

Here are five statements about bladder elimination. Consider them to test your knowledge. If you think the statement is true, circle the T; if you think the statement is false, circle the F. Change the false statements to make them true.

1. T F Urinary incontinence is the inability to control the passage of urine from the body.

2. T F The body organ that makes urine is the bladder.

3. T F The amount of fluid a person drinks affects the amount of urine the person voids (urinates).

4. T F Adult males normally stand while voiding.

5. T F Normal urine may contain small stones.

ANSWERS

1. **True.** Urinary incontinence is the inability to control the passage of urine from the body.

2. **False.** Urine is made by the kidneys and is stored in the bladder.

3. **True.** The amount of fluids taken in affects the amount of fluids voided.

4. **True.** Male patients may have a difficult time voiding if not allowed to stand.

5. **False.** Small stones or any other particles are not a normal part of urine.

BLADDER ELIMINATION

URINE
fluid that contains water and the waste products of the body

The production of **urine** by the kidneys is a delicate process that rids the blood of harmful and unneeded substances. Urine is stored in the bladder until a person is able to empty the bladder by urinating.

STRUCTURE AND FUNCTION OF THE URINARY ORGANS

The urinary system functions to regulate the fluid level in the body and to eliminate the body's fluid waste products. It also controls the amount of salt present in the body. The urinary system consists of the following structures (Figure 21–1).

KIDNEY
one of two organs that filter waste products out of the blood to be eliminated by the body

KIDNEYS   Two **kidneys,** shaped like beans, are located about halfway up the back, one on each side of the body. The kidneys filter waste products out of the blood, making urine for elimination by the body.

URETER
tube through which urine passes from the kidney to the bladder

URETERS   The **ureters** are tubes that allow the urine to drain from the kidneys to the bladder. The body has two ureters, one for each kidney.

BLADDER
the elastic muscular sac that collects urine before it leaves the body

BLADDER   The **bladder** is the collecting place for the urine before it leaves the body. Elastic muscle in the walls of the bladder allows it to stretch to hold the urine produced by the kidneys. The normal amount of fluid the bladder can hold is approximately 400 ml. Urination occurs when the bladder is stretched enough to send a message to the brain that it needs to be emptied.

URETHRA
tube that carries urine from the bladder to the outside of the body

URETHRA   The **urethra** is a tube through which the urine passes from the

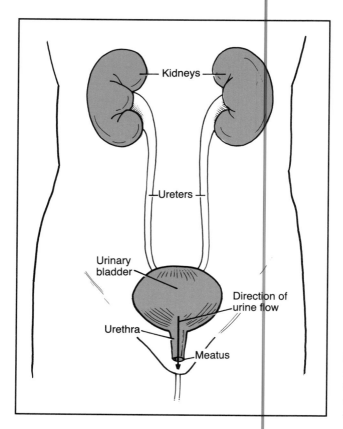

FIGURE 21–1
The structures required for urinary elimination are the kidneys, ureters, bladder, urethra, and meatus.

TABLE 21-1 OBSERVATIONS OF URINE

Observation	Usual	Unusual
Subjective		
Pattern of urination	Patients report they are voiding as frequently as usual.	Patients report an increased urinary output (polyuria) or voiding more frequently than usual.
	Patients report that urination is not painful.	Patients report pain or difficulty in urinating (dysuria).
	The patient reports no blood in the urine.	Patients report blood in the urine (hematuria).
Objective		
Color	Normally light pale yellow	Red, greenish
Odor	No odor	Foul, acetone, or other odors
Sediment	No sediment	Presence of sediment
Clarity	Clear	Cloudy
Consistency	Thin, watery	Thick
Output	1,500–1,600 ml per 24 hours	No urinary output (anuria)
		Output increased over 24 hours (polyuria)
		Output decreased or diminished over 24 hours (oliguria)

bladder to the outside of the body. The female urethra is approximately 1½ inches long. The male urethra is approximately 8 inches long. The male urethra also passes **semen** from the body.

URINARY MEATUS The **urinary meatus** is the opening of the urethra through which urine leaves the body.

HOW FLUID INTAKE INFLUENCES URINE FORMATION

Urine is formed in the kidneys. It is a fluid that contains water and waste products filtered out of the blood by the kidneys. When a person has a low intake of fluids, the kidneys save fluid by decreasing urine output. When the person has a high intake of fluids the kidneys produce more urine. Certain medications can increase urine production and output. Table 21-1 lists the normal and abnormal observations of urine and urination that you need to recognize.

CHANGES ASSOCIATED WITH AGING

Elderly persons may feel the need to **void** more often. The elderly person's bladder holds less urine than it did at a younger age. Elderly people may reduce their fluid intake in an attempt to urinate less often. Tell them that fluids are important to body functioning. Offer them fluids of their choice frequently. Six to eight glasses of fluid are recommended every day.

In addition, the elderly person may be taking a medication known as a **diuretic.** Because diuretics are designed to eliminate fluids from the body, they increase the frequency of urination. A person taking a diuretic may awaken several times during the night to empty the bladder. The physician usually tells patients to take diuretics in the morning because an evening dose interferes with sleep. See Chapter 31 for discussion of the changes in elimination function that occur with age.

SEMEN
the fluid that helps sperm move through the duct system in males

URINARY MEATUS
the opening of the urethra through which urine flows to the outside of the body

VOID
to empty the bladder

DIURETIC
a substance that causes an increase in urination

URINATION

URINATION
discharge of urine; voiding

Urination is the discharge of the body's fluid waste materials from the bladder. The term *urinate* means to empty the bladder of urine; the term *void* means the same thing. You should know how to perform the following procedures associated with urination:

- place a urinal
- give catheter care
- collect urine specimens
- test urine for glucose and acetone
- apply a condom catheter to a male patient
- measure and record urinary output

USING COLLECTION DEVICES

URINAL
a container into which a person urinates

When patients who cannot toilet themselves need to void, you need to offer them a bedpan or **urinal.** In most cases, females use a bedpan to void. Males use a urinal, because the most natural position for the male patient to void is to stand. If the patient is unable to stand or place the urinal over the penis by himself, you may need to place the urinal for him.

PROCEDURE

Placing a Urinal

If the patient is not able to place the urinal by himself, you need to do this for him.

GATHER EQUIPMENT

Urinal (plastic or metal)   Towel
Washcloth

ACTION	RATIONALE
Preparation	
1. Wash hands.	Prevents the spread of microorganisms.
2. Identify yourself and the patient.	Maintains patients' rights.
3. Provide privacy.	Maintains patients' rights.
4. Explain the procedure.	Informs patients what is happening.
Procedural Steps	
5. Assist the patient to a standing position if he is able and allowed to stand.	Standing to void is the preferred position for males.
6. When the patient is not able to stand, continue procedure while he remains lying on his back.	
7. Raise the linens and place the urinal between the patient's legs (Figure 21–2). (You should place the penis into the urinal opening if the patient cannot do so for himself.)	
8. Lower the linens and place the call signal within the patient's reach.	The patient can call you when he is finished.

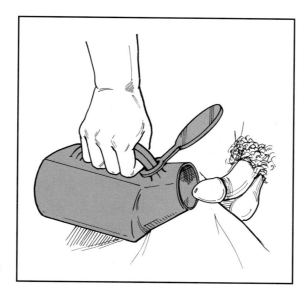

FIGURE 21-2

Position the penis so the urine is directed into the urinal.

9. Leave the patient for a short period of time.

Allows the patient to void in privacy.

10. Return in 5–10 minutes or as soon as you see the call signal.

11. Remove the urinal from beneath the linens. Be careful not to spill the contents.

12. Offer the patient a warm washcloth to wash his hands. Offer the towel for drying.

13. Place the patient in a position of comfort with the call signal within reach.

Leaves the patient with the means to communicate.

14. Take the urinal into the bathroom and observe the urine for color, clarity, and odor.

These observations are important to patient care.

15. Measure the amount of urine in the urinal if an intake and output (I&O) order has been given. Record the amount and color on the I&O record that is kept in the patient's room (see Figure 21–12).

16. If any of your observations are unusual (foul odor, thickness, or reddish color), save the specimen to show the nurse or supervisor.

May indicate the presence of disease.

17. Empty the contents of the urinal into the toilet and flush.

18. Rinse the urinal with water and empty it into the toilet.

19. Dry the outside of the urinal and return it to the patient's bedside stand.

Readies the equipment for the next use.

20. The patient may request that the urinal be placed within his reach. The urinal can be hung by the handle on the lower side rail.

Helps the patient to participate in his care.

Follow-Through

21. Wash hands.

Prevents the spread of microorganisms.

URINARY DRAINAGE CATHETERS

CATHETER

a flexible tube passed into body openings to allow fluids to enter or exit the body

When patients have no control over their urine elimination, a catheter is inserted into their bladder to take over the function of draining urine from the body. A urinary **catheter** is a flexible tube passed through the urinary meatus and the urethra into the bladder to allow urine to drain out. A catheter is inserted by a nurse or physician.

Types of Urinary Catheters

There are three types of urinary catheters (Figure 21–3).

INDWELLING CATHETER

a tube inserted into a body opening and secured in place

INDWELLING (RETENTION) CATHETER   The **indwelling (retention) catheter** is a tube inserted into a body cavity—in this case, the bladder—and secured. The

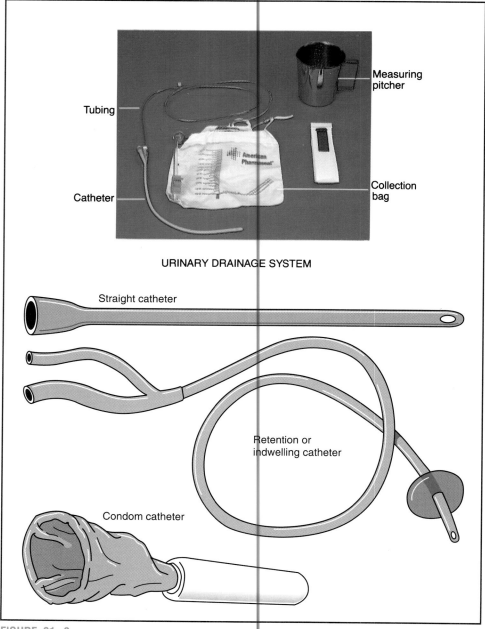

FIGURE 21–3

The indwelling and straight catheters are sterile when inserted into the patient's bladder. Because the condom catheter goes over the penis to collect urine, it is not sterile.

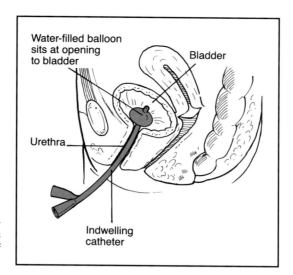

FIGURE 21–4

An indwelling catheter. The inflated balloon at the tip prevents the catheter from slipping out of the bladder.

catheter has a small balloon on the tip that is inserted into the body. The balloon is inflated when the catheter is inserted into the bladder, helping hold the catheter in place (Figure 21–4). The other end of this catheter is attached to a drainage (collection) bag that must be emptied according to the procedure of your health care institution.

STRAIGHT CATHETER A **straight catheter** is a tube inserted one time to drain urine from the bladder. After the bladder is drained of urine, the catheter is removed.

CONDOM CATHETER Used for male patients, the **condom catheter** is a sheath placed over the penis that has a tube at the bottom that allows urine to flow into a collection bag.

Catheter Care

Patients who have had an indwelling catheter inserted need special hygienic care. This type of care is called *catheter care*. Catheter care is a special way of cleaning the genital area when a person is wearing a catheter. Both male and female patients who have had an indwelling catheter inserted need catheter care at least twice a day; your institution will specify how often. When you perform catheter care, it is important to record and report any of the following observations:

- redness at the urinary meatus
- leakage around the catheter
- leakage from the catheter or drainage system
- patients' statements about pain or discomfort

STRAIGHT CATHETER
a tube inserted one time to drain urine from the bladder, after which it is removed

CONDOM CATHETER
a sheath with a tube at the bottom that allows urine from the penis to flow into a collection bag

PROCEDURE

Performing Catheter Care for Females and Males

This procedure should be performed as part of the patient's hygiene care and any time it is indicated by soiling of the area. It can be done during the care of the **perineum.**

GATHER EQUIPMENT

Bath blanket
Towel
Disposable washcloth

Basin of warm water
Disposable gloves

PERINEUM
the pelvic floor, extending from the pubic bones at the front of the body to the coccyx (tailbone) at the back

Continued on following page

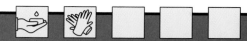

PROCEDURE

Performing Catheter Care for Females and Males
Continued

ACTION	RATIONALE
Preparation	
1. Wash hands.	Prevents the spread of microorganisms.
2. Identify yourself and the patient.	Maintains patients' rights.
3. Provide privacy.	Maintains patients' rights.
4. Explain the procedure.	Informs patients what is happening.
Procedural Steps	
5. Place a basin of warm water on the over-bed stand at the patient's bed-side.	
6. Raise the bed to the high position and lower the side rail nearest you.	Helps you maintain good body mechanics.
7. Cover the patient with the bath blanket and fold the top linens down to the foot of the bed.	Provides patient privacy.
8. Place the towel underneath the patient's buttocks.	Prevents the bottom sheets from becoming wet.
9. Put on the disposable gloves.	Offers protection while you are handling body wastes.
10. Cleanse the perineum (see the procedure for cleansing the perineal area in Chapter 13).	
11. With one hand, grasp the catheter near the urinary meatus (Figure 21–5).	Helps keep the catheter stable.

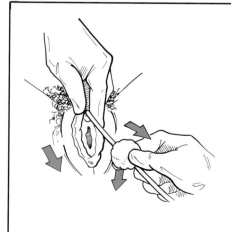
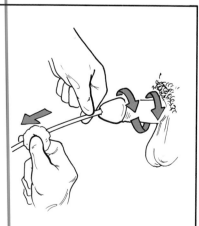

FEMALE CATHETER CARE　　　　　　MALE CATHETER CARE

FIGURE 21–5

Catheter care. It is important to clean in the direction shown so that microorganisms are not introduced into the urinary meatus.

12. *For females:* Maintain a firm grasp on the catheter while cleansing it. (Recall from Chapter 13 that it is important to use front-to-back strokes when washing the perineal area.)
    For males:
    Give a gentle tug to pull the catheter forward slightly. Maintain a firm grasp on the catheter while cleansing it. Work in a circular direction from the urinary meatus out to the edge of the glans penis (see Figure 21–5).

13. With a dampened washcloth in the other hand, wash and rinse the catheter, starting at the urinary meatus and cleansing 8 inches of the catheter.

14. Use a twisting motion as you wash.

    Friction helps loosen particles stuck to the catheter.

15. Loosen any **residue** present on the catheter tube.

    RESIDUE
    a layer of particles

16. Repeat steps 12–15.
    Note: The health care institution where you are employed may have a different procedure for catheter care; for example, you may be required to apply an **ointment** at the urinary meatus. Always follow the procedure of your institution.

    OINTMENT
    a preparation that is applied to the body's surface and contains a medication

17. Remove the towel from under the patient and bring the top linens up over the bath blanket.

18. Slip the bath blanket out from beneath the top linens.

19. Place the patient in a position of comfort.

20. Put the bed in the low position and raise the side rail.

    Ensures patient safety.

21. Place the call signal within the patient's reach.

    Leaves patient with the means to communicate.

22. Discard the disposable items and the linens appropriately.

    Helps with infection control.

23. Take the basin of water into the bathroom and pour the water into the toilet. Flush.

24. Remove gloves and dispose of them appropriately.

Follow-Through

25. Wash hands.

    Prevents the spread of microorganisms.

26. Record and report any changes observed during the procedure. Record and report the time the procedure was completed.

COLLECTION OF SPECIMENS

URINALYSIS

the most common laboratory test of urine

MEDICAL DIAGNOSIS

the decision a physician makes about a patient's illness based on information gained through a physical examination, an interview with the patient or family, a medical history of the patient, and results of laboratory and radiologic testing

GLUCOSE

sugar

ACETONE

a by-product of a certain acid; produced in abnormal amounts by persons with diabetes mellitus

RANDOM

unplanned and unexpected

FRACTIONAL

relatively small

A specimen is a small piece of body tissue or a secretion that is examined for the presence of abnormalities. Urine specimens are collected for a variety of tests. The most common urine test is a **urinalysis.** The results of a urinalysis help the physician form a **medical diagnosis.** You are responsible for collecting urine specimens to be sent to the laboratory for testing. You are also responsible for testing urine on the nursing unit to discover whether the urine contains **glucose** or **acetone.** You may be asked to collect the following types of urine specimens.

RANDOM SAMPLE   A **random** sample of urine is collected for a routine urinalysis. It can be collected any time. The sample is collected in a clean container.

FRACTIONAL SAMPLE   A **fractional** sample of urine is collected at a specific time and is used to test the urine on the nursing unit for the presence of glucose or acetone. You ask the patient to start the stream of urine, stop, and then start the stream again into a small waxed-paper or plastic cup. The patient tells you when the specimen has been collected.

DOUBLE-VOIDED SPECIMEN   The amount of glucose present in a urine sample helps the physician determine a patient's next dose of insulin. You ask the patient to void a half hour before the specimen is scheduled for collection. This is urine that may have accumulated because that patient has not emptied the bladder for a long period of time. The patient can drink water (if allowed) during the half hour. The urine from the next voiding is urine that is produced in the last half hour. The patient voids into a small waxed-paper or plastic cup and hands you the specimen for testing.

24-HOUR URINE SPECIMEN   When a 24-hour urine specimen is ordered, the patient is asked to empty the bladder. The collection of urine begins with the next voiding. The same container is used for all voidings made in the 24-hour period and is marked with the times of collection and the patient's name and room number. The urine may be refrigerated, or a preservative may be placed in the collection container. Signs should be placed in a strategic place so that the patient, family, and other care givers are aware that a 24-hour urine collection is in progress.

If you are collecting urine from a bedpan, ask the patient to have a bowel movement after voiding. Be certain that the urine is not contaminated with the feces or toilet paper.

Note the time of the last void on the laboratory slip and take the specimen to the laboratory for testing.

CLEAN-CATCH URINE SPECIMEN

a urine specimen collected after the urinary meatus and surrounding tissue have been cleansed

CLEAN-CATCH OR MIDSTREAM SPECIMEN   The **clean-catch urine specimen** is collected in sterile equipment after the urinary meatus and surrounding area have been cleansed (see the procedure for collecting a clean-catch urine specimen).

CATHETERIZED OR STERILE SPECIMEN   When a sterile urine specimen has been ordered, the sample may be collected in a catheter inserted by the nurse. The catheter is removed after the bladder is emptied, providing a specimen. The straight catheter, described earlier, is often used to obtain a sterile urine specimen. When a patient has an indwelling catheter, a sterile urine specimen can be collected from a special place in the catheter called a **port** (see the procedure for collecting a sterile urine specimen from an indwelling catheter).

PORT

an opening

STRAINER

a device that collects particles but permits fluid to pass through

STRAINING URINE   When patients are suspected of having "stones" in their urine, you may be asked to strain all of their urine specimens. To do this, ask patients to save all their urine in a container provided for them. Pour all of the urine through a special paper **strainer** that you hold over the toilet while pouring the urine through it (Figure 21–6). Report and record that the urine has

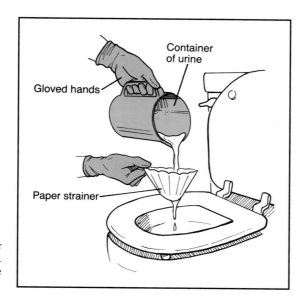

FIGURE 21-6
Pour urine through the strainer into the collection container. Check for particles in the strainer.

been strained. Do not discard any sediment, stones, or small particles that remain in the strainer; the nurse or supervisor tells you whether these particles should be sent to the laboratory for testing.

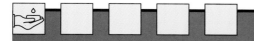

PROCEDURE

Collecting a Clean-Catch Urine Specimen

The nurse tells you when to obtain the urine specimen from the patient. It is important to explain the procedure for collecting urine to the patient so that the specimen is not **contaminated.**

GATHER EQUIPMENT

Collection container labeled with the patient's name

Packets of premoistened cleansing towels or washcloth and towel

CONTAMINATE
to soil or infect by contact

ACTION	RATIONALE
Preparation	
1. Wash hands.	Prevents the spread of microorganisms.
2. Identify yourself and the patient.	Maintains patients' rights.
3. Provide privacy.	Maintains patients' rights.
4. Explain the procedure.	Informs patients what is happening.
Procedural Steps	
5. Take the collection container to patients and ask them to use the bathroom and save a specimen of urine in the container.	
6. Explain to patients that the area around the urinary meatus should be cleansed. *For male patients:* Tell them to use the premoistened	

Continued on following page

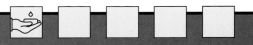

PROCEDURE

Collecting a Clean-Catch Urine Specimen
Continued

ACTION	RATIONALE
towels to cleanse from the urinary meatus out in a circular motion. *For female patients:* Tell them to use the premoistened towels to cleanse from front to back. Tell them to spread the **labia majora** while cleansing. *Note:* If patients are unable to cleanse themselves, you should complete this part of the procedure.	Removes residue that could contaminate the specimen.
7. Tell patients to start a stream of urine into the toilet, stop, and then resume the stream of urine into the collection container. Tell females to *keep the labia majora spread while urinating.* Tell patients to put the cap on the container after the urine is collected.	Ensures that the urine is from the bladder instead of the urethra.
8. Take the specimen (or have it sent) to the laboratory as soon as possible.	Specimen needs to be fresh for testing.
9. Report to the nurse that a specimen has been collected and sent to the laboratory for testing. Any specimen sent to the laboratory is accompanied by a laboratory slip that is filled out as described in Taking a Urine Specimen to the Laboratory.	

LABIA MAJORA
long outside folds of skin surrounding the urinary meatus and vagina in females

---

PROCEDURE

Collecting a Sterile Urine Specimen from an Indwelling Catheter Tube

Tell patients that you need to collect a sterile urine specimen from the tubing that is draining urine from their bladder. A specimen that is collected this way is a sterile specimen.

GATHER EQUIPMENT

Syringe with needle
Container labeled with patient's name and room number and the date and time

Disposable gloves
Two alcohol swabs

SYRINGE
instrument used to inject fluids into or remove fluids from the body

ACTION	RATIONALE
Preparation	
1. Wash hands.	Prevents the spread of microorganisms.
2. Identify yourself and the patient.	Maintains patients' rights.
3. Provide privacy.	Maintains patients' rights.
4. Explain the procedure.	Informs patients what is happening.

Procedural Steps

5. Put on the disposable gloves.

Offers protection while handling body wastes.

6. Locate the port on the tubing.

Provides entry into the drainage system without contaminating the system.

7. Open an alcohol swab and use it to clean off the port (Figure 21–7).

Reduces possibility of contamination.

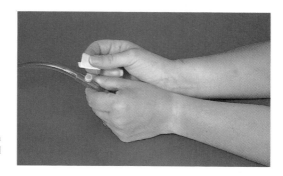

FIGURE 21–7

The port on the tubing is cleaned with an alcohol swab before the syringe is inserted and after it is withdrawn.

8. Open the syringe package.

9. Take out the syringe and remove the needle cover.

10. Place the needle into the center of the port (Figure 21–8).

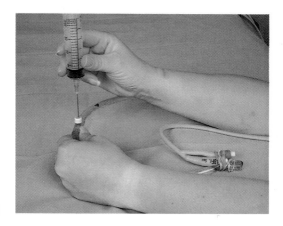

FIGURE 21–8

11. Pull the plunger back to bring urine into the syringe (Figure 21–9).

12. Collect 20–30 ml of urine and remove the needle.

13. Open another alcohol swab and clean the port.

14. Empty the urine into the sterile container.

Use of sterile equipment keeps the urine sterile.

15. Discard the syringe into the special container labeled "Sharps" in the patient's room.

An uncapped needle should never be carried out of a patient's room.

16. Remove and discard the gloves into the appropriate waste container.

Continued on following page

PROCEDURE

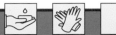

Collecting a Sterile Urine Specimen from an Indwelling Catheter Tube *Continued*

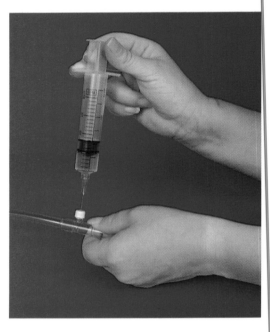

FIGURE 21-9

Follow-Through

17. Wash hands.	Prevents the spread of microorganisms.
18. Take the specimen and the laboratory slip to the laboratory or arrange to have them taken to the laboratory as soon as possible.	Specimen needs to be fresh for testing.
19. Report to the nurse that the procedure is complete.	
20. Document on the nurses' note or other appropriate place that the specimen was taken to the laboratory.	

PROCEDURE

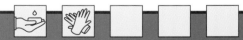

Testing Urine for Glucose and Acetone

KETONE
an acetone-like compound

This procedure is a quick test that reveals whether glucose or acetone (a chemical change caused by **ketones** in the bloodstream) is present in the urine. Directions for the test are on the bottle in which the dipsticks are stored. The test is usually done four times a day or however often the physician has ordered.

GATHER EQUIPMENT

Dipsticks   Watch
Disposable gloves

ACTION	RATIONALE

Preparation

1. Wash hands.
2. Identify yourself and the patient.
3. Provide privacy.
4. Explain the procedure.

Prevents the spread of microorganisms.
Maintains patients' rights.
Maintains patients' rights.
Informs patients what is happening.

Procedural Steps

5. Put on the disposable gloves.

Offers protection while handling body wastes.

6. Take the urine specimen to the patient's bathroom or the soiled utility room to perform the test.
7. Place the specimen cup on a paper towel on a flat surface.

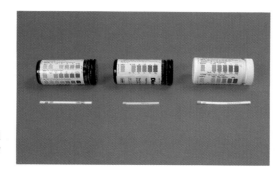

FIGURE 21–10

The dipsticks are stored in a dark-colored container that should be closed snugly after each use.

8. Open the container of dipsticks, remove one stick, and close the container (Figure 21–10).
9. Place the dipstick in the urine specimen and then remove it.
10. Begin to time the reaction occurring on the treated portion of the dipstick.
11. At the end of 10 seconds, match the reaction on the dipstick to the possible reactions shown in color on the container of dipsticks.
    Note: Read the label on the container of dipsticks to be sure of the time you must allow for the reaction; the time will vary, depending on the manufacturer.
12. Write down the result according to the scale shown on the container of dipsticks.
13. Discard the unused urine into the toilet.
14. Remove gloves and place them in a waste container.

Follow-Through

15. Wash hands.
16. Record and report the test results to the nurse or supervisor.

Prevents the spread of microorganisms.

PROCEDURE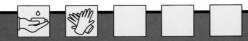

Collecting a Urine Specimen from an Infant or Child Who Is Not Toilet Trained

This procedure is used for the infant or small child who is not toilet trained or who is not able to follow directions for saving a urine specimen.

GATHER EQUIPMENT

Disposable gloves
Basin of water (105° F)
Washcloth

Towel
Plastic collection bag

ACTION	RATIONALE
Preparation	
1. Wash hands.	Prevents the spread of microorganisms.
2. Identify yourself to parents if they are present and the patient.	Maintains patients' rights.
3. Provide privacy.	Maintains patients' rights.
4. Explain the procedure.	Informs patients what is happening.
Procedural Steps	
5. Lower the side rail of the crib. Put on the disposable gloves and wash the perineum of the female and the penis of the male.	Prevents contamination of the specimen with the material from earlier elimination efforts.
6. Dry the area thoroughly.	
7. Peel off the special tape from the collection bag so that the adherent surface is ready for use. *For females:* Place the collection bag over the entire perineum. *For males:* Place the collection bag over the	The bag adheres better if the skin is dry.

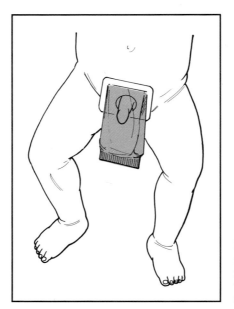

FIGURE 21–11

Disposable urine collection bag for an infant. Urine is collected in the bag and saved when a specimen is ordered.

penis and the **scrotum** (Figure 21–11).

8. Be sure that the area near the rectum is sealed securely.

9. Place a diaper over the bag.

Prevents fecal material from contaminating the urine specimen.

Prevents loosening of the bag if the infant or child kicks or pulls at the collection device.

10. Continue to give the infant or child the usual liquids.

11. Place the infant or child in a raised position (semi-Fowler's position).

12. Check the infant or child every 20–30 minutes.

13. Remove the bag gently when urine is present in the plastic collection bag.

14. Wash, rinse, and dry the perineal area.

15. Place a clean diaper on the patient. Raise the side rails of the crib.

16. Transfer the urine specimen into a clean container.

17. Remove the disposable gloves and discard them into a waste container.

Gravity helps the urine flow into the collection bag.

The weight of the urine in the bag may cause it to loosen and spill.

Prevents injury to the skin.

Follow-Through

18. Wash hands.

19. Mark the container with the patient's name and room number and the time the specimen was collected.

20. Report and record the time the specimen was collected and taken to the laboratory.

Prevents the spread of microorganisms.

> **SCROTUM**
>
> the pouch (sac) that contains the testicles and their accessory organs in males

TAKING A URINE SPECIMEN TO THE LABORATORY

Any time a specimen is taken to the laboratory, a laboratory slip must be attached to it. On the laboratory slip, write the patient's name, the room number, the kind of urine test to be performed, and the date and time the specimen was collected. For female patients, you should also note whether the specimen contains any vaginal discharge or menstrual flow. If you take the specimen to the laboratory yourself, the laboratory technicians will tell you the correct procedure for leaving a specimen in the laboratory. Generally, a timeclock is present in the laboratory, and you are asked to place the laboratory slip in the timeclock to provide a record of when the specimen arrived in the laboratory. You may also be instructed to place the specimen in the refrigerator. Never leave a specimen standing in room air, because the urine will start to break down and the test results may not be accurate.

MEASURING OUTPUT

You may be asked to measure all "output." Output includes any of the following body discharges:

Urine

Bowel movement

Perspiration
Stomach contents
Wound drainage

Remember that fluid balance in the body is important. If the patient loses too much fluid, a fluid deficit may occur and the patient may become dehydrated (see Chapter 19). The body normally eliminates fluids through urine, bowel movements, and perspiration. Fluids are also eliminated through ejection of stomach contents and drainage of wounds. Important points regarding output are as follows.

URINE OUTPUT Urine output is measured and recorded when the patient is being monitored for I&O.

BOWEL MOVEMENT The amount of the bowel movement (small, medium, or large) may be noted on the I&O record. If the patient has diarrheal (watery) bowel movements, you may be asked to measure and record the amount as output. Fecal output through a colostomy can also be measured.

PERSPIRATION Perspiration is not measurable. If the patient has a great amount of perspiration, note this by describing the perspiration as *profuse*. The bed linens and clothing of the patient who is perspiring profusely are very damp to the touch and need to be changed to keep the patient comfortable and warm.

STOMACH CONTENTS Stomach contents ejected through the mouth into an emesis basin (kidney-shaped container) can be measured and recorded when the patient is on I&O. Stomach contents may also be suctioned out through a tube inserted into the stomach through the nose. The stomach contents are suctioned into a closed container, and the amount present at the end of the shift is recorded.

WOUND DRAINAGE When wound drainage is expected after certain surgical procedures, the surgeon inserts (puts in) a drainage tube into the wound. It allows body secretions to flow from inside the body into a collection container attached to the outside end of the tube. The container (called a Jackson-Pratt container or Hemovac) can be opened and the fluid poured out for measuring and recording. The nurse is responsible for emptying the container. If you notice that it is full, inform the nurse. If the wound is draining into the dressing, inform the nurse, who will estimate the amount of drainage that is present. For example, if the dressing is thoroughly wet it will be described as *saturated*.

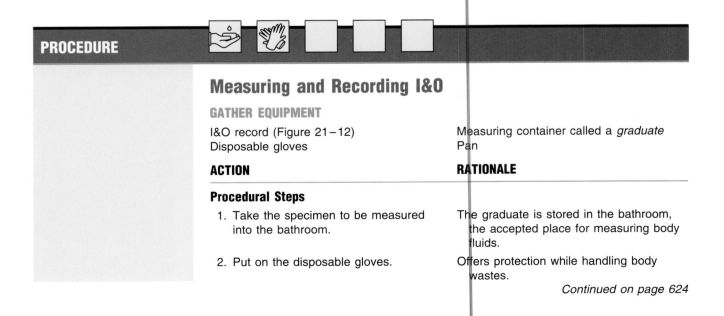

PROCEDURE

Measuring and Recording I&O

GATHER EQUIPMENT

I&O record (Figure 21–12)   Measuring container called a *graduate*
Disposable gloves   Pan

ACTION	**RATIONALE**
Procedural Steps	
1. Take the specimen to be measured into the bathroom.	The graduate is stored in the bathroom, the accepted place for measuring body fluids.
2. Put on the disposable gloves.	Offers protection while handling body wastes.

Continued on page 624

Form NS - 12

	INTAKE					OUTPUT						
Time	IV Type and Amt.	Amt. Left	Amt. Absorb.	Partial Fill IV Meds	Oral	Urine		Urinary Irrigation		Emesis	NG / IRR	
2400												
0100												
0200												
0300												
0400												
0500												
0600					240	350						350
↑ 11-7 Shift Summary					240	350					+/−	350
0800					240							
0900						250				100		350
1000					120							
1100												
1200					420							
1300												
1400						325						325
↑ 7-3 Shift Summary					780	575				100	+/−	675
1600					100							
1700						375						375
1800					360					50		50
1900												
2000					240							
2100						300						300
2200												
↑ 3-11 Shift Summary					700	675				50	+/−	725
		IV		Partial Fill IV Meds	Oral	Urine		Urinary Irrigation		Emesis	NG / IRR	
24 HOUR TOTALS					1720	1600				150		1750

DATE: *Oct 1, 1992*

FIGURE 21–12

A 24-hour record of urine output. (Courtesy of Woman's Christian Association Hospital, Jamestown, NY.)

PROCEDURE

Measuring and Recording I&O *Continued*

3. Pour the specimen into the graduate. Always use the same graduate.	Ensures that results are consistent.
4. Hold the graduate at eye level and make note of the amount (in milliliters) of specimen.	Results in the most accurate measurement.
5. If you observe anything unusual (color, odor, thickness, etc.) about the specimen, *save the specimen* and report your observation to the nurse.	May indicate a change in the patient's condition.
6. If there is nothing unusual about the specimen, dispose of it by flushing it down the toilet. *Note:* If a specimen requires special disposal, the nurse instructs you on how to proceed.	Provides for proper disposal of body fluid specimens. Never use the sink to dispose of body fluids.
7. Rinse the graduate with cold water and flush the water down the toilet.	Prepares the graduate for next use.
8. Return the graduate to storage.	
9. Remove gloves and place them in a waste container.	

Follow-Through

10. Wash hands.	Prevents the spread of microorganisms.
11. Report and record the following: • that the procedure has been done • your observations about the specimen • the amount in the correct time slot on the I&O record	Results are used to compare I&O amounts.

Reviewing the I&O Record

The figures on the I&O record are totaled at the end of the shift and every 24 hours. Review of the figures indicates one of the following situations regarding the patient's fluid balance.

FLUID BALANCE The amount of fluid taken in is similar to the amount of fluid being put out. This balance of fluids is needed for good body function. For example, water balance is adequate if the patient's total intake was 2,000 ml and the output was 2,000 ml.

INTAKE IS HIGHER THAN OUTPUT If the total intake is higher than the total output, the patient's body may be retaining (holding) fluid. You may observe edema (swelling) in the patient's body. For example, if the total fluid intake is 2,500 ml and the output is 1,500 ml, the body is retaining 1,000 ml of fluid.

OUTPUT IS HIGHER THAN INTAKE If the total output is higher than the total intake, the patient is losing fluid. You may observe dry skin and dry, cracked lips. The patient may make frequent requests for fluids. For example, if the total output is 2,800 ml and intake is 2,000 ml, the patient has lost 800 ml of fluid.

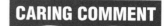

A new I&O record is placed in the patient's room every day. Before you record any intake or output, be sure you are recording on the correct I&O record by checking the patient's name on the record.

COMMON DISRUPTIONS IN URINARY FUNCTIONING

Two common disruptions in urinary function are

Urinary tract infection
Urinary incontinence

URINARY TRACT INFECTION

A **urinary tract infection** (UTI) is an infection that can occur in any part of the urinary tract. A UTI can be caused by many microorganisms.

URINARY TRACT INFECTION
infection of the kidneys, ureters, bladder, and/or urethra

Factors that Contribute to the Risk of UTI

The following factors may place a patient at high risk for a UTI.

POOR HYGIENE HABITS Most microorganisms that cause infection are from the bowel. The microorganisms enter the urinary meatus and can travel up the urethra to infect the bladder and kidneys. To prevent this type of infection, keep fecal material away from the urinary meatus. For females, always wipe the perineum from front to back. For males, wipe the penis in a circular direction away from the urinary meatus.

BLADDER CATHETERIZATION The patient who has been catheterized is at risk for a UTI. As a nursing assistant you are responsible for performing catheter care and making sure connections on the drainage system do not come apart.

URINE RETENTION Urine that stays in the bladder for a long period of time may cause infection. If necessary, assist patients to use the bathroom to empty the bladder. If the patient has a urinary catheter in place, check to be sure the catheter is draining urine.

Observations of UTI

Observe the patient for any changes from normal. The patient may tell you about the following problems with urinary elimination:

- Frequent urination
- Burning during urination
- Pain during urination
- Blood in the urine

You yourself may observe that the patient is urinating frequently or that there is blood in the urine. Observe the urine closely for any changes from usual.

Care of the Patient with a UTI

Care of the patient with a urinary tract infection consists of the following:

WARM BATHS Warm-water tub baths may relieve the patient's pain and discomfort. Bubble bath, bath salts, or oils should not be used because they may irritate the urethra and cause an infection.

HYGIENE Clean the female's perianal area from front to back to prevent further infection.

FLUIDS Encourage the patient to drink fluids to flush out the microorganisms. The patient may be offered cranberry juice because it helps make the urine acidic. Microorganisms do not thrive in an acidic environment.

TOILETING Assist or remind the patient to go to the bathroom every 2–3 hours to empty the bladder.

URINARY INCONTINENCE

URINARY INCONTINENCE
inability to control the elimination of urine

STRESS INCONTINENCE
the leakage of urine when abdominal pressure is increased, such as during a cough, sneeze, or laugh

Urinary incontinence is the inability to control the passage of urine from the body. A special muscle controls a person's ability to open and close the bladder on demand. Disease or injury can interfere with or destroy the muscle's ability to function. Urinary incontinence may be temporary or permanent.

Stress incontinence is a type of incontinence that usually occurs in females. Leakage of urine occurs when abdominal pressure is increased, such as when the patient sneezes, coughs, or picks up a heavy object. Persons who have stress incontinence may be told by the physician to perform the following exercise when emptying the bladder:

1. Start emptying the bladder.
2. Stop urinating and tighten the muscle closing the bladder.
3. Hold the muscle tight.
4. Relax the muscle and continue to empty the bladder.
5. Repeat steps 1–4 several times each time the bladder is emptied.

Care of the Patient Who Is Incontinent

The patient who is incontinent has many needs. Devices that help the patient deal with urinary incontinence are

- Incontinence pants (cloth and disposable) (see the procedure for applying incontinence pants in Chapter 20).
- Incontinence pads (cloth and disposable)
- Condom catheters
- Bowel and bladder retraining

The most important part of caring for the patient who is incontinent is keeping the skin meticulously clean. Body waste that contacts the skin can contribute to breakdown of the skin in that area. Another important part of care is to consider the patient's feelings. The patient who is incontinent has lost control of a basic body function and may react to this loss with sadness or anger. In caring for the patient who is incontinent, you

- Help the patient maintain hygiene through the use of incontinence products.
- Cleanse the skin thoroughly every time a collection device is changed.
- Participate actively with the patient in the retraining program.
- Encourage the patient and provide praise for accomplishments during the bowel and bladder retraining.
- Remain nonjudgmental.

INCONTINENCE PADS Incontinence pads are absorbent pads that are placed under the buttocks of a patient who is incontinent. Two kinds are available:

- Washable pads are made of several layers of cotton on a rubberized backing.
- Disposable pads are made of a woven absorbable material and are plastic lined.

INCONTINENCE PANTS Incontinence pants are used to contain body wastes in one area away from the patient's body. They are made of absorbable material and may be reusable or disposable. See procedure Applying Incontinence Pants in Chapter 20.

CONDOM CATHETERS A condom catheter, also known as a Texas catheter, is a catheter that is placed outside the body (as opposed to inside the body, like indwelling and straight catheters) and is worn only by males. It is a sheath placed over the penis that has a tube at the bottom that allows urine to drain into a collection bag. The condom catheter must be applied correctly and checked frequently. If it is put on too tightly, it can interfere with the circulation of blood to the penis.

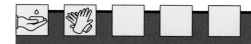

PROCEDURE

Applying a Condom Catheter

Apply the condom catheter over the patient's penis to help direct the flow of urine into a collection bag.

GATHER EQUIPMENT

Condom catheter	Disposable gloves
Collection bag for urine	Towel

ACTION	RATIONALE

Preparation

ACTION	RATIONALE
1. Wash hands.	Prevents the spread of microorganisms.
2. Identify yourself and the patient.	Maintains patients' rights.
3. Provide privacy.	Maintains patients' rights.
4. Explain the procedure.	Informs patients what is happening.

Procedural Steps

ACTION	RATIONALE
5. Raise the bed to the high position and lower the side rail nearest you.	Helps you use good body mechanics.
6. Put on disposable gloves.	Offers protection while handling body waste.
7. Fold the top linens down to the patient's knees.	Clears the work area so you can see.
8. Place the towel under the patient's thighs.	
9. Remove the condom catheter from the package.	
10. Connect the tube on the end of the catheter to the tubing of the collection bag.	Permits the urine to flow into the collection bag as soon as the catheter is in place.
11. Set the collection bag aside while applying the condom catheter.	
12. Remove the protective paper from the larger end of the condom catheter to expose the adhesive.	
13. Grasp the shaft of the penis with one hand.	Gives the stability needed to apply the condom catheter.

Continued on following page

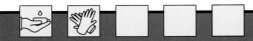

PROCEDURE

Applying a Condom Catheter *Continued*

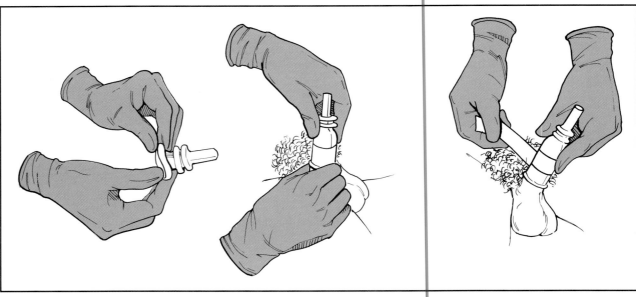

FIGURE 21–13

Applying a condom catheter. A, Roll the top of the catheter until the inner flap is exposed. B, Place the catheter over the tip of the penis. C, Roll the condom catheter down so it covers the shaft of the penis and secure it per the manufacturer's instructions.

14. Hold the condom catheter in the other hand and slip it over the penis (Figure 21–13).

15. Secure the catheter by gently pressing the adhesive to the skin at the base of the penis to form a seal. Be sure that pubic hair is not caught in the adhesive.

   If not secured, the condom will slip off the penis.

16. Tell the patient his urine will flow down a tube into the collection bag (Figure 21–14).

   Orients the patient to the presence of the condom.

17. Remove the towel from under the patient.

18. Cover the patient with the top linens.

19. Hang the collection bag below the level of the bladder on the frame of the patient's bed. Or, if a leg collection bag is used, secure it to the side of the patient's leg with the plastic straps.

   Gravity ensures drainage.

20. Remove gloves and discard them into the waste container.

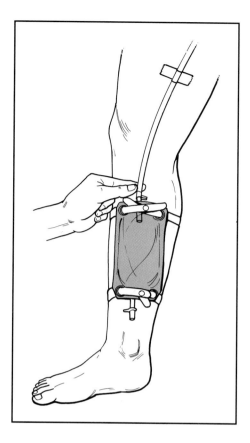

FIGURE 21–14
Check the tubing connection to the drainage bag. It should be secure to prevent urine from leaking.

Step	Rationale
21. Place the patient in a position of comfort and place the call signal within reach.	Leaves patient with a means to communicate.
22. Lower the bed to the low position and raise the side rail.	Ensures patient safety.

Follow-Through

23. Place the towel in the laundry hamper.	
24. Wash hands.	Prevents the spread of microorganisms.
25. Report to the nurse that the condom catheter was applied.	

BOWEL AND BLADDER RETRAINING A bowel and bladder **retraining program** is carried out to help patients become continent to the best of their ability. Regaining the ability to remain continent by controlling the bowels and bladder increases patients' self-esteem and feelings of independence.

The nurse may ask you to keep track of when patients urinate or have a bowel movement. The nurse uses this information to set up a schedule of activities designed to help the patient regain control of elimination functions. Activities include

- **Toileting**—During early retraining, the patient is toileted every 2 hours. The patient is encouraged to move his or her bowels in the morning after breakfast. Medication may be prescribed to help the patient in the early phase of bowel retraining.

RETRAINING PROGRAM

a program designed to help a person relearn a skill or activity

TOILETING

assisting a patient to the toilet or commode, or onto a bedpan, for the purpose of emptying the bowel or bladder

- **Fluids**—Fluids are given 30 minutes before the patient is taken to the bathroom. Urine will be in the bladder when the patient is toileted.
- **Encouragement**—Patients are encouraged to hold their urine until the specified time. As their ability to hold their urine increases, the time between trips to the bathroom is increased. This helps the bladder increase the amount of fluid it can hold.

CARING COMMENT

Remember to be patient when helping someone in a bowel and bladder retraining program. Bowel and bladder retraining takes time and effort. It should not be given up after only a few days or weeks. Control may take 2 or more months to achieve.

CHAPTER WRAP-UP

- The urinary system includes the
  Kidneys
  Ureters
  Bladder
  Urethra
- Urine is the elimination product of the urinary system.
- Fluid intake can increase or decrease urinary output.
- Common disruptions of urinary function are
  Incontinence
  Urinary tract infection
- Retraining of the bowel and bladder may help the patient become continent again.
- The following are important aspects of care of the incontinent patient:
  Observing patient's function of elimination
  Observing the urine
  Recording and reporting observations accurately
  Practicing meticulous skin hygiene
  Providing emotional support
  Participating with the patient in the bowel and bladder retraining program

REVIEW QUESTIONS

1. List the normal and unusual observations you might make when patients empty their bladder.
2. What care will you give to the patient who is incontinent?
3. Describe the difference in catheter care for females and males.
4. How is a clean-catch urine specimen collected?

ACTIVITY CORNER

How many times in a day do you void?
Recall a 24-hour period and check the times when you voided:

_____ First thing in the morning

_____ After breakfast

_____ Midmorning

_____ After lunch

_____ Midafternoon

_____ After dinner

_____ Evening

_____ At bedtime

_____ During the night

Most people follow a routine similar to yours. Thus your patients may need help with toileting at similar times. Be ready to help your patients at these times.

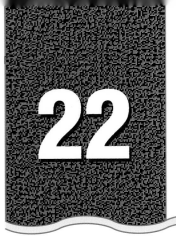

22 Learning About Human Reproduction

Objectives

AFTER YOU COMPLETE THIS CHAPTER, YOU WILL BE ABLE TO:

Identify the structure and function of the reproductive organs in males and females.

Discuss the physical and psychologic changes that occur during pregnancy.

Give a vaginal douche.

Care for patients with a vaginal infection, breast cancer, or benign prostatic hyperplasia.

Identify the sexually transmitted diseases.

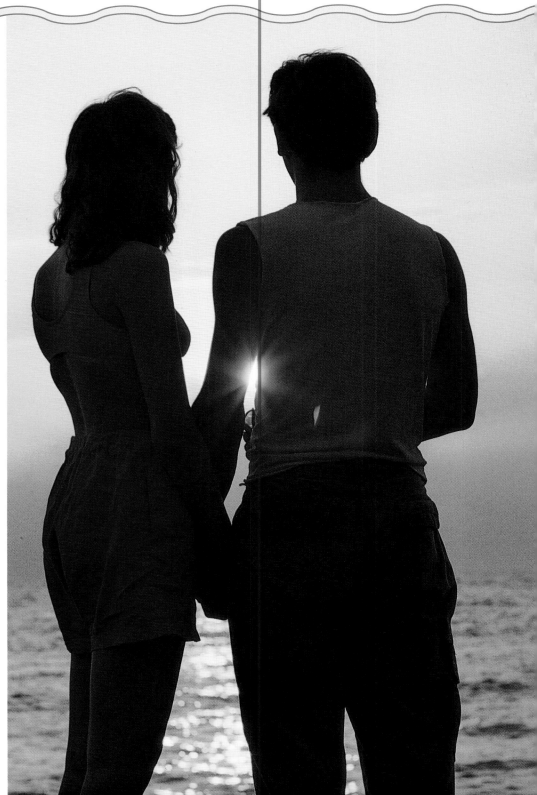

Overview A new life begins with a sperm and an egg. These join and multiply to become a fetus (an unborn baby). The miracle of birth depends on the correct functioning of the reproductive organs of the male and female.

As a nursing assistant, you care for patients who have experienced childbirth. You also provide care for patients with a disruption in the functioning of their reproductive organs. A great deal of satisfaction can be found in caring for these patients.

WHAT DO YOU KNOW ABOUT THE ORGANS OF REPRODUCTION?

Here are four statements about human reproduction. Consider them to test your current knowledge of how human life is created. If you think the statement is true, circle the T; if you think the statement is false, circle the F. Change the false statements to make them true.

1. T   F   The menstrual cycle averages 28–30 days.
2. T   F   Pregnancy is divided into 4 trimesters.
3. T   F   Acquired immune deficiency syndrome (AIDS) is transmitted only during sexual intercourse.
4. T   F   Breast cancer occurs only in females.

ANSWERS

1. **True.** The usual menstrual cycle averages 28–30 days.
2. **False.** Human pregnancy is divided into 3 trimesters.
3. **False.** AIDS can be transmitted through the use of contaminated needles or through contact with infected blood and/or body fluids. A pregnant female who has AIDS can transmit the disease to her fetus. The AIDS virus can also be transmitted during a blood transfusion, if screening procedures on the blood sample fail.
4. **False.** Breast cancer can occur in males as well as females.

EXTERNAL
outside
LABIA MAJORA
long outside folds of skin surrounding the urinary meatus and vagina in females
LABIA MINORA
small folds of skin inside the labia majora and surrounding the vaginal opening in females
CLITORIS
small organ with many nerve endings that make it sensitive to sexual arousal in females
VAGINAL OPENING
opening located between the urinary meatus and the anus in females

INTERNAL
inside
VAGINA
the canal from the cervix to the vaginal opening that stretches during intercourse and childbirth
CERVIX
birth canal; opens to allow passage of the fetus from the uterus to the vagina during childbirth
UTERUS
the womb; pear-shaped organ located above the cervix in the pelvic region of females; expands and contracts during pregnancy
FALLOPIAN TUBES
tubes located on each side of the uterus that help move the ovum from the ovary to the uterus
OVARIES
egg-shaped organs located on each side of the uterus in females; produce ovum and hormones
HORMONE
a substance that endocrine glands secrete directly into the circulating blood; the hormone travels to a designated place in the body where it is used in a chemical action
ESTROGEN
female sex hormone
PROGESTERONE
hormone that plays a major part in menstruation

STRUCTURE AND FUNCTION OF THE FEMALE REPRODUCTIVE ORGANS

EXTERNAL ORGANS

The following are the **external** organs of the female reproductive system (Figure 22–1).

- **Labia majora**—long outside folds of skin surrounding the urinary meatus and vagina in females; also known as the "outer lips."
- **Labia minora**—small folds of skin inside the labia majora and surrounding the vaginal opening; also known as the "inner lips."
- **Clitoris**—small organ with many nerve endings that make it sensitive to sexual arousal.
- **Vaginal opening**—an opening located between the urinary meatus (opening) and the anus.

INTERNAL ORGANS

The **internal** organs of the female reproductive system include the (Figure 22–2):

- **Vagina**—the canal from the cervix to the vaginal opening that stretches during intercourse and childbirth.
- **Cervix**—opens to allow the fetus to pass from the uterus to the vagina; the birth canal.
- **Uterus**—the womb; stretches during pregnancy to make room for the growing fetus.
- **Fallopian tubes**—one tube on each side of the uterus that helps move the female ovum (egg) from the ovary to the uterus.
- **Ovaries**—one on each side of the lower abdomen, produce the ovum as well as the female **hormones estrogen** and **progesterone.**

A hormone is a substance secreted by endocrine glands directly into the circulating blood—the hormone travels to a designated place in the body where a chemical action takes place.

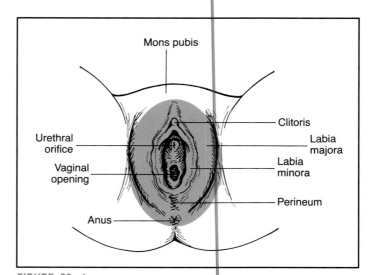

FIGURE 22–1
External organs of the female reproductive system.

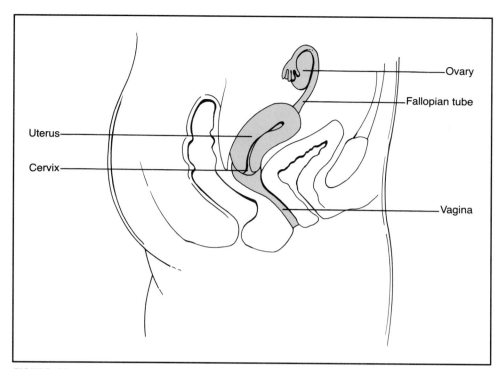

FIGURE 22-2
Internal organs of the female reproductive system.

STRUCTURE AND FUNCTION OF THE MALE ORGANS OF REPRODUCTION

EXTERNAL ORGANS

The following are the external male organs of reproduction (Figure 22-3).

- **Penis**—organ made of erectile (capable of becoming upright and hard) tissue. The glans penis (head of the penis) may be covered in some males with a loose hood of skin known as the foreskin. The removal of the foreskin is called **circumcision;** the procedure is often performed soon after birth. The penis contains the male **urethra,** which is used for the passage of both urine and sperm to the outside.
- **Scrotum**—the pouch that contains the testicles and helper organs. It is suspended behind and below the penis.

INTERNAL ORGANS

The following are the internal male organs of reproduction (Figure 22-3).

- **Testicles**—the two organs inside the scrotum that produce sperm. They also produce a male hormone called **testosterone.**
- **Duct system** (vas deferens)—small tubes that connect the testicles with the urethra so that sperm can move from inside to outside the body.

Sperm are male cells that join with the female ovum to produce a new individual. The **semen** (fluid from the helper gland) combines with the sperm from the testicles to move to the outside. Glands in the male secrete fluids that carry sperm through the urethra. The **prostate gland** is one of these glands. It is located below the bladder and surrounds the urethra.

PENIS
external organ of urination and copulation in males

CIRCUMCISION
removal of the male foreskin

URETHRA
tube that carries urine from the bladder to the outside of the body

SCROTUM
the pouch (sac) that contains the testicles and their accessory organs in males

TESTICLE
organ of the male reproductive tract that is located in the scrotum and produces sperm

TESTOSTERONE
an important male sex hormone

DUCT SYSTEM
small tubes that connect the testicles with the urethra in the male reproductive system and provide the route for sperm to reach the outside of the male's body

SPERM
the male cell that joins with the female ovum to produce a new individual

PROSTATE GLAND
the gland in males that surrounds the urethra and the neck of the bladder and secretes fluid that helps sperm move through the duct system

SEMEN
the fluid that helps sperm move through the duct system in males

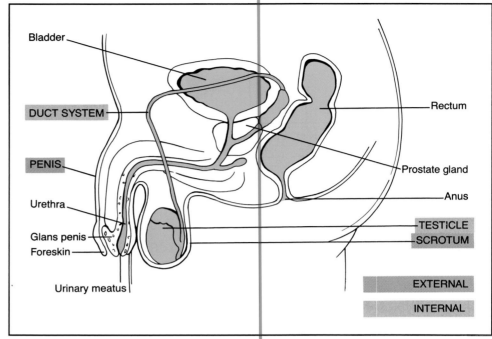

FIGURE 22-3

External and internal male reproductive organs.

FEMALE REPRODUCTIVE DEVELOPMENT

PUBERTY

the developmental and physical changes that result in adult sexual characteristics and the ability to reproduce

SECONDARY SEXUAL CHARACTERISTICS

changes in males and females that occur with puberty

MENSTRUATION

the discharge through the vagina of blood and tissue from the uterus of the nonpregnant female; also known as menses, monthly flow, and period

IMPLANTATION

the attachment of the fertilized egg to the uterine wall

MENOPAUSE

the changes that end the female's ability to bear children; also called climacteric and change of life

PREMENSTRUAL SYNDROME

symptoms including irritability, water weight gain, and breast enlargement and tenderness that occur in the female before menstruation

Reproductive development in the female begins at puberty. **Puberty** is the time of physical and developmental changes that result in adult sexual characteristics and the ability to reproduce. Hormone changes in the female begin the process. Although the rate of development during puberty varies from individual to individual, the changes that occur are the same in all females:

- secretion of hormones that prepare the ovaries, uterus, and vagina for reproduction
- appearance of **secondary sexual characteristics**, including (Figure 22–4)
    broadening of the hips
    enlargement of the breasts
    appearance of pubic and axillary (underarm) hair
- beginning of **menstruation**

During puberty, the ovaries begin to make the hormone estrogen, and the ova (eggs) begin to develop. The vagina's inner lining thickens. The uterus increases in size and weight, and an increase in the blood supply to the uterus also occurs.

These changes typically begin around the age of 11 or 12. Menstruation (also called menses and period) often occurs around this age, although some girls start to menstruate earlier and some start later. Menstruation is the discharge through the vagina of blood and tissue from the uterus of a nonpregnant female. Menstruation readies the uterus for pregnancy.

If **implantation** does not occur, the cycle begins again with the menstrual phase. The bleeding part of the cycle occurs an average of every 28–30 days. The menstrual flow (bleeding) lasts approximately 5–7 days. The menstrual cycle continues in a female's life until **menopause** (also called climacteric and change of life) occurs.

About 25% of all women who menstruate experience **premenstrual syn-**

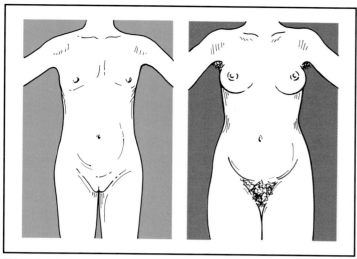

FIGURE 22-4

Secondary sex characteristics in the female include growth of hair under the arms and in the pubic area, enlargement of the breasts, and widening of the hips.

drome (PMS). PMS is believed to be caused by the changing levels of hormone (estrogen and progesterone) in the body. A woman who has PMS may experience its symptoms just before menstruation begins or during the early part of the menstrual cycle. Common symptoms of PMS are

- weight gain
- breast enlargement and tenderness
- abdominal bloating
- headache and backache
- increased appetite
- changes in behavior (mood swings, crying, depression, irritability, and difficulty sleeping)

MALE REPRODUCTIVE DEVELOPMENT

The development of the male reproductive organs, like that of the female's, begins during puberty. Changes in the male include

- appearance of secondary sexual characteristics, including (Figure 22-5)
    axillary hair
    pubic hair
    facial hair
- growth of the penis and scrotum, which becomes wrinkled and darker in color
- sperm production
- testosterone production
- ability to have and maintain an erection

HUMAN REPRODUCTION

Reproduction is the process by which a new individual is produced. Human reproduction begins with the healthy functioning of the male and female reproductive systems. **Conception** is the term used to describe the moment that the human ovum in the female is joined by the male sperm. Another term for conception is **fertilization.** The fertilization process requires very precise timing.

REPRODUCTION

the process by which a new individual is produced

CONCEPTION

the joining of the ovum and the sperm; fertilization

FERTILIZATION

joining of the ovum and the sperm; conception

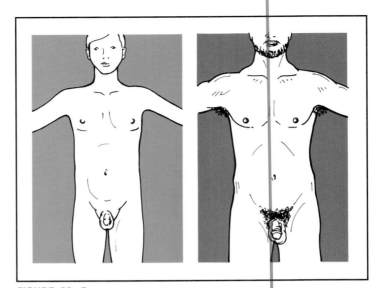

FIGURE 22-5

Secondary sex characteristics in the male include growth of axillary, pubic, and facial hair.

The sperm live only 24–72 hours, and the ovum lives only 24 hours once it is released from the ovary. A large number of sperm are produced, but only one is needed to fertilize the ovum.

Sperm are ejected through the male's urethra into the female's vagina during **intercourse.** When sperm enter the female body, they travel to the fallopian tube. If everything is functioning correctly, as soon as one sperm meets the ovum in the fallopian tubes, fertilization occurs. The fallopian tubes, which are built partially of muscle, contract and move the now fertilized ovum into the uterus.

The fertilized ovum must then attach itself to the lining of the uterus; this is called implantation. After implantation occurs, finger-like projections form. These finger-like projections form the **placenta.** The placenta is important because it performs the following functions for the fetus:

1. Supplies oxygen.
2. Supplies nutrients.
3. Removes fetal waste products.

Gestation is the period of development of the human from the time of conception until birth. The developing human is called an **embryo** from the time of fertilization until the second month. **Fetus** is the term used to refer to the developing individual in the uterus from the second month of pregnancy until birth. As it develops and grows in the uterus, the fetus is surrounded by a special fluid. This fluid, called **amniotic fluid,** performs the following functions:

1. Protects the fetus.
2. Helps control the temperature of the fetus.
3. Allows the fetus to move in the uterus.

PREGNANCY

Pregnancy is the presence of a developing embryo or fetus in a woman's body (Figure 22–6). Pregnancy is a normal event for the female; many pregnant women feel healthy and able to work throughout the 9 months of pregnancy. Physical as well as psychologic changes occur in the pregnant female. Many tests exist to confirm a woman's pregnancy. A home pregnancy test kit may be

INTERCOURSE

sexual contact between individuals

PLACENTA

forms at the site where the fertilized egg implants; provides the fetus with essential nutrients and oxygen and carries away the fetus's waste products

GESTATION

the period that starts with fertilization of the ovum and ends at birth

EMBRYO

the developing human from fertilization until the second month

FETUS

the developing human in the uterus, from the second month of pregnancy to birth

AMNIOTIC FLUID

fluid in the uterus that surrounds the fetus, protecting it from injury, allowing it to move, and maintaining its temperature

PREGNANCY

the presence of a developing embryo or fetus within a woman's body

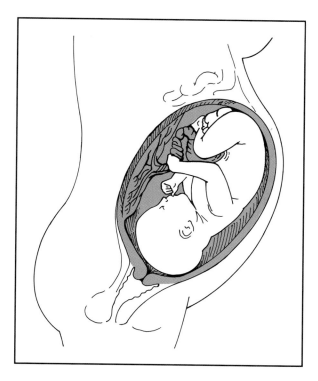

FIGURE 22-6
Side view of the developing fetus.

used, or a blood study or sonogram may be performed in the physician's office. A **sonogram** is a test that uses sound waves to make a picture of the organ being studied.

Pregnancy is divided into three distinct time periods known as trimesters. Each trimester covers 3 months of the normal 9-month pregnancy:

- **first trimester**—first–third months
- **second trimester**—fourth–sixth months
- **third trimester**—seventh–ninth months

PHYSICAL CHANGES

The most easily noticed change that occurs during pregnancy is the enlarging abdomen. This is caused by the increasing size of the uterus. The increasing size of the uterus places increased pressure on the woman's lungs and bladder. The pressure on the bladder can cause frequency and urgency in urination. Breast enlargement occurs during pregnancy because the woman's body is readying itself to provide a milk supply for the baby after birth. The mother's **pulse** rate may also increase slightly, although her blood pressure normally remains the same.

Early in pregnancy, the woman may experience **nausea** and **vomiting**. This is known as morning sickness. Later in pregnancy, **heartburn, constipation,** and **hemorrhoids** may occur. Edema (swelling) of the lower extremities may occur. The total amount of weight gained during pregnancy varies from woman to woman. Generally, the woman gains about 30–35 pounds.

PSYCHOLOGIC CHANGES

The psychologic changes begin in the first trimester of the pregnancy. The expectant mother may deny that she is pregnant. She may express the feeling that the pregnancy is not real. She begins to look for body changes that tell her

SONOGRAM
a test that uses sound waves to make a picture of an organ

PULSE
the beat of the heart as felt through the walls of the arteries
NAUSEA
an unpleasant, uncomfortable feeling in the stomach; may be experienced with vomiting
VOMIT
to eject material from the stomach through the mouth
HEARTBURN
a burning sensation in the area of the heart or the esophagus
CONSTIPATION
inability to have or difficulty in having a bowel movement
HEMORRHOID
an enlarged (swollen) vein located inside or just outside the rectum

she is indeed pregnant. During the second trimester, the fetus becomes more real to the mother, and she refers to it as the "baby." This is the time period during which the fetus begins to move and the mother realizes that motherhood is approaching. She may begin to shop for baby items as part of the preparation for the approaching birth. She now needs to wear maternity clothes to accommodate the increasing size of her abdomen. During the third trimester, the mother focuses on getting ready for the birth of the baby. A name is selected for the baby boy or girl. The mother may begin to be anxious about the birth and fearful of the pain. The mother may experience a surge of energy just before the birth occurs.

Psychologic changes may also occur in the mother during the **postpartum period.** The mother may experience depression (known as the postpartum blues). Her body is experiencing the physical changes that occur after the birth of a baby, and she may feel overwhelmed and exhausted after the birth. The new mother who is experiencing postpartum depression should be under the care of a physician.

STAGES OF LABOR

Labor is the series of muscle contractions that expel the fetus from the body. There are three stages of labor.

FIRST STAGE The first stage begins with regular **contractions** of the uterine muscles. The contractions help move the fetus out of the uterus and through the birth canal (the vagina). During this stage, the cervix thins out and opens to 10 centimeters to allow passage of the fetus. This opening of the cervix is called **dilation.**

SECOND STAGE The second stage of labor begins when the cervix has dilated to 10 centimeters. The fetus then begins its movement down through the expanding birth canal. The second stage of labor ends when the baby is delivered.

THIRD STAGE The third stage consists of the time needed for the placenta (afterbirth) to be expelled from the uterus.

When the fetus is in distress, the physician may decide to deliver the baby surgically. The surgical procedure is known as a **cesarean section.** In most cesarean sections, the mother receives a spinal anesthetic (medication injected into the spinal cord to block pain impulses); she remains awake and alert but cannot move the lower part of her body.

When the baby is born, he or she is examined, weighed, measured, and given to the mother to hold. The mother (if she is able), father (or significant other), and newborn baby are given time together to begin the bonding process. **Bonding** is creating an emotional tie. It begins with a period of close contact between the mother and the newborn in the first few hours after birth.

If the mother chooses to breastfeed her baby, breastfeeding begins as soon after birth as possible. The alternative to breastfeeding is to feed the baby prepared formula from a bottle. Whether breastfed or bottle fed the baby also receives water from a bottle.

DISRUPTIONS OF THE REPRODUCTIVE SYSTEM

VAGINAL INFECTION

Vaginal infection is a common disruption of the female reproductive system. Vaginal infection is also known as **vaginitis.** There are many causes of vaginitis.

POSTPARTUM
the first 6–10 weeks after the birth of the infant, in reference to the mother

LABOR
the series of muscle contractions that expel the fetus from the body
CONTRACTION
shortening or tightening of muscle fiber
DILATION
widening

CESAREAN SECTION
the delivery of the fetus through an abdominal incision

BONDING
creating an emotional tie with a mate or a newborn

VAGINITIS
inflammation of the vagina; a vaginal infection

One cause is sexual intercourse with an infected partner. During the sexual act, the **microorganisms** that cause an infection are transmitted from the male to the female. Poor **hygiene** is another cause. For example, after a bowel movement, the female may be wiping from the rectal area toward the vagina, a back to front wiping motion. Bacteria that are present in the stool or rectal area are thus brought into the vagina area. **Note:** T*he proper direction for female cleansing is front to back.*

Inadequate cleansing of the **perineal area** during bathing can also cause problems. Thorough cleansing of the perineal area is needed to remove all waste material and prevent the spread of infection.

Changes that occur with age, vaginal dryness, and changes in the **acidity** of vaginal fluid are three other possible causes of vaginitis. The normal balance of acidity in the vagina can be upset by frequent use of a **douche**. This upset in the balance can lead to an overgrowth of bacteria.

Common Observations of Vaginal Infection

The woman with a vaginal infection may say that her vaginal secretions

- are a different color
- smell
- are thicker
- have increased in amount

She may further report itching or burning in the vaginal area. Any combination of these observations can exist. Report your observations to the nurse.

Caring for the Patient with a Vaginal Infection

The care of the patient with vaginitis may include the use of medications and medicated douches. You may be asked to give a douche when one is ordered by the physician. (A douche may also be ordered for reasons other than vaginal infection, for example, for cleansing before certain surgeries.) A douche is a stream of water that is directed toward a body cavity to provide a cleansing action. In a vaginal douche, a stream of cleansing solution is introduced into the vagina and allowed to flow out into a bedpan. The solution loosens debris and drains it from the vagina.

A **sitz bath** is a comfort measure that can relieve the itching that accompanies a vaginal infection. As a nursing assistant, you can help the patient with a sitz bath. You should provide proper perineal care to the patient who is unable to care for herself (see Chapter 13).

MICROORGANISM

an organism so tiny it can be seen only under a microscope; capable of helping the body as well as causing disease

HYGIENE

the practice of cleanliness to promote health

PERINEAL AREA

the area between the legs, including the genitals and anus

ACIDITY

having extra acid

DOUCHE

the introduction of a fluid into the vagina for the purpose of cleansing or medical treatment

SITZ BATH

placing the hips and buttocks in water to relieve pain and discomfort of organs in the perineal area

PROCEDURE

Giving a Vaginal Douche (Nonsterile)

GATHER EQUIPMENT

Prepackaged douche kit
Cleansing solution as directed by the nurse
Cotton balls
Bath blanket
Waterproof pad

Disposable gloves (two pairs, if needed)
Washcloth
Towel
Basin of warm water
Peri-care kit
Plastic bag
Bedpan

Continued on following page

PROCEDURE

Giving a Vaginal Douche (Nonsterile) *Continued*

ACTION	RATIONALE
Preparation	
1. Wash hands.	Prevents the spread of microorganisms.
2. Identify yourself and the patient.	Maintains patients' rights.
3. Provide privacy.	Maintains patients' rights.
4. Explain procedure.	Informs patients what is happening.
Procedural Steps	
5. Offer the bedpan to the patient before beginning the douche and encourage her to empty her bladder. (Wear gloves if the patient uses the bedpan.)	A douche is more effective when the bladder is empty.
6. Empty the bedpan and prepare it for the next use. Discard the gloves.	
7. Wash hands.	Prevents contamination after handling body wastes.
8. Place the patient in the **supine** position. Put the waterproof pad under the patient's buttocks and ask her to flex her knees. The feet should be placed shoulder-width apart on the bed.	The supine position allows the solution to flow into the vagina. The waterproof pad protects the bed linens.
9. Drape the patient with the bath blanket and put on disposable gloves.	Provides warmth and privacy for the patient.
10. Place the patient on the bedpan.	The bedpan collects the returning solution.
11. Cleanse the perineal area according to the procedure suggested by your health care institution. Soap and water as well as disinfecting solutions may be used. To cleanse the perineum, use cotton balls and • always wipe from front to back • use a clean cotton ball for each stroke • cleanse the labia majora and then use your thumb and forefinger to separate the labia majora • and cleanse the labia minora • place used cotton balls in the plastic bag for disposal	Removes surface debris. Prevents possible infection. Prevents contamination of the vagina or the urinary meatus by fecal material.
12. Prepare solution and test for a temperature of 105° F. Use a bath thermometer to measure the water temperature.	A solution that is too hot can injure the lining of the vagina.
13. Remove the cover over the **elongated** tip of the douche container.	
14. Start the flow of solution by releasing the clamp before you begin to insert the tip of the douche container into the vagina. Allow the solution to flow into the bedpan. Clamp off.	Removes air so that less air enters the vagina. Air causes discomfort and may interfere with the flow of water.
15. Tell the patient you are about to insert the douche tip.	Alerts the patient to what is happening.

SUPINE
lying with the face up; lying on one's back

ELONGATED
lengthened

16. Insert the tip about 3–4 inches into the vagina and release the clamp to start the flow.

17. Rotate the tip several times.   Allows fluid to reach all parts of the vagina.

18. Use all the solution, allowing it to run out into the bedpan.   Blocking the flow can injure vaginal tissue.

19. Remove the douche tip from the vagina.

20. Help the patient to a sitting position on the bedpan.   Allows the remaining fluid to drain out of the vagina.

21. Place the empty douche container into the plastic bag.   Prevents the spread of microorganisms.

22. Ask the patient to lie down. Remove the bedpan from under the patient.

23. Wash the perineal area with the washcloth. Rinse and dry it.   Provides skin care and prevents injury from irritating solutions.

24. Remove the waterproof pad and dispose of it correctly.

25. Assist the patient to a comfortable position.

26. Observe the douche solution in the bedpan. Note its consistency, color, and odor.   Your observations help the nurse and physician plan the patient's care.

27. Discard the used douche solution according to the procedure of your health care institution.

28. Remove and discard the soiled gloves into the plastic bag. Dispose of the bag that contains the soiled materials according to your health care institution's procedure.

Follow-Through

29. Wash hands.   Prevents the spread of microorganisms.

30. Place the call signal within the patient's reach.   Allows the patient to communicate her needs.

31. Record and report to the nurse that you have completed the douche and note the time. Include appropriate observations and patient response to the douche administration. Report the presence of
    • inflammation around the vaginal opening
    • odor or discharge from the vagina

CARING COMMENTS

Make sure you give proper perineal care to your female patient. Perineal care is discussed in Chapter 13.

A **fracture bedpan** is more comfortable for the patient who is receiving a douche because it is not as high as a regular bedpan. However, a fracture bedpan should not be used for large amounts of solution because it is smaller than a regular bedpan and holds less.

FRACTURE BEDPAN

a small bedpan that slides easily under the hips, generally used for patients with a hip fracture

DISRUPTIONS IN REPRODUCTIVE FUNCTIONING

BREAST CANCER

CANCER
a disease in which certain cells of the body change into nonfunctioning cells and grow and crowd out healthy functioning cells

NULLIPARITY
never having experienced pregnancy

MAMMOGRAM
x-ray of the breast

BIOPSY
removal of living tissue and examination of it under a microscope

LUMPECTOMY
removal of a lump from body tissue, commonly the female breast

MASTECTOMY
surgical removal of the breast

Breast **cancer** is the most common type of cancer in women in the United States. Men can also develop breast cancer. The following risk factors place a woman at risk for developing breast cancer:

- family history of breast cancer (for example, mother or sister)
- history of previous breast disease
- menstrual period that started before the age of 12
- menopause (when menstrual periods stop) after the age of 50
- **nulliparity** or having borne the first child after the age of 30

Breast cancer may occur in the ducts or the lobes of the breast. It is very important for women to perform a breast self-examination (BSE) about 7–10 days after the menstrual period ends (Figure 22–7). A woman can do a BSE while in the shower. She moves the flat part of her fingers over every part of each breast. While doing this, she feels for lumps, hard knotty places, and thickening. When BSE is performed regularly, a woman is more familiar with the way her breast tissue feels and thus will notice any change very quickly.

Another way to screen for the presence of cancer in the breast is for the woman to have a **mammogram.** A first mammogram should be done between the ages of 35 and 40 so it can serve as a baseline against which later mammograms can be compared. After the age of 50, a woman should have a yearly mammogram to detect lumps that cannot be palpated (felt) during a BSE.

When a lump, hard knot, thickening, or any change is noticed, the physician may order a **biopsy** of the affected area of breast tissue.

The treatment for breast cancer is surgery. The two most common kinds of surgery for breast cancer are

- **Lumpectomy**—The surgeon removes only the cancerous tissue from the breast.
- **Mastectomy**—The surgeon may remove any combination of breast tissue and supporting muscles. The entire breast or only a portion of it may be removed.

Caring for a Patient After Surgery for Breast Cancer

You should make the observations of the postoperative patient discussed in Chapter 26. In addition, you should be aware of the psychologic effect the loss of breast tissue has on a woman. The female breast is a symbol of motherhood and sexual attractiveness.

After a mastectomy, a woman may have a feeling of loss and a change in her self-image. The woman of childbearing age may need to change her plans for bearing children in some instances. The sense of loss associated with the inability to have children may be very acute and painful.

Concern about appearance is common. In some women, further surgery may be performed to reconstruct (rebuild) the breast tissue or implant a prosthesis so that the shape and size of both breasts match. However, not all women are candidates for such surgery. Another option, after healing, is a prosthesis that can be fitted and worn in a brassiere. Prostheses are available in many shapes and sizes, and wearing one can allow a woman to look normal again.

A woman is also concerned about acceptance by her husband or other male partner. She may view the scar as ugly or as a reminder that the surgery mutilated (maimed) her. Because of this, she may feel rejected and sexually unattractive. Her self-image as a sexually attractive person is changed.

4. Move around the breast in a set way. You can choose either the circle (*A*), the up and down line (*B*), or the wedge (*C*). Do it the same way every time. It will help you to make sure that you've gone over the entire breast area, and to remember how your breast feels each month.

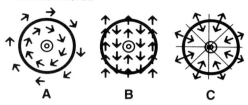

A   B   C

How To Do BSE

1. Lie down and put a pillow under your right shoulder. Place your right arm behind your head.

2. Use the finger pads of the three middle fingers on your left hand to feel for lumps or thickening. Your fingers pads are the top third of each finger.

5. Now examine your left breast using right hand finger pads.

You might want to check your breasts while standing in front of a mirror right after you do your BSE each month. You might also want to do an extra BSE while you're in the shower. Your soapy hands will glide over the wet skin, making it easy to check how your breasts feel.

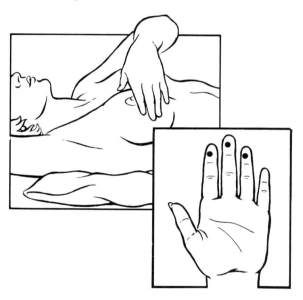

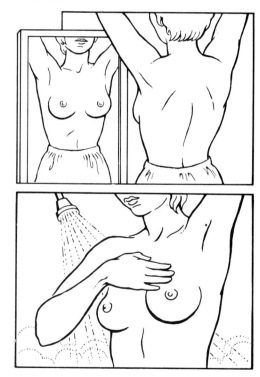

3. Press hard enough to know how your breast feels. If you're not sure how hard to press, ask your health care provider. Or try to copy the way your health care provider uses the finger pads during a breast exam. Learn what your breast feels like most of the time. A firm ridge in the lower curve of each breast is normal.

FIGURE 22–7

Performing a breast self-examination. (Courtesy of the American Cancer Society.)

As you can see, a woman who has had surgery for breast cancer has many feelings about the changes in her body. She needs continued acceptance and support from family and friends after discharge from the hospital.

CARING COMMENT

You should listen to the patient and offer your support. Report any information to the nurse or your supervisor so that steps can be taken to secure more help for the patient before she is discharged from the health care institution.

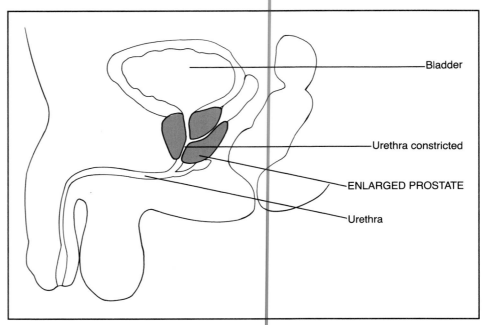

FIGURE 22-8

The prostate gland enlarges around the urethra and interferes with the man's ability to void.

PROSTATE ENLARGEMENT

As already discussed, the prostate gland is located below the bladder and surrounds the urethra in the male (see Figure 22-3). This gland commonly enlarges in males after the age of 50. The cause of the enlargement may be due to changes in male hormone levels. The medical term for this enlargement is **benign prostatic hyperplasia (BPH)** (Figure 22-8).

BENIGN PROSTATIC HYPERPLASIA
enlargement of the prostate gland

Common Observations of Benign Prostatic Hyperplasia

The observations associated with the male patient who has BPH are subjective. The patient may report the following changes:

- a decrease in the flow of urine
- a dribbling of urine instead of a steady stream
- hesitancy (difficulty in starting the flow of urine)

URINE RETENTION
accumulation of urine in the bladder because of the inability to urinate

Urine may remain in the bladder; this is called **urine retention.** When urine remains in the bladder for a long period of time, a urinary tract infection may occur because this environment (warm and dark) encourages the growth of bacteria. If the patient is not able to empty his bladder, the urine may back up and damage the function of the kidneys.

Caring for the Patient with Benign Prostatic Hyperplasia

CATHETER
a flexible tube passed into body openings to allow fluids to enter or exit the body

PROSTATECTOMY
surgical removal of the prostate gland

For the patient with BPH who has urinary retention, an indwelling urinary **catheter** is inserted by the physician or nurse (see Chapter 21). The indwelling catheter allows the urine to drain freely and decreases the risk of complications. Diagnostic studies may be made on the kidneys to ensure they are functioning normally. A patient may require the surgical procedure called **prostatectomy.** During a prostatectomy, the prostate gland is removed. When caring for a patient following a prostatectomy, you should

- Observe the catheter drainage; the drainage changes from red to pink in 24 hours.
- Observe for blood clots/red streaks in the urinary catheter. Blood clots can indicate increased bleeding.
- Report to the nurse immediately if the urine becomes more bloody (red) than the color you observed at the beginning of your care of the patient.
- Observe for body temperature increases; a fever may indicate an infection.
- *Never* use the rectal route to measure body temperature.
- Do not pull or put tension on the catheter and/or drainage tubing.
- Help the patient with activities of daily living according to his needs.
- Place the patient in a comfortable position.

CARING COMMENT

The urinary drainage in the male after prostate surgery is very bloody. The patient may be frightened when he sees the bloody drainage in the collection bag. You can listen to the patient and tell the nurse about his concerns. You should check with the nurse so that you know what color the urinary drainage should be during your shift.

PROSTATE CANCER

As a man ages, he is at increased risk for developing cancer of the prostate gland. The **tumor** is usually slow growing. The enlarged gland can be palpated (felt) by the physician during a digital examination of the rectum (a gloved finger inserted into the rectum). There are no symptoms at first; however, as the gland enlarges, the patient may have the following problems with urinating:

TUMOR
growth of tissue

- a decrease in the force of the urinary stream
- frequent urination
- a feeling that the bladder is not empty
- frequent voiding during the night
- blood in the urine

The treatment of prostate cancer depends on the kind of tumor that is present. The nurse or supervisor gives you information on how to care for the patient with prostate cancer. Listen to the patient and report the patient's concerns and feelings to the nurse or supervisor.

TESTICULAR CANCER

Cancer of the testicles occurs in men ages 20–30. The patient may notice

- an enlarged scrotum
- a feeling of fullness or pain in the scrotum
- breasts that are enlarged and painful

The physician can feel the tumor in the scrotum. The treatment depends on the kind of tumor present. The nurse or supervisor directs you in the care of the patient with testicular cancer. Patients are often concerned with their sexual function and whether or not they can father a child. When the patient talks about these concerns, take the time to listen. Be sure to report the patient's concerns to the nurse or supervisor.

SEXUALLY TRANSMITTED DISEASES

CONDOM

a sheath worn over the penis that decreases the risk of transmitting or contracting sexually transmitted diseases and has limited value in preventing pregnancy

Sexually transmitted diseases (STDs) are diseases that are acquired by participating in sexual acts with an infected partner. There are more than 20 diseases that can be transmitted in this manner (Table 22–1).

Certain behaviors put an individual at risk for acquiring an STD. These behaviors include having multiple sex partners, engaging in potentially risky sexual acts such as anal or oral sex, and not using a **condom.**

CARING COMMENT

A condom is a sheath worn over the penis. It is intended to decrease the risk of acquiring an STD. Condoms may also be used to prevent the male's sperm from entering the female's vagina and cervix. As is the case with most other forms of birth control, the use of condoms for birth control is not 100% effective.

The following are behaviors that lower an individual's risk for acquiring an STD:

- limiting the number of sexual partners
- using condoms (Figure 22–9)
- abstaining from sex (having no sexual activity)

TABLE 22–1 COMMON SEXUALLY TRANSMITTED DISEASES

ACQUIRED IMMUNE DEFICIENCY SYNDROME (AIDS)

the advanced stage of an infection by the human immunodeficiency virus, which destroys the cells of the immune system

ANTIVIRAL

an agent effective against viruses

KAPOSI'S SARCOMA

a rare form of skin cancer, associated with acquired immune deficiency syndrome

PNEUMOCYSTIS PNEUMONIA

a lung infection, associated with acquired immune deficiency syndrome

HERPES SIMPLEX

a virus that causes redness, swelling, itching, pain, and pimple-like lesions that open and crust over in the genitals

PELVIC INFLAMMATORY DISEASE

disease of the female reproductive organs

PUBIC LICE

small insects that live in pubic hair

Disease	Observations	Treatment
Acquired immune deficiency syndrome (AIDS)*	**Males and females** Vague flu-like symptoms: • fever • fatigue • weakness • cough • weight loss Symptoms of other diseases: • **Kaposi's sarcoma** • **Pneumocystis pneumonia** Increased susceptibility to infections from others	Incurable **Antiviral** drugs Treatment of symptoms
Herpes simplex (genital)	**Males and females** Genital redness and edema, along with itching and pain Pimple-like lesions that open and crust over and last about 3 weeks Recurrent Possibly flu-like symptoms	Incurable Antiviral drugs Treatment for pain Keep lesions clean and dry Use of condoms to prevent direct contact with the lesions
Pelvic inflammatory disease	**Females** Abdominal pain and tenderness Fever Vaginal discharge	Anti-infective drugs
Pubic lice	**Males and females** Redness and itching in the genital area	Special cream or lotion applied to the affected area Avoid direct contact

Disease	Observations	Treatment
	Possible presence of other sexually transmitted diseases	Avoid direct contact with clothing or linens
Gonorrhea	**Dysuria** *Males* Penile discharge *Females* Usually no symptoms A few have vaginal discharge Possible progression to pelvic infection	Anti-infective drugs
Syphilis	**Males and females** *Early stage* Chancre (sore) appears where organisms enter the body 9 days–3 months after infection Sore heals in a few weeks; the disease seems to disappear Early stage lasts 2–6 weeks *Middle stage* Begins 2–6 months after the early sore disappears; can last up to 2 years The disease may disappear by itself Low-grade fever Sore throat Headache Painful joints Rash	Anti-infective drugs, usually given by intramuscular injection, will cure syphilis in the early and middle stages
	Late stage May begin after the middle stage is complete or may remain hidden for up to 15 years If untreated, lesions occur throughout the internal organs of the body May be fatal if the heart or central nervous system is invaded If the infection involves the eyes, blindness can develop **Dementia** can occur Bones may become inflamed	Anti-infective drug, given by injection once a week for 3 weeks (given if syphilis has been present for over a year) Syphilis is more difficult to cure in the late stage

GONORRHEA
bacterial infection of the organs of reproduction and the organs of the urinary system; a sexually transmitted disease (STD)
DYSURIA
difficult or painful urination
SYPHILIS
a contagious sexually transmitted disease (STD)

DEMENTIA
changed ability to think and remember; changes in personality

* Note that AIDS may be transmitted in ways other than sexual contact.

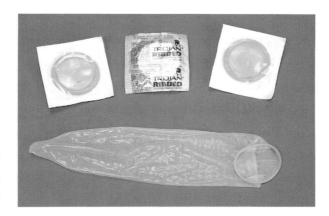

FIGURE 22–9

Condoms can be purchased in a drugstore without a prescription from a physician. Condoms may also be distributed free at some clinics and schools.

As a health care giver, you need to take actions to protect yourself from possible infection. Observations and the use of the universal precautions recommended by the Centers for Disease Control (see Chapter 11) help protect you from microorganisms that can cause infection. Use universal precautions whenever you anticipate coming into contact with drainage from body openings (vagina, penis, rectum, etc.). It is important that you wash your hands before and after any procedure you perform for a patient and that you wear gloves if drainage is present.

CARING COMMENT

STDs are spread through direct contact (usually sexual contact). Because the reason for a body drainage might not be known or patients might not suspect they have an STD, you should practice universal precautions faithfully.

CHAPTER WRAP-UP

- The female and male reproductive systems consist of external and internal organs.
- Conception is the fertilization of the ovum by the sperm. Conception occurs in the fallopian tubes. After conception, the ovum travels to the uterus and implants itself in the lining.
- Pregnancy is the presence of a growing fetus in a woman's body.
- Labor is the physiologic process of giving birth. It consists of a series of contractions of the uterine muscle, the dilation (opening) of the cervix, the movement of the fetus down the birth canal, and the delivery of the baby followed by the delivery of the placenta.
- Vaginitis is a common disruption of the female reproductive system. It is caused by a microorganism that may be transmitted to the vagina during sexual intercourse or as a result of poor hygienic care.
- A common disruption of the male reproductive system is benign prostatic hyperplasia (BPH). The treatment for BPH is surgery known as a prostatectomy.
- Sexually transmitted diseases (STDs) are diseases that are acquired through sexual contact with an infected partner. STDs can be prevented by limiting sexual contact, using condoms, and abstaining from sexual activity.

REVIEW QUESTIONS

1. Identify the internal and external organs of the female and male reproductive systems.
2. What major changes occur in the female at puberty? In the male?
3. List the physical and psychologic changes that occur in the female during pregnancy.
4. Name three ways to prevent sexually transmitted diseases.
5. What is the purpose of a douche?

6. List three observations of the male who has prostate enlargement.

7. Name six common sexually transmitted diseases.

ACTIVITY CORNER

Secretions from body openings may cause a communicable disease. How many body openings can you name?

_____

_____

_____

_____

_____

_____

_____

If you answered eyes, ears, nose, mouth, urethra, vagina, and anus, you are correct. Another correct answer is a wound that is the result of surgery or an accident.

Helping in Special Situations

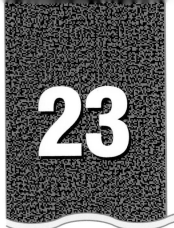

23 Admitting Patients

Objectives

AFTER YOU COMPLETE THIS CHAPTER, YOU WILL BE ABLE TO:

Describe the admission process.

Prepare a room for a newly admitted patient.

Assist with admitting a patient.

Understand the patient's and family's feelings about the patient's being admitted to a health care institution.

Assist with transferring a patient.

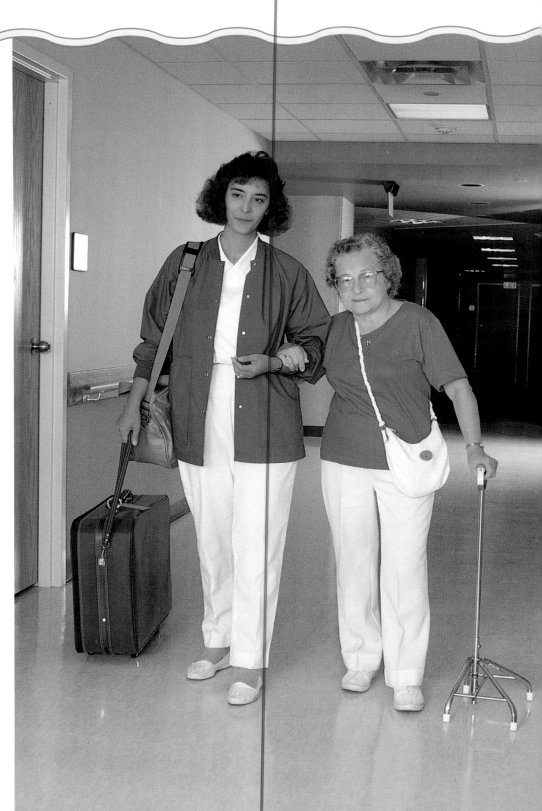

Overview Being admitted to a health care institution for care can be a frightening experience for an individual. The admitting personnel and the nurses ask the patient or a family member for a lot of information. On their first admission to a hospital, patients may be fearful of the unknown. You can help by answering their questions about their room and trying to make them feel comfortable and welcome.

WHAT DO YOU KNOW ABOUT ADMITTING A PATIENT?

Here are three statements about admitting patients to a health care institution. Consider them to test your current ideas about the admission process. If you think the statement is true, circle the T; if you think the statement is false, circle the F. Change the false statements to make them true.

1. T F Showing the patient the room and bathroom facilities is part of the admission process.

2. T F Patients receive an identification bracelet when they arrive on the nursing unit.

3. T F Patients are allowed to keep their medications in case they are needed.

ANSWERS

1. **True.** The patient needs to be oriented (shown) to the new surroundings.

2. **False.** Patients receive an identification bracelet in the admitting office or emergency room of the institution.

3. **False.** Medications are sent home with a family member or stored according to the institution's procedure. Medications are never kept in the patient's room.

ADMISSION TO A HEALTH CARE INSTITUTION

ADMISSION

letting someone or something into someplace

Admission to a health care institution is the process by which the patient enters the health care system. Admission may be planned or may be an emergency. The patient may or may not be ill or in pain. The patient may be fearful and uncomfortable about the admission. The family may have feelings of concern about their loved one. You should do everything you can to make the admission process as pleasant and comforting as possible for the patient and those who arrive with the patient.

TYPES OF ADMISSIONS

The patient may be admitted into a hospital or into a long-term care facility. A person being admitted to a hospital may be coming from any number of places:

- home if the admission is elective (planned)
- the emergency room if the admission is unexpected

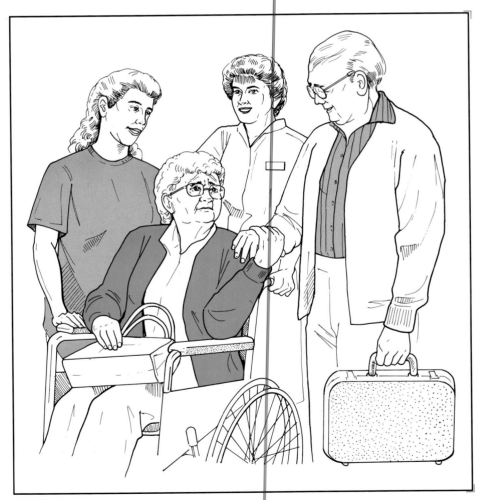

FIGURE 23–1

The patient may arrive on the unit in a wheelchair. One or more family members may accompany the patient.

- another unit in the hospital (this type of admission is also called a transfer)
- a long-term care setting

Someone being admitted to a long-term care facility may be coming from

- home if the individual needs help with self-care
- a hospital if care is needed for an injury or illness

ADMISSION PROCESS

The **admission process** begins in the admitting office or emergency room of the institution. During the admission process, the following steps are systematically performed:

- The patient is asked for information. Personnel in the admitting office or the emergency room perform this function. They question the patient or family and record the answers on the admission record. The admission record becomes a permanent part of the patient's chart. After questioning, the patient is taken to a room on the nursing unit.
- The patient is admitted to a room on the unit. The nurse performs a nursing history and a physical examination of the patient as part of the admitting process. The nursing assistant helps by orienting the patient, helping the patient unpack, and measuring the vital signs and performing any other tasks that might be assigned.
- The paperwork (consent form, intake and output record, nurses' notes, etc.) that will be used during the admission is generated.
- The patient is given information about the health care institution.

The patient receives an identification bracelet in the admitting office or in the emergency room if admitted from there. The patient arrives on the nursing unit with the identification bracelet in place.

ADMISSION PROCESS
the process by which the patient enters the health care system

ADMISSION TO THE NURSING UNIT

Care of patients begins when they are admitted to the nursing unit (Figure 23–1). The registered nurse begins the plan of care as soon as the nursing history and physical examination are completed (Figure 23–2). The physician's orders are part of the admission process. They tell the nurse and members of the health care team what diagnostic studies, medications, and diet are ordered and what activities are permitted.

When a new patient is expected, you will be told the patient's name and assigned room number. You may also be told the expected time of admission. You need to prepare for the patient's arrival.

PREPARING FOR THE PATIENT

When a new patient is expected, the room must be made ready. Getting the room ready for the patient is your responsibility. Find out the following information from the nurse:

- whether the patient is expected to arrive in a wheelchair, on a cart, or on foot
- whether any **specimens** need to be collected

SPECIMEN
sample; small piece of body tissue or secretion used for examination

9/91	LUIS RAMEZ 39 M
W.C.A. HOSPITAL	0-1-672-543
NURSING HISTORY & ASSESSMENT	DR. CHANG ROOM 601
	Addressograph

Physician: _Chang_   Date of Admission: _03-05-93_   Time: _0145_

VITAL SIGNS: T _99.8_   AP _100_   R _18_   BP _142/90_   (R) ✔   (L) _____   WT _149_   HT _5' 2"_

ADMITTED FROM: Admissions _____   E.R. _____   Direct Admit _✔_   O.R. _____

MODE: Ambulatory _____   W/C _✔_   Walker _____   Stretcher _____

HISTORY/INFORMATION OBTAINED FROM: _Patient_   RELATIONSHIP: _—_

PRESENT COMPLAINT: _Abdominal pain_

    Location: _upper right side_   Onset: _5 hours ago_   Frequency: _constant_

    Precipitating Factors: _ate 5 pieces of pizza and a lot of chocolate candy_

    Duration: _Since supper last nite_   Relief Achieved by: _Antacid doesn't help_

DNR: ( ) Yes   (✗) No   Health Care Proxy: ( ) Yes   (✗) No

ALLERGIES

DRUGS/FOODS/OTHER	REACTION
No known allergies	

PRESENT DIET: (List Restrictions): _None_

Present Appetite vs. Usual Appetite: ( )SAME   ( )BETTER   (✗)WORSE

Difficulty Swallowing: ( )YES   (✗)NO   COMMENTS: _____

Difficulty Chewing: ( )YES   (✗)NO   COMMENTS: _____

IMMUNIZATIONS: (14–18 years old)   Up-to-date: (✗)Yes   ( )No

MEDICAL HISTORY   KEY: M=Mother F=Father S=Sister B=Brother

Medical History	Self	Onset	Treatment	Family Member
Heart Disease				M
Hypertension				M
Diabetes				F
Kidney Disease				
Arthritis				M
Seizures	S	age 2	Takes Dilantin	S
Sleep Disorders				
CVA				M
Respiratory Disease				
Cancer				
Emotional Illness				
Congenital Anomalies/Handicap				
Other Serious Illnesses				

SURGERIES (List/Date): _T and A as a 5 yr. old_

SMOKING: (✗)No   ( )Yes   Amount _____   # Years _____   Quit Smoking: ( )Yes   How Long Ago: _____

ALCOHOL: ( )Never   (✗)Occasionally   ( )Regularly   What do you drink: _____

DRUGS: Type/Frequency: _____   Type/Frequency: _____

FIGURE 23–2

A sample nursing history and assessment form. (Courtesy of Woman's Christian Association Hospital, Jamestown, NY.)

W.C.A. HOSPITAL

NURSING HISTORY & ASSESSMENT

– Page 2 –

PRESENT MEDICATIONS (Prescription and Over-The-Counter)

*CODE: A=Sent Home,   B=Not Brought In,   C=Kept on Unit

Name	Dosage	Times	Last Dose	Purpose (Pt. Perception)	*Code
Dilantin	*100 mg*	*2 X / day*	*3/4/93*	*seizures*	*β*

SOCIAL: Living Alone _____ Spouse __*X*__ Children _____ (Ages _____)   Other: _____

Do you take care of anyone else?   No __*X*__ Spouse _____ Children _____   Other: _____

Who manages their care while you are unable? _____

HOME PHYSICAL LAYOUT: (*X*) 1 Floor   ( ) 2 Floors   Location of BR *1st fl* _____ Location of Bedroom _*1st fl*_

MEDICAL EQUIPMENT IN HOME: (*X*) None   ( ) Crutches   ( ) Cane   ( ) Walker   ( ) Wheelchair   ( ) Hospital Bed

   ( ) Commode   ( ) O_2 ( ) Lifeline   ( ) Other: _____

PREADMISSION HOME SERVICES NOW IN USE: (*X*) None   ( ) Nursing   ( ) Homemaker   ( ) Personal Care Aide

   ( ) P.T.   ( ) Meals on Wheels   ( ) Hospice   Agency: _____

NEW NEEDS: (*X*) Nursing   ( ) Personal Care Aide   ( ) Meal Preparation   ( ) Transportation   ( ) Placement

   ( ) Other: _____

In the event that I need help in planning for my hospital discharge, please contact:

CARA RAMES	*SPOUSE*	*520 SARAH CT.*	*250-6431*
Name	(Relationship)	Address	Phone

HAS THE PATEINT BEEN ORIENTED TO: **WAS FAMILY NOTIFIED OF ADMISSION?**   (*X*) Y   ( ) N

Patient Bill of Rights (*X*) Y   ( ) N   No Smoking Policy (*X*) Y   ( ) N   Bed Operation (*X*) Y   ( ) N   Television (*X*) Y   ( ) N

Intercom   (*X*) Y   ( ) N   Menu   (*X*) Y   ( ) N   Roommate   (*X*) Y   ( ) N   Siderails   (*X*) Y   ( ) N

Visiting   (*X*) Y   ( ) N   Call Bell   (*X*) Y   ( ) N   Telephone   (*X*) Y   ( ) N   Bathroom (*X*) Y   ( ) N

Chaplaincy Program (*X*) Y   ( ) N

NAME AND PHONE NUMBER OTHER THAN THOSE LISTED ON FRONT SHEET: _____

PROPERTY/VALUABLES/JEWELRY

(*X*) Dentures–( ) Full/ (*X*) Partial ↓   ( ) Glasses   ( ) Contacts   ( ) Hearing Aid–( ) Right/ ( ) Left

(*X*) Electric Razor   ( ) Money: $ *5.—* (Bedside *5.—* Safety Deposit Receipt _____)   ( ) Watch _*yellow color*_

( ) Rings _*None*_ (How Many?___)   Other: _____

( ) Clothing (Describe: *Black shoes, white socks, black slacks and shirt,* _____)

( ) Other: _*underpants & T-shirt (white). Maroon jacket.*_

"Do you understand that we are not responsible for any clothing or personal effects that you will keep in your hospital room, or for any articles that might be sent or brought to you during your hospital stay?

Yes (*X*) _____*Luis Ramez*_____   _*Self*_

           Signature of Patient or Relative   (Relationship)

History taken by: _____*Sharon Davis, RN*_____   Signature/Title

FIGURE 23–2
Continued

PROCEDURE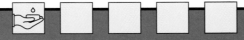

Preparing the Patient's Room

GATHER EQUIPMENT

Admission checklist (if used in your institution)
Pen
Admission kit
Gown or pajamas
Clothing list
Valuables envelope
Sphygmomanometer and stethoscope

Thermometer
Urine or stool specimen container
Equipment not included in the admission kit—bedpan, urinal, wash basin, emesis basin, tissues, a water pitcher and glass, and portable scale (when this equipment is included in an admission kit, it is usually disposable)

ACTION	RATIONALE
Preparation	
1. Wash hands.	Prevents the spread of microorganisms.
Procedural Steps	
2. Open the bed by fanfolding the covers to the foot of the bed (Figure 23–3).	Shows that a patient has been assigned to the bed.

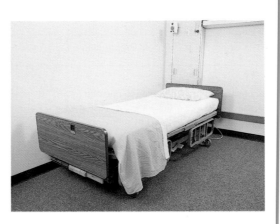

FIGURE 23–3
The open bed tells patients they are expected.

3. Fold the hospital clothing at the foot of the bed.	Readies it for the patient's arrival.
4. Unpack the equipment from the admission kit and store it in the patient's bedside stand.	Readies it for use.
5. Place the admission checklist (Figure 23–4), pen, stethoscope, sphygmo-	Saves time—equipment is ready to use.

ADMISSION CHECKLIST

Patient's name: _____ Age: _____

Room number: _____ Time of admission: _____

Reason for admission: _____

Accompanied by _____

FIGURE 23–4
Some institutions use an admission checklist similar to this one.

Allergies _____

(Fill in every blank. Use yes and no as appropriate.)

Identification bracelet on _____

Temp. _____ Pulse _____ Resp. _____ BP _____ Time _____

Height _____ Weight _____

Marks on body: Bruising _____ Rash _____ Decubitus ulcer _____

Scars _____ (Fill in Head, Chest, Back, Arm(s), Leg(s), Buttocks and indicate
right or left side)

Dentures: Full upper _____ Full lower _____

            Partial upper _____ Partial lower _____

Glasses: With patient _____ Wears all the time _____

                        Reading only _____

Contacts: _____ Able to insert own _____ Needs help _____

Hearing aid: With patient _____ Right ear _____ Left ear _____

Other prostheses: Braces _____ Crutches _____

                    Artificial limb _____ Other _____

Jewelry: Ring _____ Watch _____ Earrings _____ Other _____

Instructions given on:

        Drinking fluids _____ Withholding fluids _____

        Call signal _____

        Bed controls _____

        Bathroom/tub/shower facilities _____

        Television/radio _____

        Menu and mealtimes _____

        Specimen collection _____

        Visiting hours _____

Forms completed:

        Valuables form _____

        Clothing sheet _____

        Other _____

Medications: Given to nurse _____

               Given to family member _____
               (Fill in names)

Checklist completed by _____

               Date _____ Time _____

FIGURE 23-4
Continued

manometer, and thermometer on the
over-bed stand.

6. Lower the bed if the patient is walking   Prepares for a safe transfer to bed.
   or arriving in a wheelchair. Raise the
   bed if the patient is coming on a cart.

7. Attach the call signal to the linens at
   the head of the bed.

Follow-Through

8. Wash hands.   Prevents the spread of infection.

GETTING THE PATIENT SETTLED IN THE ROOM

After the admission to the health care institution is complete, the patient arrives on the nursing unit. In many institutions, a volunteer accompanies the patient to the nursing unit. The patient brings admission papers from the admission office; these are given to the nurse in charge.

When you see the patient has arrived, you should introduce yourself and tell the patient your job title. Smile when you greet patients and shake hands with them and their family members or whoever else might be accompanying the patient.

Ask patients their name and check their identification bracelet to verify that this is the patient you are expecting for admission.

Take patients to their assigned room and complete the admission following the procedure that your institution uses.

PROCEDURE

Admitting the Patient

ACTION	RATIONALE
Preparation	
1. Wash hands.	Prevents the spread of **microorganisms.**
Procedural Steps	
2. Assist the patient to the bed or chair.	Maintains patient safety.
3. Introduce the patient to any roommates.	Shows courtesy and consideration.
4. Ask the family members to wait in the hall or the waiting room while you finish admitting the patient. Close the door or pull the privacy curtain.	Provides privacy.
5. If the patient has any valuables, they should be listed according to your institution's procedure.	Provides for safekeeping.
6. Ask the patient to change into the hospital garment or personal pajamas.	Makes the patient comfortable.
7. Weigh the patient and measure the patient's height if the patient is able to stand. Write down the measurements.	Gives baseline information about height and weight.
8. Ask the patient to put personal items in the drawer of the bedside stand. If the patient is unable, you should do this. If the patient brings any medications, give them to the nurse or your supervisor.	Places personal articles close by. Follows the policy of the institution and is safer for the patient.
9. Assist the patient into bed, place the patient in a position of comfort, and pull the covers up over the patient. Raise the side rails when indicated. (The nurse will tell you whether a patient is allowed to sit in a chair.)	Provides for patient comfort and safety.
10. Take the patient's **vital signs** and write down the measurements.	Provides baseline information.
11. Place the patient's clothing and large articles in the closet or dresser	

MICROORGANISM
an organism so tiny it can be seen only under a microscope; capable of helping the body as well as causing disease

VITAL SIGNS
the signs of life: temperature, pulse, respirations, and blood pressure

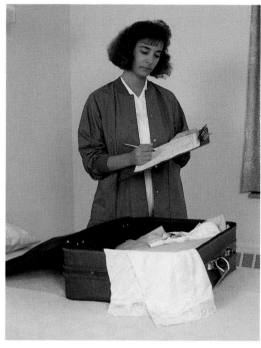

FIGURE 23-5
Complete the clothing sheet as you unpack.

drawers if you are working in a long-term care setting. Fill out a clothing sheet if required to do so by the institution (Figure 23-5).

12. Find out from the nurse whether the patient is **NPO** or is permitted to drink **fluids.** If fluids are permitted, fill the water pitcher with fresh water and place it within the patient's reach.

Ensures that the physician's orders are carried out.

13. Show the patient the **call signal** and make sure it is within the patient's reach. Explain that the call signal is connected to an intercom at the nursing station. Encourage the patient to practice using the call signal. Explain how the TV/radio controls work.

Helps orient patients to their new surroundings.

14. Show the patient how to work the controls on the bed, if the bed is electric. Elevate the back of the bed and adjust the **knee gatch,** if allowed.

Same as step 13.

15. Explain the times meals are served. Assist the patient in filling out a menu for the next day's meal if this is part of the procedure in your institution.

Same as step 13.

16. If the patient is able to walk, show the bathroom. Point out the emergency call signal in the bathroom and explain that it may be used if help is needed in the bathroom.

Same as step 13.

17. If a urine or stool specimen has been ordered, explain how the patient should use the special containers that are placed in the bathroom.

Ensures that the patient provides specimens needed for laboratory testing.

18. If the patient is on bed rest, weak, or dizzy, raise the side rails.

Provides for patient safety.

NPO
abbreviation for nothing by mouth
FLUIDS
liquids
CALL SIGNAL
a communication tool used by patients who must remain in bed or in a chair; also called a call light or call bell

KNEE GATCH
equipment that helps raise the lower part of the bed so the legs are elevated

Continued on following page

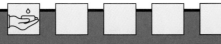

PROCEDURE

Admitting the Patient *Continued*

19. Open the privacy curtains and the door.

20. Call the family from the hall or waiting room to the patient's room.

Shows courtesy and consideration for the patient and family.

21. Explain the visiting hours.

Follow-Through

22. Wash hands.

Prevents the spread of microorganisms.

23. Before you leave the room, check that the

Ensures patient safety and helps maintain patients' rights.

   • bed is in low position with the side rails raised, when indicated
   • call signal, water, and personal items are within reach
   • patient is covered
   • patient looks neat and comfortable
   • patient's needs are met (by asking if anything else is needed before you leave).

24. Complete the admission checklist, if your institution uses one (Figure 23–6).

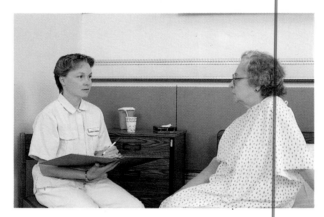

FIGURE 23–6
Fill out the admission checklist after the patient is changed and comfortable.

25. Report the following to the nurse or your supervisor:
   • That the admission procedure has been complete.
   • That the patient is in a chair or in bed. Report whether the side rails are raised.
   • That the vital signs and height and weight have been completed. If an admission checklist is used, report that it is complete.
   • Your observations of the patient. (Include any important information the patient or family may have told you. Include anything unusual you may have noticed.)

The call signal is secured with a clip to the bed linen near the patient's hand. If the patient is unable to use the call signal, you may instruct any family members present about its use.

TAKING CARE OF THE PATIENT'S PERSONAL BELONGINGS

A patient may bring personal belongings into the health care setting. Personal belongings include items such as toilet articles, reading material, clothing, footwear, and a purse or wallet.

Valuables such as money and jewelry should be sent home with family members or stored in the safe provided by the institution. If valuables are stored in the safe, the valuables sheet/envelope is filled out and also placed in the safe. When you write about the patient's valuables, describe the jewelry in common terms. Do not identify metal as silver or gold. Use the words "white metal" or "yellow metal." For jewelry with stones, do not use terms such as "diamond" or "ruby"; instead, describe the stone as "white" or "red." For example, write down "A yellow metal ring with a white stone" for an engagement ring. Sign the sheet or envelope before you take it to the safe. The personnel who place the valuables in the safe give you a receipt. The receipt is placed on the patient's chart. The items are returned when the receipt is taken to the safe at discharge.

Clothing is listed on the clothing sheet. If your patient is being admitted to a long-term care setting, check to make sure all personal belongings are marked with the patient's name. **Indelible** ink should be used so that the name does not wash off. When you describe what appears to be valuable clothing use general terms; for example, to describe a fur coat, use the term "fur" instead of "sable" or "mink coat." Sign the clothing sheet when you are finished. The clothing sheet also becomes a part of the patient's chart.

INDELIBLE
can't be erased or washed out

Personal belongings such as dentures, glasses or contact lenses, watches, razors, and TVs or radios are kept at the bedside. The items are listed on the admission checklist. The admission checklist, if your institution uses one, becomes part of the patient's chart. The patient may want to keep a small amount of money to purchase items such as the daily paper, a snack, or something on the gift cart. Advise the patient not to keep a large amount of money in the room. When the patient decides to keep cash, the amount should be recorded in the chart. When cash is sent to the safe, the patient or family should count the money in your presence. You should *not* handle the patient's money.

Personal belongings are the patient's property. You should always ask the patient's permission before you open a drawer, cabinet, or closet in which the patient keeps personal belongings. This maintains patients' right to privacy.

HELPING THE PATIENT DRESS AND UNDRESS

In a nursing home, the patient may wear street clothes every day. In a hospital, the patient may need to change into a hospital gown or pajamas or personal pajamas shortly after admission. Patients may need help with dressing and undressing (Figure 23–7), or you may have to complete a patient's change of clothing yourself. The following chart provides some guidelines.

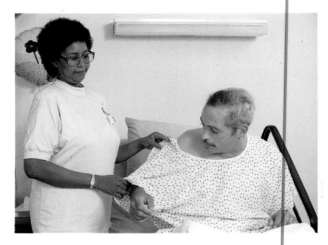

FIGURE 23–7
The patient should help as much as possible when dressing and undressing.

GUIDELINES FOR DRESSING AND UNDRESSING PATIENTS

- Find out from the patient or family member how much help the patient needs dressing or undressing. The nurse can also tell you how much help to give.
- Provide privacy. Be sure to keep the patient covered. Close all window curtains and doors. If more than one patient is in the room, pull the privacy curtain around the bed.
- Encourage the patient to assist as much as possible. Allow extra time for the very young or older patient. Anyone in pain may also take longer to dress and undress.
- Take clothing off the patient's strong side first.
- Put clothing on the weakest side first.
- Make sure the clothing being put on belongs to the patient. Clothing should not be shared.
- Place soiled clothing in the proper container. In the hospital, soiled clothing is sent home for laundering. In a long-term setting, patient laundry is placed in specially marked containers and washed separately from linens.

UNPACKING THE PATIENT'S BELONGINGS

The patient may need help unpacking. Ask patients how they want their belongings arranged in the drawer, cabinet, or closet. When you unpack, check to see whether clothing is marked with the patient's name if you are working in a nursing home. Fold the clothing neatly and place it where the patient directs. Hang dresses, jackets, and coats. Place personal articles in a drawer or on the top of the dresser or bedside stand. The clothing checklist can be filled out at this time.

THE PATIENT'S FEELINGS ABOUT ADMISSION

Patients may tell you about their feelings of fear, anxiety, anger, or unhappiness. The health care institution is a strange place to the newcomer and has many rules that the patient may not understand. A child, for example, may feel abandoned if the parent(s) leave for the night. You should hold and comfort children, if they are allowed out of bed. Your presence in the room may help calm and reassure the child. An elderly person may feel a sense of loss when entering a long-term care institution. This loss is very real because all personal possessions are kept in just one room or even a half of a room. The patient needs a period of adjustment. You should be a good listener and encourage the patient to talk. Report the patient's feelings and concerns to the nurse.

CARING COMMENT

Always be considerate of the patient's feelings and do what you can to make the adjustment period as comfortable as possible.

PATIENT TRANSFERS

A transfer is the moving of a patient from one room to another in the same institution or from one institution to another. A transfer may be performed for several reasons:

- The patient requests a transfer. The patient may request a private or semiprivate room when admitted. If such a request cannot be granted, the patient is admitted to whatever room is available and is transferred when the requested room becomes available.
- The patient's condition changes. If the patient's condition changes, the patient may be transferred to or from a specialty unit, such as the intensive care unit.
- Another health care institution is desired because it provides more specialized treatment or is closer to home.

When a transfer is planned, patients may speak of the same feelings they felt on admission—fear, anger, etc. A transfer may mean the patient must learn new routines. It could mean that the patient's condition is not getting any better. You should tell the patient that the transfer to another room is beneficial and important in getting well. Listen to the patient's comments and report any fears and concerns to the nurse.

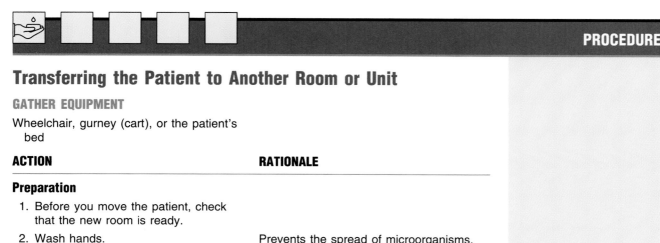

PROCEDURE

Transferring the Patient to Another Room or Unit

GATHER EQUIPMENT
Wheelchair, gurney (cart), or the patient's
  bed

ACTION	RATIONALE
Preparation	
1. Before you move the patient, check that the new room is ready.	
2. Wash hands.	Prevents the spread of microorganisms.
3. Identify the patient.	Maintains patients' rights.

Continued on following page

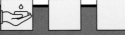

PROCEDURE

Transferring the Patient to Another Room or Unit
Continued

Procedural Steps

4. Provide privacy by asking visitors to wait in the hall or waiting room.

Maintains patients' rights.

5. Explain the procedure.

Informs patients what is going to happen.

6. Collect all personal belongings in a transfer bag or place them in the patient's luggage. Take equipment as per the institution's procedure.

Ensures that all belongings are moved with the patient.

7. Transfer the patient.

Ensures patient safety.

   • Wheelchair transfer: Wheel the patient to the new room (Figure 23–8). (Patients may be able to hold a few items in their lap. A family member or another staff member may be able to help carry belongings.)

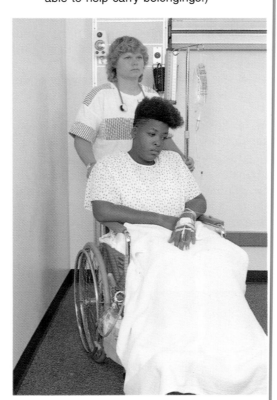

FIGURE 23–8
Cover the patient with a bath blanket or a spread during transfer to another room.

   • Cart/stretcher transfer: Make sure side rails are raised. Most carts/stretchers have a bottom shelf that holds personal items or equipment.
   • If there are many personal belongings, place them on a cart for transfer. Do not attempt to carry belongings with you when you transfer the patient.

8. When you arrive in the new room, introduce the patient to the new roommate(s), if it is not a private room.

Helps the patient feel welcome.

9. Introduce the new staff member who will be caring for the patient.

Helps the patient feel welcome and identifies who can be called for help.

10. Provide privacy while transferring the patient to the new bed.

Maintains patients' rights.

11. Lower the bed and raise side rails when indicated.

Ensures patient safety.

12. Cover the patient and place in a position of comfort.

13. Place the call signal within patient's reach.

Leaves the patient with means to communicate.

14. Place personal belongings in the drawer, cabinet, or closet.

15. Open the privacy curtains.

16. Ask the patient if anything is needed.

Gives the patient an opportunity to express needs.

Follow-Through

17. Wash hands.

Prevents the spread of microorganisms.

18. Report to the nurse on the new unit that the patient is in the room.

19. Return to your assigned unit and
   • Report to the nurse that the patient transfer has been completed. Report the time of the transfer and your observations of the patient during the transfer.
   • Follow the procedure for cleaning the room after a patient discharge.

Communicates that patient has been safely transferred.

20. Wash hands.

Prevents the spread of microorganisms.

CHAPTER WRAP-UP

- The patient may be admitted to a health care facility from a variety of settings.
- Prepare the room before the patient arrives on the unit.
- Admit the patient according to the procedure of your health care institution.
- Teach the patient about the
    Call signal
    Bed controls
    Bathroom/tub/shower safety
    Television and radio
    Menu and meal times
    Visiting hours
- Consider the patient's and family's feelings about the patient's being admitted to a health care institution.
    Be a good listener.
    Encourage communication.
    Be considerate of the patient's and family's feelings.
- Patients may be transferred because a change in their condition requires it or they requested a room change.

REVIEW QUESTIONS

1. What is done to prepare a room for a newly admitted patient?
2. List the feelings patients may have about being admitted to the health care institution.
3. List the reasons for a patient transfer.

ACTIVITY CORNER

You may need to tell a patient about hospital beds, call signals, and other things that help make a stay in a hospital or nursing home comfortable. You need to become familiar with patient rooms and the equipment in them so you are confident about using them. How many of the following activities can you do comfortably?

_____ Raise and lower the side rails.

_____ Raise and lower the head of the bed.

_____ Place the bed in the high or low position.

_____ Ring the call signal and use the cancel button.

_____ Locate the emergency call signal in the bathroom.

Practice if you cannot complete any of these activities.

Discharging Patients 24

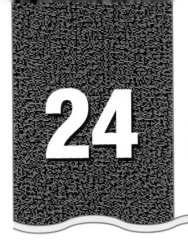

24 Discharging Patients

Objectives

AFTER YOU COMPLETE THIS
CHAPTER, YOU WILL BE ABLE TO:

State the types of information
   included in a discharge plan.
Help with a patient's discharge.
State the importance of
   discharge instructions.

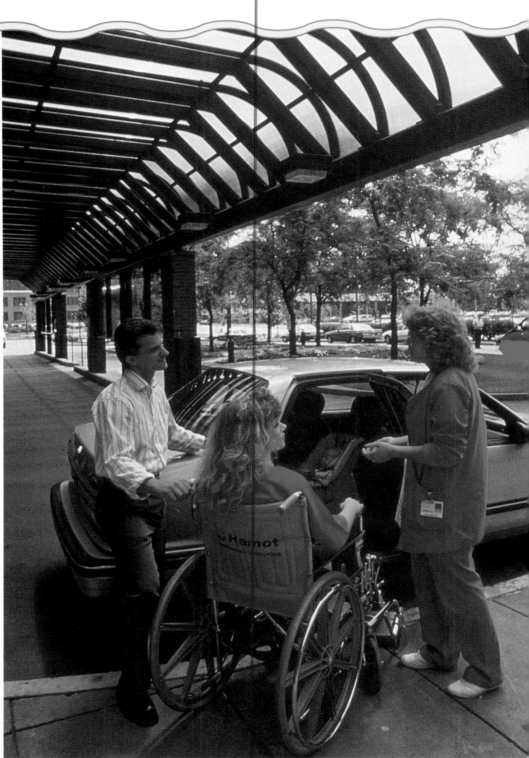

Overview Most people look forward to being discharged from a health care institution. Getting a person ready to leave is a team effort. The nursing assistant plays an important role in the safe discharge of the patient.

WHAT DO YOU KNOW ABOUT DISCHARGING A PATIENT?

Here are three statements about discharging patients. Consider them to test your current ideas. If you think the statement is true, circle the T; if you think the statement is false, circle the F. Change the false statements to make them true.

1. T F A discharge plan starts when the patient is discharged.
2. T F Patients are taught about the medications they will take after discharge.
3. T F Patients leave the health care institution with a written set of instructions about care.

ANSWERS

1. **False.** A discharge plan starts when the patient is admitted.
2. **True.** The nurse teaches patients how their medications work, how to take them, and what side effects to expect.
3. **True.** The nurse gives a set of discharge instructions, which are a summary of the main points of the discharge plan, to patients on the day they are discharged.

DISCHARGE
the process that prepares a patient to leave a health care institution

DISCHARGE PLAN
a written plan of teaching that prepares a person to perform self-care after discharge from the health care institution

HEALTH CARE TEAM
the group of people who have the education necessary to provide care to patients

Discharge is the process that prepares a patient to leave the health care institution. Patients need to be able to care for themselves or find someone to help with their care after discharge. They may need to enter a long-term care institution for a while before going home.

DISCHARGE PLAN

The nurse develops a **discharge plan** for the patient (Figure 24–1). While all members of the **health care team** are responsible for preparing the patient for discharge, other professionals of the team contribute to the plan. For example, a **social worker** may refer a patient or the patient's family to a community agency that can help meet some of the patient's needs, such as an agency that

NURSING DISCHARGE PLANNING

DATE	INITIAL	QUESTIONS TO ASK THE PATIENT/SIGNIFICANT OTHER	RESPONSE
		1. In the event the patient will need assistance, who will: a. make or prepare the meals? b. do the laundry? c. clean the house? d. purchase the groceries? 1. Is food available in the home now? e. drive patient to appointments? f. change patient's dressings (if applicable)? g. check on patient at least daily? h. assist with patient's ADLs? 1. Will patient be independent? 2. Will patient be dependent? a. How much assistance is needed? i. j. k. 2. In the event that the patient will need assistance, where is the a. bedroom located? b. bathroom located? 3. Teaching: What does this patient/significant other need to know prior to discharge? a. Physician instructions b. See appropriate teaching flowsheets and provide copy of Discharge/Patient Information sheets, if applicable c. Are discharge teaching plans progressing smoothly? d. If NO, have plans been made to include family/significant others for discharge teaching? e. If NO, has social work been contacted for assistance?	 YES or NO YES or NO YES or NO N.A. N.A. YES or NO YES or NO YES or NO

INITIAL	SIGNATURE AND TITLE	INITIAL	SIGNATURE AND TITLE

FIGURE 24–1

Assessment of patient's discharge needs. ADLs, activities of daily living. (Courtesy of Woman's Christian Association Hospital, Jamestown, NY.)

provides meals for people who are unable to buy food or cook their own meals. The physician might refer the patient to a **physical therapist** who will teach the patient special exercises that ease pain.

The discharge plan includes

- teaching patients activities that help them begin the process of returning to good health (special exercises, ambulating, etc.)
- teaching patients about their treatment (wound care, diet, medications, etc.) so that they can continue after discharge

The nurse begins the discharge plan when the patient is admitted. Complications in the patient's condition may be prevented when the members of the health care team explain to the patient the reasons for certain activities and treatments included in the plan.

Nowadays, the discharge plan is especially important because changes in the health care system have reduced the length of time a patient can stay in the hospital. The introduction of the DRG (diagnosis-related groups) system of insurance payments to health care providers has led to major reductions in the lengths of patients' stays in health care institutions. Patients spend more time **convalescing** at home after discharge.

By the time of discharge, the teaching specified in the discharge plan should be completed. Patients are taught about their

- disease or illness
- treatment
- activity
- diet and nutrition
- medications
- future appointments
- resources

DISEASE AND ILLNESS

Patients have the right to know about their **disease** or **illness.** The more knowledge patients have about their disease, the more they cooperate in their care. The physician teaches patients about their disease, and the nurse reinforces this information and answers any questions patients have. Patients are taught the following about their disease before discharge:

- the name of their disease
- the **etiology** of their disease
- the changes in their body function caused by the disease
- usual and unusual signs and symptoms associated with the disease
- possible complications

TREATMENT

A **treatment** is a procedure, such as a dressing change or an application of ointment, that should be continued for a period of time after discharge. The physician orders the treatment, and the nurse or other professional teaches the patient how to continue the treatment. The procedure is explained and demonstrated for the patient. The patient is given a chance to practice performing the procedure, with the nurse watching to make sure it is done correctly. Patients are taught the following about the treatment of their condition:

- the purpose of the treatment
- how often the treatment must be performed
- how to perform the treatment
- what supplies are needed to perform the treatment
- what to report to the physician

SOCIAL WORKER
a professional who helps patients and their families deal with psychosocial problems

PHYSICAL THERAPIST
professional who helps ease the pain of muscle, bone, nerve, or joint injury or disease

CONVALESCE
to recover health and grow stronger gradually after an illness

DISEASE
sickness; a condition of the body or one of its parts that causes a change in the body's functioning

ILLNESS
sickness; a condition different from the normal health state; any change, temporary or long-lasting, in a person's physical, emotional, or spiritual health and well-being

ETIOLOGY
cause

TREATMENT
a procedure, such as a dressing change or application of ointment, which can be done by a doctor or a nurse, or performing eye surgery, which can be done only by a surgeon

ACTIVITY

Patients are usually anxious to return to their previous level of activity. Following the physician's orders, the nurse, along with the physical therapist, teaches the patient the following information about activity:

- the date the patient can expect to return to normal activity
- progression to normal activity (rest as needed; return to light duty [type of work] in 2 weeks)
- type and amount of activity (no driving for 2 weeks; walking permitted; no aerobics for 3 weeks)
- what special exercises need to be done and how often
- the use of crutches, canes, braces, and walkers
- restrictions on lifting, driving, and climbing stairs

DIET AND NUTRITION

DIETICIAN
professional who promotes good
health through proper diet

Proper diet and nutrition are important to healing. The physician orders a special diet for the patient, which must be followed after discharge, and the **dietician** teaches the patient the changes that are required to fulfill the physician's orders. The nurse answers any questions the patient may have and reinforces information about

- foods that are allowed and foods that are not allowed
- the purpose of the special diet
- dietary **supplements** (healthy snacks or commercial preparations added to the diet)
- counting **calories** to monitor weight gain or loss

SUPPLEMENT
to complete or add to
CALORIE
a measure of energy produced by
the breakdown of food in the body

MEDICATION

MEDICATION
a drug

The patient may need to take **medication** to regain and maintain health. It is important for the patients on medication to know why medication has been ordered, how and what time to take it, and what side effects to expect. After the physician orders the medication, the nurse teaches the patient

- the name of the medication
- how often the medication should be taken
- how much medication to take in a dose
- the purpose of the medication
- the side effects of the medication and when to notify the physician of problems
- precautions such as taking the medication with food or water or not driving or operating heavy equipment after taking the medication

FUTURE APPOINTMENTS

Follow-up care is necessary so that the patient's progress can be monitored. The patient is taught about the importance of future appointments. After the physician specifies when the patient should be seen after discharge, the nurse provides the patient with the following information:

- the purpose of the follow-up appointment
- the date and time of the appointment
- the name of the physician or other health care provider

DISCHARGE INSTRUCTIONS

Complete all sections.

Diet: _____ *Soft diet for 1 week. Then resume usual eating pattern.* _____
_____
_____
_____

Activity: _ *May climb stairs. Drive in 10 days.* _____
_____
_____
_____

Medications (include name of medication, dose, times to be taken, expected side effects, restrictions): _____
_____
_____ *For pain—Tylenol 325 mg. every four hours* _____
_____
_____

Treatments (dressing change, skin care, etc.): _____
_____
_____ *Do not remove dressing. Call if blood or other drainage soaks through.* _____
_____
_____

Restrictions: _ *No showers for 1 week.* _____
_____
_____
_____
_____

Appointment (name of physician(s), address, telephone number, date, time): _____
_____
Appointment in 1 week – October 10, 1992 at 2 pm.
Dr. Jim Kelly   619 Main St.   Phone – 642-6420
_____

Other: _ *Call if nauseated or if you have pain not relieved by Tylenol.* _____
_____
_____
_____

Discharge Instructions _ *Julie Roomer, RN* _____ RN Signature

_____ *Oct. 3, 1992* _____ Date

Copy given to patient _ *Yes* ___ or family _____ or not given _____

FIGURE 24-2

Discharge instructions.

- the address and phone number of the physician or other health care provider

In addition, the nurse writes down this information on the discharge instruction form and gives it to the patient.

RESOURCES

Patients should always have a resource (another person or an agency in the community) to call on if they have questions about care or changes in their condition or if problems arise with treatment, medications, or diet. The patient is informed of resources by the nurse, with help from a social worker when needed. The following information is given to the patient:

- the name and phone number of the physician
- the name and phone number of a dietician
- the services, names, addresses, and phone numbers of home health care services and community support groups

DISCHARGE INSTRUCTIONS

SUMMARY
briefly repeating the main points of a discussion

A successful discharge plan prepares the patient for care at home. At the time of discharge, the patient is given discharge instructions to be followed during recovery (Figure 24–2). The discharge instructions form is a form on which the nurse writes down a **summary** of the main points of the discharge plan that has been in operation during the patient's stay in the health care institution. The nurse reviews all that has been taught, and the patient is given time to ask questions before leaving. The nurse and patient sign the discharge instructions form, and the patient receives a copy to take home.

DISCHARGE PROCEDURE

When the physician writes the discharge order, you may be asked to carry out the patient's discharge procedure. The nurse in charge assumes responsibility for all activities included in the discharge procedure. You assist under the supervision of the nurse. Be sure to clarify with your institution what you can and cannot do as part of helping with the discharge procedure.

PROCEDURE

Discharging the Patient

You should become familiar with the discharge procedure of your health care institution. A physician's order is always needed for a patient discharge. Proceed with discharging the patient only under the direction of the nurse or supervisor.

GATHER EQUIPMENT

Wheelchair or stretcher   Discharge slip

ACTION	RATIONALE
Preparation	
1. Wash hands.	Prevents the spread of microorganisms.
2. Identify yourself and the patient.	Maintains patients' rights.

3. Provide privacy.   Maintains patients' rights.

4. Explain the procedure.   Informs patients what is happening.

Procedural Steps

5. Help the patient pack belongings.   Ensures that the patient has all personal
   Check all cabinets and drawers for the   belongings.
   patient's personal items.

6. Check for valuables that have been in
   storage in the safe. Follow your institution's procedure for returning valuables to the patient.

7. The nurse returns any medications
   brought from home to the patient.

8. Check that the discharge instructions   Verifies that a copy of the discharge in-
   are with the patient's belongings.   structions has been given to the patient
                                             by the nurse.

9. Assist the patient with dressing, if
   necessary.

10. Obtain a wheelchair (Figure 24–3).   Prevents tiring of the patient during the
                                          discharge procedure.

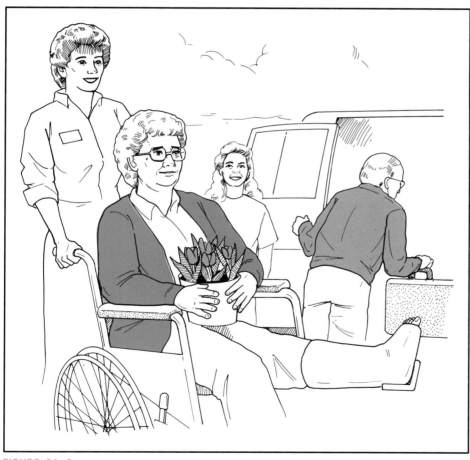

FIGURE 24–3

A wheelchair makes discharge more pleasant for the patient who cannot walk a long distance.

11. Assist the patient into the wheelchair.

12. Stop at the nurses' station for the dis-   The slip informs discharge personnel that
    charge slip before you take the patient   the patient has indeed been discharged
    off the unit.   by the physician.

Continued on following page

PROCEDURE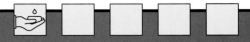

Discharging the Patient *Continued*

13. Wheel the patient and all the patient's belongings to the designated place for discharge according to your institution's procedure:
    • cashier
    • discharge desk
    • business office
    Note: A family member may take the patient's belongings to the transport vehicle while the discharge paperwork is being completed.

    Provides time for paying the bill, signing papers, and finalizing the discharge.

14. Follow your institution's procedure to complete the discharge.

15. Wheel the patient to the front door and assist the patient into the car or other vehicle used for transport.

    Provides safety until the patient is in the transport vehicle.

16. Say good-bye to the patient and close the door of the vehicle.

Follow-Through

17. Return to the unit with the wheelchair and the discharge slip.

18. Clean the wheelchair as directed by your health care institution and return it to the storage area on the unit.

    Prepares equipment for the next use.

19. Return discharge slip, as directed by your institution, to the appropriate person on the unit (for example, the unit secretary or ward clerk).

    Signifies that discharge is complete.

20. Return to the patient's room and strip the linens from the bed or notify other personnel as designated by your institution. Place linens in soiled laundry hamper.

    Prepares the room for cleaning by designated personnel.

21. Wash hands.

    Prevents the spread of microorganisms.

22. Notify the appropriate personnel that the room is vacated and ready for cleaning.

    Allows personnel to schedule cleaning and preparation of the room for the next patient.

23. Report the following to the nurse or supervisor:
    • That the patient has been discharged
    • Time of discharge
    • The type of transportation used for discharge (car, van, or ambulance)
    • The person(s) who accompanied the patient during discharge (for example, spouse, child, or friend)
    • That discharge instructions were with the patient
    • How the patient tolerated the discharge procedure
    • Observations of the patient during discharge

DISCHARGE FORM

Cashier stop: Yes   No

Date: _____   Discharge Time: _____

Discharge to:

    1. Home (routine) (adult home) _____

    6. Home or adult home with organized home health care (VNA, etc.)

    _____

  24. Home with IV therapy provided by an agency _____

    2. Another acute care hospital _____
       (prospective payment facility)

    3. Residential health care facility _____

    5. Non PPS health care facility _____
       (JMHC rehab, medical and alcohol or JMHC adult or adolescent psychiatric
       units)

    9. Against medical advice (self discharge)

    8. Expired

PROCEDURE:

    a) discharge order obtained
    b) call Cashier, 188 (admissions off hours)
    c) mark "Yes" if patient or family needs to stop at cashier
    d) mark the appropriate discharge code (see list on back) and write in name if
       to another facility or circle if JMHC
    e) note date and time of discharge
    f) TAKE this completed form to the cashier or admissions immediately on
       patient discharge. This form should *not* be mailed.

CASHIER HOURS:
    Monday–Friday 0730 to 1730
    Saturdays–0800 to 1600
    Sundays–0800 to 1430
    Holidays–0800 to 1300

FIGURE 24–4

You may be required by your health care institution to complete a discharge form. (Courtesy of Woman's Christian Association Hospital, Jamestown, NY.)

- That you have given the discharge slip to the designated person on the unit
- That appropriate personnel have been notified that the room is ready for cleaning

24. Complete any forms your health care institution requires to fill out as part of the discharge process (Figure 24–4).

CHAPTER WRAP-UP

- Planning for discharge begins when the patient is admitted to a health care institution.

- The discharge plan includes teaching the patient and/or family members about the patient's care after discharge.
- The discharge procedure is carried out after the physician writes the order for discharge.

REVIEW QUESTIONS

1. Identify the steps of the discharge procedure.
2. What kind of information is included on the discharge plan?

ACTIVITY CORNER

Use this activity to help you make sure personal belongings are not left behind when you help with a patient discharge. Write down all areas you need to check for the patient's personal belongings:

_____

_____

_____

_____

_____

_____

_____

_____

Caring for the Preoperative Patient **25**

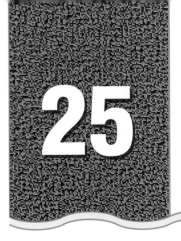

25 Caring for the Preoperative Patient

Objectives

AFTER YOU COMPLETE THIS CHAPTER, YOU WILL BE ABLE TO:

Describe the physical and psychologic needs of the patient about to have surgery.

Describe the preoperative care given by the nursing assistant.

Use a preoperative checklist to complete the routine care of a patient before surgery.

Respond to patient and family needs before surgery.

Help prepare a patient for surgery.

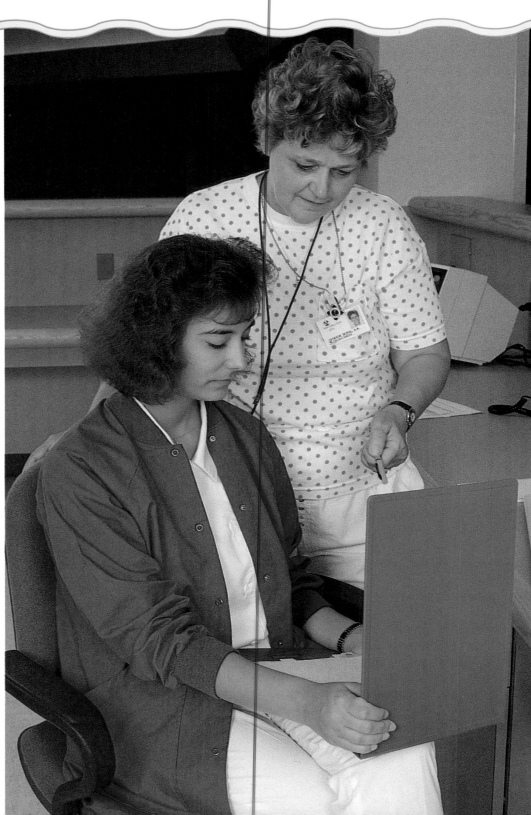

Overview **Surgery** is one of the methods physicians use to treat patients. Surgery is a procedure in which an opening is made into the body. It can be done on any part of the body. Surgery may range from a simple (removal of a wart) to a complex (brain surgery) procedure. It is performed to cure or control the spread of disease, decrease or remove pain, repair the body, transplant a body organ, or make a change in the patient's appearance. No matter what the reason for the surgery, most patients experience stress and anxiety.

The nursing assistant plays an important role in the care of patients who are about to have surgery. These individuals have special needs that you can meet once you are properly trained. For a patient to get well after surgery, you must provide the best possible care from the time of the patient's **admission** into the health care institution.

SURGERY
operation

ADMISSION
letting someone or something into someplace

WHAT DO YOU KNOW ABOUT THE PREOPERATIVE PATIENT?

Here are seven statements about the preoperative care of patients. Consider them to test your current ideas about preoperative care. If you think the statement is true, circle the T; if you think the statement is false, circle the F. Change the false statements to make them true.

1. T   F   *Appendectomy* means repair of the appendix.
2. T   F   Anxiety may be a problem for the patient scheduled for surgery.
3. T   F   The patient needs to give informed consent before surgery.
4. T   F   The perioperative period is the time before surgery.
5. T   F   The nursing assistant is responsible for helping complete the preoperative checklist.
6. T   F   An elective surgery occurs in an emergency.
7. T   F   Patients who have received general anesthesia during surgery remain unconscious for 24 hours after surgery.

ANSWERS

1. **False.** The ending *ectomy* means removal; thus *appendectomy* means the removal of the appendix.
2. **True.** Anxiety and stress are common problems prior to surgery.
3. **True.** The patient or the patient's guardian must sign a consent form before surgery can begin.

4. **False.** The perioperative period includes the time before, during, and after surgery. The preoperative period is the time before the surgical procedure.
5. **True.** The nursing assistant is responsible for helping complete the activities listed on the checklist and checking them off as finished before surgery.
6. **False.** Elective surgery is planned ahead of time.
7. **False.** The patient wakes up in the recovery room a short time after the surgery is over. The patient may be drowsy after surgery but can be aroused easily.

THE PREOPERATIVE PERIOD

PREOPERATIVE PERIOD
the period of time between the decision for surgery and surgery

The **preoperative period** is the time before surgery during which the patient is prepared for a surgical procedure. There are two types of surgery.
- **Elective surgery**—optional surgery (the patient chooses whether or not surgery will be done)
- **Emergency surgery**—surgery that is made necessary by the patient's condition or injury

THINGS THAT NEED TO BE DONE IN THE PREOPERATIVE PERIOD

Preparation of the patient before surgery includes some or all of the following.

Diagnostic Studies

DIAGNOSTIC STUDY
a procedure or examination that helps the physician diagnose a disease or illness

The physician may order special **diagnostic studies,** such as a blood test or an x-ray examination, in order to have a measurement of certain body functions before the surgical procedure begins. Diagnostic studies are performed by specially trained technicians.

Special Preparations

The physician is the one who orders any special preparations for surgery. You may be asked to do such things as

ENEMA
a solution that loosens fecal material and stimulates peristalsis of the intestines

- Give an **enema.**
- Shave the surgical site.
- Help the patient bathe with a special soap.
- Keep the patient from drinking fluids.

Informed Consent

INFORMED CONSENT
when a person is informed of (told about) a procedure or treatment and agrees (gives consent) to having the procedure or treatment done

The registered nurse or physician is responsible for obtaining **informed consent** from the patient or the patient's guardian before the surgical procedure is performed.

Teaching the Patient About the Surgery

The physician is responsible for helping the patient and the patient's family understand the reasons for surgery. The registered nurse explains the procedure when the patient or family need more information. When patients or their family members tell you they do not understand something, tell the nurse or your supervisor. Do not offer explanations or answer questions about the patient's surgery.

CARING COMMENT

Do not try to answer the patient's or family member's questions about a surgical procedure because you may not be giving accurate information. It is the physician's and nurse's responsibility to provide this information.

Patients need to be taught about special activities that they will need to perform after the surgical procedure. The registered nurse is responsible for teaching patients these activities. You are expected to remind the patient to cough and to breath deeply after the surgical procedure and to help the patient **ambulate** (see Chapter 26).

AMBULATE
walk

THE PREOPERATIVE PATIENT'S NEEDS

The patient who is scheduled for a surgical procedure has psychologic, physical, and educational needs.

PSYCHOLOGIC NEEDS

Whether the surgery is elective or an emergency, the patient and family may experience anxiety. Patients may be anxious about a variety of things:

- how soon they can return to their usual routine
- the possibility that the surgery might not be successful
- whether they will return to their previous level of function
- the loss of finances because they have to take time off from work
- changes in their body as a result of the surgery, such as a scar or the loss of a body part (this affects their **body image**)

BODY IMAGE
the feelings and thoughts individuals have about their body

Patients' anxiety may be observed in behaviors such as crying, pacing, sadness, lack of appetite, inability to sleep, or changes in vital signs. To help decrease the patient's anxiety, you should:

- Remain calm.
- Attend to the patient's needs.
- Listen to the patient's concerns and convey them to the nurse.
- Touch the patient's arm or shoulder as a gesture of concern and caring (Figure 25–1).
- Report the patient's anxious behaviors to the supervisor or nurse.

CARING COMMENT

It's likely that a patient who is about to undergo emergency surgery will experience more anxiety and stress than a patient who is having elective surgery.

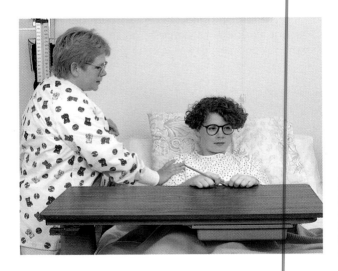

FIGURE 25-1
Because surgery is a stressful event, listen to the patient and let the nurse or supervisor know if the patient expresses fears or concerns.

PHYSICAL NEEDS

To help make sure that the patient is physically ready for the surgical procedure, you should look for and report any of the following to the nurse or supervisor:

- chest pain
- elevated temperature
- nausea or vomiting
- signs of respiratory problems (cough, sniffles, sneezing, or difficulty breathing)

If a patient is experiencing any of these symptoms, surgery may be dangerous and therefore postponed.

Patients are given medication 30–60 minutes before surgery. This preoperative medication can cause confusion and unsteadiness. **Safety** is a very important consideration after the patient has been medicated. You can help by keeping the side rails raised and reminding the patient not to get out of bed alone. Place the call signal nearby so that the patient can call for assistance.

SAFETY
the status of being safe from experiencing or causing hurt, injury, or loss

CARING COMMENT

The call signal is placed near the patient's hand and secured with a clip to the bed linen. In the event the patient is unable to use the call signal, you should instruct any family member present how to use it.

EDUCATIONAL NEEDS

Every health care institution has a preoperative plan for patient education. The nurse is responsible for educating the patient and family members what to expect before, during, and after the surgical procedure. Knowing what is expected and what can happen lessens patients' fear. All care givers participate in getting the patient ready for surgery. The nurse or supervisor tells you how you can help. Before surgery, the patient and family are taught:

- How to cough and breathe deeply and the reason for doing so
- How to move and turn and the reason for doing so
- About PRN (as needed) medications and asking for them
- How to splint an incision when moving or coughing and breathing deeply
- The reason for the preoperative shave
- The reason for remaining on an NPO (nothing by mouth) order
- The need for insertion of a urinary **catheter**
- The need for a preoperative enema (or enemas)

CATHETER
a flexible tube passed into body openings to allow fluids to enter or exit the body

PREPARING THE PATIENT FOR SURGERY

During the preoperative period, you may be asked to

- Assist in admitting the patient to the nursing unit.
- Measure, record, and report the patient's vital signs (Figure 25–2).
- Measure, record, and report the patient's height and weight.
- Provide care and comfort to the patient.
- Encourage the patient to get enough rest.
- Assist the patient with personal needs (bathing, toileting, etc.).
- Assist in activities to prepare the patient for surgery (enema, skin preparation, etc.).

Before the patient leaves the nursing unit for the operating room, certain activities must be completed. You may be asked to assist with some of the following activities the evening before or the day of the surgery.

Rest and Sleep

The patient needs a good night's rest before surgery. You can help the patient rest by keeping the environment dim and quiet. Visitors may be asked to leave early the night before surgery so the patient can sleep.

Bowel Elimination

The physician may order an enema for the patient before surgery. You may be requested to do this procedure. The enema helps clean out the bowel and decreases constipation in the patient after surgery (see Chapter 20).

BOWEL ELIMINATION
the way the body gets rid of its solid waste, produced in the bowel

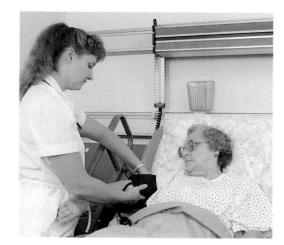

FIGURE 25-2
Measuring vital signs is an important part of patients' preoperative and postoperative care.

BLADDER ELIMINATION
discharge of the body's liquid waste from the bladder; same as urination and voiding

URINAL
a container into which a person urinates

NUTRITION
the study of food's relationship to health; the act of providing food to nourish the body

Bladder Elimination

The physician may order the insertion of a urinary catheter before surgery. This procedure is done by the nurse. You are responsible for making sure the catheter tubing is free of kinks and looped on the bed and that the drainage bag is below the level of the bladder.

The patient who has not had a urinary catheter inserted needs to void in the bathroom. Voiding must be completed before the nurse administers any preoperative medication. If patients need to urinate after receiving medication, ask them to use the bedpan or the **urinal** because the medication can cause patients to become dizzy upon standing.

Nutrition

The physician writes an NPO order for the patient (Figure 25–3). The patient may be kept NPO for 6–12 hours before the surgical procedure. Patients who are kept NPO before surgery tend to have less nausea and vomiting after surgery. You may be asked to place the patient's empty water pitcher and glass inside the bedside stand or in the bathroom at midnight so the patient doesn't accidentally drink water.

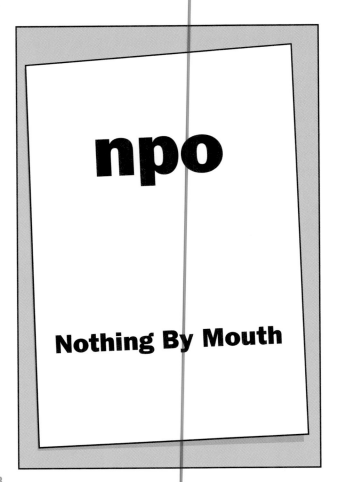

FIGURE 25–3
A health care institution may use reminders such as this NPO sign. Staff who come in contact with the patient will realize that the patient should not take in anything by mouth.

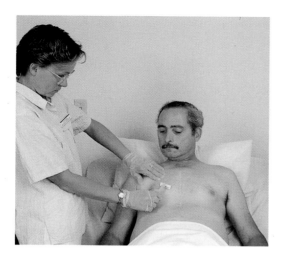

FIGURE 25-4

The nursing assistant helps prepare the patient for surgery by shaving the area where the incision will be made by the surgeon. This patient's chest will be operated on.

Skin Preparation

Skin preparation is an important part of the physical preoperative preparation of the patient. The hair on the skin in the operative area is shaved off the evening before or on the day of surgery. This is called a shave prep. The area to be shaved is determined by the type of surgery and the physician's order (Figure 25-4). The nurse explains to the patient why the shave prep is necessary. (The removal of body hair prevents infection of the site after surgery.)

In some institutions, the shave prep is completed by personnel when the patient arrives in the holding area of the operating room. In other institutions, you may be responsible for shaving the skin after the patient has been bathed or has taken a shower with special soap. The nurse tells you what area of the body to shave (Figure 25-5). Before you shave the skin, inspect it for

Rashes
Scars
Moles or growths
Pimples
Reddened areas
Bruises
Abrasions

ABRASION
a wound that results from rubbing or scraping the skin

CARING COMMENT

Any open areas in the skin may allow **microorganisms** to enter the body and cause an infection. Report any open areas in the patient's skin to the supervisor or nurse before shaving the skin.

MICROORGANISM
an organism so tiny it can be seen only under a microscope; capable of helping the body as well as causing disease

In some health care institutions, one nursing assistant may be assigned to perform shave preps on all the patients who are scheduled for surgery. A prepackaged kit may be available; if not, you can assemble the equipment you need from the supplies available on the unit. Follow your health care institution's procedure.

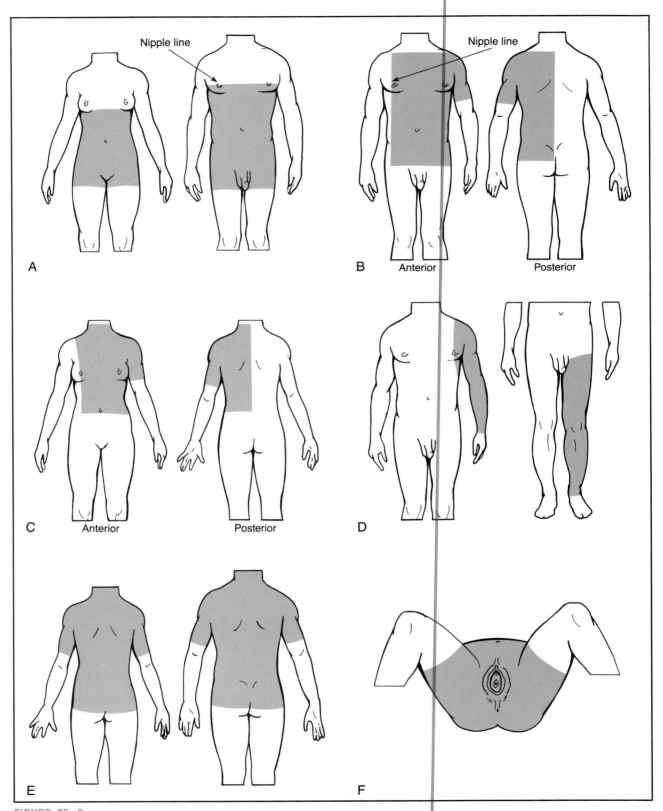

FIGURE 25-5

See legend on opposite page

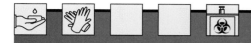

Performing a Shave Prep

Hair provides a place for microorganisms to grow; shaving it off reduces the chances that the surgical incision will become infected. Always inspect the skin before you start shaving.

GATHER EQUIPMENT

Prepackaged soap sponge
Disposable razor
Basin of warm water
Towel
Washcloth

Waterproof pad
Disposable gloves
Use prepackaged preoperative prep kit if available.

ACTION	RATIONALE
Preparation	
1. Wash hands.	Prevents the spread of microorganisms.
2. Identify yourself and the patient.	Maintains patients' rights.
3. Provide privacy.	Maintains patients' rights.
4. Explain the procedure.	Informs patients what is happening.
Procedural Steps	
5. Raise the bed to the high position and lower the side rail nearest you.	Helps you maintain good **body mechanics.**
6. Place the waterproof pad under the patient.	Keeps patient comfortable by protecting the linens.
7. Position the patient so that the area to be shaved is easy to reach.	
8. Put on the disposable gloves.	Protects you in the event the skin is nicked or cut, bringing you in contact with body fluids.
9. Moisten the soap sponge by placing it in the basin of warm water.	
10. Apply the shaving solution to the skin and work up a lather (Figure 25–6).	Softens the skin and decreases discomfort from the razor.
11. Keep the skin damp and hold it taut (stretched) with one hand. Holding the razor in the other hand, shave the skin.	Smooths out the skin so it can be shaved close. Helps prevent damage to skin while shaving.

BODY MECHANICS
the use of the body to lift, push, or pull objects

Continued on following page

FIGURE 25–5

A, Abdominal prep. Shave from the nipple line (males) or from below the breasts (females) down to the pubic area. The procedure of the health care institution may specify that the pubic area be shaved. Shave across the entire width of the body from side to side. B, Chest prep. Shave from the nipple line of the unaffected side across the front of the body to the other side. Shave down to the pubic area. Shave over the shoulder and about 3 or 4 inches down the arm. On the back, shave from the shoulder area down to the buttocks on the affected side. C, Breast prep. The shave prep for breast surgery is similar to the prep for chest surgery, with these exceptions: Shave above the shoulder to the chin in front and the hairline in the back, and shave only as far as the patient's waistline. D, Extremity prep. For surgery on an extremity, shave the skin of the entire arm or leg. E, Back prep. Shave the entire back. Start at the patient's hairline and shave down to the middle of the buttocks. Include the axillary area (under the arms). F, Groin prep. For any surgery in the groin area, shave the entire area, front and back. When instructed to, shave as high as the waistline in the front and the back. Shave down around each leg about 6 inches.

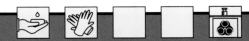

PROCEDURE

Performing a Shave Prep *Continued*

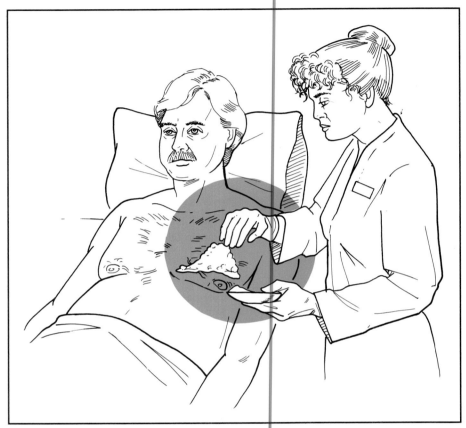

FIGURE 25-6

Apply the shaving solution to the skin and work up a lather.

12. Place the razor at a 45° degree angle and shave in the direction the hair grows (Figure 25-7).	Reduces damage to the skin.
13. When the area has been shaved, wash the skin with soap and warm water, rinse, and dry.	Removes soap and hair.
14. Check the skin closely to be sure that no hair remains.	Hair provides a place for microorganisms to grow.
15. Remove the waterproof pad and place the patient in a position of comfort.	
16. Raise the side rails and place the bed in the low position.	Ensures patient safety.
17. Remove the disposable gloves and place them in the waste container.	
18. Empty the water into the toilet; wash, dry, and store the basin.	Readies equipment for next use.
19. Discard the razor into the sharps container.	Prevents injury to others.

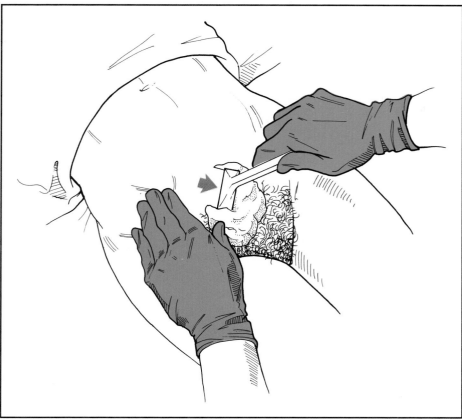

FIGURE 25-7

Keep the skin taut (stretched) with one hand and shave the skin with the razor held in the other hand.

Follow-Through

20. Wash hands.	Prevents the spread of microorganisms.
21. Report to the nurse • that the procedure has been completed • whether there are any cuts or razor nicks in the skin • whether any skin changes are present	Keeps the nurse informed of the patient's preparation for surgery.
22. Record that the procedure has been completed and place a check at the appropriate place on the preoperative checklist.	Provides a record that the procedure was completed.

Additional Preparations

Other preparations for surgery may be completed by the nurses in the patient's room or in the operating room area. These preparations may include

- insertion of a urinary catheter
- start of an intravenous solution
- injection of the preoperative medication
- insertion of a nasogastric (from nose to stomach) tube

Preoperative Checklist

		Initials
Blood pressure	*124/78*	*JR*
Temperature	*98.6*	*JR*
Pulse	*76*	*JR*
Respirations	*18*	*JR*
Allergies	*None*	*JR*

Lab results   WBC *9,000*   HCT *40*   HGB *9*

CXR *NEG*   EKG *NORM*   T & C *—*

Other _____

Circle when completed: Initials

			Initials
NPO	(Yes)	No	*JR*
Preop teaching	(Yes)	No	*SB*
History & physical	(Yes)	No	*SB*
Consent signed	(Yes)	No	*SB*
Identification bracelet	(Yes)	No	*JR*
Prostheses out (dentures, etc.)	(Yes)	No	*JR*
Capped teeth	(Yes)	No	*JR*
If Yes: Location	*all molars*		
Voided	(Foley)	Yes No	*JR*
Cap on	(Yes)	No	*JR*
Skin prep	(Yes)	No	*JR*
Enema	Yes	(No)	*JR*
Makeup/polish removed	(Yes)	No	*JR*
Rings	(Taped)	Removed	*JR*
Family present	(Yes)	No	*JR*

Family directed to wait in _*Surgical waiting room*_

Medicated with _*Demerol 100 mg Im @ 1045 SB*_

Time _*1045*_   Signature _*Shirley Brown RN*_

To operating room at _*1100*_   Signature _*Shirley Brown RN*_

	Initials	Signature
BRACKER, MARCIA A. 34	*JR*	*Julie Rowe N.A.*
1-0001-02 ROOM 424	*SB*	*Shirley Brown RN*
DR. JOHNSON		
Patient Stamp		

FIGURE 25–8

A completed preoperative checklist. The nursing assistant may be responsible for completing the patient checklist. WBC, white blood cells; HCT, hematocrit; HGB, hemoglobin; CXR, chest x-ray study; EKG, electrocardiogram; T&C, type and crossmatch (of blood specimen); NPO, nothing by mouth. (Courtesy of Woman's Christian Association Hospital, Jamestown, NY.)

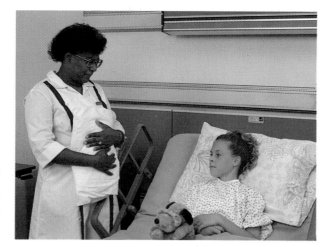

FIGURE 25-9
Teaching the patient to use a pillow to press against an incision is a part of preoperative teaching. The procedure may be taught by the nurse and reinforced by the nursing assistant.

PREOPERATIVE CHECKLIST

The **preoperative checklist** is a record that shows that the activities required for preparation of the patient for surgery were completed (Figure 25-8). The nurse tells you what activities on the preoperative checklist are your responsibility. You may be asked to sign the checklist to show that you completed your activities. The nurse also gives you the following information:

- What the patient has been taught about the surgery.
- How you should respond to the patient's and family members' questions.
- The approximate time by which your duties should be completed.
- Whether you should teach the patient about coughing and deep breathing exercises or reinforce them if they have already been taught (Figure 25-9).
- What care you should give before surgery (shave prep, enema, etc.).
- To report any anxious behaviors the patient may have.

PREOPERATIVE CHECKLIST
a record that shows that the activities required to prepare the patient for surgery have been completed

CARING COMMENT

Some of the duties on the preoperative checklist are the responsibility of other care givers. Always check with the nurse to verify the duties for which you are responsible.

PREOPERATIVE ROUTINE
activities that are performed to prepare the patient for surgery; usually the 24-hour period before surgery

Together, the activities that are performed for the patient about to have surgery are referred to as the **preoperative routine**. The preoperative routine is usually completed in the 24-hour period before surgery. It includes all the activities listed on the preoperative checklist.

PROCEDURE

Completing the Preoperative Checklist

The checklist is used so that the completion of each preoperative preparation is documented in the same place and so that the operating room staff can be informed that all procedures were completed. The nurse is responsible for making sure that the preoperative checklist is completed before the patient leaves for the operating room. You are responsible for the tasks the nurse or your supervisor has assigned you.

Continued on following page

PROCEDURE

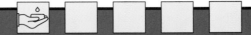

Completing the Preoperative Checklist *Continued*

GATHER EQUIPMENT
Preoperative checklist
Pen

ACTION	RATIONALE
Preparation	
1. Bring the preoperative checklist and a pen to the patient's room.	
2. Wash hands.	Prevents the spread of microorganisms.
3. Identify yourself and the patient.	Maintains patients' rights.
4. Provide privacy.	Maintains patients' rights.
5. Explain the procedure.	Informs patients what is happening.
Procedural Steps	
6. Place the water pitcher and glass inside the patient's bedside stand.	Removes the possibility that the patient may accidentally drink a glass of water.
7. Measure vital signs and record them on the checklist.	Provides the operating room staff with baseline vital signs.
8. Check that the patient is wearing an identification bracelet. Record that information on the checklist.	Allows identification of the patient by the operating room staff.
9. Remove all prostheses (except hearing aids): • dentures • glasses • contact lenses • artificial limbs	Prevents damage or loss of **prosthesis.** Removal of dentures prevents obstruction of the airway.
10. Remove all the patient's clothing and put a clean gown on the patient.	Provides access in case other treatment or procedures become necessary.
11. Assist the patient to remove makeup and nail polish. Record removal of makeup and nail polish on the checklist.	Allows operating room staff to observe for changes in the skin and nails during surgery.
12. Remove rings or place tape over them (Figure 25–10). Remove all other jewelry. Record removal of jewelry on the checklist or that rings are taped.	Prevents loss or damage of jewelry.

PROSTHESIS
an artificial replacement for a missing part of the body

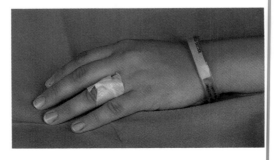

FIGURE 25–10
Be certain that the ring is covered by tape so that it does not fall off while the patient is in the operating room.

13. If the patient has a hearing aid, leave it in and record that it was left in on the checklist.

Allows patients to hear what the operating room staff say to them.

14. Complete the duties the nurse has assigned you, check off each duty, and sign your initials on the checklist to show that you have completed your duties.

Follow-Through

15. Wash hands.

Prevents spread of microorganisms.

16. Give completed checklist to nurse or supervisor in charge.

CARING COMMENT

Patients who wear dentures may ask to keep their dentures in until it is time to leave for the operating room. Check with the nurse or supervisor to make sure this is permissible. The dentures may be allowed to remain in place to help patients maintain their **self-image.**

SELF-IMAGE
your idea of who you are and what your role in life is

THE CONSENT FORM

Patients must give consent (permission) for a surgical procedure to be performed on their body. The physician explains the surgical procedure to the patient and invites questions. When patients have been fully informed about their surgery, they are asked to sign a consent form (Figure 25–11).

The consent form includes the following information:

- Patient's name
- Date of surgery
- Name of the surgery
- Name of the surgeon
- Statement that the patient has been informed of the surgery and gives permission for the surgery to be performed
- Signature of a witness (a person who watches the patient sign the consent form)

The physician or registered nurse is responsible for asking the patient to sign the consent form. By signing the form, the patient gives permission for the surgery to be performed as the physician explained it. When the patient is unable to sign the consent form, the patient's next of kin or legal guardian takes the responsibility of signing so that the surgery can be performed. After the form has been signed by the patient or guardian, the physician or nurse signs it as a witness.

General Consent for Surgery and Other Procedures

Date of Surgery __11/3/92__

1. I authorize the performance upon _____*Lawrence J. Brooks*_____
                                                            (state "myself" or name of pateint)

    of the following: _____*Appendectomy*_____
                                              (state name of operation and/or procedure)

    _____

    to be performed by or under the direction of Dr. _____*Charles T. Tooley*_____ .

2. I have been advised of the possible consequences of not having this procedure done. I have also been advised of any practical alternative methods of treatment.

3. The risks and possible consequences of the operation/procedure are: _____

    _____*hemorrhage, postoperative wound infection*_____

    _____

    _____

4. I authorize the above-named doctor, and any other persons as may be needed to assist the doctor, to give me a blood transfusion(s) and/or blood conponents. The doctor has explained to me that I need or may need this/these for the following reasons:
              low red blood cell count

    The doctor has explained to me, in general, what a transfusion is and the procedures that will be used. He/she has also explained to me, and I understand, that there are possible risks involved with blood transfusion(s) and/or blood components, including infectious hepatitis, unexpected blood reactions, fever, chills, hives, and acquired immune deficiency syndrome. No guarantees have been made to me about the outcome or the fitness or quality of the blood to be used. Blood from volunteer donors screened by currently acceptable procedures will be used.

5. I understand that the explanation that I have received is not exhaustive and that other, more remote risks and consequences may arise. I have been advised that if I desire a more detailed and complete explanation of any of the foregoing, such explanation will be given me.

6. Additionally, I consent to the performance of operations and procedures in addition to or different from those now contemplated, whether or not arising from presently unforeseen conditions which the above-named doctor(s) or his/her associates may consider necessary or advisable during the course of the operation.

7. I acknowledge that I have received no warranties or assurances with respect to the benefits to be realized or consequences of this procedure.

8. For the purpose of advancing medical education, I consent to the admittance of observers to the operating room.

9. I consent to the disposal by hospital authorities of any tissues or body parts that may be removed.

10. I consent to the photographing or recording of the operations or procedures to be performed, including appropriate portions of my body, for medical, scientific, or educational purposes, provided my identity is not revealed by the pictures or by descriptive texts accompanying them.

11. I acknowledge that I have read this document in its entirety and that I fully understand it and that all blank spaces have been either completed or crossed off prior to my signing.

12. If D.N.R. orders are in effect, they will be rescinded for the perioperative period unless extended by the surgeon.

13. I have been afforded full opportunity by my doctor, whose signature appears below, to ask any and all questions I have regarding the above.

    (CROSS OUT ANY OF THE ABOVE PARAGRAPHS THAT DO NOT APPLY)

    _____*Lawrence J. Brooks*_____
                    Patient's Signature

    _____*11/3/92*_____   _____*0732*_____
            (Date)   (Time)

    _____*Charles T. Tooley, M.D.*_____
                    (Physician's Signature)

FIGURE 25–11

Consent form for surgery. (Courtesy of Woman's Christian Association Hospital, Jamestown, NY.)

Nursing assistants do not have the authority to sign the consent form as a witness.

The time just before surgery is very stressful for the patient. The patient may express concerns such as

- fear of the surgical procedure and receiving **anesthesia**
- how long the surgery will last
- whether the surgery will be successful
- how much pain there will be after surgery
- the effects of the anesthesia
- what the diagnosis will be, if diagnostic testing is performed during the surgical procedure
- whether the surgeon will talk to family members following the surgery

Let the nurse know of the patient's concerns before the patient leaves the unit for the operating room.

ANESTHESIA

a loss of feeling or sensation in one part of the body or all of the body caused by an anesthetic medication

TRANSFERRING THE PATIENT TO THE OPERATING ROOM

After the nurse has given the patient preoperative medication, raise the bed to the high position and raise all side rails. The bed is placed in this position because the cart from the operating room is high. Moving the patient onto the cart will be more comfortable for the patient if the bed is in the high position. If the time to take the patient to the operating room is delayed, you may need to place the patient's bed in a low position.

When the patient is ready for transfer onto the operating room cart, make sure there is enough staff available to help with the transfer. Remember that the patient has been medicated and may be unable to help during the transfer.

You can direct the patient's family or significant others to a cafeteria or other place to eat, to restrooms, or to the chapel. In addition, tell them where the surgical waiting room is located. Encourage the family or significant others to ask questions and let the nurse know they have questions.

You may hear the term "**perioperative**" used. This refers to the time before, during, and after a surgical procedure.

PERIOPERATIVE

the period before, during, and after a surgical procedure

Many hospitals now provide a special waiting area for the families and friends of patients in surgery. Nurses may be available to report on the progress of the surgery. This practice helps decrease the anxiety and stress of waiting for a loved one's surgery to be completed.

ANESTHESIA

When patients arrive in the operating room, they are given a medication to cause a loss of sensation in one part of the body or in the entire body. This loss of sensation is called *anesthesia*. The anesthetic (the medication that produces anesthesia) is given by a physician who specializes in giving such medication. The physician is called an *anesthesiologist*. An *anesthetist* is a registered nurse who is certified to administer anesthetics under the direction of the physician. The patient receives one of the following types of anesthesia:

General anesthesia
Local anesthesia
Spinal anesthesia

GENERAL ANESTHESIA

GENERAL ANESTHESIA
loss of feeling or sensation in the entire body caused by an anesthetic medication introduced into the blood

During a lengthy or complex surgery, the patient receives an anesthetic that blocks sensation in the entire body.

General anesthesia is a deep sleep. A general anesthetic causes this effect because it is introduced into the blood. A general anesthetic is used for patients who have surgery on body organs such as the heart, liver, or kidney. It is also used in joint (for example, hip or knee) replacement or special tests. A general anesthetic affects many body functions (see chart on The Effects of General Anesthesia on Body Functions).

THE EFFECTS OF GENERAL ANESTHESIA ON BODY FUNCTIONS

Thinking Function

- The patient may experience mental confusion, sleepiness, or agitation because the anesthesia affects the brain. The patient may also be slow to respond to questions.

Respiratory Function

- The patient's respiration rate may slow down because the anesthetic affects the brain's breathing control center.
- Respiratory complications can occur if
    the surgery involves the chest or upper abdominal area
    a disease of the lungs was present before surgery
    the patient is overweight
    the patient is elderly
    postoperative activities such as coughing and deep breathing
        are not done

Circulatory Function

- The patient's inactivity and slower blood flow may cause circulatory problems such as the formation of blood clots.
- Changes in blood pressure after surgery may cause dizziness.

Protective Function of the Skin

- The patient's skin may become dry in the hospital environment. Dry skin breaks down easily.

- The patient may discover that lying in one position decreases pain or discomfort. By lying in one position, however, the patient can develop decubitus ulcers over bony areas of the body.
- Patients who are at risk for skin complications after surgery are those:
    with nutritional problems
    with circulation problems
    who do not turn in bed
    who have had skin problems in the past

Gastrointestinal Function

- General anesthesia slows down the movement of food through the gastrointestinal tract. This can cause constipation.
- The general anesthetic used may cause nausea and vomiting.

Urinary Function

- When anesthesia affects the bladder, the bladder may not empty completely. Urinary retention can result in urinary infection.
- Insertion of an indwelling catheter as part of preoperative preparation also increases patients' risk for bladder infection.

Activity Function

- The patient may be weak and move slowly after surgery. The patient may not move the part of the body on which the surgery was performed. The lack of movement causes the muscles to atrophy (shrink).

Fluids

- The patient's fluid balance may change after surgery. Patients who experience nausea and vomiting after surgery lose fluids. They will receive fluids intravenously (through the vein) until they are able to take fluids by mouth.

LOCAL ANESTHESIA

When a patient undergoes **local anesthesia**, an anesthetic is injected directly into the surgical area where the loss of sensation is needed. For example, when a wound needs sutures (stitches), local anesthesia blocks the pain that would be caused by the needle going through the skin. As the local anesthetic wears off, sensation returns to the affected area.

A local anesthetic may also be applied directly to the skin or mucous membrane. For example, an anesthetic ointment can be applied to gums in the mouth to relieve the feeling of soreness.

The patient remains awake when a local anesthetic is used. During some surgical procedures in which a local anesthetic is used, the surgeon may order a medication to help the patient relax. This medication does not produce the deep sleep that a general anesthetic does.

LOCAL ANESTHESIA
loss of feeling or sensation in the part of the body in which an anesthetic medication has been injected or applied on the skin

SPINAL ANESTHESIA

For **spinal anesthesia**, the anesthetic is injected into the spinal canal and produces a loss of sensation from the point of injection down to the toes of

SPINAL ANESTHESIA
loss of feeling or sensation in the body parts below the area of the back where anesthetic medication was injected

both feet. The impulses from the nerves in the spinal cord are blocked so that the brain no longer receives a message of pain from the areas served by the nerves. The patient remains awake and alert during the surgical procedure but cannot move the lower extremities or feel anything below the area of the injection. A medication that relaxes the patient and decreases anxiety may also be ordered. As the spinal anesthetic wears off, sensation returns to the lower extremities.

Spinal anesthesia is commonly used in surgeries performed on the male genital organs. For the mother who is about to give birth, spinal anesthesia helps decrease the pain caused by contractions of the uterus. Spinal anesthesia is also used for surgical procedures on the lower back.

CHAPTER WRAP-UP

- During the preoperative period, the patient is prepared for a surgical procedure.
- Certain activities must be completed before the patient goes to the operating room. Completion of these activities is documented on the preoperative checklist.
- The patient who is awaiting surgery has physical (safety and comfort) and psychologic (decreased anxiety and stress) needs.
- As a nursing assistant, you may be asked to assist with the preparation of the patient for surgery by
  Providing a restful environment
  Helping the patient with bowel or bladder elimination
  Helping the patient meet nutritional requirements
  Preparing the patient's skin (shaving)
  Completing the preoperative checklist

REVIEW QUESTIONS

1. What duties are listed on the preoperative checklist?
2. Why is the preoperative checklist important?
3. Explain the shave prep procedure.
4. Tell why an enema might be needed before surgery.
5. Why are makeup and nail polish removed before surgery?
6. List the three types of anesthetics that may be given before a surgical procedure.

ACTIVITY CORNER

Find two persons who have had an operation. Ask them what feelings they had *before* the operation. Which of the following feelings did they have? If you have had an operation, check which feelings you had before surgery in the third column.

	First Person	Second Person	Yourself
Fear of pain	_____	_____	_____
Fear of not waking up	_____	_____	_____
How long the operation would last	_____	_____	_____
How soon food would be served	_____	_____	_____
How long it would be necessary to stay in bed	_____	_____	_____
How soon discharge would occur	_____	_____	_____
How long it would take to return to normal	_____	_____	_____

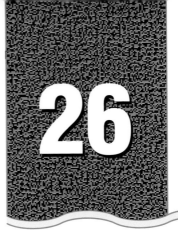

26

Caring for the Postoperative Patient

Objectives

AFTER YOU COMPLETE THIS CHAPTER, YOU WILL BE ABLE TO:

List the activities you perform when the patient returns from the recovery room.

Describe how the patient's postoperative activities prevent complications after surgery.

Explain why vital signs are monitored during the postoperative period.

Assist with the care of the postoperative patient.

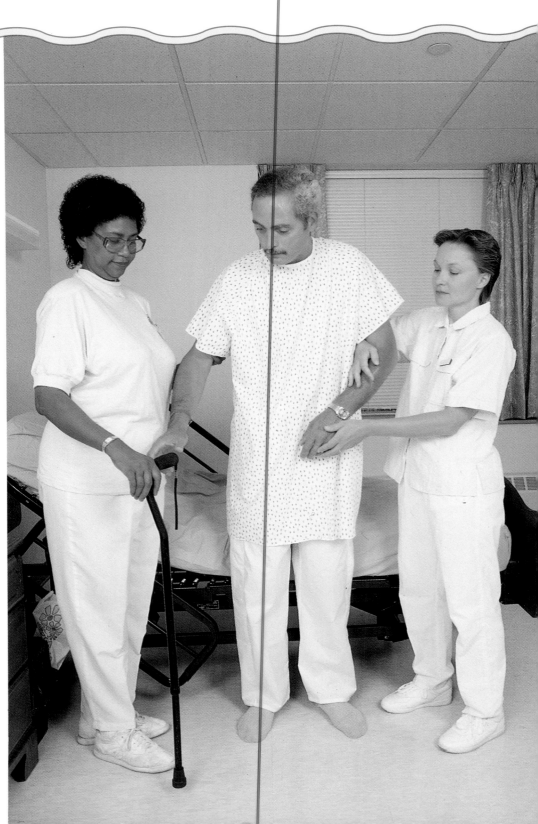

Overview After surgery, patients require skilled care to recover. Patients go to the recovery room immediately after surgery and remain there for a short time. Patients are transferred to the nursing unit when they are awake and responding to people and have stable vital sign measurements. When patients come to the unit, you will assist the other nursing staff with their postoperative care.

WHAT DO YOU KNOW ABOUT POSTOPERATIVE CARE?

Here are six statements about the postoperative care of the patient. Consider them to test your current ideas about postoperative care. If you think the statement is true, circle the T; if you think the statement is false, circle the F. Change the false statements to make them true.

1. T F Patients are safe once they have had surgery.
2. T F Patients need assistance with activities of daily living for a week after surgery.
3. T F Measuring vital signs is the nursing assistant's only responsibility after surgery.
4. T F The word *ostomy* means that a body part was removed during surgery.
5. T F The pulse is normally fast after surgery.
6. T F Patients should be encouraged to cough and take deep breaths after surgery.

ANSWERS

1. **False.** The postoperative period is a critical time.
2. **False.** Patients are encouraged to care for themselves as soon as possible after surgery.
3. **False.** The nursing assistant is also responsible for helping the patient with personal care and keeping a safe environment.
4. **False.** *Ostomy* means an opening; *ectomy* means the removal of.
5. **False.** The pulse is usually slow after surgery, because the anesthesia slows down body function.
6. **True.** Coughing and deep breathing help patients remove the anesthetic from their lungs.

IMPORTANCE OF POSTOPERATIVE CARE: PREVENTING COMPLICATIONS

COMPLICATION
the occurrence of another disease or problem in addition to the original disease or problem

The most important reason for giving care after surgery is to prevent **complications.** Complications delay the patient's return to good health. When you provide good postoperative care, you help patients maintain life and function. The care you provide can help prevent common complications that may occur following a surgical procedure. The Common Postoperative Complications chart lists common complications and the reasons why they might occur.

COMMON POSTOPERATIVE COMPLICATIONS	
Complication	Reason
Infection	May occur at the site of the incision (cut) if sterile technique is broken in the operating room or if the patient has had a poor diet and cannot heal properly.
Pneumonia	May occur if the patient does not move the extremities or cough and deep breathe.
Blood clots	May occur if the patient does not move the extremities while in bed or does not walk soon after surgery.
Constipation	Can occur if the patient does not take enough fluids because the anesthetic slows down the activity of the intestines.
Decubitus ulcers	May occur if the patient does not relieve pressure on the skin by moving and turning or walking.
Urinary retention or infection	May occur if an indwelling catheter was inserted before the surgery, if the patient does not take fluids, or if the patient does not move and turn or walk soon after surgery.

PNEUMONIA
acute inflammation or infection of lung tissue

CONSTIPATION
inability to have or difficulty in having a bowel movement

DECUBITUS ULCER
a bedsore; a sore caused by continual pressure on the body parts of a patient who must stay in one place

URINARY RETENTION
accumulation of urine in the bladder because of the inability to urinate

THE POSTOPERATIVE PERIOD

POSTOPERATIVE
after surgery; used to refer to the period of recovery

RECOVERY ROOM
a room near the operating room where the patient is observed immediately after surgery

EXTREMITY
a limb of the body; an arm or leg

The **postoperative** period begins as soon as surgery is completed. Patients are transferred from the operating room to the **recovery room.** The staff in the recovery room observe patients until the vital signs become stable. The recovery room staff test patients' ability to respond by calling patients' name, issuing commands such as "Wiggle your toes," and moving their **extremities.** Patients' responses tell the staff whether patients can hear and respond to a command correctly. When patients can respond appropriately and have stable vital signs, they are ready for transfer to the nursing unit.

Your care of patients begins when they are brought to the nursing unit

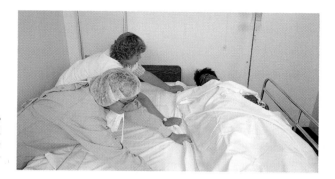

FIGURE 26-1
Care givers transfer a patient to the bed by using a sheet to pull the patient onto the bed. The bed is placed in the high position before the transfer begins.

after surgery (Figure 26-1). You must have certain skills and knowledge to care properly for postoperative patients. Most patients receive the same type of care after surgery.

Note: The recovery room may also be referred to as the PARR (Post-Anesthesia Recovery Room) or the PACU (Post-Anesthesia Care Unit).

PREPARING THE POSTOPERATIVE ROOM

If patients are scheduled to return to their room after surgery, the room is prepared for postoperative care. After the patient is taken to the operating room, prepare the patients' room for their return as follows:

- Make the bed so that the top linens can be pulled over patients after they have been transferred to the bed. Place the bed in the high position (Figure 26-2).
- Place an intravenous pole near the bed so that the intravenous fluid bag can be hung after patients have been transferred to their bed.
- Move the over-bed table and all chairs out of the way so that the cart on which patients are brought from the operating room can be wheeled close to the bed for the patient transfer.
- Clean off the bedside stand and the over-bed table so that a clean surface is available for supplies.

The following supplies are needed in the patient's room after surgery (Figure 26-3):

- an **emesis** basin and a box of tissues on the bedside stand
- a postoperative vital signs **flow sheet** and pencil (Check that the flow sheet is stamped with the patient's name and room number.)

EMESIS
stomach contents brought up and expelled from the mouth; vomitus
FLOW SHEET
a record of a series of measurements and observations made at frequent intervals during a specific time period

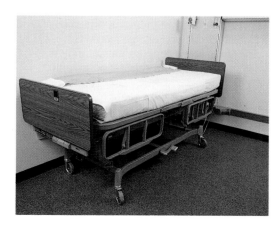

FIGURE 26-2
An operating room bed is ready for the patient's return from surgery.

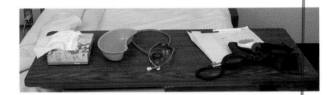

FIGURE 26–3

Basic supplies are needed for the care of the patient returning from surgery.

STETHOSCOPE

an instrument used to hear and amplify the sounds of an internal organ (heart, lungs, or bowels)

- a sphygmomanometer (blood pressure cuff) and a **stethoscope** on the bedside stand or over-bed table

While you are giving care to other patients, watch for the return of your patient from surgery so you can help get the patient settled into the room.

THE PATIENT'S ARRIVAL ON THE UNIT

The recovery room nurses accompany patients to their room. You and other staff who are available help transfer patients to their bed. Certain activities are performed at this time to keep patients safe and comfortable.

PROCEDURE

Caring for Patients from the Recovery Room

ACTION	RATIONALE
Preparation	
1. Identify the patient.	Ensures that the patient who has arrived is the one you are expecting.
Procedural Steps	
2. Help transfer the patient from the stretcher to the bed.	Having several care givers help provides for a safe and comfortable transfer.
3. Make the patient comfortable by placing in correct body alignment and placing a pillow under the head, if permitted.	Gives the patient a feeling of security and helps decrease pain.
4. Raise the side rails, lower the bed, and place the call signal within reach.	Ensures patient safety. Leaves the patient a means to communicate.
5. Stay with the unconscious patient.	Ensures patient safety.
6. Ask the nurse if there are any special instructions you should follow.	Ensures that you know what additional care is required.
• Understand that the patient may remain sleepy for several hours after returning.	Ensures that you provide for the patient's safety.
• Realize that the patient may respond when called by name.	The general anesthesia makes the patient sleepy, but as it is eliminated from the body, the patient begins to return to consciousness and is more able to respond.
7. Provide extra blankets if the patient is cold.	Provides warmth. The patient may be cold because of the cold temperature maintained in the operating room.
8. Begin taking vital signs as directed.	Helps monitor body functions affected by the general anesthesia.

9. Observe the patient's level of consciousness: unresponsive, drowsy, or responds to commands or name.

Helps determine that the patient is reacting as expected from the general anesthesia.

10. Observe for pain.

Assists the nurse in deciding whether pain medication should be given.

11. Make sure all tubing is connected and unobstructed. (Tubing should not be pinched in the side rails or underneath the patient.)

Helps keep tubing connections sterile. Ensuring that tubing is not pinched allows substances to flow in or out as needed.

12. Check dressing for amount and type of drainage.

The nurse adds more dressings if needed.

13. Check that the **intravenous** fluids are running. Be sure that the drops are falling into the drip chamber.

Helps in monitoring the intravenous delivery of fluids and in preventing possible complications.

INTRAVENOUS
through the vein

14. Report any unusual observations to the nurse.

Helps prevent complications.

15. If vomiting occurs, turn the patient's head to one side, support the patient's head, and hold the emesis basin to collect the vomitus. Use a washcloth and towel to wash the patient. Before you offer water for patients to rinse their mouth, ask the nurse whether the patient is permitted to rinse the mouth.

Prevents aspiration of vomitus that can occur because the patient is not fully conscious.

16. Observe and record the amount, color, and thickness of the vomitus.

Note: If your patient has had a spinal anesthetic, ask the nurse for special instructions.

Helps you assist the patient in recovering with complications.

• Many patients are required to lie flat on the back for 8–12 hours following spinal anesthesia.

Helps prevent the headaches that may occur if the patient changes position.

• Move the patient at least every 2 hours.

Relieves pressure and helps circulation.

• Keep the body in correct body alignment.

Provides for patient comfort.

COMING OUT OF ANESTHESIA

Each type of **anesthesia** results in a different patient response. Recall the three types of anesthesia from Chapter 25:

- **General anesthesia** affects all body functions because it is introduced into the patient's circulation.
- **Local anesthesia** affects only a small area of the body and does not affect body functions.
- **Spinal anesthesia** affects the lower extremities from the area of injection down to the toes. The body functions temporarily affected are feeling and sensation below the level of the injection, the ability to move the lower extremities, and bowel and bladder control.

RESPONSE AFTER GENERAL ANESTHESIA

During the postoperative period, patients are very sleepy, but can respond when you call their name. Patients may experience nausea and **vomiting.** Over

ANESTHESIA
the loss of sensation in one part of or all of the body caused by an anesthetic medication

GENERAL ANESTHESIA
loss of sensation in the entire body caused by an anesthetic medication introduced into the blood

LOCAL ANESTHESIA
loss of sensation in the part of the body in which an anesthetic medication has been injected or applied on the skin

SPINAL ANESTHESIA
the loss of sensation in the body parts below the area of the back where anesthetic medication was injected

a period of about 12–24 hours, patients become more awake and aware of their surroundings. You may be responsible for attending to patients' needs and providing for their safety once they return from the recovery room.

RESPONSE AFTER LOCAL ANESTHESIA

The amount of time that a local anesthetic affects body tissues may be 1 or more hours. Feeling and sensation return as the medication wears off. Patients are awake and alert and able to eat. There is no vomiting or nausea. In some situations, you may be asked to participate in care by applying ice or elevating a body part.

RESPONSE AFTER SPINAL ANESTHESIA

During the first 12 hours after surgery in which spinal anesthesia was used, patients must remain flat on their back. During this period, you check for return of sensation to the lower extremities. Patients are able to eat and drink fluids and do not experience nausea and vomiting.

VOMIT
to eject material from the stomach through the mouth

CARING COMMENT

General anesthesia affects patients' sensory (seeing, hearing, tasting, and smelling) functions and thinking. This raises their risk for injury immediately after surgery. Be sure to place the bed in the low position, put up the side rails, and place the call signal within patients' reach.

THE TWO TYPES OF PATIENT NEEDS AFTER SURGERY

The patient who has had surgery has two types of needs: physical and psychologic. The needs must be satisfied to help the body heal. The person may be weak as a result of the surgery itself and the effects of the anesthesia received during the surgery.

PHYSICAL NEEDS

For many patients, the first day after surgery is the day they require the most assistance with physical needs. They may require assistance to meet the most simple needs:

- **hygiene** (bathing, oral care, and grooming)
- ambulation (walking)
- turning and positioning their body
- nutrition
- **elimination**
- comfort and safety

You should encourage patients to participate in their care as soon as the nurse tells you what is included in patients' plan of care.

HYGIENE
the practice of cleanliness to promote health

ELIMINATION
the way the body rids itself of unusable food and fluid; the discharge of the waste products created by the body's metabolism

PSYCHOLOGIC NEEDS

Patients have many worries about how their body will function after surgery. However, calm and relaxation are necessary so the body can focus its energy on healing and recovery. Some common concerns of postoperative patients follow.

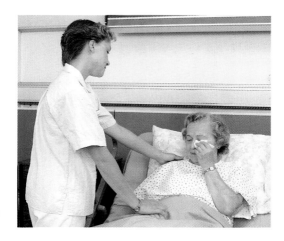

FIGURE 26-4

Crying may be an expression of a patient's psychologic needs.

- Some patients are very relieved after surgery because they are glad it is over.
- Patients may be anxious about the future if there are things that they can no longer do. For example, the person who has had a limb amputated worries about the loss of function.
- Patients may have problems with self-image if the surgery will leave a scar. For example, a woman who has had a breast removed may not feel like a desirable woman. Patients may cry or look sad. Encourage patients to express their feelings. When you tell the nurse or supervisor about a patient's feelings, use the patient's words. Examples are "I don't think I can live like this" and or "I'm feeling depressed." You can then add your own observations about how the patient is behaving, such as crying, looking away when spoken to, and not answering questions (Figure 26-4).

CARE OF THE POSTOPERATIVE PATIENT

The care of the postoperative patient is very important. As a nursing assistant, your role is to help meet the physical and psychologic needs of the patient. The following are your responsibilities:

- Measure vital signs.
- Remind the patient to **cough** and do **deep breathing.**
- Provide patient safety.
- Orient the patient.
- Help the patient move and turn.
- Care for the skin.
- Provide fluids as needed.
- Help with urinary elimination.
- Provide patient comfort.
- Care for tubes when present.

COUGH

sudden expulsion of air from the lungs

DEEP BREATHING

the intake of air deep into the lungs, followed by a slow release of air from the lungs

MEASURING VITAL SIGNS

One of the most important responsibilities you have when caring for the postoperative patient is to measure the vital signs (temperature, pulse, respiration, and blood pressure). Vital signs are affected by the general anesthetic used during surgery. A change in vital signs may signal a change in the patient's condition. Keeping a record of vital signs helps the nurse and physician monitor the patient for possible early complications.

POSTOPERATIVE VITAL SIGNS FLOW SHEET

Time	Blood Pressure	Temperature	Pulse	Respirations	Initials
0945	110/62	36.4	70	16	ER
1000	110/62	36.3	70	16	ER
1015	110/64	36.4	72	16	ER
1030	110/64	36.6	70	18	ER
1100	112/64	36.6	72	18	ER
1130	114/66	36.6	76	16	ER
1230	114/66	36.9	76	18	JB
1330	114/68	36.9	76	18	JB
1430	116/68	36.9	78	18	ER

Initials	Signature	Initials	Signature
ER	Elaine Revers, NA		
JB	June Bender, LPN		

Teresa Melonis
Room 2419

Patient Stamp

FIGURE 26–5

An example of a postoperative flow sheet.

Many health care institutions have what is known as a postoperative flow sheet (Figure 26–5). The flow sheet is used to document information about vital signs after the patient returns to the nursing unit. It is your responsibility to maintain the flow sheet and to report to the nurse immediately any changes in vital signs. The nurse tells you how often to measure the patient's vital signs and where to document the results. Most health care institutions follow the following schedule (or one like it) to check the vital signs of the postoperative patient:

Every 15 minutes for the first hour after return to the unit
Every 30 minutes for the second hour
Every hour for the next 3 to 4 hours
Every 4–8 hours for the rest of the patient's stay in the hospital

Tell the nurse if any of the vital signs increase or decrease since the last time you measured them. For example, if the respirations drop to 10 breaths

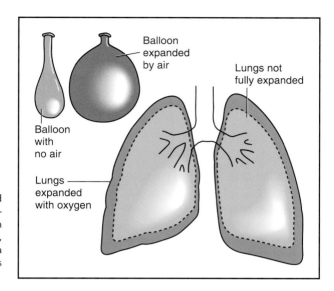

FIGURE 26-6

Balloons illustrate how expanded lungs make more oxygen available to the body's tissues. When enough oxygen is breathed in, the lungs fully expand just like a balloon does when enough air is blown in.

per minute, notify the nurse immediately. Tell the nurse if you observe that patients' skin feels warmer than usual or patients tell you they feel hot. Also report a pale or ashen color to the skin.

ENCOURAGING THE PATIENT TO PRACTICE COUGHING AND DEEP BREATHING

The nurses teach the patient to cough and breathe deeply before the surgical procedure, because the patient needs to work to expand the lungs after surgery. The patient may not cough and breathe deeply because of pain from the surgical procedure or weakness from the anesthetic medication. It is important to remind the patient to cough and breathe deeply because these exercises:

- Help the lungs expand (Figure 26-6).
- Provide oxygen to the body.
- Loosen lung secretions.
- Help prevent the hypostatic pneumonia that can occur if lung secretions stay in one place.

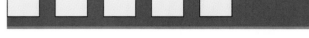

PROCEDURE

Assisting the Patient with Deep Breathing

The patient is asked to take deep breaths so that the lungs expand and fill with air. Deep breathing helps with the oxygen–carbon dioxide exchange in the lungs. *Note:* Your institution may arrange for you to observe a respiratory therapist (a professional skilled in caring for patients with breathing problems) help a patient with deep breathing and coughing.

ACTION	RATIONALE
1. Position the patient in an upright position.	Increases expansion of the lungs.
2. Tell the patient to take a slow deep breath.	

Continued on following page

PROCEDURE

Assisting the Patient with Deep Breathing
Continued

ACTION	RATIONALE
Preparation	
3. Ask the patient to hold the breath for about 3 seconds.	Helps get air to all areas of the lungs.
4. Ask the patient to breath out slowly.	
5. Tell the patient to repeat this procedure two or three times every hour.	

PROCEDURE

Assisting a Patient to Cough

Coughing and deep breathing are often done at the same time. If the patient does not have mucus pooling in the lungs, the nurse may tell you that coughing is not necessary. *Note:* After certain surgical procedures, such as eye surgery or the repair of a hernia, the patient *may not be allowed to cough.* Check the patient's care plan to be sure of the order.

ACTION	RATIONALE
1. Tell patient to take a deep breath.	
2. Tell patient to cough a few times when breathing out.	Helps loosen mucus so it can be brought up from the lungs.
3. Splint the incision with a pillow; this may help the patient who has had chest or abdominal surgery breathe easier (Figure 26–7).	Decreases pain and discomfort that coughing can cause.

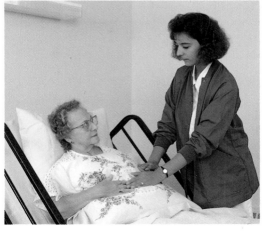

FIGURE 26–7
The patient should use both hands to hug a pillow toward the incision. If the patient is too weak, place your hands on the pillow, and provide pressure while the patient coughs.

4. Ask the patient to cough only enough to bring up the mucus.	Too much coughing can make the patient tired.

Some patients need to be encouraged or reminded often to cough and deep breath. Provide praise when the patient follows through correctly.

Do not automatically tell patients to do coughing and breathing exercises. Follow the nurse's directions about coughing and deep breathing exercises because these procedures are performed only when ordered by the physician.

To get children to perform the coughing and deep breathing exercises, give them a teddy bear or some other stuffed animal to hold against the incision while they do the exercises.

PROVIDING SAFETY AND ORIENTATION

Patients who are confused or weak after surgery have safety and orientation needs. Help patients stay safe and gain their cooperation by doing the following:

- Orient patients to person, place, time, and day.
- Raise the side rails when patients are weak. This includes the young child and frail elderly patient.
- Place the call signal within patients' reach and tell them where it is. Remind patients how to use the call signal.
- Assist patients in getting out of bed (Figure 26–8) and in ambulating.
- Check on patients frequently.
- When patients are in the bathroom stay in their room so that you can hear them if they call for help.
- Keep the room quiet and allow patients to rest.
- Plan your care so that you are not constantly disturbing patients.

PREVENTING BLOOD CLOTS

Patients who have circulatory risks after surgery have the need for protection against the formation of blood clots. When blood **circulation** is not normal, blood pools (stays in one place) and can cause a blood clot, which can be a very serious condition. To prevent this from happening, perform the following:

CIRCULATION

the movement of blood through the body caused by the heart's pumping action

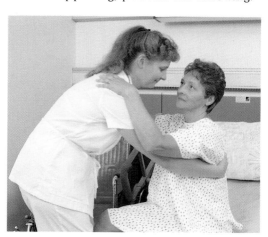

FIGURE 26–8

When you help patients get out of bed, allow them to move at their own pace.

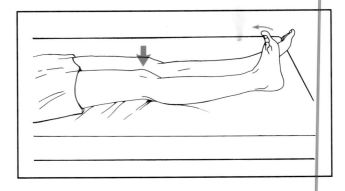

FIGURE 26–9

The patient should tighten the quadriceps muscle before ambulating. The patient should straighten the leg and push the kneecap toward the bed.

QUADRICEPS EXERCISE

a leg exercise performed by the patient in bed to help the circulation of blood

- Monitor vital signs on the schedule set up by the health care institution in which you work. A change in vital signs may signal a problem with circulation or breathing.
- Ask patients to change position every 2 hours. If the patient is unable to turn independently, assist the patient to change position if this is allowed by the physician's orders. Movement helps the circulation and thus prevents blood clot formation.
- Ask patients to move their legs up and down a few times every 2 hours, if this is allowed by the physician's orders, to stimulate the circulation.
- Remind patients to do the leg exercises they were taught by the nurse before surgery. Leg exercises help increase circulation. These leg exercises are also referred to as **quadriceps exercises** (Figure 26–9). Every 2 hours, the patient should

    Press down on the bed with the back of the knee.
    Point the toes toward the head of the bed.
    Tighten the thigh muscles.

- Assist patients with ambulation (Figure 26–10). Many patients are out of bed the same day or the day after surgery. Encourage patients to walk a little farther each time they are up. Stay nearby or beside them, depending on their condition. Follow the institution's established ambulation schedule.
- As patients' strength returns, the nurse will tell you whether they should use a wheelchair for moving about the unit or should walk alone or with the assistance of care givers (Figure 26–11).

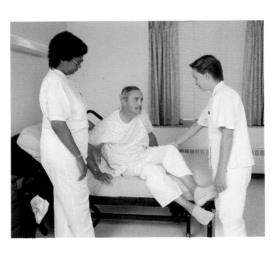

FIGURE 26–10

Until the patient becomes stronger, two care givers may be needed to help the patient walk.

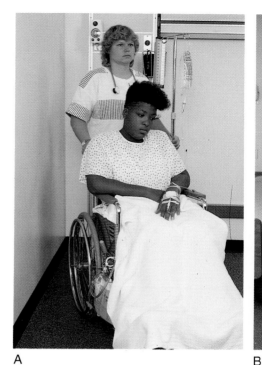

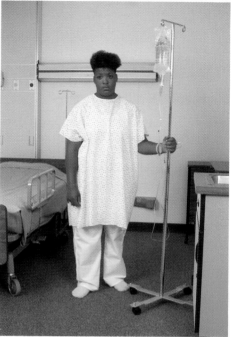

A   B

FIGURE 26-11

A, The patient may need to use a wheelchair until strength returns. B, When patients ambulate, they can hold onto the intravenous pole to steady themselves.

- In the first few days after surgery, tell patients to change position slowly. Patients should be told to use special care when sitting up or lying down from a standing position. Quick moves and changes in position can cause **orthostatic hypotension** and falls.
- If patients are nauseated or vomiting, position them on their left side, when possible (Figure 26-12), to prevent inhalation of **vomitus.** If a patient inhales vomitus into the lungs, a condition called **aspiration** can occur. The aspiration may result in a life-threatening pneumonia. Remember to check with the nurse to be sure that a side-lying position is allowed for a patient.
- Observe the patient for any bleeding or changes in vital signs; report changes to the nurse or supervisor.
- Apply antiembolic stockings, if ordered.

ORTHOSTATIC HYPOTENSION
a dizzy feeling caused by a fall in blood pressure; occurs when a person sits or stands too quickly
VOMITUS
results of vomiting; material ejected from the stomach through the mouth
ASPIRATION
the act of inhaling vomitus, mucus, or a small object into the respiratory system; may occur in persons who are unconscious, under the effects of general anesthesia, or having difficulty swallowing

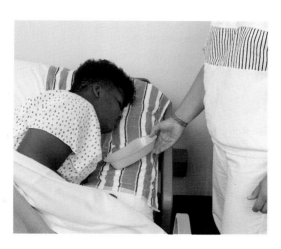

FIGURE 26-12
The left side-lying position helps prevent the patient from inhaling vomitus into the lungs.

Positioning the patient on the left side decreases the risk of aspirating vomitus into the lungs.

Antiembolic Stockings

ANTIEMBOLIC STOCKINGS

elastic stockings worn to prevent the formation of an embolus

The use of **antiembolic stockings** decreases the risk of blood clot formation. These stockings help blood return to the heart by keeping steady pressure on the muscles of the lower extremities. The application of elastic stockings requires the physician's order. Check the plan of care or ask the nurse if your patient requires elastic stockings. Remember that even though the patient is wearing these special stockings, moving the legs up and down in bed or walking is still necessary.

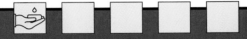

PROCEDURE

Applying Antiembolic Stockings

The nurse measures the patient's legs and orders the appropriate elastic stockings. Stockings may be knee high or thigh high. Elastic stockings are removed during the patient's bath. They should also be removed at least twice daily so that legs can be cleaned and checked for problem areas such as redness and swelling.

GATHER EQUIPMENT

Elastic stockings   Talcum powder

ACTION	RATIONALE
Preparation	
1. Wash hands.	Prevents the spread of microorganisms.
2. Identify yourself and the patient.	Maintains patients' rights.
3. Provide privacy.	Maintains patients' rights.
4. Explain the procedure.	Informs patients what is happening.
Procedural Steps	
5. Elevate the bed to a comfortable working position.	Reduces strain on your back muscles.
6. Place the patient in the supine (back-lying) position for a half hour before applying the stockings.	Prevents the veins from becoming distended (swollen) with blood. The veins should not be distended when stockings are put on.
7. Apply a small amount of talcum powder to legs, which should be clean.	Helps the stockings go on easier.
8. Gather the material of the stocking from top to bottom in your hands (Figure 26–13).	
9. Place bottom opening over toes and heel. Adjust for a smooth fit.	Wrinkles interfere with circulation.
10. Continue to pull the stocking toward the knee or thigh, removing all wrinkles.	

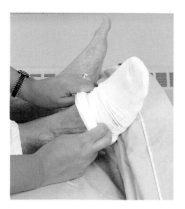

FIGURE 26-13

11. Repeat with other stocking when the nurse tells you to put the elastic stockings on both legs. (If only one elastic stocking is ordered, be certain you apply it to the correct leg.)

In certain medical conditions, the patient may have an elastic stocking ordered for only one lower extremity.

12. Check the band at the top of each stocking to be sure it is not binding.

Tightness interferes with circulation.

13. Tell the patient not to wear the stockings rolled down.

Creates tightness that interferes with circulation.

14. Observe the stockings for smoothness. If wrinkles or binding are present,
    • Remove the stocking.
    • Check the toes for warmth.
    • Check the leg for signs of irritation and/or swelling.
    • Report the observations to the nurse.
    • Replace the stockings as directed by the nurse.

Follow-Through

15. Record and report
    • the time stockings were applied
    • observations of skin condition before the stockings were applied

CARING FOR THE SKIN

The skin protects the body against entry of harmful microorganisms and injury. You play an important role in keeping the skin intact. It is your responsibility to

• Apply lotion to the skin to keep the skin moist. Pay particular attention to the elbows, heels, hips, and back.
• Turn and position the patient at least every 2 hours to prevent the formation of decubitus ulcers.
• Inspect the skin for any reddened areas that do not go away after the pressure is removed. A red area that stays after pressure is removed may be an indication that a decubitus ulcer is forming.

Other measures that help prevent decubitus ulcers are discussed in Chapter 13.

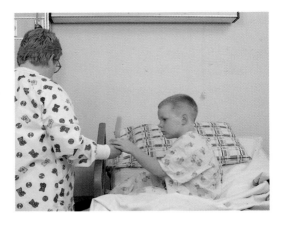

FIGURE 26–14
A popsicle provides important fluids after surgery.

PROVIDING FLUIDS

The effects of general anesthesia include the slowing down of gastrointestinal functioning, which may cause discomfort to the patient. The following points are important to remember when providing postoperative care to patients who underwent general anesthesia for surgery.

- Do not give patients food or fluid until the nurse tells you to do so. If you give patients food or fluids too soon, nausea, vomiting, or intestinal blockage may occur.
- After patients are permitted to have food and fluids they usually progress very quickly from a liquid diet to a soft diet to a regular diet (Figure 26–14). (For more information about diet, see Chapter 19).
- Encourage patients to drink fluids when the order is changed from NPO (nothing by mouth) to clear liquids. This can help relieve the dry mouth and **dehydration** that can occur after general anesthesia.
- Fluids also help make lung secretions more liquid so patients can cough them up.

DEHYDRATION

condition resulting from a loss of body fluid

HELPING WITH URINARY ELIMINATION

Patients with a urinary catheter may feel like they need to urinate but be unable to do so. You should explain that the feeling is created by the pressure of the catheter.

After the catheter is removed, the patient may have difficulty urinating. The following measures may help relax the urinary meatus, which allows the patient to empty the bladder.

- Run water in the bathroom sink while patients are sitting on the bedpan or commode.
- Place patients' hands in a basin of warm water while they are sitting on the bedpan or commode.
- Give patients a glass of water with a straw in it and ask them to blow bubbles in the water by blowing air through the straw. Patients should do this while attempting to urinate.

PROVIDING PATIENT COMFORT

Patients may be in pain after surgery. Observe for signs of pain such as facial grimacing, gasping, clenched fists, or crying. Ask patients if they have pain and report their responses and your observations to the nurse. The nurse administers medications to relieve pain.

Patients who have had an **abdominal** incision may be uncomfortable and in pain when they move. The physician may order a binder to be applied. Two kinds of binders are available:

ABDOMINAL
pertaining to the abdomen

- Elastic binder with Velcro closures
- Binder made of washable cotton material (scultetus binder, T-binder)

The binder may be applied to

- Make the patient more comfortable.
- Hold a dressing in place.
- Provide support when the patient moves and turns.

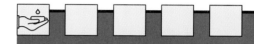

PROCEDURE

Applying a Binder

The binder is applied after the daily bath. It should remain on the patient until the nurse tells you to remove it. If it becomes soiled, a fresh binder should be reapplied. If the binder becomes loose, it should be resecured.

GATHER EQUIPMENT

Binder

ACTION	RATIONALE
Preparation	
1. Wash hands.	Prevents the spread of microorganisms.
2. Identify yourself and the patient.	Maintains patients' rights.
3. Provide privacy.	Maintains patients' rights.
4. Explain the procedure.	Informs patients what is happening.
Procedural Steps	
5. Ask patients to turn on their side or assist them to turn.	The binder is usually applied when the patient is in the bed.
Scultetus binder:	
6. Place the binder on the bed and center it. Tuck one edge of the binder close to patients' back.	Patients automatically lie in the correct spot when they return to the supine position.
7. Return patients to the supine (back-lying) position (Figure 26–15) and pull binder through.	

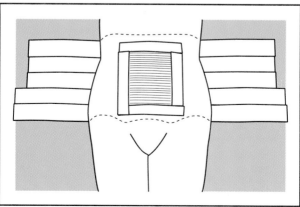

FIGURE 26–15

(Redrawn from Sorensen KC, Luckmann J: Basic Nursing: A Psychological Approach, 2nd ed. Philadelphia, W. B. Saunders Company, 1986.)

Continued on following page

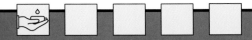

PROCEDURE

Applying a Binder *Continued*

ACTION	**RATIONALE**

Preparation

8. Starting at the bottom of the binder, bring each tail across the abdomen. Smooth each strip and pull it taut (Figure 26–16).

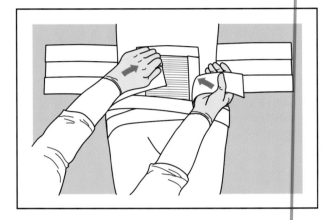

FIGURE 26–16

(Redrawn from Sorensen KC, Luckmann J: Basic Nursing: A Psychological Approach, 2nd ed. Philadelphia, W. B. Saunders Company, 1986.)

9. Secure binder at the top with a pin (Figure 26–17). The binder should be snug but not too tight.

A snug binder is comfortable and supporting. A tight binder is uncomfortable for the patient.

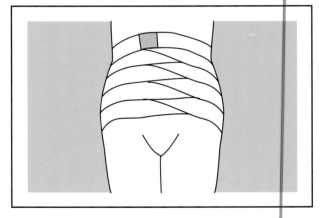

FIGURE 26–17

(Redrawn from Sorensen KC, Luckmann J: Basic Nursing: A Psychological Approach, 2nd ed. Philadelphia, W. B. Saunders Company, 1986.)

Elastic binder:

10. Repeat steps 5–7.

11. Secure the binder with the Velcro strips. The binder should be snug but not too tight.

T-binder:

12. Bring strap between legs and pin to the waistband. T-binders are used to keep perineal dressings in place (Figure 26–18).

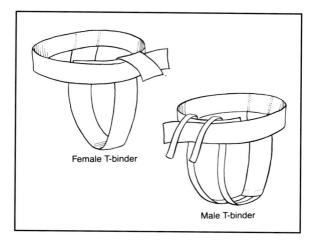

Female T-binder

Male T-binder

FIGURE 26–18

T-binders. (From Sorensen KC, Luckmann, J: Basic Nursing: A Psychological Approach, 2nd ed. Philadelphia, W. B. Saunders Company, 1986.)

Follow-Through

13. Record and report that the binder has been applied. Report any patient statements about comfort or discomfort.

Provides a legal record that the procedure was done.

CARING FOR PATIENTS' TUBES

Tubes are placed in the body to carry substances into the body (for example, tubing may carry intravenous fluids and oxygen into the body) and carry drainage away from the body (for example, a urinary catheter drains urine out of the bladder and a drain in an incision carries debris away from the operative site).

Tubes that carry substances into the body include

- Intravenous tubing—carries fluids into the circulation. Patients need this kind of fluid because their ability to swallow is lost until the effects of the general anesthetic wear off.
- Oxygen tubing—supplies oxygen to the lungs through the nose or mouth. Patients may have previous breathing problems or may have developed a problem with oxygen and carbon dioxide exchange during or after the surgery. Remember that cells need oxygen for proper functioning.

Tubes are needed to carry material away from both natural and artificial body openings. Tubes that carry drainage away from natural body openings include

- **Nasogastric tubing**—inserted through the nose into the stomach. Secretions are drained away, observed, and measured. Certain surgeries and patient conditions result in the need to keep secretions out of the stomach. When necessary, substances such as medication and liquid food can be given through this type of tubing.
- Urinary **catheter**—permits the drainage of urine from the bladder. The physician may order the removal of the tubing unless close monitoring of urinary output is necessary.

Tubes that carry material away from artificial body openings include

- Tubes that promote drainage of body secretions from the operative site. A **Penrose drain** is an open-ended tube that allows secretions to drain out onto a dressing. In another type of drain, drainage from the opera-

NASOGASTRIC TUBE

tube inserted through a nostril into the stomach

CATHETER

a flexible tube passed into body openings to allow fluids to enter or exit the body

PENROSE DRAIN

a drain placed in the body during surgery that allows secretions to flow out of the body into an absorbent pad

JACKSON-PRATT DRAIN
a drain placed in the body during surgery that allows secretions to flow out of the body into a collection container

HEMOVAC DRAIN
a drain placed in the body during surgery that allows secretions to flow out of the body into a collection container

tive site flows into a collection container. Examples of collection-type drains are the **Jackson-Pratt drain** and the **Hemovac drain.**

If a large artificial opening is created, a pouch-like collection container may be placed over the site to collect secretions.

It is important that you follow special guidelines when caring for postoperative patients who have tubes inserted (see Guidelines for Caring for a Postoperative Patient with Tubes Chart).

GUIDELINES FOR CARING FOR A POSTOPERATIVE PATIENT WITH TUBES

Action	Rationale
Check all tubing connections and report any breaks to the nurse immediately.	Prevents injury to the skin caused by some body secretions.
Check that all tubing is free from obstruction caused by pinching by side rails or the patient's body.	Pinched tubing stops the flow of fluids and oxygen into the body and the flow of secretions out of the body.
Observe all collection containers for color, thickness, and amount of drainage. Record your observations.	To monitor the function of the body's organs.
Monitor the levels in the intravenous containers and the water bottle connected to the oxygen tubing.	The nurse must be notified when levels are low. In some institutions, you may be permitted to put distilled water in the bottle that provides humidity for the oxygen.
Monitor levels of collection containers. If the urine collection bag fills up, empty it and measure and record the amount of urine. You may be permitted to empty other collection devices, depending on the policy of your institution.	Alerts you to possible problems if secretions are more than normal.
Keep the skin around all openings clean.	Prevents injury to the skin and helps with patient comfort.
Do not raise collection containers above the drainage site.	Prevents the backup of secretions into the body.
Keep all tubing clear when moving or turning the patient.	Prevents an obstruction that could interfere with the flow into or out of the body.
Never disconnect any tubing.	Interferes with treatment. Also, a break can introduce harmful microorganisms and cause infection.
Record and report Color, amount, and thickness of drainage Any pain, swelling, or discoloration around the tubes	Provides a legal record. Keeps the nurse informed about the patient's condition.

CARING COMMENT

If the patient has an indwelling urinary catheter inserted after surgery, remember to perform catheter care (see Chapter 21).

CHAPTER WRAP-UP

- The postoperative period begins as soon as the surgical procedure is complete.
- The time spent in the recovery room is part of the postoperative period.
- The postoperative complications that must be prevented are
    Infection
    Pneumonia
    Blood clots
    Constipation
    Decubitus ulcers
    Urinary retention or infection
- Postoperative complications may be prevented by
    Reminding the patient to cough and deep breathe at least every 2 hours to help expand the lungs.
    Offering fluids as soon as they are permitted to keep the body hydrated.
    Assisting the patient to ambulate to help the blood circulate so that blood clots do not form.
    Helping the patient move and turn to loosen secretions in the lungs.
    Placing the patient in a position of comfort so that the body gets the rest it needs to heal.
    Ensuring patient safety by raising side rails to prevent falls when the patient is confused or weak.
- Attend to patients' physical and psychologic needs after surgery:
    Physical needs are the greatest immediately after the surgery is completed.
    As patients gain strength, encourage them to do as much for themselves as possible.
    Help patients perform the activities that prevent postoperative complications.
    Psychologic needs are important when there is a change in body image caused by the surgical procedure.
    Listen to patients and report their concerns to the nurse or supervisor.

REVIEW QUESTIONS

1. What is done to prepare the room for the arrival of the patient from the recovery room?
2. List the measures you are responsible for taking to prevent complications in the postoperative patient.
3. Describe how general anesthesia affects each body function.
4. What increases patients' risk for complications after surgery?

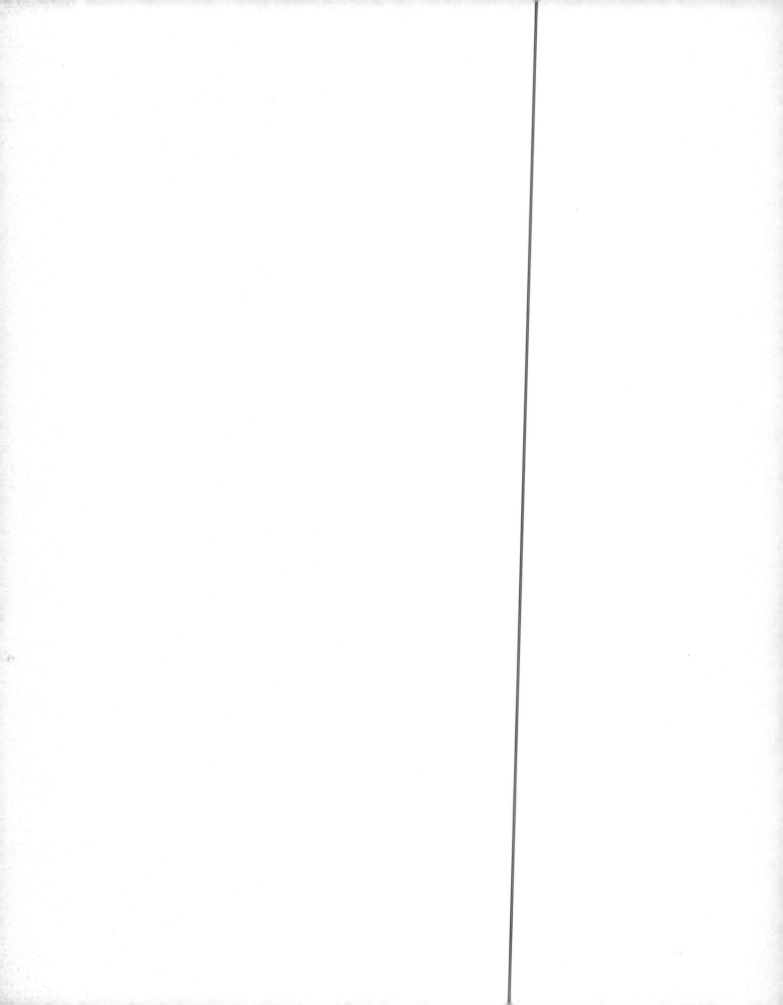

UNIT SEVEN

Considering the Whole Person

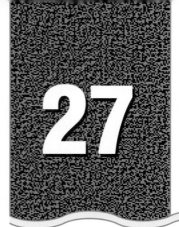

27 Understanding Psychologic Development

Objectives

AFTER YOU COMPLETE THIS CHAPTER, YOU WILL BE ABLE TO:

Define the term *developmental tasks*.

Describe developmental needs across the life span.

Explain how you can help patients continue to meet their developmental needs while in the health care institution.

Describe how support systems help the patient.

Describe the person with anxiety.

Care for patients with anxious behaviors.

Describe the person with depression.

Care for patients who are depressed.

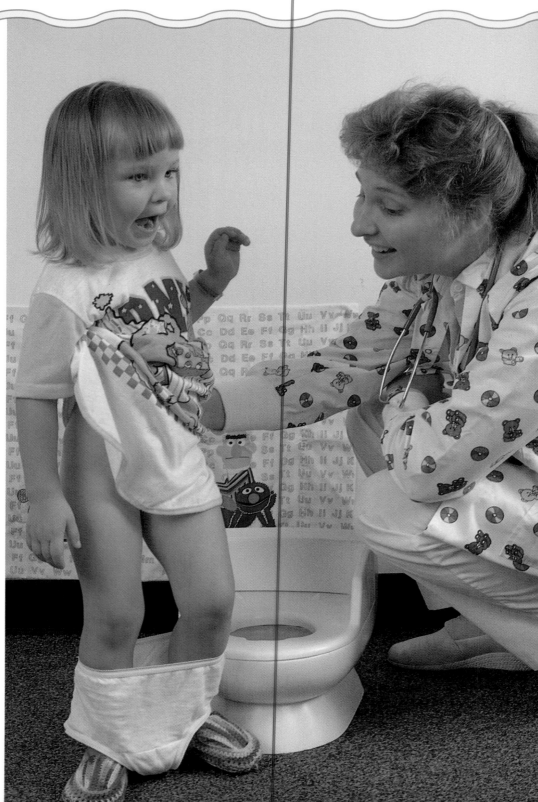

Overview Psychologic development is very important to growth and maturity. Each person has developmental needs that must be met. When developmental needs are met, the person can approach life with a sense of self-esteem and accomplishment along with the feeling that life is good. If you are caring for elderly patients, you will listen to many stories about the past. Older people need to talk about their past life, and you can help meet this need by listening and encouraging patients to reminisce. As a nursing assistant, you will find many opportunities to help people meet their psychologic needs.

WHAT DO YOU KNOW ABOUT PSYCHOLOGIC DEVELOPMENT?

Here are seven statements about psychologic development. Consider them to test your current knowledge of how a person develops psychologically. If you think the statement is true, circle the T; if you think the statement is false, circle the F. Change the false statements to make them true.

1. T F As individuals mature and develop, they learn to think and problem-solve.

2. T F Once persons are mentally ill, they can never be cured.

3. T F Infants learn to trust others when their basic needs are met.

4. T F Marriage can be considered a milestone in life.

5. T F Older people who reminisce about their life may be considered mentally ill.

6. T F Anxiety is a feeling that is common to all people.

7. T F The person who is depressed may talk and move slowly.

ANSWERS

1. **True.** Thinking and problem-solving begin early in life and become mature skills for most people when they become adults.

2. **False.** Mental illness can be temporary or long term. Many forms of mental illness can be treated with medication or counseling.

3. **True.** The infant who is fed, kept clean and dry, touched, and loved learns to trust that the world is a good place to be.

4. **True.** Marriage is an important milestone of young adulthood.

5. **False.** Reminiscing is an important and expected part of psychologic development.

6. **True.** Anxious behaviors may be displayed by a person. A little anxiety helps one function better, but too much anxiety interferes with functioning.

7. **True.** Depression causes the functions of the body to slow down.

PSYCHOLOGY
the study of mental development, mental processes, and behavior

BEHAVIOR
the manner of conducting oneself

PSYCHOLOGIC DEVELOPMENT

Psychology is the study of the mind and **behavior.** As people develop, they begin to use their brain to think, solve problems, and make decisions. Over

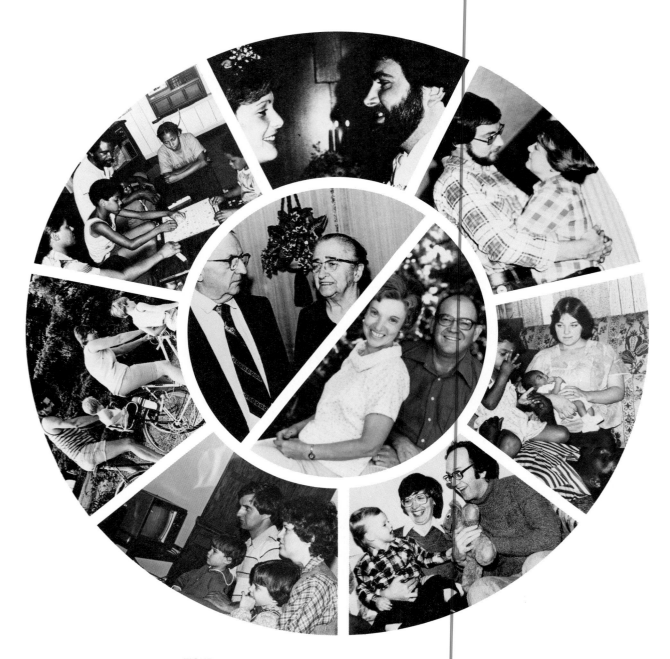

FIGURE 27–1

The cycle of growth and development. (From Foster RLR, Hunsberger MM, Anderson JJT: Family-Centered Nursing Care of Children. Philadelphia, W. B. Saunders Company, 1989.)

time, the mental processes become mature. The road to adulthood consists of many changes that a person must master. Most persons build on experience and strive to behave in ways that are acceptable to society (Figure 27–1). Psychologists who have studied the **development** of the mind and the way people behave have been able to identify the steps to adulthood and maturity. Their studies have enabled people in the health care professions to support the developmental needs of patients.

DEVELOPMENT
growth from a lower to a higher state of functioning

ERIKSON'S THEORY OF PSYCHOSOCIAL DEVELOPMENT

Psychosocial development refers to the influence of society on people's mental development and behavior. One of the most important explanations of psychologic development of this century was made by Erik Erikson. He identified 8 **developmental stages** in the life of human beings (see chart) and identified what developmental behaviors occur as the individual progresses through each stage across the life span. These behaviors are called **developmental tasks.** An individual must accomplish a certain group of developmental tasks in one developmental stage to progress to the next stage and begin the developmental tasks associated with it. The tasks do not have to be accomplished in any specific order.

A **milestone** is an event that marks something special. Examples of milestones are

PSYCHOSOCIAL
referring to the influence of society on mental development and behavior
DEVELOPMENTAL STAGE
stage during which certain behaviors are expected of an individual
DEVELOPMENTAL TASK
an expected accomplishment that helps a person develop as an individual
MILESTONE
a significant point in development

- an infant's first steps
- a child's first day of school
- a young adult's marriage
- a middle adult's change of job or career
- an older adult's retirement

A milestone for you might be completing your nursing assistant program and beginning to work as a care giver.

As a nursing assistant, you can help patients meet their developmental needs in each stage of life (see Stages of Development chart).

ERIKSON'S EIGHT STAGES OF DEVELOPMENT	
Stage	**Developmental Need**
Infancy (birth to 1½ years)	Trust
Toddler (1½–3 years)	Beginning independence
Preschool age (3–6 years)	Control over self and environment
	Discovery of outer world
School age (6–12 years)	Close friends
	Success at home and school
	Praise and recognition
Adolescence (12–18 years)	Identify with body changes
	Make transition from child to adult
Young adult (18–40 years)	Relationships
	Commitment
Middle age adult (40–65 years)	Guide the next generation
Older adult (65+ years)	Feel good about how life was lived
	Reminisce

HELPING PATIENTS MEET THEIR DEVELOPMENTAL NEEDS

As a nursing assistant, you can help patients continue to meet their developmental needs in the health care institution. It is necessary to help with these needs even though a person is ill. It is important for you to know each patient's developmental level. Observe patients' current functioning to determine their level of development. Methods for helping patients meet their developmental needs are described in the following sections.

The Infant's Developmental Needs

INFANT

the person at the beginning of life (from birth to 1½ years), for whom all needs are met by others

Infants learn to trust others and feel that the world is a safe place when basic needs like food and warmth are met (Figures 27–2 to 27–4). Infants believe the world revolves around them and do not understand if no one responds to their demands.

You can help infants develop and maintain trust when you care for them. Each response to a need builds trust between the infant and whoever is giving care (for example, parent or other relative or care givers). Give your attention to infants by touching them, talking to them, and making eye contact with them when caring for them. Be consistent in giving care. For example, always check the infant who is crying to find out what is needed.

Infants cry when they are hungry, wet, uncomfortable, or in pain. Respond to the need for nutrition by feeding the infant formula, other fluids, and solids as ordered. Try to anticipate the infant's need for food and fluid. Do not keep the infant waiting when hunger is evident.

Check the infant's clothing and diaper for dryness. If the diaper is soiled, remove it, cleanse the skin, and apply a dry diaper immediately. Put clean, dry clothing on the infant when needed.

In addition to needing to be fed and diapered, the infant might need to

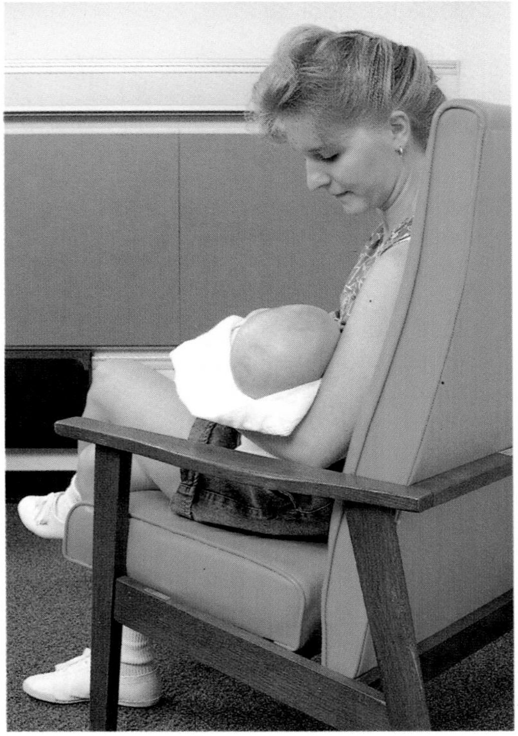

FIGURE 27–2
A mother holds her infant close while breastfeeding.

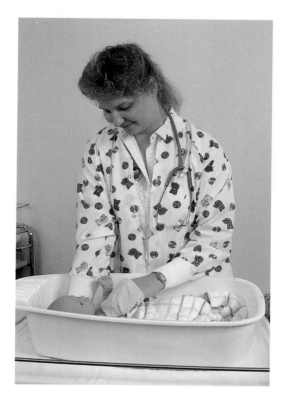

FIGURE 27-3

Monitor the newborn's body temperature and keep the baby warm, because the body does not regulate temperature well at birth.

be held and comforted. Rocking seems to comfort many infants. Talk or sing to infants, because they like to hear the comforting sound of another person's voice. When placing an infant in a crib, remember to change positions from back to side to stomach. Keep the infant warm and comfortable with a small blanket.

These measures help the infant develop the resources needed for continued healthy psychologic development. If basic needs are not met, the infant grows to mistrust and be suspicious of others.

The Toddler's Developmental Needs

The **toddler** begins to gain independence but still needs the support of others (Figure 27-5). Toddlers learn to control themselves as well as others around them. Independent behaviors such as feeding, walking, dressing, and controlling bowels and bladder are learned (Figure 27-6).

TODDLER

the young child from 1½ to 3 years of age

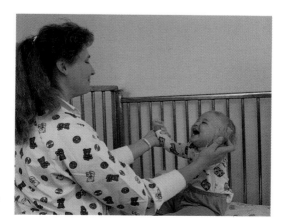

FIGURE 27-4

Communicate by talking, singing, smiling, and touching to help fill the need for social interaction.

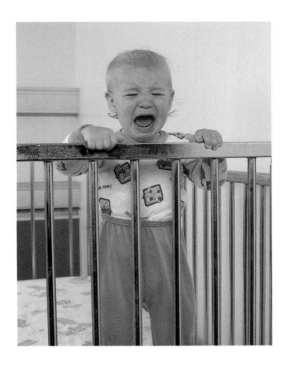

FIGURE 27-5
Respond quickly to crying or other signs of discomfort.

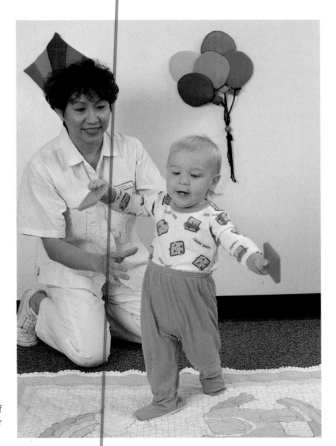

FIGURE 27-6
Toddlers develop a sense of control by trying to do things for themselves.

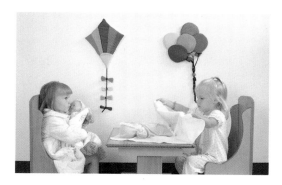

FIGURE 27-7

Preschool-age children explore the world more and begin to take more control over themselves and their environment.

Toddlers are self-centered and think they are the most important part of the world. You should realize that toddlers want to succeed but become frustrated and doubt their own ability.

When toddlers become ill or are hospitalized, their behavior may regress (go backward). They may choose to be dependent for a while. Do not shame or scold toddlers when they do not do things they have already learned. For example, a toddler who has learned to control bowel and bladder may soil the bed or underpants. Treat the situation matter-of-factly by changing the bed linens and helping the toddler change into clean clothing. When things are back to normal for the toddler, the soiling should stop.

You should allow toddlers in your care to do as much for themselves as possible. Do not do everything for them. However, do not expect more from toddlers than they can do. Check with the parent or nurse to find out what the toddler is capable of doing.

Set limits for toddlers, because independent behaviors should develop in a secure environment. Setting limits helps toddlers learn how to control their behavior. Encourage toddlers to be independent, but remember that they have not yet developed a sense of responsibility and still need adult direction. For example, during playtime, toys might be restricted to a specific area on the unit where the toddler is permitted to play. You may need to remind the toddler who has taken a toy from the area that toys are permitted only in that area. You may need to take the toddler by the hand and together return the toy.

As health returns, provide opportunities for feeding, dressing, and toileting and encourage toddlers to resume their independent behaviors at the previous level of functioning. This sense of independence prepares the toddler to enter the preschool age and continue psychologic development in a positive way.

The Preschool-Age Child's Developmental Needs

Preschool-age children are eager to learn and explore, which they do by playing, keeping busy, and learning to control their environment (Figure 27-7). Preschool-age children like to take charge and let others know their demands and wishes.

PRESCHOOL AGE
the child from 3 to 6 years of age

When your patient is a preschooler, you should give the child the lead in self-care activities. Encourage the child to do as much as allowed (Figures 27-8 and 27-9). Give sincere praise when the child performs successfully.

The child at this age is very curious and may have many questions for you. Answer as truthfully as you can. For example, if children ask you about a stethoscope, you can let them handle the **stethoscope** and listen to their own heart beat. Explain how the stethoscope works in a simple manner, such as, "The sound from your heart goes through the tubes to your ears."

STETHOSCOPE
an instrument used to hear and amplify the sounds of an internal organ (heart, lungs, or bowels)

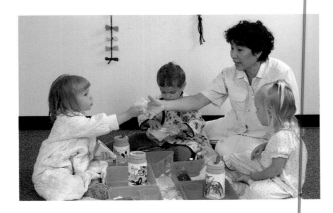

FIGURE 27–8
Supervise the play activities of young patients.

When you support the preschool-age child with learning and exploring experiences, the result is self-confidence and a feeling of goodness.

The School-Age Child's Developmental Needs

SCHOOL-AGE
the child from 6 to 12 years of age (the years before adolescence)

PEER
an equal; one who belongs to the same group (age, school, etc.)

INTERACTION
a communication between two or more people

School-age children expand their horizons to the outside world. **Peers** are very important to the development of self. Children of the same age group may be gathered together for games and **interaction.** You should encourage patients to join in as soon as their physical conditions allow it. The telephone is a major source of communication with friends and family. School-age children should be encouraged to use the telephone to keep up with news of school and home as well as to talk about their needs and feelings.

These are busy years, when the child is full of energy and wants to succeed at home and school. Help direct the child's energy so that success can

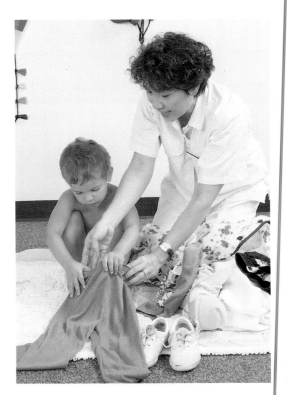

FIGURE 27–9
Reward appropriate independent behavior.

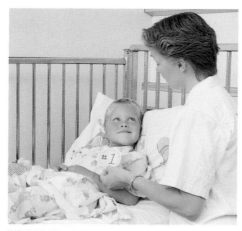 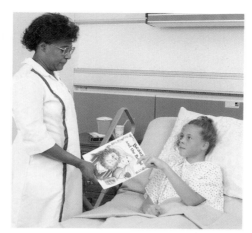

FIGURE 27–10
Reward a child who has been cooperative.

occur. Because ill children may not have the energy needed to keep up with usual routines, plan for rest periods before starting a procedure (bathing, dressing, walking, etc.) that might tire them.

Encourage and **reinforce** appropriate behaviors. Praise and other rewards are effective with the school-age child. You can praise children when they successfully complete a procedure in which their cooperation was important. For example, if a child stays in a certain position until an important test is finished, you can offer a reward. A reward can be something as simple as a sticker or other small item that may be kept on the unit (Figure 27–10).

Your actions can add to the school-age child's feelings of **self-esteem.**

The Adolescent's Developmental Needs

During the adolescent years (ages 12–18), the child grows into adulthood. Peers are very important to children in this age group (Figure 27–11). As for the school-age child, the telephone is an important means of maintaining contact with friends. Encourage this activity when permissible.

Adolescents are keenly aware of the changes in their body. They may be sensitive about their body, so privacy is important. Protect the adolescent's

REINFORCE
to strengthen by giving extra support

SELF-ESTEEM
how confident and satisfied a person feels

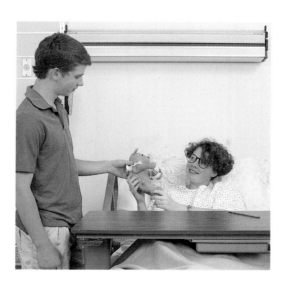

FIGURE 27–11
Adolescents need support and encouragement from peers.

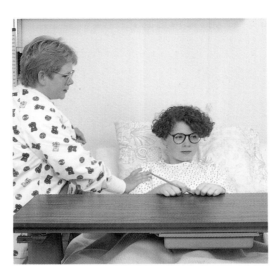

FIGURE 27–12
Take time to talk with and comfort an adolescent who is feeling afraid or angry.

privacy as you would any patient's. Make sure gowns are securely tied at the back and, whenever possible, provide bottoms for the patient.

During the teen years, the adolescent swings back and forth between child-like and adult behaviors. When the demands of the adult world become too much to handle, the adolescent reverts (goes back) to the safe and known world of childhood. In this case, he needs clear expectations about how he should act.

You should treat the adolescent as an adult, not as a child. For instance, if the patient is angry and afraid and throws something on the floor, you should take time to talk about feelings. You might say something like, "You seem to be angry. Let's take a few minutes to talk about what might be bothering you" (Figure 27–12). Do not **criticize** the patient. Criticizing results in feelings of guilt and does not make the patient feel any better.

CRITICIZE
to find fault

The Young Adult's Developmental Needs

Young adults (ages 18–40) need to develop close relationships with persons of both sexes (Figure 27–13). Sexual intimacy also develops at this age. Illness or injury may interrupt this important developmental need. Provide young adults with quiet, uninterrupted time to spend with significant others. When distance

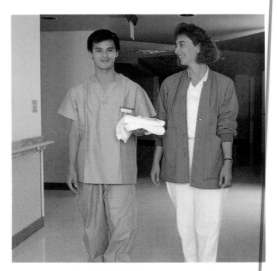

FIGURE 27–13
Close friendships may develop in the workplace between people of the opposite sex.

is a problem, the telephone can be used to communicate with friends and family.

Business and social relationships are important to the young adult's self-esteem. These relationships may need to be suspended while the person is in the health care setting. You should realize that illness or injury may disrupt patients' plans for family and career. Patients may wish to talk about themselves or about family, friends, work, and school. Encourage patients to talk about their feelings and concerns, and report pertinent information to the nurse or supervisor.

The Middle-Aged Adult's Developmental Needs

During middle age (40–65 years), a person nurtures and guides the next generation. Concern for the next generation is not limited to one's own children. It can extend to children of others and to children and young people one has met through being a volunteer in a community agency.

Middle-aged adults may be helping their children through school and may be attending school themselves as part of a midlife career change. Illness and injury can disrupt important plans, causing feelings of loss and uncertainty about the future. You can be supportive of middle-aged patients by allowing them to talk about frustrations and feelings as well as accomplishments and dreams. Report any pertinent information to the nurse or supervisor.

The Older Adult's Developmental Needs

Older adults (65 years and over) need to feel positive about themselves and the achievements of a lifetime. They need to feel that life is worth living. **Reminiscing** is a healthy behavior in which the person shares the unique experiences of a lifetime (Figure 27–14).

REMINISCE
to think or talk about past events

As a nursing assistant, you can listen to the patient who talks about past experiences. The patient's reminiscing can provide you with a wealth of information and help you get to know the patient (Figure 27–15). Persons who are happy with the way they lived their life have no regrets and look forward to spending their older years secure in the knowledge that life was good. If dissatisfaction with life is expressed, the person may be experiencing a loss for what might have been. The person may need to resolve some problems and may feel frustrated because illness or injury is interfering.

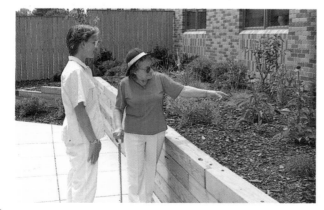

FIGURE 27–14
Older adults take pride in their past achievements and need to continue to feel that their life is worthwhile.

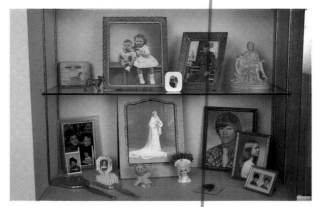

FIGURE 27-15
A memorabilia cabinet in a long-term care institution can help a patient reminisce about the past.

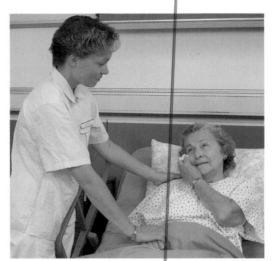

FIGURE 27-16
You can support the patient by using touch and listening.

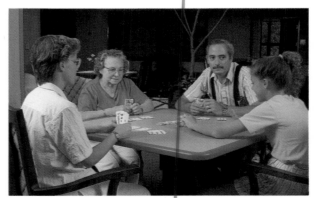

FIGURE 27-17
Interacting with others is important.

THE HELPING ROLE OF SUPPORT SYSTEMS

Having **support systems** is particularly important for patients, because the individuals in the support system are available whenever patients express a need for psychologic support. Support systems may be informal, including families, friends, co-workers, and pets; or formal, such as Alcoholics Anonymous.

You can be part of a patient's support system by interacting with the patient's family members, friends, and other visitors (Figure 27–16). People who are important to the patient should be important to you. Work with the nurse to help identify patients' support systems. You should

- Talk with patients and report to the nurse whether they mention supportive people or groups.
- Observe interactions between patients (Figure 27–17).

SUPPORT SYSTEM
the individuals a person can turn to for help

CARING COMMENT

If patients appear to have little support, discuss this with the nurse. The nurse will start a referral to a social worker. The social worker can assist patients while they are in the health care institution and can arrange for supportive services to be provided when patients are discharged.

COMMON DISRUPTIONS IN PSYCHOLOGIC FUNCTIONING

MENTAL ILLNESS

Mental health is emotional wellness. Persons who are emotionally well are able to function and interact with others and the environment. They are able to care for themselves and others. In some situations, a mentally healthy person may be physically unable to provide self-care.

Mental illness is the opposite of mental health. The mentally ill patient loses the sense of emotional well-being that is needed to function in a healthy manner. Mental illness may be either temporary or long-lasting.

MENTAL ILLNESS
disruption in psychologic functioning

CARING COMMENT

Do not use labels such as "crazy," "nuts," or "out of it" to refer to the person who is mentally ill. Use the terms "mentally ill" and "mental illness" when discussing the person whose mental or emotional well-being is threatened.

You can play an important role in the care of the person who has a disruption in psychologic functioning. The nurse will tell you what is wrong with the patient's psychologic functioning. You should understand that how you interact with the patient can affect how the patient feels. Be sure to report all changes in the patient's behavior to the nurse. Changes can appear in

- **Physical functioning:** for example, lack of sleep or loss of appetite or overeating
- **Psychologic functioning:** for example, feeling sad, worthless, or helpless; a sudden change in behavior; or withdrawal

ANXIETY

ANXIETY

an uneasy feeling that comes from
something that is going to happen
or an individual believes might
happen

CONFLICT

a struggle; a disagreement between
what is happening to the individual
and what is expected

Anxiety is an uneasy feeling. Anxiety in response to an event perceived as
threatening is a common human experience. Your patients may demonstrate
anxious behaviors in response to

- illness
- surgery
- diagnostic studies
- hospitalization
- **conflict**
- separation

Anxiety may also be caused by events in the environment, such as destructive
weather, war, or economic hardship. Anxiety may also result from events within
the individual (Figure 27–18), such as pregnancy, divorce, or a conflict in
values. The behavior exhibited by the individual may indicate the level of
anxiety the individual is experiencing. There are four levels of anxiety:

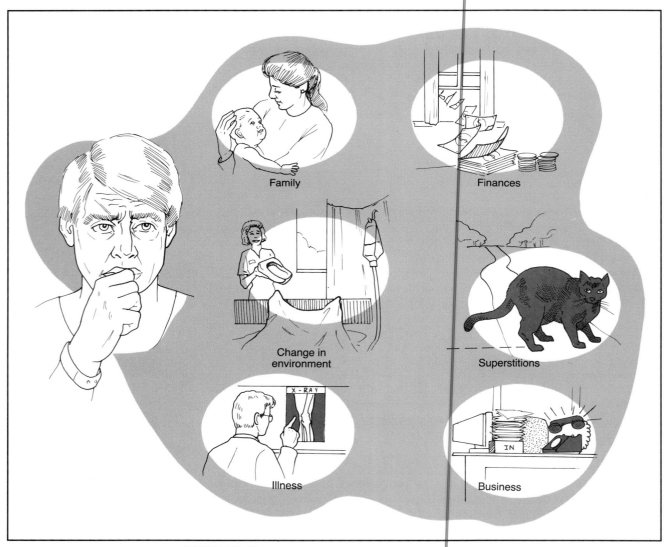

FIGURE 27–18

Many events in a person's life can cause anxiety. (From DuGas BW: Introduction to Patient Care: A
Comprehensive Approach to Nursing, 4th ed. Philadelphia, W. B. Saunders Company, 1983.)

MILD ANXIETY   This is the most common level of anxiety. When people experience mild anxiety, they have an increased awareness of what is happening around them. The person functions as normal or even better than normal. Mild anxiety is often helpful to the person.

MODERATE ANXIETY   Persons with moderate anxiety begin to pay less attention to things around them. They may need help in focusing their energy so they can function.

SEVERE ANXIETY   In severe anxiety, the things and events in the person's life are out of focus. The person cannot concentrate and solve problems. Comments such as "I can't think" or "I don't know what to do" are often made. The person who has severe anxiety needs some help and direction in order to function.

PANIC   The person in a state of panic is helpless and suffers a loss of control. This person is not able to tell what is real from what is not. The person must be protected from injury and helped to return to a state of lessened anxiety.

Observations of the Patient with Anxiety

Anxiety affects a person's functioning. The patient who is anxious may display physical as well as psychologic behaviors.

PHYSICAL BEHAVIORS

In the anxious person the following sequence of physical behaviors may be observed. At first there is

- Slight rise in vital sign measurements
- Slight muscle tension

If the anxiety is not relieved, other physical behaviors may be

- Increased pulse, respirations, and blood pressure
- Increased muscle tension
- Diaphoresis (sweating)
- Frequent urination
- Frequent changes in body position
- Verbalization of
    dizziness
    headache
    feeling that heart is pounding
    flushed feeling

If the anxiety is still not relieved, you may observe

- Continued increase in vital sign measurements
- Exhaustion

PSYCHOLOGIC BEHAVIORS

The psychologic behaviors the patient may exhibit include the following. At first the patient

- Appears calm
- Exhibits enhanced ability to problem-solve

If the anxiety is not relieved, the patient may

- Appear preoccupied
- Be inattentive to surroundings
- Feel helpless
- Worry a lot
- Cry or forget things

If the anxiety is still not relived, the patient may display

- An inability to learn or problem-solve appropriately

- Inappropriate behaviors
- Intense feelings of terror and doom

It is important for you to record your observations and report them to the nurse as soon as you observe something new or different about a patient's behavior.

CARING COMMENT

Anxiety upsets a person's sense of well-being. Persons may not always be aware that they are anxious, however.

Caring for the Patient with Anxiety

The patient who is anxious is not able to respond appropriately to others or to the environment. Be able to recognize the signs of anxiety and report them to the nurse. When you care for anxious patients, you should

- Remain calm. If they sense you are uncomfortable, their anxiety may increase.
- Be aware of your own unspoken communication. Patients can sense if you are not genuinely interested in them.
- Use simple, easy-to-understand words so that persons can understand you and follow your directions when necessary.
- Provide a quiet atmosphere to help calm patients.
- Sit with patients so that you can be a support system and help prevent injury.

DEPRESSION

DEPRESSION

sadness and a decrease in the usual behaviors associated with daily functioning

Depression is sadness and hopelessness along with a decrease in usual behaviors associated with daily functioning. If a person is unable to cope with depressed feelings, they may become long-lasting. Depression may interrupt behaviors that help the person to function at home, school, and work. Persons with depression may withdraw from interaction with other people and the environment and may be unable to care for themselves. They may not be able to continue working or going to school because they have no energy or interest in doing these everyday functions.

The following are some of the causes of depression:

- Medications
- Lack of a certain substance in the brain
- Inherited tendency (in some families, more than one person may experience depression)
- The feeling of helplessness about a situation, an illness, or an event

Observations of the Patient with Depression

The person with depression exhibits physical as well as psychologic behaviors. You might observe the following physical behaviors in the patient:

- Poor appetite or lack of appetite
- Change in sleep patterns (the person may sleep all of the time or may not be able to sleep)
- Constipation
- Lack of energy (the inability to complete activities of daily living)

The psychologic behaviors you might observe include

- Feelings of hopelessness—the patient may say, "No one can help me now"
- **Apathy** about the self; the patient may say, "There is nothing I can do about it anyway"
- Poor self-esteem; the patient may say, "I'm not good for anything"
- **Rejection** of family and friends

APATHY
lack of interest

REJECTION
not wanted by or not satisfied with someone or something

Caring for the Depressed Patient

Because depressed persons may do little for themselves, you may need to help them until they are able to take responsibility for their own needs. The chart below shows some of the actions you can take to help the person and the reasons the actions are needed.

HOW A NURSING ASSISTANT CAN HELP A DEPRESSED PATIENT	
Action	**Reason**
Keep a record of food and fluid intake	Poor overall intake by mouth
Encourage the patient to eat	Lack of appetite
Encourage exercise and activity	Lack of interest in self and surroundings
Encourage daytime wakefulness	Allows for a night's sleep
Spend time with the patient	Shows that you have not abandoned patient
Listen to what the patient says	Shows an interest in the patient

When you take care of a patient with depression, it is important to remember that the person does not have the energy to function normally. Even activities of daily living (eating, dressing, studying, etc.) may become too difficult or almost impossible for the depressed person to perform (Figure 27–19).

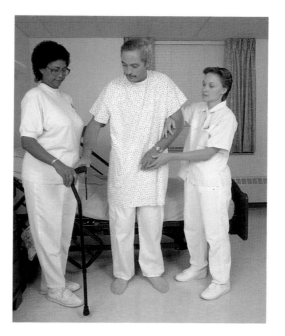

FIGURE 27–19
The patient who is ill may become depressed and need encouragement to exercise.

Health team members develop very specific guidelines for the care of the depressed patient. Check the patient's care plan or ask the nurse about helping the patient with activities of daily living.

For the deeply depressed patient you may need to

- Assist with activities of daily living by setting up equipment needed for bathing, dressing, grooming, and eating.
- Plan enough time so the patient can complete a task.
- Offer encouragement and praise when the patient successfully completes an activity.
- Allow enough time for the patient to respond to your questions or directions.

As the depression lifts, the patient is expected to take more responsibility for self-care. Your role is to continue to offer support and encouragement to help the patient with self-esteem needs.

CARING COMMENT

When you care for the depressed patient, be prompt in reporting and recording any change in the patient's behavior to the nurse or supervisor.

CHAPTER WRAP-UP

- Psychology is the study of the mind and behavior.
- You can help patients complete their developmental tasks by helping them meet their physical and psychologic needs:
  - Help meet patients' physical needs by providing hygiene and other basic needs when patients cannot meet these needs themselves.
  - Help meet patients' psychologic needs by showing support (listening, talking, etc.).
- A support system is the individuals a person can call on for help.
- A person who is mentally healthy has emotional well-being. A threat to emotional well-being may result in mental illness.
- Mental illness can be temporary or long-lasting.
- Anxiety is an uneasy feeling and is a response to a threat. There are four levels of anxiety:
  - Mild anxiety
  - Moderate anxiety
  - Severe anxiety
  - Panic
- Depression is sadness and hopelessness along with a decrease in usual behaviors associated with daily functions.
- Observations of the patient with anxiety or depression include noting physical as well as psychologic changes.
- Care of patients with anxiety or depression is directed at helping them meet their basic needs when they cannot. Another important nursing assistant role is offering support to patients by sitting and talking with them and listening to them.

REVIEW QUESTIONS

1. What is the best way to help persons meet their developmental needs at each stage of life?
2. What kind of observations are important when you care for the patient with mental illness?
3. What behaviors would you observe in the patient with moderate anxiety?
4. Describe the behaviors of the person who is depressed.
5. How can you help the patient who is anxious? The patient who is depressed?

ACTIVITY CORNER

Reminiscing is important for an elderly person. Set aside about 10 minutes for reminiscing with an elderly person. What were the highlights of the person's past life? Examples might be some of the following: marriage, spouse, family, children, siblings, school days, life's work, and hobbies. List the highlights that the person talked about during the reminiscence.

Highlights

_____

_____

_____

_____

_____

_____

Does the person feel good about life? Yes _____ No _____

What causes anxious feelings? Check the situations that make you anxious.

_____ Feeling ill

_____ Looking for a job

_____ Not understanding instructions

_____ Being involved in an accident

_____ Waking up late on a school or work day

_____ Uncomfortable situation/communication in the workplace

_____ Separation from children (for example, due to day care or school)

_____ Separation from spouse (for example, due to illness or employment)

_____ Losing money (any amount, large or small)

Your patients may experience some of the same situations, so you should recognize that common ordinary events can cause anxiety.

28 Understanding Social and Cultural Development

Objectives

AFTER YOU COMPLETE THIS CHAPTER, YOU WILL BE ABLE TO:

Describe socialization and its importance to development across the life span.

Define the term *culture*.

Define the term *ethnicity*.

Tell how culture affects our role in society.

Tell how culture influences patient care.

Define the term *spirituality*.

Explain how spirituality helps in patient healing and comfort.

Use the concepts of socialization, culture, and spirituality when giving care to patients.

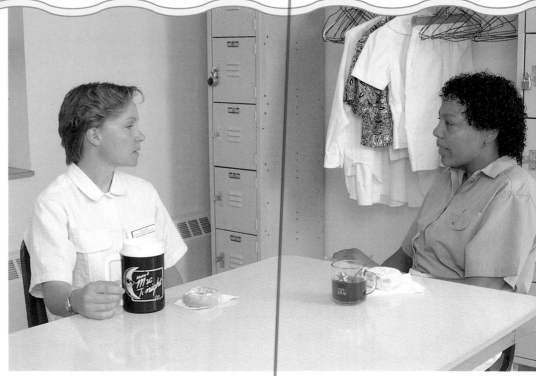

Overview The physical growth of an individual can be seen by even the most untrained eye. This chapter, however, introduces you to the less visible social and cultural aspects of the individual's development. Being aware of patients' social and cultural influences will help you give better care. Social and cultural influences affect how the patient reacts to you, other health care givers, family, and friends. In addition, you will understand yourself better when you realize that some of your feelings and actions are based on your own social and cultural development.

WHAT DO YOU KNOW ABOUT SOCIAL AND CULTURAL DEVELOPMENT?

Here are six statements about social and cultural development and spirituality. Consider them to test your ideas about them. If you think the statement is true, circle the T; if you think the statement is false, circle the F. Change the false statements to make them true.

1. T   F   A person is a member of many social groups.
2. T   F   An infant is a social being.
3. T   F   Language, diet, and tradition are part of one's culture.
4. T   F   Having a stereotype of a person can help you take better care of the person.
5. T   F   Hispanic people value youth over age.
6. T   F   Belief in a higher power can help the ill individual better cope with illness.

ANSWERS

1. **True.** Each person is a member of a variety of social groups, including family, church, school, and work groups.
2. **True.** The first social group to which an infant belongs is the family.
3. **True.** Culture includes language, diet, and tradition, as well as religion and values.
4. **False.** A stereotype is a label that can interfere with the way you interact with another person.
5. **False.** Hispanics value age over youth.
6. **True.** The belief in a higher power can give a person strength in coping with illness.

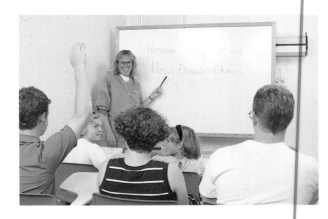

FIGURE 28–1

Young patients who learn about their health needs are part of a social group.

SOCIALIZATION

SOCIALIZATION
participation in a social group
INFANT
the person at the beginning of life (from birth to 1½ years), for whom all needs are met by others
FAMILY
a group of people (not necessarily related) having a relationship
TODDLER
the child from 1½ to 3 years of age
PRESCHOOL AGE
the child from 3 to 6 years of age
SCHOOL AGE
the child from 6 to 12 years of age (the years before adolescence)
PEER
an equal; one who belongs to the same group (age, school, etc.)

Socialization is participation in a group and is a learned behavior (Figure 28–1). Socialization begins at birth and continues throughout the lifetime. For the **infant**, socialization occurs basically within the **family** unit (Figure 28–2). In the **toddler** and **preschool-age** years, children expand their horizons to the world outside. The groups in which toddlers and preschoolers participate include day care, preschool, and the immediate neighborhood. In the **school-age** years, socialization includes friendship with same-sex **peers**, participation in school activities, and membership in groups such as the scouts.

The **adolescent** places high value on interacting with peers. Friends are often more important to adolescents than family, and participation in peer group activities and peer acceptance are most important. With the passage into young adulthood, the social structure is extended to the workplace and marriage and children. During the middle adult years, the family expands to include grandchildren. **Spouses** often rediscover each other after the children leave home, when they have more leisure time together and fewer responsibilities. Some may also extend their social contacts by rejoining the work world or social clubs. In the later years of **maturity**, the possibilities for socialization

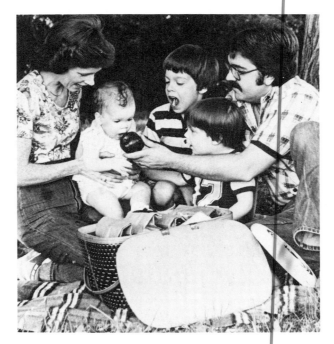

FIGURE 28–2

The family is a person's first social group. (From Foster RLR, Hunsberger MM, Anderson JJT: Family-Centered Nursing Care of Children. Philadelphia, W. B. Saunders Company, 1989.)

begin to decrease as a result of losses associated with **aging** (death of family and friends, loss of work, decreased **self-esteem,** and loss of financial security).

Older persons who are in good health can maintain or increase their socialization by helping others in the community.

SOCIALIZATION GROUPS

A person may belong to and participate in a variety of groups. A person becomes socialized to various groups throughout life.

Family

Socialization begins with the **nuclear family.** The nuclear family consists of parents and children. The nuclear family may also include others (such as grandparents, aunts, or uncles) who belong to the same **household.**

A blended family consists of all persons who belong to the same household as part of a joining of families. For example, when a widowed man with two children marries a divorced woman with two children and they all move into the same house, the result is a blended family.

An extended family includes relatives and close friends who influence a family but do not live in the same house.

Within the family, each person learns to behave within the standards adopted by the family.

Friends

Children learn to interact with the world beyond the family when they develop social relationships with friends. A friend is a companion. Friends share trust, joy, and sorrow. Some friendships begin in childhood and are lifelong (Figure 28–3). In the early stages of a person's development, friends are usually of the same sex. During adolescence and adulthood, friends may be of either sex.

Friendship can take the form of either a one-to-one relationship or a larger group of people who share common ground. Friendship helps people learn about and accept beliefs and values not present in their own family.

Activities

When people participate in activities such as sports or belong to a club, they are socializing. A club or team may have certain rules that the member must accept. Activities such as sports teach the concept that goals can be accomplished when people work together. Belonging to a club gives people access to other people who share a common interest (for example, birdwatching or golfing).

Religious Organizations

Each religious group (Christian, Muslim, etc.) offers guidelines for a certain way of life. Everyone in that faith has basically the same beliefs. A person may be born into a family that follows a certain faith and may follow the teachings of

ADOLESCENT
the child who is maturing; teenager

SPOUSE
married person (husband or wife)
MATURITY
state of full development
AGING
the physical and psychologic changes that occur as life continues
SELF-ESTEEM
how confident and satisfied a person feels

NUCLEAR FAMILY
family group consisting of parents and children
HOUSEHOLD
those who live under one roof and make up a family

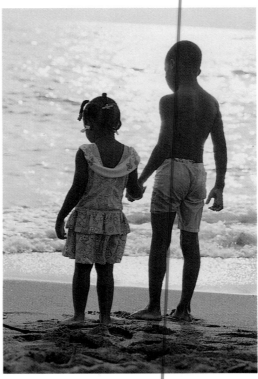

FIGURE 28-3
Having a friend to rely on is an important part of a child's social life.

that faith for a lifetime. In some cultures, children are exposed to a variety of religions and permitted to choose a faith when they come of age. Individuals may also investigate different religions on their own and join the religious group of their choice.

Workplace

WORKPLACE

the place (such as a factory or office) where work is done

The **workplace** socializes a person to the expectations in a field of endeavor. People also learn to work together as a team. Many friendships in adulthood begin in the workplace (Figure 28–4).

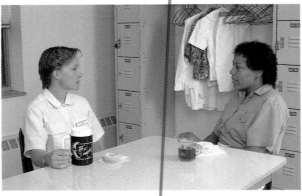

FIGURE 28-4
Social interactions in the workplace are one part of a person's socialization.

Ethnic Groups

A person's **ethnic** group provides for socialization with others with the same cultural background. Ethnic heritage may influence practices of daily life (such as dressing and eating) as well as rituals (such as marriage and death). Belonging to an ethnic group contributes to a person's sense of identity.

Socialization occurs as a person goes through the developmental stages of life, as described in Chapter 27. The tasks that Erikson identified tell how a person defines him or herself and this in turn helps define who a person is in relationship to others (socialization).

ETHNIC

referring to the customs, language, and values of a group, especially a minority group

CULTURE

Culture refers to the beliefs, social expectations, and characteristics of a racial, religious, or social group (Figure 28–5). The values and customs people learn in their culture influence their interactions with others (Figure 28–6). These cultural expectations are often passed from generation to generation. Culture may include any combination of the following:

Traditions
Diet
Language
Values
Religion

CULTURE

the beliefs, social expectations, and characteristics of a racial, religious, or social group

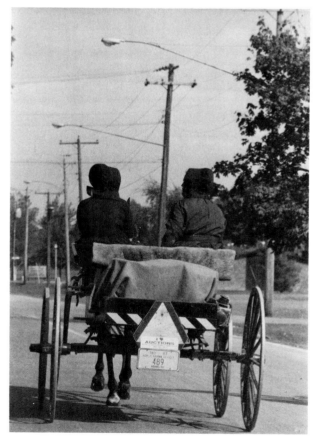

FIGURE 28–5
Traditions and values are passed on to the new generation of followers. (Courtesy of Dr. Margaret M. Andrews, Rochester, NY.)

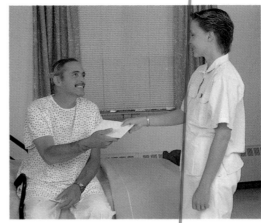

FIGURE 28–6
Sending a get-well greeting is a tradition that helps cheer up a patient.

TRADITIONS

TRADITION
a practice that is handed down from generation to generation

Traditions or customs are practices that are handed down from generation to generation, for example, eating turkey and stuffing on Thanksgiving day. Honoring traditions gives stability and security to families and other groups. A person or family group can invent a tradition and pass it on to future generations.

DIET

DIET
the total amount of food eaten by an individual

Special dietary practices are part of every culture. Sometimes these dietary choices are based on a religious teaching. For example, matzo, an unleavened bread, is eaten by Jews during the eight days of Passover. Passover is celebrated to remember the flight out of Egypt during which unleavened bread was eaten. Hindus will not eat beef because the cow is sacred in their religion. Preparing and eating the foods associated with one's cultural group can give one comfort and a sense of belonging.

LANGUAGE

Certain groups use the language of their ethnic group to communicate. For example, most Hispanic groups speak Spanish instead of English. Some people are able to communicate in more than one language.

VALUES

VALUE
something or someone of importance or worth

Values are learned through the family, cultural group, and religious organizations. Often people lead their lives on the basis of these learned values.

RELIGION

ILLNESS
sickness; a condition different from the normal health state; any change, temporary or long-lasting, in a person's physical, emotional, or spiritual health and well-being

Individuals may belong to the same religion as others in their cultural group. Members of a religious group are often a great source of support to one another. Belief in a higher power often gives a person strength to cope with the problems of daily life as well as with **illness** and death.

ETHNIC GROUPS

The human race is composed of four basic races:

- Black (African)
- White (Caucasian)
- Yellow (Asian)
- Red (Native American)

Ethnic groups develop within these races. These groups are formed on the basis of a common language, religion, or geographic location. Members of an ethnic group keep the customs, language, and values of the group to which they belong. **Ethnicity** refers to certain qualities associated with an ethnic group. Note that a person may be a member of more than one ethnic group (for example, the child of an interracial marriage). The person often learns about the values and beliefs of both groups and adopts one group, or the person may be socialized to only one of the groups.

ETHNICITY
certain qualities associated with a member of an ethnic group

THE INFLUENCE OF CULTURE AND ETHNICITY ON THE INDIVIDUAL

A person's cultural and ethnic backgrounds influence the way they view themselves and other people. It can also affect the way people interact with each other. Some people who experience interactions with members of a certain cultural or ethnic group in a particular way expect all other members of the group to behave in the same way. This is **stereotyping** people. A stereotype may have no basis in fact, may be a judgment, or may be an oversimplified opinion of a particular group. The following are some examples of stereotypes.

STEREOTYPE
an image one has of members of a group

COMMON STEREOTYPES	
Observation	**Stereotype**
Wrinkles	Aging
Bloodshot eyes	Alcoholic
Stethoscope	Doctor or nurse
Overweight	Eats too much
Unkempt child	Neglect
Temper tantrum	Poor self-control

CARING COMMENT

Be aware of the stereotypes you may have about groups of people. A stereotyped belief can affect the way you interact and give care to your patients.

CONSIDERING CULTURE AND ETHNICITY IN GIVING CARE

You must first understand yourself before you can understand another person's culture and ethnicity. You should explore what your own culture and ethnicity have taught you about other cultures' and ethnic groups' practices. You may have learned negative images that can interfere with positive interaction and acceptance of others. When you experience problems in accepting a patient's culture and ethnicity, you may want to talk to the nurse about your feelings.

Your health care institution may have a program to help you understand more about different cultures and ethnic groups and to be more accepting of them.

CARING COMMENT

To provide the best care possible, you must accept each individual as a person worth valuing. You must respect other people's beliefs and values even though they are not the same as your own.

To change your negative outlook on different cultures and ethnic groups,

- Learn about the cultures and ethnic groups who are living in the area served by your health care institution.
- Question yourself about valuing the rights of others to have their own beliefs, practices, and traditions.
- Get to know each patient as an individual.
- Avoid stereotyping others.
- Accept that cultural and/or ethnic practices are resistant to forced change.

CARING COMMENT

Sharing beliefs, traditions, values, and practices with other people is a positive way for others to learn about you and for you to learn about others.

SPECIFIC CULTURAL GROUPS

The cultural aspects of development influence the views a person has on family life, religion, present and future feelings about life, and health care. There are many different cultural groups. The common cultural groups that you may serve in your role as a nursing assistant can include

- African Americans—persons whose ancestors lived in Africa
- Hispanics—persons of Spanish, Mexican, or Puerto Rican heritage
- Whites—persons belonging to the Caucasian race
- Asians—persons whose ancestors lived in Asian countries such as China, Japan, or Korea
- Native Americans—persons whose ancestors lived in North America before it was settled by people from other countries
- Arabians, Arabs—persons whose ancestors lived in Middle Eastern countries such as Saudi Arabia, Iran, Iraq, and Kuwait

AFRICAN AMERICANS

In African-American culture, the family is an extended family that is very supportive of its members. The family includes "aunts" and "uncles" who may not be related by blood but come from the neighborhood or religious groups. Black Americans are spiritual and worship in a variety of religious groups.

Those black individuals who are faced with meeting day-to-day needs may

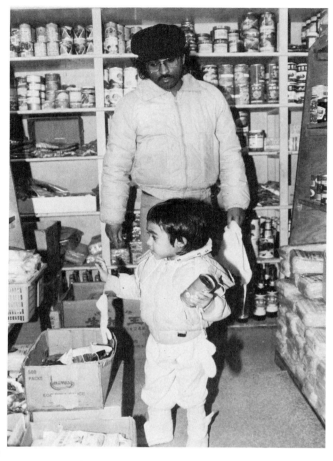

FIGURE 28–7

This young father is acting as a positive role model for his child. (From Foster RLR, Hunsberger MM, Anderson JJT: Family-Centered Nursing Care of Children. Philadelphia, W. B. Saunders Company, 1989.)

be focused mainly on the present and may not plan for future needs. Education in some African-American communities may be limited because of poverty, discrimination, and the absence of positive role models (Figure 28–7). There is a higher incidence of hypertension (high blood pressure) in blacks. Today most of the people in this culture depend on health care professionals to provide for health care needs, although some rely on **folk medicine** practices.

HISPANICS

In Hispanic culture, Spanish is the primary language. Mexican, Cuban, and Puerto Rican people are part of the Hispanic culture. For Hispanics who are recent **immigrants** to the United States and for those who have never learned the English language, communication with people outside the Hispanic culture may be difficult. The family is very important among Hispanics. The father is considered the head of the family and traditionally worked outside the home, while mothers were expected to work in the home. However, many Hispanic women now hold jobs. Hispanic culture values age over youth. The passage of time is not important in this culture; some individuals may not be interested in even the time of day. Religion (usually Roman Catholic) plays a central role in the life of the Hispanic. When illness occurs, it may be viewed as a punishment from God. Hispanic people usually seek the services of a **folk healer** before seeking health care from licensed health care professionals.

FOLK MEDICINE
a tradition of medicine practiced by nonprofessionals, for example, using parts of plants for treatment

IMMIGRANT
a person who arrives in a country with the intent of living there

FOLK HEALER
nonprofessional person who is consulted about health care and healing

WHITE CULTURE

To most people of the white middle class, family closeness is important. Youth is valued over age. The focus of this group tends to be on the future. The roles of the male and female in the home may not be traditional. In many families, the man helps with household tasks and child care. The choice of religion is very individual. Many white people use over-the-counter medications available in pharmacies when an illness occurs. They may attempt to self-diagnose an illness. A health care professional is usually consulted, however.

ASIANS

Asians represent diverse cultural groups from many different Asian countries: China, Japan, Vietnam, Laos, Cambodia, and Korea, for example (Figure 28–8). In general in Asian culture, the family is considered more important than the individual. The father is the undisputed head of the family. There is a deep respect for elder persons as well as for ancestors. Some religions are based on **ancestor** worship. The people of Asian cultures value education and hard work.

ANCESTOR
one from whom a person is descended

Health may be viewed as a balance between yin and yang. Yin is seen as female, negative, and cold, while yang is male, positive, and warm. When illness is present, the yin and yang are believed to be out of balance. The balance between cold and warm is seen as essential to health. In order to regain health, the Asian works to restore the yin–yang balance in the body. Asians also believe there is a flow of energy in the body. They believe that acupuncture (inserting a needle into the body at a specified point) is valuable in interrupting or restoring the flow of energy within the body. Asians may use herbs for healing. Help from health care professionals is often sought, however.

NATIVE AMERICANS

The Native American culture consists of many individual tribes with practices unique to each specific tribe. The family is important and may include indivi-

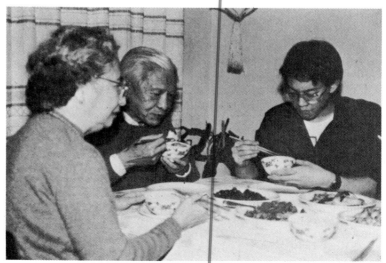

FIGURE 28–8
People of Asian descent use special tools (chopsticks) for eating. (From Foster RLR, Hunsberger MM, Anderson JJT: Family-Centered Nursing Care of Children. Philadelphia, W. B. Saunders Company, 1989.)

duals who are not related by blood. The aged members of this society are highly valued. The Native American lives in the present and tends to finish one thing before going on to something else. Special ceremonies may be performed to cure an illness. The medicine man (shaman) continues to be a source of health care for Native Americans. However, they seek health care from professional sources when it is available.

ARABIANS

Arabs believe that humans cannot control things in life; some things depend on God. Their beliefs are influenced by Islam, their religion. Arabs show a great love of family and consider distant relatives as close family members. They are quick to make friends and do favors for others; they are concerned about the impression they make on others. Arab society demands conformity (obedience) from its members. For example, arranged marriages and dress codes are still practiced by many Arabs.

The education of females and health care practices in Arab countries are changing from traditional practices. Arabs in America may choose to adopt modern ways while still keeping traditions they hold important. Health care professionals are consulted when necessary.

CARING COMMENT

When caring for patients, it is all right to ask them about preferences about care that might be based on their culture. The patient or a family member is often willing to share information that will help you give the care the patient needs. You can ask questions such as, "Is it all right to shave your beard?" or "Do you want this (religious) medal pinned on your gown?"

CULTURE AND PATIENT CARE

The culture a person is associated with can influence how you give care for that individual person. It is important for you to acknowledge different cultures and learn to respect each for the contribution it makes to society (Figure 28–9).

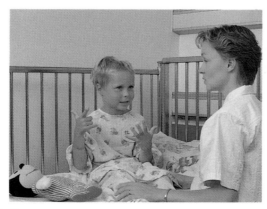

FIGURE 28–9
The feelings a patient expresses about health are part of the patient's culture.

Being aware of a person's beliefs about family, religion, time, and health is essential to caregiving. You need to be flexible and accepting of belief systems that are different from your own when you care for people of other cultures.

SPIRITUALITY

SPIRITUALITY
belief in or sensitivity to religious values

RELIGION
an organized set of beliefs about a higher power

ATHEIST
person who denies the existence of a god

Spirituality is the way a person interacts with a higher power. A person may do this through belonging to a religious group and practicing a **religion.** Persons may follow the religion of their culture, or they may choose a different one. The person who believes in a higher power may show increased spiritual needs when an illness occurs. The person who denies the existence of a god is called an **atheist.**

TYPES OF RELIGION

Many different religions exist in the world today.

Christianity

CHRISTIANITY
religion based on the teachings of Jesus Christ

Christianity is a religion with many followers, called Christians (Figure 28–10). Christians believe in the teachings of Jesus Christ. There are two general types of Christian denominations

BAPTISM
a Christian initiation ritual marked by the use of water

COMMUNION
an act of sharing; in this context, "Holy Communion" (bread and wine)

PROTESTANT DENOMINATIONS   Protestant denominations include the Lutherans, Presbyterians, Baptists, and Methodists. Some of these groups believe in **baptism** of an infant, whereas others believe in adult baptism. The water of baptism is used to purify and initiate a person. Followers of these religions take **communion.** Bread and wine are taken during communion to commemorate the death of Christ. A member of the clergy is called a minister, reverend, or pastor.

CATHOLIC DENOMINATIONS   The Catholic denominations include Roman Catholic and Greek or Russian Orthodox religious groups. Episcopalians (Anglicans) consider themselves "catholic." Followers believe in sacraments including baptism, communion, confession, and sacrament of the sick. A member of the clergy is called a priest. Nuns are women in the church who give themselves to a life of service to others.

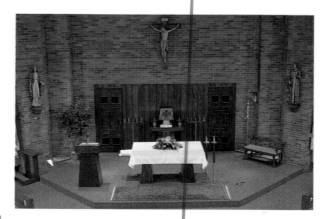

FIGURE 28–10
A chapel in a health care institution is designed to accommodate patients of different religious groups.

Judaism

A large group of people follow the teaching of **Judaism.** The groups in Judaism include the Reformed, Orthodox, Conservative, and Reconstructionist groups. Followers may adhere to certain dietary restrictions as part of the practice of the religion. A member of the clergy is known as a rabbi.

JUDAISM
religion developed by ancient Hebrews

Other Religions of the World

Islam, Hinduism, Confucianism, and Buddhism are other major world religions. The followers of Islam are called Muslims. They believe in the teachings of Allah and his prophet, Muhammad. Worshippers are called to prayer five times a day. Muslims are forbidden to eat pork or drink alcohol. In India, Hinduism is a major religion. Hindus may follow certain dietary limitations and observe special rites when a member dies. Confucianism is common in China, and followers follow the teachings of Confucius. Buddhists are found in China and other Asian countries. They hold life in very high regard and follow the teachings of Buddha.

ISLAM
Muslim; religion based on the teachings of Allah and his prophet, Muhammad

SPIRITUAL COMFORT DURING ILLNESS

The belief in a higher power can influence patients' perception of their illness. The patient may view illness as a

- punishment from God
- trial or test from God

The belief in a higher power can

- provide strength in coping with the illness
- bring hope of healing or cure (which helps a person cope with illness)

CARING COMMENT

Many people believe in the spiritual power of prayer. Patients may ask you to pray with them. You can do this if you feel comfortable about praying. It will help patients to know that you can pray for them.

ACCEPTING OTHERS' SPIRITUALITY

Your culture and your family often are the basis for your beliefs about a higher power. You will observe different religious practices among your patients and their families during illness and death. You need to show them

- understanding
- acceptance
- a **nonjudgmental** attitude

To help patients meet their spiritual needs, you can

- Provide quiet time for patients and their families to observe their religious practice.
- Ask patients or family members if they would like to see a member of the clergy.
- Tell the nurse or supervisor of patients' or family members' desire for a visit from the clergy.
- Remember that the need for spiritual comfort often increases during the time of illness and dying.

NONJUDGMENTAL
not passing judgment on someone whose beliefs are not the same as yours

CHAPTER WRAP-UP

- Socialization is a learned behavior.
- Socialization is a lifelong process.
- Each person becomes socialized to many different groups, including family, friends, co-workers, and religious groups.
- Culture is the system of beliefs, social expectations, and characteristics of a racial, religious, or social group. It includes a combination of traditions, dietary choices, language, values, and religion. Individuals are influenced by their culture.
- Each person is a member of an ethnic group. Different ethnic groups have different customs, languages, and values.
- A stereotype is an image one has of members of a group.
- You should understand that patients' culture and ethnicity may affect their interaction with care givers.
- Spirituality is a belief in or sensitivity to religious values.
- Support patients' spirituality by displaying understanding, acceptance, and a nonjudgmental attitude.

REVIEW QUESTIONS

1. Define the terms *socialization*, *culture*, *ethnicity*, *spirituality*, and *stereotyping*.
2. During a child's infancy, how does the family influence socialization? What are the positive effects of this socialization? The negative effects?
3. What task of adolescents has an impact on their socialization with others?
4. How can socialization improve the self-worth of the older adult?
5. How can having a stereotype interfere with providing good patient care?
6. How do each of the following ethnic groups seek health care? Africans, Hispanics, whites, Asians, Native Americans.
7. How can you help patients meet their spiritual needs?

ACTIVITY CORNER

What is your cultural heritage? _____
Ask two people in your school or workplace what their cultural heritage is.

_____

_____

Does culture make a difference in the following?

How people dress? Yes _____ No _____ Sometimes _____

How people eat? Yes _____ No _____ Sometimes _____

How people treat illness? Yes _____ No _____ Sometimes _____

Are you able to interact with people from other cultures? Yes _____ No _____
If no, what can you do to help increase understanding of other persons' cultures?

_____ Asking persons about their culture

_____ Reading about a culture different from yours

_____ Other _____

Do other people understand your culture? Yes _____ No _____

If no, are you willing to tell others about your culture? Yes _____ No _____

List a few things about your culture that another person might like to know.

_____   _____

_____   _____

29

Understanding Sexuality

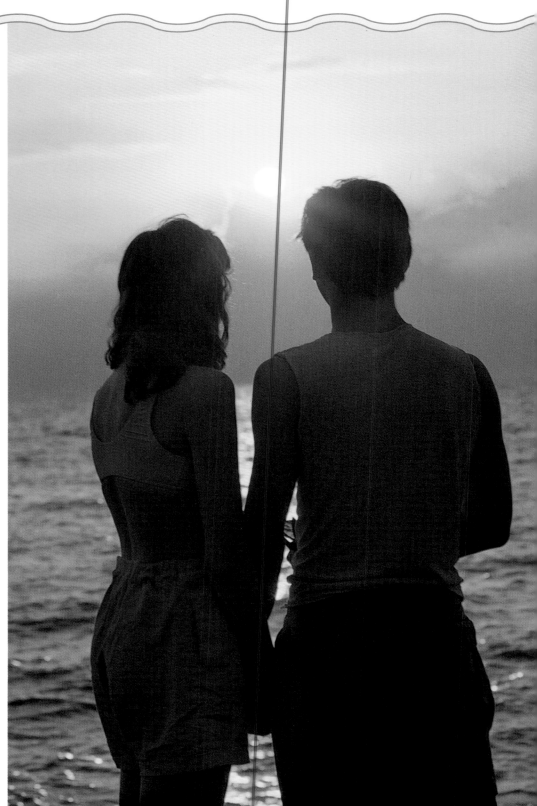

Objectives

AFTER YOU COMPLETE THIS CHAPTER, YOU WILL BE ABLE TO:

List the factors that affect a person's sexuality.

Identify three kinds of sexual preference.

List observations of the patient who is a victim of rape.

Care for a patient who is a victim of rape.

Overview Sexuality begins at birth. As we grow, we develop a sense of being either male or female. Our sexuality develops and changes as we age.

WHAT DO YOU KNOW ABOUT SEXUALITY?

Here are three statements about sexuality. Consider them to test your current ideas about sexuality. If you think the statement is true, circle the T; if you think the statement is false, circle the F. Change the false statements to make them true.

1. T F Sexuality ends around age 65.
2. T F A homosexual person is attracted to persons of the opposite sex.
3. T F Sexual well-being is an important part of life.

ANSWERS

1. **False.** Sexuality begins at birth and ends with death.
2. **False.** A homosexual is attracted to persons of the same sex.
3. **True.** Sexual well-being helps a person lead a happy, healthy life.

WHAT IS SEXUALITY?

SEXUALITY
the sense of being male or female; the intimacy that exists between two people

Sexuality is the sense of being male or female. It is the intimacy that exists between two people. It includes sexual attitudes and behaviors. Individuals' sexuality may be influenced by a number of factors in their environment. These factors include

- religious beliefs
- cultural behaviors
- **ethnic** background
- physical attributes
- age
- health

ETHNIC
referring to the customs, language, and values of a group, especially a minority group

Sexuality has two components:

- Psychologic (feelings)
- Physical (the sexual act)

PSYCHOLOGIC
relating to psychology; mental
INTIMACY
closeness

The **psychologic** part consists of the development of the sex role by the child as well as the closeness and **intimacy** between individuals. The psychologic aspect of sexuality is very important. It includes the sexual self-image that individuals develop while they are growing up. People may express their psychologic sexuality in a variety of ways, for example, by writing poetry or playing music.

The physical expression of sexuality involves the body's organs, nerves, and hormones. In addition, the five senses contribute to a person's awareness of sexuality. Hugging, holding hands, cuddling, and kissing are some expressions of sexuality. Sexuality is influenced by a person's continued good health; injury and disease may interfere with a person's sexual well-being.

SEXUALITY ACROSS THE LIFE SPAN

Infancy

INFANCY
the time from birth to 1½ years, during which all needs must be met for a person

During **infancy,** a baby responds to a loving environment. This is provided by the people (especially the parents) who care for the baby. Infants are influenced by how other people treat them. The family often casts the infant in a girl or boy role early in life. Baby girls are often cuddled more than baby boys. The cuddling leads to the expectation of softness from the female infant. Clothing and colors may be used to help identify the sex of the infant. Girls' clothing is often made with ruffles and ribbons, and boys' clothing is often decorated with kites, cars, and sport designs.

Toddlerhood

TODDLER
the young child from 1½ to 3 years of age

Toddlers begin to identify themselves as a boy or girl. They become interested in their body. A child of this age begins to imitate the parent of the same sex (Figure 29–1). A strong preference for typical girl/boy toys emerges. Girls often show a preference for soft toys, dolls, and toys that reflect the home, while boys often prefer cars, trucks, and tools.

Preschool Age

PRESCHOOL AGE
the child from 3 to 6 years of age

During the preschool years, the child forms an emotional attachment to the parent of the opposite sex. Children love to pretend and play "dress up" in adult's clothing. Another form of play is interest in and exploration of each other's genitals. The **preschool-age** child learns about the physical differences between a girl and boy. The natural curiosity of this age group leads to many questions about the differences between boys' and girls' bodies as well as differences between the adult male and female bodies.

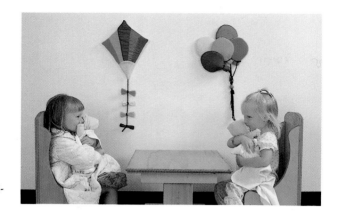

FIGURE 29-1
Toddlers often imitate the activities of their same-sex parent.

School Age

The **school age** child may talk about the physical aspects of being a girl or boy. At this age, the child prefers the company of other children of the same sex.

The latter part of school age brings about the physical changes **(puberty)** associated with the development of **secondary sexual characteristics.** This physical development increases children's awareness of their own sexuality (Figure 29-2).

Adolescence

As discussed earlier (see Chapter 22), hormonal changes initiate the development of the secondary sexual characteristics in the **adolescent.** There may be serious discussions about the size of the sexual features (the breasts in females and the penis in males). The adolescent is attracted to adolescents of the opposite sex and begins to develop close relationships. The body continues to mature physcally. The male is able to **impregnate** the female, and the female is capable of becoming pregnant and giving birth. "Crushes" may occur as the adolescent starts to become more intimate in a psychologic as well as a physical way. The psychologic and physical intimacy that is important in adulthood begins during adolescence.

Young Adulthood

The young adult may choose to develop an intimate relationship through marriage or cohabitation (living together). The body matures physically, and the

SCHOOL AGE
the child from 6 to 12 years of age (the years before adolescence)
PUBERTY
the developmental and physical changes that result in adult sexual characteristics and the ability to reproduce
SECONDARY SEXUAL CHARACTERISTICS
changes in males and females that occur with puberty
ADOLESCENT
the child who is maturing; teenager
IMPREGNATE
to make pregnant

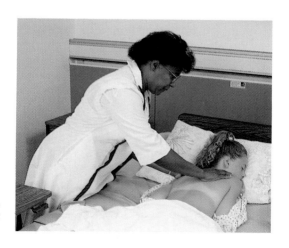

FIGURE 29-2
Growing children are very aware of the changes in their body. You should respect children's need for privacy.

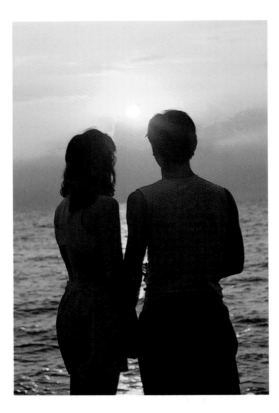

FIGURE 29–3
Hand-holding is one way a couple expresses a sense of intimacy.

VALIDATE
to confirm; make sure

changes that occurred during adolescence are accepted by the adult. In addition, the sex role becomes well defined. Young adults **validate** their sexuality by choosing to have a significant other (a spouse or life partner) (Figure 29–3). A couple may think about starting a family and raising children during the young adult years. Some couples want to experience the joy and anticipation of pregnancy. A couple may choose to adopt a child. For example, if an inherited disease is present in one of the persons or if the female cannot become pregnant or the male cannot impregnate his mate, the couple may choose to adopt a child to complete the family.

The Middle Years

Many physical changes occur during the middle years. Physical and sexual activity may decrease in frequency. The changes in sexual activity may cause middle-aged persons to question their identity as a sexual being. Changes occur in the home environment because children leave home and the couple may be alone and not needed by children for the first time in many years. A period of psychologic adjustment for both partners occurs as a result of the "empty nest" syndrome.

The Later Years

ELDERLY
a term frequently used to refer to older adults, usually individuals over age 65

IMPOTENCE
inability of the male to achieve and maintain the rigid erection needed for successful sexual intercourse

As a result of the aging process, the **elderly** adult faces many changes in sexual function. The person may feel "sick," tired, or sexually unattractive. As age increases, sexual intercourse generally decreases. Changes related to aging may include dryness of the vagina in females, resulting in painful sexual relations. **Impotence** may occur in males. Certain medications (taken at any age) may interfere with the desire for sexual activity or may affect the male's ability to achieve erection.

The physical aspects of sexuality may require the acceptance of new techniques and alternatives. For example, a person with arthritis may find that bearing weight with the hands and knees during intercourse is too painful. In such a situation, the person may need to adopt a position that is less painful.

The absence of a partner is a barrier to sexual activity. When a couple is separated by death, the surviving partner needs to make a choice about further sexual activity. Because females often outlive males, they may live out their days in loneliness or may seek out others of similar age and circumstances for caring and closeness. When a couple is separated by the need for one partner to live in a nursing home, choices again must be made. Remember to provide privacy during visits so that sexual needs can be expressed and met.

CARING COMMENT

Sexuality is a quality that is present throughout the life span, and as a nursing assistant you need to be aware of a person's sexuality (Figure 29–4).

SEXUAL ORIENTATION

Sexual orientation is the sex of persons with whom one prefers to have sexual activity. The three kinds of sexual orientation are

- Heterosexual—an attraction for persons of the opposite sex.
- Homosexual—an attraction for persons of the same sex.
- Bisexual—an attraction for persons of either sex. The person who is bisexual may participate in heterosexual and homosexual relationships.

CARING COMMENT

Be aware of your feelings about sexuality and sexual orientation. *Do not* judge a person's sexuality just because it is different from your own.

SEXUALITY AND WELL-BEING

Knowing that patients have sexuality needs can help you work to increase their self-esteem and sexual self-image. You can observe for patients' behavior. Remember that illness can change how a patient behaves.

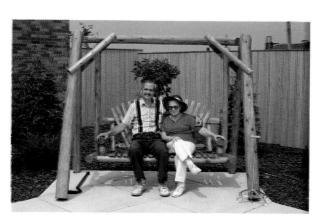

FIGURE 29–4

A middle-aged man and an elderly lady who are residents in a nursing home are comfortable with their sexuality.

CARING COMMENT

Remember that sexuality includes closeness, physical contact, and intimacy as well as the sexual act.

Statements such as the following may alert you to a patient's sexuality concerns:

"How come he is different from me?"

"I don't want anyone to see this awful scar across my breast."

"When is it okay to have sex again?" (This may be asked, for example, by the husband or wife after the birth of a child or by a person who has experienced a heart attack.)

"You must look pretty sharp in a bathing suit."

"I'm not as attractive to the opposite sex as I used to be."

Patients' behaviors may indicate that they have sexuality concerns. You may observe

MODESTY
being shy, humble, or moderate

- more than the usual amount of **modesty**
- giggling and flirting with patients of the opposite sex
- embarrassment when personal care items (such as sanitary napkins and belts) are displayed
- socially unacceptable public behaviors such as a male's touching a female's breasts or buttocks
- attempts to kiss a care giver

Illness or treatment may cause a change in patients' body image that can affect their sexuality. Some conditions that may change body image and therefore sexuality include

- burns and their resulting scars
- surgery and resulting scars or changes in body function
- the aging process (for example, dryness of the vagina)
- decreased or absent ability to perform the sexual act
- certain medications

Record and report your observations to the nurse or supervisor, who will plan the appropriate approach to take.

CARING COMMENT

As a nursing assistant, you can best help by accepting patients as a person and recognizing their feelings about sexuality.

THE PATIENT WITH SEXUAL NEEDS

A patient may make sexual advances to you as a care giver. A sexual advance may be physical or verbal. The patient may make physical advances by touching your body inappropriately. Kissing on the lips or caressing and groping body parts such as the penis, breasts, or buttocks is not acceptable behavior. You should step away from the patient and keep calm. Do not giggle or laugh. Use a matter-of-fact tone of voice to tell the patient that the behavior is unacceptable. You might use a statement such as

"I like you as a person, but I do not like what you are doing."

"What you are doing is not acceptable."

A patient's verbal sexual advances may take the form of suggestive comments while you are giving care. The patient may comment on your attractiveness or question your availability. Examples of suggestive comments are

"We could do great things together."
"You look like you would be good in bed."
"Will you meet me in the patient lounge later tonight?"

You need to decide if the statement is a sexual advance. If the patient's tone of voice, gestures, or touch indicate a sexual advance, you should respond matter-of-factly. You might respond to suggestive statements by saying

"I understand how frustrating your illness can be, but such a comment is not acceptable to me."

Be sure to report any patient's sexual advances, whether physical or verbal, to the nurse or supervisor. If a patient is known to display unacceptable suggestive behaviors, the nurse will give you further direction.

A male patient may have a penile **erection** while you are giving care. A female patient may have an erection of the clitoris and the nipples. An erection may be caused by

- Stimulation—from your touch while you are giving care or from **erotic** thinking, reading, or television programming
- Medication—for example, a general anesthetic

If your patient has an erection, you should understand that the patient may not have control over the situation. Be matter-of-fact and do not judge the patient. Make sure the patient is safe (lower the bed to the low position, raise the side rails, and place call signal within reach) and provide privacy. You can tell the patient that you are leaving and what time you will return. An appropriate statement for you to use is

"I'll leave now for a little while. I'll be back in about 10 minutes to check on you. If you need anything before then, please use the call signal."

If the erection occurs when the patient is recovering from general anesthesia, you can say:

"A person recovering from general anesthesia may have an erection. I'll let you rest for about 10 minutes, and then I'll come back to take your blood pressure."

A patient may express a desire for privacy with a spouse or other sexual partner. Report such requests to the nurse or supervisor and follow directions. Whenever possible, arrangements should be made to provide privacy according to the policy of the health care institution.

ERECTION
when erectile tissue fills with blood and becomes rigid

EROTIC
pertaining to sexual desire

CARING COMMENT

Know your own feelings about sexuality, because you will encounter a wide variety of sexuality needs and preferences in your patients. When you are secure in your feelings, you are more able to recognize the sexuality needs of others.

RAPE

Rape is a criminal act of sexual assault without the consent of the victim. Rape includes the **penetration** of the vagina or anus. The victim of rape may be male or female. The rape victim suffers physical as well as psychologic **trauma.**

RAPE
the criminal act of having sex with someone without that person's consent

PENETRATION
passing into or through

TRAUMA
injury

LACERATION

cut in the skin caused by a sharp object

PHYSICAL EVIDENCE   The physical evidence of rape may include

- discharge from the vagina or anus
- bruises or **lacerations** in the genital area
- discomfort or pain
- the presence of blood, hair, or semen (fluid that contains sperm)

PSYCHOLOGIC TRAUMA   The psychologic trauma of rape includes

- anger
- disbelief
- crying
- **hysteria**
- fear of the
   return of the rapist
   possibility of pregnancy
   possibility of contracting a sexually transmitted disease

HYSTERIA

extreme emotional agitation

CARE OF THE RAPE VICTIM   When you care for the victim of rape, you should

- Remain calm and speak in a quiet, confident voice. Your calmness is a support to the patient.
- Stay with the patient in a quiet place, because he or she may be frightened that the attacker will come back.
- *After* all tests have been completed, help the patient with oral and personal hygiene care. If the person bathes and showers too soon, valuable evidence might be destroyed.
- Listen while the patient expresses fears or concerns. The victim needs to be able to talk openly and confidentially with someone.
- Accept the person without making judgments, to let the victim feel accepted, that he or she is still a good person.

The nurse directs you in the care of the rape victim. The two especially important qualities you need to show in caring for the rape victim are nonjudgmentalness and confidentiality. Be sure to remain nonjudgmental when you give care. Report any feelings the patient shares with you to the nurse or your supervisor. Do *not* share information with anyone except those involved with care, however. This maintains confidentiality. Confidentiality is the patient's right.

CHAPTER WRAP-UP

- Sexuality is the sense of being male or female. Sexuality begins at birth, continues throughout life, and ends at death.
- The elderly person's sexuality needs may be disrupted by the inability to perform the sexual act or by the lack of a close partner.
- Patients' statements and behaviors can indicate that they have concerns about their sexuality.
- Rape is a violent act of crime that can cause physical and psychologic trauma in the victim.

REVIEW QUESTIONS

1. What factors help sexuality develop?
2. Define the terms *heterosexual*, *homosexual*, and *bisexual*.
3. What would you observe in the person who is a victim of rape?

ACTIVITY CORNER

Choose a 2-hour time period and observe for various expressions of sexuality in the world around you. Observe while watching television, shopping at the mall, strolling at the zoo, or watching any activity where people gather. Observe for the following and fill in the blanks by checking how you felt about the behaviors.

	Comfortable	Uncomfortable	Embarrassed
Hugging	_____	_____	_____
Holding hands	_____	_____	_____
Kissing	_____	_____	_____
Flirting	_____	_____	_____
Sitting close	_____	_____	_____

Realize that sexuality is expressed in many ways across the life span.

Caring for Special Groups of People

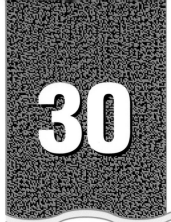

30

Caring for Infants and Children

Objectives

AFTER YOU COMPLETE THIS CHAPTER, YOU WILL BE ABLE TO:

Outline the normal changes in the growth of infants and children.

Describe the safety, comfort, and play needs of infants and children.

Discuss the needs of hospitalized children.

Diaper an infant.

Feed an infant and a child.

Weigh and measure an infant.

Bathe an infant and a child.

Define *diarrhea*.

Care for the infant and child with vomiting or diarrhea.

Define *communicable diseases*.

Care for the infant and child with a communicable disease.

Define *failure to thrive*.

Care for an infant or child who fails to thrive.

Care for an infant or child who is a victim of abuse.

Care for an infant or child with a physical disability.

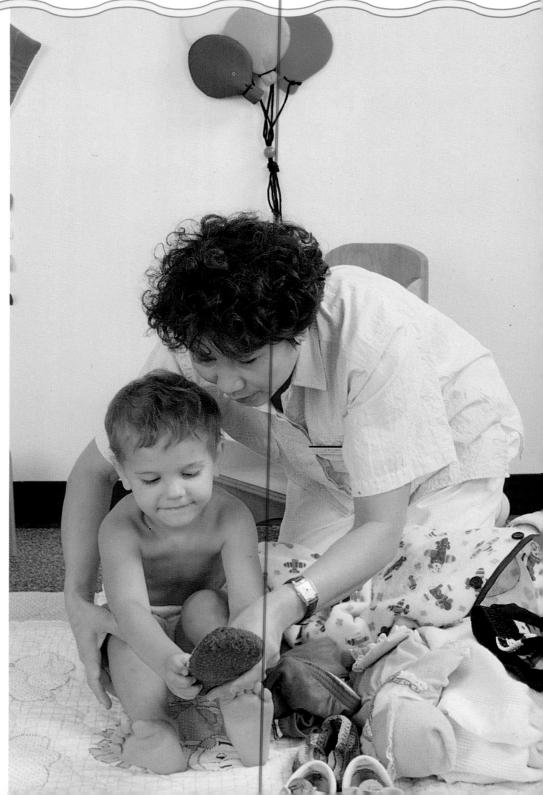

Overview Infancy and childhood are times of great change. Infants and children grow physically and mentally at very fast rates. Their needs are different from those of adults. Needs include physical care and the need for play and learning. You can help children meet these needs while they are in the health care institution.

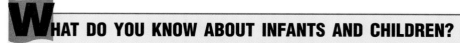

WHAT DO YOU KNOW ABOUT INFANTS AND CHILDREN?

Here are seven statements about infants and children. Consider them to test your current knowledge of the young. If you think the statement is true, circle the T; if you think the statement is false, circle the F. Change the false statements to make them true.

1. T F The human infant is completely helpless at birth.
2. T F The infant can sit unassisted at about 4 months of age.
3. T F The best food for the human infant is breast milk.
4. T F Most children are toilet trained (potty trained) by about 1½ years of age.
5. T F The permanent teeth appear during the school years.
6. T F Diarrhea may cause a loss of body fluids that can result in dehydration.
7. T F Many communicable diseases can be prevented by immunizations.

ANSWERS

1. **True.** All needs (warmth, safety, nutrition, etc.) of the human infant must be provided by others.
2. **False.** The infant learns to sit unassisted at 6–8 months of age.
3. **True.** The infant thrives very well on breast milk because it is specifically formulated for humans.
4. **False.** The child is usually not mature enough physically to control bowel and bladder elimination until about 2½ years of age.
5. **True.** The permanent teeth come in during the school-age years.
6. **True.** Diarrhea can cause the water balance of the body to change. The lost fluid must be replaced.
7. **True.** When the guidelines for immunization are followed, the infant and child are protected from diseases that are transmitted from one person to another.

THE INFANT'S DEVELOPMENT

INFANT

the person at the beginning of life (from birth to 1½ years), for whom all needs are met by others

The human **infant** is helpless at birth. All of the infant's needs must be met by others. Comfort, warmth, safety, food, and love are the important ingredients that help the human grow and develop (Figure 30–1). The period of **infancy** extends from birth to 1½ years of age. By the age of 1 year, however, most humans have begun to walk, talk, and feed themselves. Infants understand body language as well as the language of touch. They begin to respond to the world around them, yet protection and care are still necessary.

VITAL SIGNS

VITAL SIGNS

the signs of life: temperature, pulse, respirations, and blood pressure

PULSE

the beat of the heart as felt through the walls of the arteries

RESPIRATION

the exchange of oxygen and carbon dioxide between the air and the body cells

BLOOD PRESSURE

pressure caused by the blood circulating against the arteries

The **vital signs** of the infant are very different from the normal vital signs of the adult. Infants have a higher pulse rate and respiration rate because the speed with which they are growing demands a high level of energy from their body. The ranges for vital signs during the first year of life are as follows:

Pulse:	120–160 beats per minute
Respirations:	30–60 breaths per minute
Blood pressure:	74/50–100/70

PHYSICAL GROWTH

FONTANELLE

soft spot on the infant's skull where the bones do not meet; closes as the infant grows

The physical growth during infancy is the fastest of any stage of life.

- The infant's length increases by 50% in the first year of life. For example, infants who measure 20 inches in length at birth may reach a length of about 30 inches at 1 year.
- The infant's weight doubles by 5 months of age and triples by 1 year of age. For example, infants who weigh 7 pounds at birth may weigh 14 pounds by the time they are 5 months old and 21 pounds at 1 year.
- The **fontanelles** at the back of the skull close up at about 3–4 months, and the fontanelles at the front of the skull close up by about 18 months of age. The fontanelles are present at birth to allow the head to mold during a vaginal delivery. Closing of the fontanelles ensures that the brain is more fully protected by the bones of the skull.
- The first teeth erupt at about 6–7 months of age. The first tooth can appear as early as a few weeks or as late as 10–12 months of age (Figure 30–2).

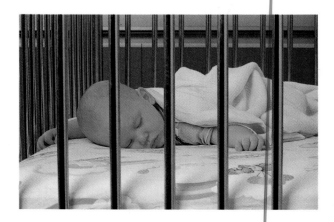

FIGURE 30–1
The care giver provides comfort, warmth, and safety for the infant.

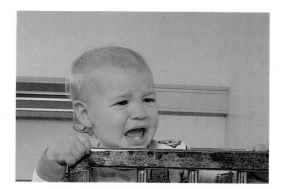

FIGURE 30–2
By about 1 year, the infant has 6 teeth.

CARING COMMENT

Infants have the need to suck. They may suck on their thumb (Figure 30–3). Other choices might be a piece of soft cloth, such as the edge of a blanket, or a **pacifier.** The health care agency may keep a supply of pacifiers available for infants to use.

PACIFIER
a nipple-shaped device used by babies to satisfy sucking needs

As infants grow, they begin to become active and move on their own. At first, the activity and movement of the infant are not meaningful. Activity progresses quite rapidly, however, and can be noted on almost a month-by-month basis.

2–3 MONTHS Infants are able to raise their head and chest off a flat surface. They can hold a small object if it is placed in their hand. If you place your finger on their palm, they grasp it. Their hand may bump or strike an object that is nearby. These movements are known as **reflexes.** Infants' neck muscles are becoming stronger and they are beginning to control their head movements.

REFLEX
an automatic response to a stimulus

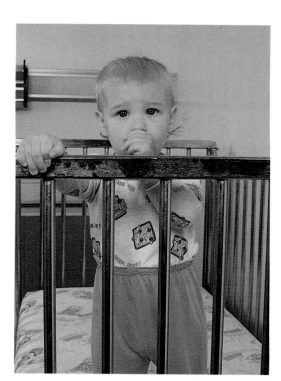

FIGURE 30–3
Infants find comfort in sucking their thumbs.

4 MONTHS   Infants can hold an object and put it in their mouth. They may discover their hands and feet and spend time watching them. They begin rolling from side to side.

5–6 MONTHS   Infants can sit if supported by a pillow. By 6 months of age, they may be able to sit up without help. They are able to move objects from one hand to another.

8 MONTHS   Infants begin to crawl, and at first find it easier to crawl backwards. As they become stronger, they crawl forward. They may pull themselves to a standing position as early as 8 months of age.

9 MONTHS   The thumb and fingers are used to pick up objects. This movement is known as the pincer grasp. Prior to using the **pincer grasp**, infants use their whole hand to grasp objects.

PINCER GRASP

movement of the thumb and fingers to pick up objects

1 YEAR   Infants can stand and may begin to walk without support. By climbing, they exercise their large muscles.

"Cruising" is the walking a child does while holding onto furniture. This activity provides support and muscle strengthening before actual walking begins.

PSYCHOLOGIC, SOCIAL, AND COGNITIVE GROWTH

As in physical growth, great strides are made in **psychologic**, social, and **cognitive** growth during infancy. One of the first psychologic events is bonding. Bonding is the creation of an emotional tie between newborns and their parents. It is a period of close contact in the first few hours after birth.

PSYCHOLOGIC

relating to psychology; mental

COGNITIVE

pertaining to cognition, one's awareness and judgment of something

1 MONTH   Infants can tell the difference between objects and the human face. They respond to discomfort by crying.

2 MONTHS   Cooing sounds begin, and smiling is a response to a social situation. A moving object is followed with the eyes.

3 MONTHS   Infants begin to laugh and are interested in the things going around them. They respond to sound by turning and looking in the direction of the sound.

4 MONTHS   Infants know who their mother or chief care giver is and are beginning to recognize familiar faces.

5 MONTHS   Imitation is important, and vowel sounds are verbalized.

6 MONTHS   Infants enjoy playing, and their speech consists of babbling and beginning use of consonants (the letters *g*, *d*, *k*, etc.). They respond to their name by smiling or briefly paying attention.

7–8 MONTHS   Infants display **stranger anxiety.**

STRANGER ANXIETY

a fear of strangers in which the infant may cry, hide, and refuse to go to an unfamiliar person

9 MONTHS   Infants are interested in searching for hidden objects and enjoy a game of peek-a-boo.

10 MONTHS–1 YEAR   Infants cry when separated from their parents. They can make their needs known by using two or three words together.

PLAY

Play is important in the life of the infant. During infancy, play is singular; that is, the infant does not actively play with another infant or child. Play helps the infant learn many things:

• How to socialize with the family group

- How to explore the surrounding environment
- How to control the head, hands, and feet

From birth to about 3 months, infants experience very little play growth. From 3 to 6 months of age, infants play alone and discover their body parts. The hands and feet are convenient play objects. Soft toys, made of cloth or plush material, are preferred. The infant at this age may develop a preference for certain toys. The parents are the preferred playmates from 6 to 9 months. Pat-a-cake is a popular activity.

At 1 year, the infant uses activity boxes and tries to play with the box to bring forth sound or activity. The infant may be interested in looking at books and show a beginning interest in toys that can be pushed and pulled.

CARING COMMENT

Choosing a toy for a young child is an important responsibility. Be certain toys are age appropriate and have no loose or sharp parts.

NUTRITION

Nutritional growth progresses from breast milk or formula feeding to self-feeding ability in the first year of life. Solid foods such as strained vegetables, meats, and cooked cereals are introduced at 4–6 months of age.

When teething begins, infants begin to feed themselves with finger foods. They may prefer finger foods over baby foods at about 6 months of age and may begin to use a cup to drink liquids. At 1 year, they begin to use a spoon to feed themselves and may be interested in eating some table foods.

Sources of Nutrition

The sources of **nutrition** available to the human infant are the following:

BREAST MILK Breast milk helps infants meet their **protein, calorie,** and **vitamin** needs during the first 6 months of life. It also contains special factors (**enzymes** and **antibodies**) that help prevent **infection** in the infant. The normal infant is born with enough iron stored in the body to last until 6 months of age. After the age of 6 months, infants may obtain their **iron** needs from supplemental food. The mother makes the decision about how long she will breastfeed her infant.

COMMERCIALLY PREPARED FORMULA Commercially prepared **formulas** provide the same nutrients that breast milk does. The bottle-fed infant does not receive protection against infection like the breast-fed infant does. Commercially prepared formulas are available in iron-fortified formulas. After 6 months of age, the physician may recommend cow's milk for infants who are receiving about one-third of their calories from other sources.

SOLID FOOD The ideal time to begin an infant on solid food is controversial. The physician may recommend the infant be started on solid food at 4–6 months of age. The first solid food introduced is usually rice cereal because most infants are not allergic to it. After the infant has accepted the rice cereal, strained fruits and vegetables may be offered.

Feeding

You may observe the mother breastfeeding her child. The infant should grasp the mother's nipple and the areola (the darkened area of tissue that surrounds

NUTRITION
the study of food's relationship to health; the act of providing food to nourish the body

PROTEIN
a material needed for cell growth; used in muscles

CALORIE
a measure of the energy produced by the breakdown of food in the body

VITAMIN
an organic substance that is essential in small amounts to the body's health

ENZYME
a protein substance made by the body that helps break down chemicals in the body

ANTIBODY
a substance that helps protect the body; part of the body's immune system

INFECTION
the body's response to invasion by harmful microorganisms and their multiplication in the body

IRON
a dietary substance that is necessary for the replacement of red blood cells

FORMULA
milk mixture that is fed to babies

the nipple) when sucking. This helps prevent cracking and soreness of the nipples. In the beginning, the infant should be allowed to suck on each breast for 5 minutes at each feeding. The amount of time the infant feeds can be lengthened each day. If the mother's nipples become sore and cracked, the mother can

- Expose the nipples to air.
- Apply a soothing cream to the nipples between feedings.

As a nursing assistant, you also may

- feed an infant a bottle of commercially prepared formula
- feed an infant or toddler baby food

Be sure you know your institution's procedure for feeding infants and children. Regardless of whether you or the mother is feeding the infant, make sure you provide a calm environment. If you are feeding the infant, do not rush. Speak in a soft voice and hold the infant securely.

PROCEDURE

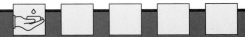

Feeding Infants from a Bottle

Feeding from a bottle should be a restful and relaxing time for infants. Infants should always be held for bottle feeding.

GATHER EQUIPMENT
Bottle of infant formula, juice, or water

ACTION	RATIONALE
Preparation	
1. Wash hands.	Prevents the spread of microorganisms.
2. Identify yourself and the patient.	Maintains patients' rights.
3. Provide privacy.	Maintains patients' rights.
4. Explain procedure to parent when appropriate.	Informs parent what is happening.
Procedural Steps	
5. Test the fluid for temperature. (Follow your health care institution's procedure for checking the fluid's temperature. Many institutions require that infant formula be given at room temperature.)	Hot fluid can burn mucous membranes of the mouth.
6. To feed a bottle of fluid to infants, hold them in your arms while you are in a sitting position (Figure 30–4). Support infants' head and shoulders in your arms. The infant's body can rest in your lap.	Gravity helps the fluid go down. Holding promotes bonding. Infants take fluid better when they are in a comfortable position.
7. Place the nipple in infants' mouth so they can close the mouth around it and suck out the fluid.	Having the mouth closed around the nipple forms a seal that keeps air out.
8. Keep the bottle upright so that fluid is in the nipple.	Decreases the amount of air in infants' stomach. (Air causes discomfort.)
9. Permit infants to feed at their own pace.	

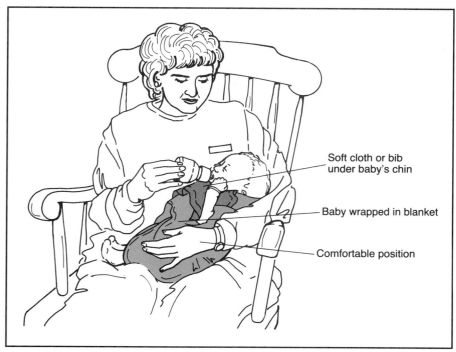

FIGURE 30–4

The infant is always held for feeding. If the infant is in lying position while feeding, fluid can enter the eustachian tubes and cause an ear infection.

10. At regular periods, remove the nipple from infants' mouth and **burp** them (Figure 30–5).

Permits infants to rest and release any air that is trapped in the stomach.

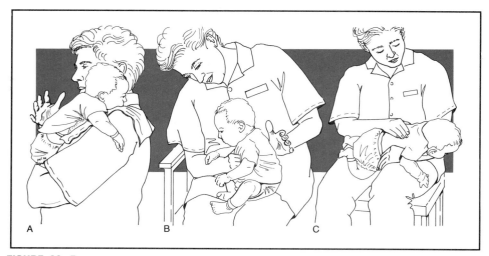

FIGURE 30–5

Positions for burping. A, Shoulder. Place a diaper across your shoulder. Hold the infant upright against your shoulder and pat the back gently for several moments to allow trapped air to escape. B, Sitting upright in lap. Hold infant sitting upright in your lap and support with one arm while patting back with the other hand. C, Across the lap. Lay infant across your lap and gently pat the back.

11. After infants have burped, resume the feeding and repeat the feeding/burping sequence until the feeding is completed or infants are satisfied.

Burping helps a baby expel gas from the stomach through the mouth by patting the back.

BURP
to help a baby expel gas from the stomach through the mouth by patting the back

Continued on following page

PROCEDURE

Feeding Infants from a Bottle *Continued*

ACTION	RATIONALE
12. Talk to infants and use eye contact during the feeding.	Encourages socialization and security.
13. When the feeding is complete, wash, rinse, and dry any evidence of fluid from infants' face and neck.	Removes fluid residue from the skin.
14. Place infants in their crib or infant carrier. The nurse will recommend the proper position (side-lying or back).	Permits infants to rest while fluid is digesting.

Follow-Through

ACTION	RATIONALE
15. Record the kind and amount of fluids taken in. Record the time of the feeding. Report the information about the feeding to the nurse.	Provides a record of the fluid intake.
16. Place the soiled linens in the linen hamper.	
17. In the health care institution, discard the bottle and nipple. In the home setting, bottles and nipples are reused after cleaning. The used bottle and nipple are cleaned thoroughly with a bottle brush in hot soapy water. Clean and rinse until all milk **residue** is removed. The physician will tell the mother whether the bottles and formula should be **sterilized.**	Prevents the spread of microorganisms. Prevents contamination of formula by harmful microorganisms.
18. Wash hands.	Prevents the spread of microorganisms.

RESIDUE
a layer of particles
STERILIZE
to kill all harmful microorganisms on an object by placing it in an autoclave or in boiling water

---

PROCEDURE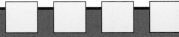

Feeding Infants or Toddlers Baby Food

In the health care setting, infants and toddlers are fed the kind of food to which they are accustomed. The nurse will tell you whether infants are to receive strained or junior foods. As much as possible, hold infants during feeding.

GATHER EQUIPMENT

Strained or junior baby foods in cereals, vegetables, fruits, and meats
Dishes
Spoons
Bib
Towel
Washcloth
Infant carrier seat or a high chair

ACTION	RATIONALE

Preparation

ACTION	RATIONALE
1. Wash hands.	Prevents the spread of microorganisms.
2. Identify yourself and the patient.	Maintains patient's rights.
3. Provide privacy.	Maintains patients' rights.
4. Explain procedure to parent.	Informs parent what is happening.

Procedural Steps

5. Open the jars of baby food and warm them in a pan of warm water.

   Warm foods taste better to infants.

6. Test the temperature of the baby food. A temperature of 105° F is acceptable.

   Food or fluid that is too hot can burn the mucous membranes of the mouth.

7. Pour the baby food onto a dish and stir. (Your health care institution may permit infants to be fed directly out of the jar.)

   Stirring removes hot spots that may be caused by heating.

8. Wash, rinse, and dry infants' face and hands.

9. Place infants in a sitting position.

   Gravity helps the food go down into the stomach.

10. Secure the bib or other protection around infants' neck.

    Protects clothing from spills.

11. Fill the teaspoon about half full of food. (If you are using a special infant spoon [smaller than a teaspoon], it may be filled level with food.)

    Prevents you from placing too much food in infants' mouth for them to swallow safely.

12. Feed infants one half-teaspoonful at a time, and offer a variety of food. Allow time to swallow between spoonfuls.

    A variety of food is needed so that infants receive the vitamins, minerals, and calories they need.

13. Talk to infants during the feeding.

    Eating is a social time, and communication helps infants feel a sense of belonging.

14. Continue to feed infants until they indicate they are finished (Figure 30–6).

    Infants know when they are full.

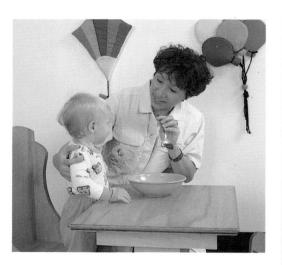

FIGURE 30-6

Infants may turn their face away from the oncoming spoon. They may keep their lips together or spit out unwanted food.

15. When finished, wash, rinse, and dry infants' face and hands.

    Removes food residue from the skin.

Follow-Through

16. Place soiled linens in the linen hamper. Discard jars in the appropriate container. Return used dishes to the kitchen.

17. Wash hands.

    Prevents the spread of microorganisms.

CARING COMMENTS

Strained foods are foods that have been blended to a smooth, thick liquid consistency. Junior foods are a thicker consistency and contain small pieces of food the toddler can chew. Make sure the child is old enough to be eating junior foods.

A microwave oven may be available to warm strained or junior foods. Stir food after removing it from the microwave to prevent hot spots. Remember to test the food for temperature before beginning feeding, because the container may feel cool to the touch but the food may be hot. Follow your health care institution's guidelines for microwave use.

HYGIENE

BACTERIA

microorganisms that reproduce by cell division; also called germs

Bathing the infant removes **bacteria**, waste material, and surface contaminants from the skin. Bathing is the ideal time to observe the infant's skin condition. Guidelines for giving a bath are as follows:

- Give the bath in a warm environment.
- Grasp infants gently and securely to lift them up (Figure 30–7).
- Never leave young patients while they are being bathed.
- Follow the sequence of washing, rinsing, and drying from head to toe.
- Pay particular attention to skin folds.
- Infants may be given a bath in a changing table, crib, or portable plastic tub. A crib may be used for children.
- Keep infants warm and covered, because their bodies do not regulate heat loss and heat production well.

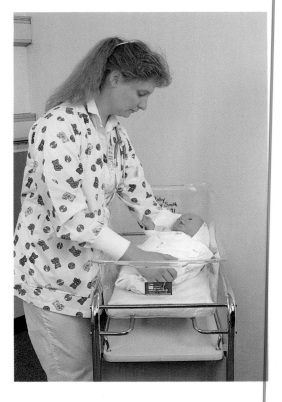

FIGURE 30–7

Infants need to feel safe and secure when they are lifted.

- If permitted by your health care institution, allow the parent or other adult caretaker to participate in giving **hygiene** care to the young patient.

All hygienic care must be done for infants. Use a gentle touch and talk to infants while you provide care. You may be responsible for

- Bathing infants
- Measuring and weighing infants
- Diapering infants

HYGIENE

the practice of cleanliness to promote health

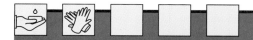

PROCEDURE

Bathing Infants and Toddlers

GATHER EQUIPMENT

Basin of warm water
Washcloths
Cotton balls
Alcohol swab (if umbilical cord care is required)
Towel
Mild soap

Lotion
Comb
Set of clean clothing
Diaper
Small blanket
Disposable gloves

ACTION	RATIONALE
Preparation	
1. Wash hands.	Prevents the spread of microorganisms.
2. Identify yourself and the patient.	Maintains patients' rights.
3. Provide privacy.	Maintains patients' rights.
4. Explain procedure (when children are old enough to understand).	Informs patient what is happening.
Procedural Steps	
5. Moisten a cotton ball with warm water and wipe the eye from the inner to outer **canthus.** Discard used cotton ball. Repeat cleansing on the other eye with a clean, moistened cotton ball. Discard the used cotton ball.	Removes any eye discharge that has accumulated.
6. Wet and squeeze the washcloth. Do not use soap. Wash one side of the face from forehead to chin and then wash the other side of the face in the same way. Dry face with the towel.	Clear water does not irritate the skin.
7. Pick up infants and support them one arm. The head should be supported by your hand; place your thumb and middle finger over infants' ears (Figure 30–8).	Placing your thumb and finger over the ears prevents water from entering them.
8. Wash the scalp with soap, rinse, and dry.	
9. Wash the neck and ears. Pay particular attention to the skin folds on the neck.	
10. Be certain all soap is removed; rinse and dry.	Soap residue may irritate the skin.

CANTHUS

the angle created by the eyelids in either corner of the eye; the inner canthus is the corner near the nose; the outer canthus is the outer corner

Continued on following page

PROCEDURE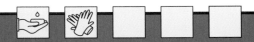

Bathing Infants and Toddlers *Continued*

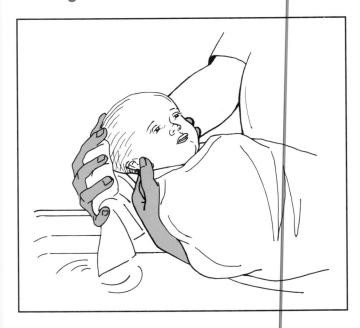

FIGURE 30–8

UMBILICUS

navel; scar that marks the connection of the umbilical cord to the fetus

UMBILICAL CORD

the cord that connects the growing fetus to the mother's uterus through which oxygen, carbon dioxide, fluids, and other nutrients are exchanged

GENITALIA

the external organs of the reproductive system

LABIA

folds of skin surrounding the urinary meatus (opening) and vagina in females

PENIS

external organ of urination and copulation in males

SCROTUM

the pouch (sac) that contains the testicles and their accessory organs in males

ANUS

the posterior opening of the body through which waste materials are expelled

RETRACT

to pull back

FORESKIN

a fold of skin that covers the tip of the penis in males who are not circumcised

11. Remove shirt and wash the trunk, arms, hands, and fingers. Wash between the fingers.

12. Cover infants with the towel before rinsing.

13. Rinse and dry the washed areas. Cover infants with towel between washing, rinsing, and drying.

14. Place infants on their side and wash, rinse, and dry the back.

15. Lift the towel from the lower part of the body and remove the diaper. Wash, rinse, and dry the abdomen and around the **umbilicus.** Wash, rinse, and dry each leg down to the foot. Pay attention to cleansing the skin folds and between the toes.

16. Clean around the **umbilical cord** with an alcohol swab. Discard the swab.

17. Put on the disposable clean gloves. Cleanse **genitalia** with moistened cotton balls.
    For females:
    Spread the **labia** and cleanse in a front-to-back motion. Use a clean, moistened cotton ball for each stroke.
    For *males:*
    Wash with moistened cotton balls from the tip of the **penis** down to the **scrotum** and **anus.** (Do not **retract the foreskin** in the male infant.)

Removes the small particles of dirt that accumulate between the fingers.

Prevents heat loss.

Protects you from contamination by body wastes.

In most male infants, the foreskin cannot be retracted until about 3 years of age.

18. Wash, rinse, and dry the anus, the buttocks, and folds in the skin that infants may have at the thighs.

19. Rediaper infants. Remove and discard the disposable gloves.

20. Finish dressing infants, wrap them in a small blanket, and place them in the crib or isolette.

Conserves infants' body heat.

21. Discard soiled disposables into the appropriate waste container. Place soiled linens and clothing in laundry hampers.

Follow-Through

22. Wash hands.

Prevents the spread of microorganisms.

23. Report and record the condition of infants' skin. The usual observations include
    • Tiny milia (whitish marks) over the nose and chin that disappear during the first 2 weeks of life
    • Peeling of the skin during the first few weeks of life
    • A yellow tinge to the skin that may appear during the first week of life
    • Forceps marks on the head (if instruments were used during birth)

Provides a legal record of infants' skin condition. Alerts the nurse if anything unusual is noticed.

WEIGHING AND MEASURING

Infants' and toddlers' weight and height are measured at admission. Daily weights may be ordered and should be performed at the same time of day on the same scale. Infants and toddlers should be weighed and measured while they are undressed.

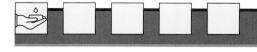

PROCEDURE

Weighing and Measuring Infants and Toddlers

Take children to the room where the weigh table is located to weigh and measure them.

GATHER EQUIPMENT

Baby scale   Pencil
Waterproof pad   Paper

ACTION   **RATIONALE**

Preparation

1. Wash hands.   Prevents the spread of microorganisms.
2. Identify yourself and the patient. Maintains patients' rights.
3. Provide privacy.   Maintains patients' rights.
4. Explain procedure to parent.   Informs parent what is happening.

Continued on following page

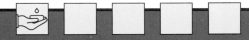

PROCEDURE

Weighing and Measuring Infants and Toddlers
Continued

Procedural Steps

5. To weigh infants or toddlers, carry them to the weigh table, usually located in the treatment room. Undress children on the table (unless they were undressed back in the room and carried in a blanket to the table; if so, uncover them).

6. Place the waterproof covering on the table and adjust the scale to zero.

    A fresh cover is placed on the table for each patient who is weighed and measured.

7. Place children on the table in the supine (back-lying) position.

8. Secure the safety belt or keep one hand on children's abdomen so that they do not roll over (Figure 30–9).

    Prevents injury from falls.

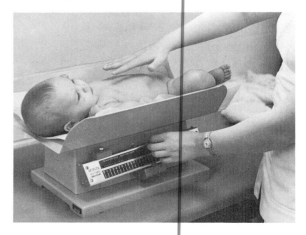

FIGURE 30–9
Keep infants safe while they are on the scale. (From Bonewit K: Clinical Procedures for Medical Assistants, 3rd ed. Philadelphia, W. B. Saunders Company, 1990.)

9. Move the pointer at the right until it balances in the middle.

    Scales work on the principle of balancing weights.

10. Read the number indicated at the arrow on the scale.

11. Write down the weight and slide the pointer back to the zero marker.

    So you have the measurement when it is time to record it.

12. To measure children's length, place the feet against the bottom of the scale. Make sure the body is straight. Read the number that corresponds to the top of the child's head. If there is a measuring bar on the equipment, it can be brought down and placed against the top of the child's head. The number where the measuring bar stops is read.

    The child is measured from head to foot.

13. Write down the child's height.	So you have the measurement when it is time to record it.
14. Return the measuring bar to the original position before you lift patients from the table scale.	
15. Dress children or wrap them in a blanket.	Provides warmth and comfort.
16. Lift children from the table and remove the waterproof pad.	Prepares the scale for the next use.
17. Place the used pad in the appropriate container (laundry hamper if the pad is cloth; waste container if it is disposable).	

Follow-Through

18. Take children back to their crib or parent.	
19. Record and report the weight and length and the time the measurements were made.	Provides a record of measurement.
20. Wash hands.	Prevents the spread of microorganisms.

DIAPERING

The frequency with which diapers need to be changed varies from child to child. Infants should be changed as frequently as needed. Check infants' diapers often for dampness or the presence of a bowel movement. If disposable diapers are used, be sure the correct size is available. Cloth diapers can be folded down to fit an infant or a toddler. The equipment needed for diapering in a health care institution is usually assembled in one area in the patient's room.

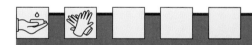

PROCEDURE

Diapering Infants and Toddlers

Lay infants and toddlers on a safe surface when changing their diaper.

GATHER EQUIPMENT

Disposable gloves
Fresh diaper (disposable or cloth)
Pins if a cloth diaper is used
Disposable washcloth
Basin of warm water (105–110° F)

Soap, if required by your health care institution
Towel
Waterproof changing pad
Container for disposal of the soiled diaper

ACTION

RATIONALE

Preparation

1. Wash hands.	Prevents the spread of microorganisms.
2. Identify yourself and the patient.	Maintains patients' rights.
3. Provide privacy.	Maintains patients' rights.
4. Explain procedure (when children are old enough to understand).	Informs patient what is happening.

Continued on following page

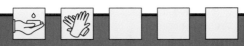

PROCEDURE

Diapering Infants and Toddlers *Continued*

Procedural Steps

5. Lower the crib side rail nearest you and place patients in the back-lying position. If using a changing table lay patients in the back-lying position on the table and secure the safety belt.

   The safest position for a diaper change is the supine (back-lying) position. The safety belt prevents children from falling from the changing table.

6. Place a waterproof changing pad under patients.

   Prevents soiling of bed linens.

7. Put on the disposable gloves.

   Protects you from contamination from body waste.

8. Loosen the adhesive tabs or unpin the pins on each side of the diaper.

9. Bring the top part of the diaper down between the thighs.

10. Grasp the ankles and lift the buttocks (Figure 30–10).

    Prevents injury from friction caused by pulling from under infants.

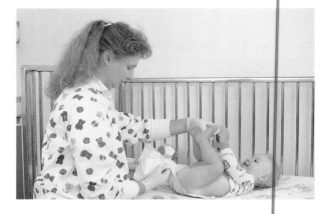

FIGURE 30–10
Remove the diaper when you lift the buttocks.

11. If a bowel movement is present in the diaper, use a dry corner of the diaper to wipe the waste material from the skin of the buttocks. Remove as much of the bowel movement as possible.

    Helps with skin care of the buttocks.

12. Place the soiled diaper at the edge of the waterproof changing pad and out of patients' reach.

    Young patients may reach for a soiled diaper merely because it is there.

13. Dip the washcloth into the water, use soap if permissible, and wash, rinse, and gently dry the genitals and **perianal area** (Figure 30–11). Remember to wash from front to back.

    Cleansing removes all waste (liquid and solid) from the skin. Gentleness is needed when skin has been irritated by many bowel movements. Washing from front to back prevents the spread of microorganisms.

14. Place the clean diaper under the buttocks by grasping the ankles and lifting the buttocks high enough to place the clean diaper under the patient.

PERIANAL AREA
the area around the anus

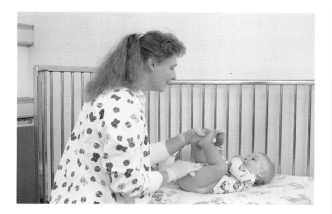

FIGURE 30–11

Repeat the rinsing procedure until all soap is removed.

15. If a special cream, powder, or **oint- ment** has been ordered, apply it at this time (Figure 30–12).

Protects the skin and helps it heal.

OINTMENT
a preparation that is applied to the body's surface and contains a medication

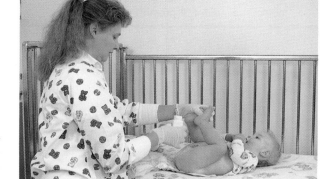

FIGURE 30–12

Special cream, ointments, or powder may be ordered to protect the skin in the diaper area from moisture or to help healing.

16. Bring the loose part of the diaper up between the thighs and adjust the diaper so that it fits the patient snugly.

    Note: On a newborn, fold the front of the diaper away from the umbilical cord.

17. Secure the diaper by using the adhesive strips on a disposable diaper or pins if a cloth diaper is used. (Be extra careful to keep pins out of patients' reach.)

18. Remove all equipment and raise the side rail of the crib. Or transfer infants from table to crib if a changing table was used. Put up side rails.

19. Wash, rinse, and dry the basin. Dispose of the washcloth.

20. Place soiled towel and waterproof changing pad in the linen hamper.

21. Dispose of the soiled diaper according to the procedure of your health care

A snug diaper is comfortable and stays in place, preventing leakage.

Avoids friction on the umbilical area.

Infants and children are curious and may injure themselves if they handle a pin.

Prevents falls from the crib.

Readies equipment for the next use.

Continued on following page

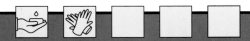

PROCEDURE

Diapering Infants and Toddlers *Continued*

institution. Disposable diapers may be placed in a designated container.

22. Cloth diapers, if soiled with a bowel movement, must be rinsed before being placed in a designated container.

Cloth diapers cannot be laundered properly if fecal material is not removed.

Follow-Through

23. Remove the disposable gloves and place them in the waste container.

24. Report and record the following:
    - time diaper was changed
    - condition of infant's skin
    - application of cream or ointment if ordered
    - amount, color, and consistency of bowel movement, if present

Provides a legal record that procedure was done, that bowel and bladder were emptied, and that skin condition was noticed.

CARING COMMENT

While providing care to infants and toddlers, remember to talk to them, maintain eye contact, and touch them to enhance their social development while in the health care institution.

THE TODDLER'S DEVELOPMENT

TODDLER
the young child from 1½ to 3 years of age

The **toddler** years end at about 3 years of age. Some experts identify the toddler years as from 1½ to 3. Toddlers are interested in exploring the nearby world. They still rely on others to provide for comfort, warmth, safety, food, and love and belonging. In addition, they are beginning to make their needs known to others. Toddlers are quick, impulsive, and inquisitive. They are prone to **accidents** and have a special need for protection. The changes experienced during infancy continue.

ACCIDENT
unforeseen or unplanned event

VITAL SIGNS

Vital signs change in the toddler years from what they were in infancy. The pulse and respirations are slower, and the blood pressure is higher. The ranges for vital signs in the toddler years are as follows:

Pulse: 90–140 beats per minute
Respirations: 24–40 breaths per minute
Blood pressure: 80/50–112/80

PHYSICAL GROWTH

Height increases, but weight is not gained at the same rate as the infant. Sight becomes sharper. Activity patterns become more meaningful and continue to progress.

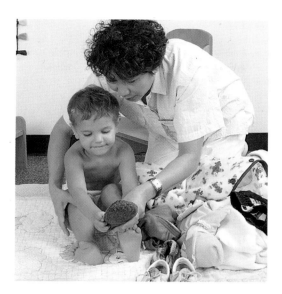

FIGURE 30-13
Toddlers show independence when they try to dress themselves.

1½ YEARS Toddlers experiment with running and at times do not watch where they are going. They find great pleasure in undressing themselves (Figure 30-13).

2 YEARS At this age, toddlers can jump in place and kick a ball and may be willing to perform on command. They begin to put on clothing, but the clothes may be put on backwards or inside out or may not match in color.

2½ YEARS The development of large muscles continues with the ability to stand on tiptoe, and the toddler may try to hop on one foot. The ability to control the movement of the hands and fingers is important, and the toddler practices this activity by drawing pictures. The pictures may have meaning to the toddler but look like a series of large strokes and curves to anyone else. Toddlers are very curious and may prefer to do things for themselves.

3 YEARS Toddlers can learn to ride a tricycle; this activity involves the large and small muscles as well as the kind of thinking necessary to steer and control a tricycle. They may be able to copy simple shapes and draw a primitive stick person (the stick person may not have body parts or clothing).

PSYCHOLOGIC, SOCIAL, AND COGNITIVE GROWTH

1½ YEARS Toddlers can use the word "no" appropriately and the word "mine" to show possession of an object. They can speak 10-20 words. A beginning understanding of time is apparent, especially in relation to bedtime. The toddler may express a fear of the dark.

2 YEARS Toddlers believe the world revolves around them. **Temper tantrums** occur when the toddler is frustrated. Toddlers know their own name and may use short sentences made up of two or three words. The 2-year-old may play with another toddler for short periods of time. In some 2-year-olds, toilet training may be started even though the child's body functioning is not yet mature enough for the **bowels** and **bladder** to be controlled.

3 YEARS Imitation of the parent of the same sex occurs. A few bright colors may be identified. **Vocabulary** shows a dramatic increase, and by 3 years the toddler may know about 800 words.

TEMPER TANTRUM
display of behavior in which children may throw themselves on the floor and kick and scream
BOWEL
the intestine
BLADDER
the elastic muscular sac that collects urine before it leaves the body
VOCABULARY
the collection of words or phrases used by a person

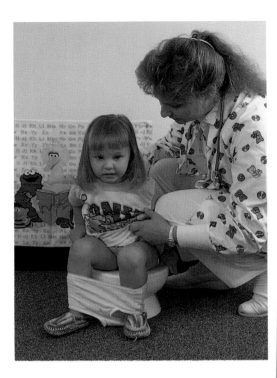

FIGURE 30–14

If the child is able, toilet training should be continued in the health care institution.

CARING COMMENT

Toilet training is an important milestone in the life of a child. You can help young children by encouraging them to use the potty when they are allowed to be out of bed (Figure 30–14).

PLAY

During play, the toddler begins to learn the concept of sharing. Most toddlers play alongside each other rather than with each other (Figure 30–15). By age 3, some toys may be shared with others. The development of hand-eye coordination continues, and the toddler finds coloring with crayons particularly enjoyable (Figure 30–16). Toddlers may not yet understand that coloring is done on

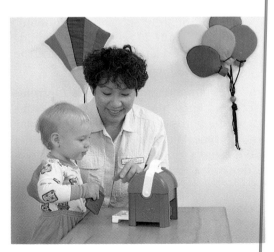

FIGURE 30–15

Large, colorful toys are attractive to toddlers. At this age, play needs to be supervised.

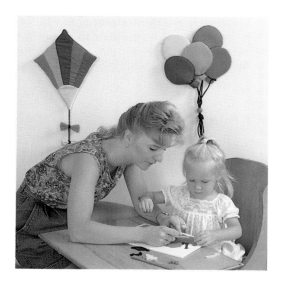

FIGURE 30-16

Toys that require hand-eye coordination are important to the toddler's cognitive development.

paper, and may find the wall or floor just as attractive a place on which to color. Although they like to color, they may not understand the use of color. For example, they may color the grass blue or whatever color of crayon they have in their hand. The 3-year-old has not developed enough hand-eye coordination to stay within the lines if a coloring book is used.

Play with other children continues to increase, and more verbal interaction takes place. Simple wooden puzzles may be put together and taken apart many times. This seems to be a challenge that allows the toddler to be successful. Toddlers are very possessive and may grasp an object tightly to their body and use the word "mine" quite emphatically.

NUTRITION

Although the rate of weight gain is slower in the toddler years than in infancy, a well-balanced diet is needed to provide the energy needed for physical growth and activity. Three meals a day and healthy snacks are important. Toddlers can communicate the feeling of hunger.

By the age of 2, toddlers can feed themselves efficiently and may be able to handle a drinking cup or glass with little assistance. They may show a strong preference for one kind of food and may want to eat the same food for a number of days. For example, peanut butter may be a choice for 2 or 3 days, after which it might not be requested for a while.

The toddler progresses from eating finger foods to eating almost all table foods by the age of 3. Teeth continue to erupt, and by age 3 most of the first teeth are in. These are known as **deciduous** teeth because, like the leaves on a deciduous tree, they fall out. They are replaced by permanent teeth.

DECIDUOUS
subject to falling out or being shed

HYGIENE

The toddler needs to be given hygienic care by a care giver. Follow the procedure for bathing an infant presented earlier. In some hospitals and long-term child care facilities, a raised tub may be available. When bathing a toddler in a tub, follow these guidelines:

- Follow the procedure for bathing an infant. Umbilical cord care is not necessary, but you should use the corners of a washcloth to clean the umbilical area thoroughly.

- N*ever* leave the toddler alone in a tub.
- N*ever* allow the toddler to stand in the tub.
- N*ever* allow the toddler to touch the water faucets.
- Wrap a towel around the toddler to provide a firm grip when lifting the toddler from the tub.

THE PRESCHOOLER'S DEVELOPMENT

PRESCHOOL AGE
the child from 3 to 6 years of age

The changes that occur during the **preschool age** (3–6 years) reflect the needs of the body: The rate of growth slows, and this is reflected in a lower intake of food. The preschooler's psychologic, social, and cognitive growth are important as the young child's world expands beyond home.

VITAL SIGNS

The changes in the growing child's vital signs continue. The ranges of vital signs for the child during the preschool years are as follows:

Pulse:	80–100 beats per minute
Respirations:	20–30 breaths per minute
Blood pressure:	82/50–110/78

PHYSICAL GROWTH

The preschooler grows taller and stands up straight. Weight gain slows down to about 5 or 6 pounds per year.

4-YEAR-OLD   Four-year-olds can hop on one foot and catch a ball. They are able to dress and undress themselves without help. More control of a pencil or crayon is evident. They can draw shapes and complete a stick person made of three parts (head, torso, limbs).

5-YEAR-OLD   At 5 years, children may begin to roller-skate and can tie their shoelaces quite well. They are beginning to print words and are interested in signing their own name. Hand dominance (right or left) is also determined.

6-YEAR-OLD   The 6-year-old is able to hold a pencil and print words. The child has more control over body movements. The child is growing stronger and is less likely to show fatigue.

PSYCHOLOGIC, SOCIAL, AND COGNITIVE GROWTH

Praise is very important to psychologic, social, and cognitive growth. Preschoolers know if they have done something wrong. Imaginary friends play a role in helping a child socialize (Figure 30–17). The ability to count shows that the thinking processes are developing; the preschool-age child is attracted to coins and shows a beginning knowledge of the worth of pennies, nickels, and dimes.

PLAY

Preschoolers' social life is promoted through play. They play well with other children. Playing house and other pretend games help preschoolers learn skills necessary to function in the world outside the home. Action toys that have multiple uses are especially attractive at this age.

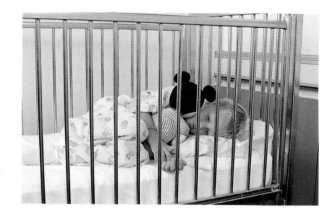

FIGURE 30-17
A preschooler may use a stuffed toy for comfort and companionship.

NUTRITION

Preschoolers can feed themselves completely and show preferences for certain foods.

FEEDING A CHILD

In the health care institution, children are fed when they are too young or too weak to be able to feed themselves. You may be responsible for feeding a child. Remember to allow children to choose their food whenever possible. Children can indicate what food they want by nodding their head in answer to your questions. This allows them some control over what is happening.

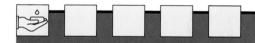

PROCEDURE

Feeding Children

All equipment should be placed on the over-bed table.

GATHER EQUIPMENT

Food from the diet as ordered
Silverware
Napkins

Warm washcloth
Towel
Bib or other protective cover

ACTION	RATIONALE
Preparation	
1. Wash hands.	Prevents the spread of microorganisms.
2. Identify yourself and the patient.	Maintains patients' rights.
3. Provide privacy.	Maintains patients' rights.
4. Explain procedure.	Informs patients what is happening.
Procedural Steps	
5. Wash the patient's face and hands before the feeding begins.	Helps the patient feel refreshed.
6. Place the patient in the semi-Fowler's or high Fowler's position.	Gravity helps the food or fluids go down into the stomach. Helps prevent choking.

Continued on following page

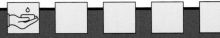
Feeding Children *Continued*

7. Place the tray with the food on the over-bed table. Open all food containers.	Makes procedure more convenient for you.
8. Lower the side rail on the side nearest you.	Allows for easy reach.
9. Place the bib or protective pad on the patient's chest.	Protects clothing from soiling if food is dropped.
10. Cut table foods into small bite-size pieces.	Allows for easier swallowing by the patient.
11. Place food on the teaspoon and offer it to the child by placing the spoon on the tongue.	
12. Allow time for the child to swallow the food.	Lets the child enjoy the taste of the food.
13. Continue feeding by offering different foods that are on the tray.	Rotating foods helps the child enjoy the meal.
14. Offer fluids during the meal.	Helps wash down food.
15. When feeding is complete, remove the protective cover from the patient's chest and wash, rinse, and dry the patient's face and hands.	The covering is no longer needed and may be soiled.
16. Lower the back of the bed to a flat or low Fowler's position. Place the patient in a comfortable position and raise the side rail.	
17. Place call signal within reach.	Leaves patients with the means to communicate.
18. Remove the tray from the room and place it in the designated place for return to the kitchen.	The trays are cleaned and prepared for the next meal.

Follow-Through

19. Wash hands.	Prevents the spread of microorganisms.
20. Report and record the amount of food and fluids the patient has eaten.	Provides a legal record of patient's intake.
21. Record intake on the intake and output (I&O) record if the nurse has told you to measure the amount of food and fluids taken in by the patient.	The I&O record shows the amount of food and fluid taken in over a period of 24 hours.

HYGIENE

Assistance with bathing is still needed. Preschoolers may be able to wash their face and hands but need help with shampooing their hair and bathing the rest of their body.

THE SCHOOL-AGE CHILD'S DEVELOPMENT

PEER
an equal; one who belongs to the same group (age, school, etc.)

During the school-age years, children still need the security of the family. They also form **peer** relationships that help meet their needs for security and belonging. Their peers have similar interests and activities.

VITAL SIGNS

The vital signs in the school-age child are still changing. The ranges are as follows:

Pulse: 75–100 beats per minute
Respirations: 20–30 breaths per minute
Blood pressure: 84/54–120/80

PHYSICAL GROWTH

Physical change continues, with a growth rate of 1–3 inches a year and a weight gain of 3–6 pounds a year.

- Vision is normally 20/20 at this age and is similar to the expected visual range of the adult.
- During school age, the permanent teeth begin to erupt.
- Muscle strength doubles during this age period. The child participates in active sports that require the use of the developing muscles of the body.
- The ability to write is developed, and drawings become more **intricate** and complete.

  INTRICATE
  complex

- The child's vocabulary increases, along with the ability to use more complex sentence structures.
- Early in this period, the child recognizes time on a clock and is conscious of the passage of time. For example, the child is able to identify the seasons and understands such concepts of time as hour, month, and year.

PSYCHOLOGIC, SOCIAL, AND COGNITIVE GROWTH

Cognitive growth is promoted by attendance at school. Psychologic and social development continue as the child learns to make and keep friends. Play fosters the concept of team participation. Playmates continue to be primarily of the same sex.

NUTRITION

Good nutrition may be threatened because school-age children may be so busy that they forget to eat. They need to be reminded to eat. They also need to be

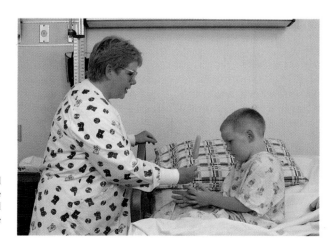

FIGURE 30–18

The school-age child who is ill needs food and fluids. Creative approaches such as offering fluid in the form of a popsicle may be necessary.

encouraged to eat nutritional food rather than junk food. The increase in activity makes a high caloric intake necessary; the child may ingest (eat) about 2,500 calories of food in a typical day (Figure 30–18).

THE ADOLESCENT'S DEVELOPMENT

Adolescence (13–18 years) is a period of intense physical, psychologic, social, and cognitive growth. The **adolescent** is preparing for adulthood.

VITAL SIGNS

During adolescence, the vital signs stabilize to the ranges of the normal adult measurements.

Pulse:	60–90 beats per minute
Respirations:	12–16 breaths per minute
Blood pressure:	94/62–140/88

PHYSICAL GROWTH

Physical growth and stature become those of an adult.

- The adolescent growth spurt occurs, and adolescents may add 25% to their height.
- Weight gain occurs: 15–60 pounds in boys and 15–50 pounds in girls.
- The **secondary sexual characteristics** appear during this period of growth. In girls, the breasts develop and **menstruation** begins. In boys, the voice deepens and facial hair develops. The growth of pubic hair occurs in both sexes. The release of **hormones** stimulates the appearance of these secondary sexual characteristics.

PSYCHOLOGIC, SOCIAL, AND COGNITIVE GROWTH

For an adolescent, friends assume more importance than family. The parental influence decreases as the adolescent practices for the lifetime role of adult. The adolescent may become sexually active. In early adolescence the self is very important to the child. As development continues, the search for an identity continues.

PLAY

Team sports are important. The adolescent may participate in as well as watch sports. Interactions with the opposite sex are enhanced by dances and other school- and community-sponsored activities.

NUTRITION

The adolescent is a very busy person who continues to enjoy junk foods. The growth spurt associated with adolescence means that a high intake of calories is important.

ADOLESCENT
the child who is maturing; teenager

SECONDARY SEXUAL CHARACTERISTICS
changes in males and females that occur with puberty

MENSTRUATION
the discharge through the vagina of blood and tissue from the uterus of the nonpregnant female; also called monthly flow, menses, and period

HORMONE
a substance that endocrine glands secrete directly into the circulating blood; the hormone travels to a designated place in the body where it is used in a chemical action

THE INFANT AND CHILD IN A HEALTH CARE INSTITUTION

Infants and children each have special needs when they are cared for in a health care institution.

CARING FOR INFANTS

Caring for infants who are ill or injured or who have a chronic disease that requires assistance is a very important part of being a nursing assistant. The infant is completely helpless. You are responsible for bathing, feeding, dressing, grooming, diapering, and positioning infants. In addition, you must provide safety and security. Your skill in observing and reporting changes from normal is also important. This skill will help you respond to the needs an infant expresses through behaviors such as crying, eating, and sleeping.

Infancy is a time of bonding with parents. Therefore separation of the infant from the parents can cause irritability and interfere with the development of a trust relationship with the parent. Infants may show signs of regression (return to an earlier state of development) when separated from their parents. For example, they might stop crawling and prefer to be carried while ill. The parents may be affected by the separation just as much as the infant.

Whenever you have a few spare moments, you should spend time with the infants and other young children in your care. Use touch by gently rubbing the infant on the arms, legs, or back or letting the infant hold your hand. You can talk and sing to an infant. Humming a tune helps relax an infant. If the infant is allowed out of the crib, you can hold and rock the infant. Even a few minutes of attention lets infants and young children know that they are important. These actions help them develop a sense of trust that the world is a good place to be.

You should be understanding and supportive of the parents, allow them to participate in the infant's care, and encourage them to visit. The nurse will tell you when the parents can participate directly in the infant's care.

CARING FOR TODDLERS

Toddlers are not as helpless as infants and want to do many things for themselves. They are quick and may do things without thinking. Your role is to ensure safety while allowing the toddler a small degree of independence. For example, toddlers may want to wash their face and hands before meals. You can prepare a washcloth and direct the toddler in washing. If they ask for assistance in toileting, you can help them pull their underpants down and back up again. You should provide for the toddlers' safety and security and be certain to plan time to play. Give lots of praise, hold the toddlers, and be certain all needs are met.

Toddlers who are ill and in the health care institution fear abandonment (being left alone). They are not sure that their parent(s) will return. Regression may occur: They may stop feeding themselves and, although toilet-trained, may become **incontinent**. Toddlers may be afraid of the care giver. The parent(s) is encouraged to visit often and participate in care as much as the child's physical condition allows.

INCONTINENT
unable to respond to the urge to eliminate the waste products of the body

CARING FOR PRESCHOOLERS

The preschooler is a delightful person who can do many things independently. As their good health returns, preschoolers begin to help you with their care.

MUTILATION

destroying or crippling a part of the body

Because safety is still a major concern, the preschooler should be monitored while out of the crib. You should respond whenever possible when the preschooler requests something special such as a treat, calling home on the telephone, or watching a favorite television show. The preschooler responds to kind words and praise and is eager to cooperate and please care givers.

The preschooler fears **mutilation.** Play therapy helps these children understand and work through their feelings about what might happen to their body. Explain what you are doing when you are giving care and be honest in your communications with the child. Children of this age have not learned to control their feelings or how they behave. They may cry or not want their body touched because they don't understand what is happening.

The inability to sleep and rest may interfere with a return to health. The parent(s) may want to spend the night to be near the child. If the institution permits this, the parent(s) should be encouraged to stay overnight.

CARING COMMENT

NONJUDGMENTAL

not passing judgment on someone whose beliefs or activities are not the same as yours

Accept the preschooler's behavior and remember to stay **nonjudgmental** when you are responsible for giving care.

CARING FOR SCHOOL-AGE CHILDREN

School-age children can do most of their self-care except when very ill. Most children begin helping in their care as soon as they are able. Be sure to provide privacy during bathing, dressing, and toileting because a child may be very modest. Try to respond to the child's wishes whenever possible, but set limits when necessary. Remember that a school-age child has more understanding than the preschooler and may be able to listen to reason.

A child this age is usually permitted by the institution to use an adult-size twin bed. Safety is a concern because children are used to their own bed and may try to get up during the night without calling for assistance. Be sure to show children how to use the call signal. Give them confidence in using it by encouraging a practice session. Give verbal praise whenever appropriate.

The school-age child is fearful of possible pain. Explanations, honesty, and encouragement to participate in care whenever possible help decrease the fear of pain. Sometimes, children see their illness as a punishment for misbehaving. Let them know that they did not do anything to cause the illness.

Friends from school are missed. When permissible, encourage the child to attend play groups that are scheduled on the unit. You may be responsible for organizing play groups.

CARING COMMENT

When you have a spare moment, make the effort to give a child attention and join in the child's play.

CARING FOR ADOLESCENTS

Independence is important to the adolescent, and this quality is lost to a certain degree when a person is in a health care institution. Encourage adoles-

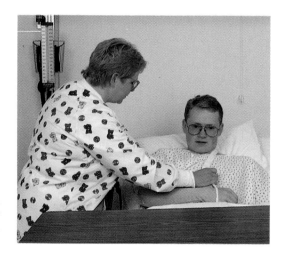

FIGURE 30–19

Injuries to muscle or bone may result when adolescents are active in sports. This may disrupt their image of themselves as an active, independent person.

cents to participate in decisions about their health care. Be honest when adolescents voice fears and concerns. Encourage them to talk about their fears, and inform the nurse or supervisor about them. Your role as a listener is important to the adolescent.

Adolescents are forming a new **body image**, and any possibility of change is a threat. You should be aware of this if treatment may cause a change in the patient's body (Figure 30–19). If it can be arranged, the adolescent should be given a room with another adolescent patient to help meet the need for peer relationships.

BODY IMAGE
the feelings and thoughts individuals have about their body

COMMON DISRUPTIONS IN CHILDREN

Common disruptions in the functioning of infants and children are

- vomiting and diarrhea
- communicable disease
- failure to thrive
- child abuse
- physical disability

VOMITING AND DIARRHEA

Vomiting and **diarrhea** are symptoms of common childhood diseases, such as gastritis (inflammation of the stomach lining). Vomiting may occur when otitis media (inflammation of the middle ear) is present. In addition, vomiting or diarrhea can cause **dehydration** because of the fluid loss associated with each. Important substances needed by the cells, such as **sodium** and **potassium**, are also lost as a result of vomiting and diarrhea.

Vomiting can be caused by infection of the gastrointestinal system and other diseases. Diarrhea can be caused by

- infection
- bowel disease
- difficulty in absorbing foods in the intestinal tract
- **lactose intolerance**

VOMIT
to eject material from the stomach through the mouth
DIARRHEA
frequent, watery stools
DEHYDRATION
condition resulting from a loss of body fluid
SODIUM
a chemical element found in the body's fluids
POTASSIUM
a chemical element required for cell function
LACTOSE INTOLERANCE
inability to digest milk because of the lack of the enzyme that breaks down a sugar found in milk

Observations of the Infant or Child with Vomiting or Diarrhea

There are important observations to make when the infant or child is experiencing vomiting and diarrhea. Observe for the amount and frequency of the

SPECIMEN

sample; a small piece of body tissue or a secretion or excretion used for examination

EXCORIATION

a scratch or abraded (rubbed off) area of the skin

vomiting and diarrhea. The appearance of the vomitus or diarrhea is also important; report the presence of any red liquid or particles to the nurse. The nurse may ask you to test the **specimen** for occult (hidden) blood. If the child is losing fluid, you should also check that the mucous membranes of the mouth are moist. You may also be asked to measure the patient's temperature.

For the infant or child with diarrhea, observe the perineal skin for any redness, **excoriation,** or rashes. The following questions will help you with observations of the infant or child experiencing vomiting or diarrhea.

- How does the patient look? Does the patient appear ill? Are the eyes bright and clear? Is the patient active and alert?
- Is body temperature elevated?
- Is the patient experiencing pain? Are there behaviors that could indicate that pain is present, such as lying still and not permitting anyone to touch a body part, crying or moaning, or drawing up the knees? Can the child tell you where the pain is?
- What is the patient's weight? Is there a weight loss?
- What is the patient taking in for nourishment?

Care of the Infant or Child with Vomiting or Diarrhea

The care of the infant or child with vomiting or diarrhea focuses on three areas:

- To maintain fluid balance, provide fluids as ordered by the physician. The nurse or supervisor will tell you what kinds of fluids the patient is allowed to have. Flavored fluids that include important substances such as sodium and potassium may be ordered. Crushed ice that is flavored may also be offered.
- To maintain nutrition, encourage the patient to eat the foods served. Offer foods the child likes that are within the prescribed diet. The parent(s) are a primary source for information on the child's dietary preferences.
- To prevent skin breakdown, wash, rinse, and dry the infant or child's perianal area after each bowel movement. You can use a mild soap if the child has no soap **allergies.** Use a gentle touch. You may be asked to apply a cream or ointment that is prescribed by the physician. Observe the skin carefully and report and record any problems as soon as changes are noted.

ALLERGY

an abnormal response caused by exposure to an allergen (for example, dust or food); hypersensitivity

The following are additional care responsibilities:

- After the patient has vomited, swab the mouth with a wet washcloth. Children who are old enough to cooperate may be willing to rinse their mouth with water.
- Be sure to remove the vomitus or bowel movement from the room so the air smells fresh. Also be aware certain smells in the environment may trigger the vomiting reflex.

Vomiting or diarrhea may appear to be a simple problem at first. However, an infant or small child can become severely ill and dehydrated when fluids are lost and not replaced quickly. Dehydration can be life-threatening, and the infant or child is often cared for in a health care institution until the vomiting or diarrhea stops.

COMMUNICABLE DISEASE

VIRUS

a microorganism that needs living tissue in order to reproduce

Communicable diseases are diseases that are caught from another person. Bacteria and **viruses** are common causes of communicable diseases. Many communicable diseases can be prevented. The following chart shows communicable diseases that occur in infants and children.

COMMUNICABLE DISEASES

Diphtheria—Diphtheria is an infection of the tonsils, pharynx, larynx, or nose. A false membrane forms in the throat and can cause problems. Diphtheria is caused by a bacterium.

Pertussis—Pertussis is also known as whooping cough. It is caused by a bacterium. The disease begins with an irritating cough that progresses to a violent, crowing cough that ends with a "whoop."

Tetanus—Lockjaw is a common name for tetanus. This disease causes the muscles to become painful and rigid. Tetanus is caused by a bacterium.

Polio—Polio is caused by a virus. Polio can lead to paralysis.

Measles—A virus causes measles to occur. A dusky red rash appears first on the face and then on the rest of the body. The child with measles may have an elevated body temperature.

Mumps—Mumps is caused by a virus. The area from the front of the ear to below the jaw swells. An elevated body temperature is also present.

Rubella—Another name for rubella is German measles. Rubella is caused by a virus. A rash is present on the body, and an elevated body temperature may be present.

Influenza—A virus is responsible for influenza. A severe infection, caused by bacteria, may result.

Chicken Pox—Chicken pox is caused by a virus. A rash appears, followed by open spots that crust over in 6–7 days. The child experiences itching wherever the rash is present. A lowered body temperature may be present.

Immunization

Many of the communicable diseases of childhood are preventable by **immunization.** Immunization offers protection against a particular disease. The parent or caretaker is responsible for following a schedule of immunizations for the infant or child. In some states, parents must show proof of immunization when the child is registered in school. Before immunizations were developed, the communicable diseases of childhood were responsible for lifelong problems or death. The schedule for immunization is shown in the chart below.

IMMUNIZATION

a procedure that helps the body develop an antibody against a specific harmful microorganism

SCHEDULE FOR IMMUNIZATIONS

Diphtheria, tetanus, and pertussis (DTP)
Immunizations (DTP) are given at 2, 4, and 6 months of age, with a booster given at 15–18 months. Another dose is recommended at 4–6 years of age. Immunization (DT) for tetanus and diphtheria is recommended at age 14–16 and then every 10 years throughout life.

Oral Polio Vaccine
The vaccine is given at 2, 4, and 6 months of age, with a booster at 18 months of age. Another dose is recommended at 4–6 years of age.

Continued on following page

SCHEDULE FOR IMMUNIZATIONS *Continued*

Measles, mumps, and rubella (MMR)
Immunization is given at approximately 18 months of age and prior to entering school.
Haemophilus influenza type b
One of two schedules is used: at birth, 1–2 months, and 6–18 months; or at 1–2 months, 4 months, and 6–18 months.
Hepatitis B
This immunization is given at birth, 1–2 months, and 6–19 months; or at 1–2 months, 4 months, and 6–19 months. Though recommended, it is optional and parents may refuse the immunization of their infants.

Care of the Infant or Child with a Communicable Disease

LETHARGIC
abnormally drowsy and indifferent

The infant or child with a communicable disease may be tired and **lethargic.** Make the patient as comfortable as possible. Place the child in a position of comfort and provide a quiet environment. If body temperature is elevated, the patient should be dressed in light clothing. The temperature of the room should be kept at a comfortable level and not overly warm. Fluids are important when body temperature is elevated, because persons with elevated temperatures may be too ill to take in extra fluid or may refuse extra fluids. The nurse will give the infant or child a medication to lower the body temperature if such a medication has been ordered by the physician.

CARING COMMENT

SUSCEPTIBLE
unable to resist

Hand washing is of critical importance when you give care to the infant or child with a communicable disease. Hand washing helps prevent the transmission of germs to other children or adults who may be **susceptible** to the communicable disease.

FAILURE TO THRIVE

Failure to thrive is a disruption in the infant's or child's nutritional functioning. It is the failure to gain weight. Normal physical growth is interrupted and the infant or child appears very thin for age and size. Failure to thrive has several possible causes:

- Physical defects—The child may not be able to eat or may not be able to use the nutrients taken in. Poor sucking ability or a problem in the stomach or intestines may be interfering with the child's ability to absorb nutrients or gain weight.
- Environmental problems—The parents or other caretaker may not have enough knowledge about an infant or child's nutritional needs. The infant or child may not be receiving a balanced diet. The parent may not be concerned about the child's nutritional needs.

DEPRIVATION
lack of something

- Emotional **deprivation**—There may be a problem with parent-child interactions.
- Combination—Failure to thrive may be caused by a combination of physical defects, environmental problems, and emotional deprivation.

The infant or child who fails to thrive is lethargic. The child assumes a passive role regarding needs. Unlike other children, the child may not reach out for toys. You may observe the child rocking on all fours for long periods of time.

The child may stare at care givers as if starved for attention.

Parent-child **interactions** may be different from the usual interactions you observe between parents and children (talking, smiling, touching, etc.). You should observe the interactions of the mother and/or father while they care for the infant or child. Critical observations include:

- Do the parents look at the infant or child?
- Do the parents talk to the child during care and at other times?
- Do the parents hold the child?
- When held, is the child held close to the body or at arm's length?
- Do the parents smile at the child?
- Is there eye contact between the child and parents?
- Do the parents call the child by name?

INTERACTION

communication between two or more people

Report and record your observations. The health care team uses them in planning the care of the child and education of the family. Your documentation (also called charting) is important. Be objective when you record the interactions between the parents and child. Write down the behaviors you see. The child's height and weight also are important.

Care of the Child with Failure to Thrive

Nutrition is an important part of care. Feeding the child may be difficult if the sucking reflex is poor (the child cannot suck on a nipple hard enough). Because the infant lacks the strength to suck for any length of time, more frequent feeding may be required. The physician will gradually order an increase in the frequency of feeding.

Allow the infant enough time to eat and encourage food and fluids. The infant or child requires extra attention, including being held and cuddled and talked and sung to. Continue to observe the interactions between the child and the parents. Intake and output records are essential because they are used to determine the child's progress or lack of it.

CARING COMMENT

The infant or child with failure to thrive should not be permitted to quit eating after only a few bites of food. Because **fatigue** may affect the amount of food taken in by the child, plan extra time to feed the child.

FATIGUE
tiredness; weariness

CHILD ABUSE

Child **abuse** is mistreatment of a child. It is a breach of ethics (see Chapter 3). A child of any age, from birth through adolescence, may be abused. A child may be abused by a caretaker such as the mother, father, or guardian, as well as a friend or relative. Many states have passed laws that require professionals such as doctors, nurses, and clergy to report any cases of suspected child abuse.

ABUSE
improper use; mistreatment

Observations

A child who is a victim of abuse may have physical evidence of abuse or may display behaviors that result from abuse. Some of the following may be observed in an abused child:

- marks on the child's body such as bruises, cuts, abrasions, or burns, caused by objects such as belts, hands, or cigarettes

- vacant staring or intense watchfulness
- extraordinary quietness
- lack of eye contact
- fear of adults
- aggressive behavior
- hyperactive (abnormally increased) behavior
- statement of who did the abuse; the child may also express guilt

When you notice anything unusual it is important that you report the observations to the nurse or supervisor.

Preventing Child Abuse in the Health Care Institution

Child abuse can be verbal, physical, or psychologic abuse. Verbal abuse includes shouting at young patients, saying mean things, or using swear words. Always speak in a calm voice and never use swear words with any patient. If you feel you cannot handle a situation, ask for help from the nurse or supervisor.

Physical abuse includes hurting a child's body in some manner. Spanking, feeding the child fluids that are too hot, bathing the child with water that is too hot, and handling the child in a rough manner are all examples of child abuse. Always test the temperature of fluids before feeding a child or giving a bath or enema. N*ever* strike a child for any reason. Always hold a child securely but gently.

Psychologic abuse include threats of harm, such as telling children they will get a spanking if they do not do something. Rather than threatening a spanking you should sit and talk quietly with the child. If the child is too young to discuss a problem, try to distract the child from the undesirable behavior. For example, if toddlers cry and kick their feet, hold them and talk quietly to them. You can try to offer a soft, cuddly toy.

Never tease or make fun of a child. Never make children feel like they are worthless. Children need to hear positive remarks from care givers. For example, they like to hear that they have done a good job. You should remember to give praise for desirable behavior. Use emphasis in your comments, speak directly to the child, and use the child's name. Use statements like the following, emphasizing the underlined words:

"You did such a <u>good</u> job washing your face [combing your hair, etc.], Johnny."

"Oh Mary, what a grown-up thing to do! You should be <u>proud</u>."

"You helped make the procedure go better when you didn't move. I admire <u>your courage</u>."

Caring for the Abused Child

An abused child may be admitted to a health care institution for an illness or emergency as well as for investigation of abuse. Follow these guidelines when you care for an abused child:

- Maintain confidentiality.
- Observe for development that is considered normal for the child's age.
- Observe for unusual behaviors not caused by the medical condition.
- Use gentle touch and a calm voice during your interactions with the child.
- Communicate positively with the child, family members, and other visitors.
- Offer praise and encouragement.

PHYSICAL DISABILITY

The term **handicap** may mean that a physical disability is present. A handicapped child may not be able to do the normal things expected of a child. Other terms for handicapped include *disadvantaged* or *exceptional*. Because of illness or injury, the child may not be able to talk or do activities of daily living. The child may have missing or misshapen body or limbs, facial **deformities**, or other changes that cannot be hidden by clothing.

HANDICAP
disability

DEFORMITY
abnormal part

Treat handicapped persons the same as any other patient in your care. If any adjustments in care are necessary, you will receive this information from the nurse or supervisor. You can also check the nursing care plan for information on special care. Follow these guidelines when you care for a handicapped child:

- Know what the child is capable of doing.
- Use touch to show your acceptance.
- Use eye contact when you communicate.
- Be nonjudgmental when you give care.
- Accept the child with whatever disabilities are present.
- Be gentle when you handle body parts that may be painful to the child.
- Spend time with the handicapped child, even when it seems like the child does not realize you are present.
- Encourage the child to do as much as possible.
- Give praise and encouragement.
- Encourage the child to play with other children in the same age group whenever possible.
- Be supportive of parents who may be working through feelings about their handicapped child. Listen to them and report your observations to the nurse or supervisor.

CHAPTER WRAP-UP

- The human infant needs warmth, safety, nutrition, and love. These needs must be met by the parent or other adult caretaker.
- During the first year of life, the pulse and respirations are high and the blood pressure is low.
- The rate of growth (length and weight) slows down from 1 to 3 years of age. Activity is important to the development of the muscles concerned with movement.
- The preschool-age child (age 3 to 6 years) experiences growth in height and weight. As the child's world expands beyond the home, psychologic, social, and cognitive growth become important.
- The years from 6 to 12 are known as the school-age years. The pulse and respiratory rates are slowing down and the blood pressure is increasing; all vital signs are nearing the levels of an adult.
- The teen years (from 13 to 18) are known as adolescence. The vital signs become similar to those of adulthood.
- When infants and children are ill, they have special needs. It is important to help them meet their needs for warmth, safety, nutrition, and love.
- Vomiting and diarrhea are common disruptions in infants and children. Dehydration can be a complication of vomiting or diarrhea because fluid is lost and cannot be replaced as normal.
- Many communicable diseases are preventable by immunizations. The

parent or other adult caretaker is responsible for following a schedule of immunizations.

- Care of the patient with failure to thrive includes the encouragement of food and fluids. Touch, eye contact, and communication are important parts of care.
- Child abuse may be verbal, physical, or psychologic.
- Treat handicapped persons the same as any other patient in your care.

REVIEW QUESTIONS

1. Describe the changes in vital signs that occur during infancy; the toddler, preschool, and school-age years; and adolescence.
2. Explain how play and activity affect the physical and social growth of the infant and child.
3. What weight and height changes are expected during the first year of life? During adolescence?
4. What complication occurs when an infant or child loses fluids because of vomiting or diarrhea?
5. What care is important for the infant or child who is vomiting or has diarrhea?
6. What are the common communicable diseases of childhood? How can these communicable diseases be prevented?
7. List three causes of a child's failure to thrive.

ACTIVITY CORNER

You have been asked to organize a play activity for three children in your care. The toy chest has a large metal dump truck, a coloring book and crayons, a baby doll, a puzzle with large pieces, and a set of dominoes. Which toy would you give each of the following children who are recovering from an illness?

A 10-year-old _____

A 6-year-old _____

A 3-year-old _____

Caring for Elderly Patients 31

31

Caring for Elderly Patients

Objectives

AFTER YOU COMPLETE THIS CHAPTER, YOU WILL BE ABLE TO:

Describe the normal changes that occur with aging.

Describe the communication, nutrition, elimination, comfort, activity and mobility, protective, and psychologic needs of the older adult.

Give examples of reality orientation and fantasy validation.

Explain how relocation affects the older adult.

Define Alzheimer's disease, Parkinson's disease, and cancer.

Give care to patients with Alzheimer's or Parkinson's disease or cancer.

Describe hospice care.

Discuss death and dying.

Care for the body after death.

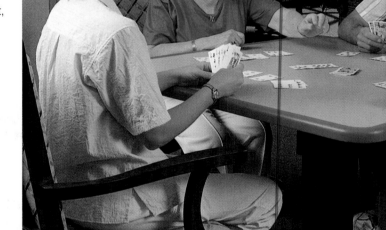

Overview Medical advances, improved nutrition, and the emphasis on keeping fit have all combined to increase the human life span. Twelve percent of all individuals in the United States are over the age of 65. For many, this is the time to retire and pursue interests. For others, it marks the beginning of major life changes and a time of health problems.

As a nursing assistant, you care for elderly people with a wide range of needs. This chapter discusses the normal changes of aging as well as disruptions in human functioning that may occur.

WHAT DO YOU KNOW ABOUT THE ELDERLY?

Here are seven statements about the elderly. Consider them to test your current ideas about aging. If you think the statement is true, circle the T; if you think the statement is false, circle the F. Change the false statements to make them true.

1. T F To be called elderly, an individual must be over the age of 70.
2. T F Most elderly persons live in nursing homes.
3. T F Alzheimer's disease affects the brain.
4. T F Older adults have a decrease in hearing function.
5. T F The elderly patient's pulse is usually 60 beats per minute or less.
6. T F The elderly person hears high-pitched sounds more easily than low-pitched sounds.
7. T F Reality orientation is used for all disoriented patients.

ANSWERS

1. **False.** There is a common belief that after the age of 65 a person may be called elderly.
2. **False.** Only 5–10% of Americans over the age of 65 live in nursing homes.
3. **True.** Alzheimer's disease short-circuits the message centers in the brain.
4. **True.** Although hearing ability changes in all older adults, each person has a different degree of hearing loss.
5. **False.** Because of a stiffening of the blood vessels, the pulse is usually greater than 60 beats per minute.
6. **False.** Low-pitched sounds are easier to hear for the patient with age-related hearing loss.
7. **False.** Reality orientation is useful for the majority of patients. Other patients can benefit from fantasy validation.

NORMAL CHANGES IN AGING

ELDERLY

a term frequently used to refer to older adults, usually individuals over age 65

AGING

the physical and psychologic changes that occur as life continues

VITAL SIGNS

the signs of life: temperature, pulse, respirations, and blood pressure

A decrease in the efficiency of the body's functioning begins in early adulthood. The changes occur slowly and many people do not feel different until they are in their late 50s or early 60s. The years after age 65 are known as late adulthood. The person who is 65 or older may be referred to as an older adult or **elderly.**

Aging refers to the physical and psychologic changes that occur as life continues. Aging cannot be defined simply by naming a certain number of years of life. Some physical changes, such as graying hair, wrinkled skin, and stooped posture, affect a person's outward appearance (Figure 31–1), but they do not affect the individual's health or the ability to function in society. On the other hand, some physical changes cause safety or health concerns. For example, people with a decreased ability to walk, see, or hear are at increased risk for injury. Psychologic changes can include feeling hopeless, taking a longer time to answer questions, and finding it difficult to accept the changes that occur with aging.

As a person ages, the changes that occur in the person's body functioning can be observed by others. As a nursing assistant, you will observe changes in the following functions in your elderly patients:

- **vital signs**
- protective (skin and immune protection)
- the senses
- activity and mobility
- sleep patterns
- nutrition and metabolism
- digestion and elimination
- psychologic state
- cognition

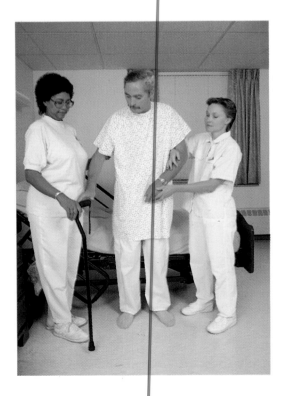

FIGURE 31–1
Physical changes in the elderly person include wrinkles, graying hair, and changes in ambulation.

VITAL SIGN CHANGES

Body Temperature

The body's temperature-regulating system is less efficient. In the elderly patient, a temperature measured by mouth may be lower than 98.6° F, the average for most people. The best way to determine a person's normal **body temperature** is to measure and record the body temperature for several days. This shows the range of body temperatures that can be expected for the patient. Any body temperature above or below the expected range can indicate a problem for the patient.

Detecting a **fever** in an older adult may be difficult. A temperature of 98.6° by mouth for a patient whose usual temperature range is 97.8–98° by mouth may indicate that a fever is present. Report changes in any vital sign measurement to your supervisor or the nurse in charge.

Taking an axillary temperature on an older adult may result in inaccurate results. If the patient is underweight, there may not be enough body tissue in the **axilla** to give an accurate body temperature measurement.

BODY TEMPERATURE
the degree of body heat or coldness measured by a clinical thermometer

FEVER
above-normal body temperature; also called pyrexia

CARING COMMENT

AXILLA
the armpit

Pulse Rate

Changes in pulse rate occur as a result of changes in the blood vessels and in the heart. In young persons, the blood vessels are elastic (stretch easily) and smooth on the inside walls. With age, the blood vessels work less efficiently because of

Atherosclerosis
Arteriosclerosis

The inability of the blood vessels to dilate (widen) or constrict (become narrow) causes the heart to work harder. The **pulse** may be bounding (you are not able to **obliterate** the pulse at the wrist), because the heart is working much harder to deliver **oxygenated** blood to the cells of the body. Because of changes in the blood vessels, the pulse may also be weak and difficult to count in the extremities. Locating the pulse may be difficult because of the blood vessel stiffness. Think about the difference between feeling a pen (a stiff vessel) and a straw (a soft vessel); it would be easier to feel blood moving through the straw than the pen.

ATHEROSCLEROSIS
a bumpiness of the walls of the blood vessels due to fat deposited there

ARTERIOSCLEROSIS
a thickening and stiffening of the walls of the blood vessels; also called "hardening of the arteries"

PULSE
the beat of the heart as felt through the walls of the arteries

OBLITERATE
erase

OXYGENATED
carrying oxygen

Blood Pressure

The **blood pressure** may become elevated because the heart is working much harder to pump blood through the blood vessels that are no longer elastic and smooth. **Hypertension** is a common problem in older adults. There are many possible reasons for this change. A blood pressure measurement greater than 140/90 indicates the heart is working less efficiently than usual. A single high measurement indicates a possible problem with heart function. The physician will ask for three or more measurements taken over a period of time to help in the diagnosis of hypertension.

BLOOD PRESSURE
the pressure caused by the blood circulating against the arteries

HYPERTENSION
persistently high blood pressure

Respirations

The lungs lose their efficiency because of changes that occur as a result of the aging process or disease. In addition, changes in the spine and rib cage that result from aging or disease can affect how the lungs expand. The respiratory rate is affected by the reduced efficiency of the lungs. It may be higher or lower than what the patient's range was in earlier years.

CHANGES IN PROTECTIVE FUNCTION

Normal aging of the skin is influenced by factors such as

- age and **heredity**
- **diet**
- **health** status
- **environment**

The skin becomes drier and more fragile with age due to the loss of moisture. Wrinkles and lines appear, and the skin may sag. Use gentleness when you care for the person with fragile skin, because the skin can tear easily and provide an entrance for harmful microorganisms into the body.

Along with the changes in the skin, the hair becomes thinner, especially in males. There is a loss of the **subcutaneous fat** that offers insulation against cold. The older adult may feel cold more often than a younger person. You should provide elderly patients with enough covering (sweaters, blankets, etc.) to keep them warm and comfortable.

Because their **immune system** is less efficient, older persons may be more prone to diseases caused by harmful microorganisms. The immune system can be helped, for example, when the older adult is protected by an injection of a **vaccine** against influenza. Practice hand washing faithfully to prevent the spread of **microorganisms** (Figure 31–2).

CHANGES IN THE SENSES

Vision

With age, the eye becomes less able to focus on objects that are near. This condition is called **presbyopia.** The ability to read a book or watch television is decreased (Figure 31–3). Prescription glasses or **contact lenses** can correct presbyopia. If your patient wears glasses or contact lenses, keep them clean and available for the patient to use.

The eye's ability to adapt to a change from light to dark decreases with age. When elderly persons go from a brightly lit room into a dark room, their eyes take longer to adjust to the reduction of light and see what is in the darker room. Turn on lights before you take a patient into a darkened room to prevent injury that could be caused by the patient's inability to see well.

HEREDITY
the physical and mental traits you receive from ancestors; inheritance

DIET
the total amount of food eaten by an individual

HEALTH
any state of physical, emotional, and social well-being felt by the individual

ENVIRONMENT
the conditions, circumstances, or objects that surround a person

SUBCUTANEOUS FAT
an inner layer of skin that insulates the body

IMMUNE SYSTEM
the body's defense system against harmful microorganisms

VACCINE
a preparation that is administered to produce or artificially increase immunity to a particular disease

MICROORGANISM
an organism so tiny it can be seen only under a microscope; capable of helping the body as well as causing disease

PRESBYOPIA
a visual condition in which the eye is unable to focus on near objects

CONTACT LENSES
prescription lenses that float on the cornea, to help correct a defect in vision

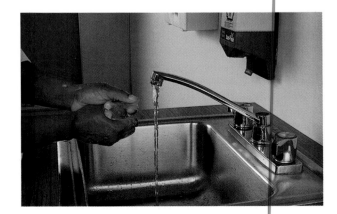

FIGURE 31–2

Hand washing is very important when caring for elderly patients. Because their immune system is weak, they are prone to contagious diseases.

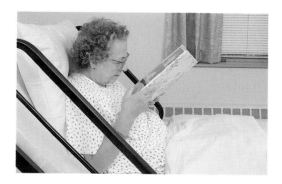

FIGURE 31-3

This patient is holding the family photo album too close. She needs to have her vision checked.

With age, the eyes also become sensitive to glare. Glare from sunlight, highly polished floors, or mirrors may be painful to the elderly person's eyes. Encourage the patient who is affected by glare to wear sunglasses outdoors or indoors (Figure 31-4).

Changes in peripheral vision (the ability to see to the sides) also occur (Figure 31-5). The range of vision narrows with age. The eyes may also become dry as part of the aging process. If you make this observation in a patient, report it to the supervisor or the nurse so that action can be taken.

To understand what peripheral vision is, look straight ahead. Do not move your body or head. Use your eyes to look first to the right and then to the left. Normally, if you put your hands and arms straight out at your sides, you should be able to see your hands. Peripheral vision allows us to see danger that may not be directly in front of us.

Hearing

Hearing becomes less acute as a person ages. High-pitched sounds become difficult to hear; low-pitched sounds and voices are easier to hear. Use a low pitch when you speak to patients.

A **hearing aid** may help many people who have a hearing problem hear sounds in their environment. Encourage patients who have a hearing aid to wear it. Older persons may lose the ability to tell from which direction a sound is coming. They may also find it difficult to distinguish sounds, so you may need to repeat words until your patients can understand what you are saying (Figure 31-6).

The accumulation of **cerumen** in the ear may affect the elderly person's ability to hear sounds clearly. Cerumen can be removed by irrigating (washing out) the ear; the doctor or nurse performs the irrigation when it is necessary.

HEARING AID
a device that makes sounds louder for persons who are hard of hearing

CERUMEN
earwax

Touch

The sense of touch may also be reduced in normal aging. An older person may be unable to determine the temperature of objects. You need to be especially aware of the possibility of an accidental burn when an older patient is unable

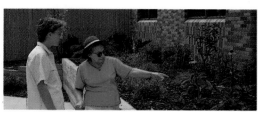

FIGURE 31-4

Solutions to the elderly person's sensitivity to glare include wearing sunglasses and hats with brims.

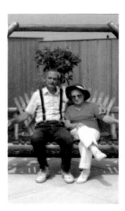

FIGURE 31-5
When patients lose peripheral vision, their view of the world looks like this.

to feel whether water or coffee is extremely hot. You may need to place an ice cube in a hot drink to cool it enough for the patient to drink. In addition, be sure water for bathing is at the correct temperature.

The ability to detect and feel cold may also be impaired. As discussed earlier, the older body's temperature-regulating system is not as efficient, so cold weather can be harmful. A condition called **hypothermia** can occur. Again, be sure to provide sweaters or extra blankets to help elderly patients keep warm.

HYPOTHERMIA
body temperature lower than normal

Taste

Taste, another of the five senses, helps us to enjoy our food. An older adult may tell you that "food doesn't taste the way it used to." This change can be part of the normal aging process. **Taste buds** decrease in number as well as in their ability to recognize the normal taste sensations. Many older adults add a variety of spices to their diet in the attempt to satisfy their need for taste satisfaction. Smoking also interferes with the ability to taste food.

TASTE BUDS
cells on the tongue that distinguish salty, sweet, sour, and bitter tastes

CARING COMMENT

Changes in taste may also be due to disease or medications. Be sure to report patients' subjective observations to the nurse.

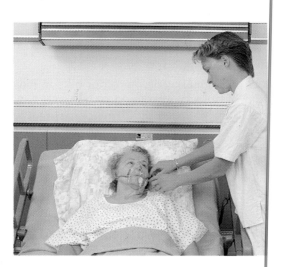

FIGURE 31-6
Be sure to face the patient who has difficulty hearing when you are explaining procedures.

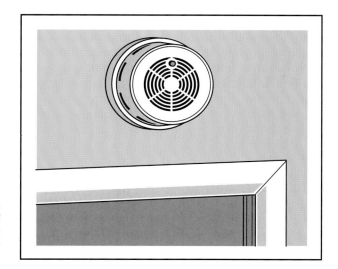

FIGURE 31-7

The inability to smell smoke can lead to disaster and the loss of life for the elderly patient. Encourage elderly persons to have smoke detectors in the home.

Smell

A decrease in the sense of smell may affect the way food tastes. The decrease in the ability to smell also can be a safety concern. The inability to smell smoke from a fire or a gas leak in the home can lead to tragedy for the older adult. A smoke detector is an excellent, low-cost safety device that can be used in the home or health care institution (Figure 31-7). The detector sets off a shrill alarm when it senses smoke. The alarm continues until someone locates and extinguishes (puts out) the source of the smoke.

CHANGES IN ACTIVITY AND MOBILITY

The ability to be active and mobile changes to a different degree in each aging person. People may find over the years that they do things such as get in and out of bed and walk more slowly.

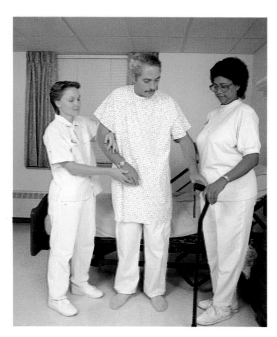

FIGURE 31-8

Make sure there are no hazards in the patient's environment that could cause injury.

BONE

the hard, rigid connective tissue that makes up most of the skeleton

OSTEOPOROSIS

disease in which calcium leaves the bones and enters the bloodstream

FRACTURE

a break in the bone at any point or place

ACTIVITIES OF DAILY DIVING (ADLs)

activities used to accomplish tasks such as toileting and grooming on a daily basis

ASSISTIVE DEVICE

an item a person uses to accomplish a task

ARTHRITIS

inflammation of a joint.

A person's **bones** and muscles change with age. Some of these changes result in a shorter stature (reduced height). Older persons may appear stooped over when they stand, and this makes their extremities appear longer. Bones can become brittle due to a condition called **osteoporosis.** When bones become thin and brittle from loss of calcium, **fractures** can occur more easily. You need to be aware of the safety hazards in the environment so you can take action to prevent injury to your patient. Hazards in the environment include loose throw rugs, chairs, waxed floors, and dim lighting (Figure 31–8).

Muscle strength and tone are affected by a decrease in activity and mobility. Walking and performing the **activities of daily living (ADLs)** can cause fatigue. Patients may require the use of **assistive devices** such as canes or walkers to help them move around (Figure 31–9). The assistance of a care giver may also be required so that patients can walk and perform their ADLs safely.

Joint stiffness, especially in the early morning, can be a problem for the older adult. This stiffness may be due to **arthritis.** This discomfort can limit movement in the affected extremities. It may be difficult and painful for the person to hold a cup of coffee or open a door. Allow more time for the patient with arthritis to complete tasks.

Patients who have joint stiffness and pain require your assistance in completing ADLs, getting in and out of bed, and walking. Some patients may require your help only in the morning, when the stiffness and pain are at their highest level (Figure 31–10).

A good way for patients to exercise their muscles and joints is to be able to attend to self-care needs such as bathing, eating, and toileting. Patients' self-worth and sense of accomplishment are also increased when they are active and mobile enough to provide as much care for themselves as possible. You can encourage your patients to do as much of their bath as they can. Be sure to check with the nurse or the patients' care plan to be sure how much a patient can do.

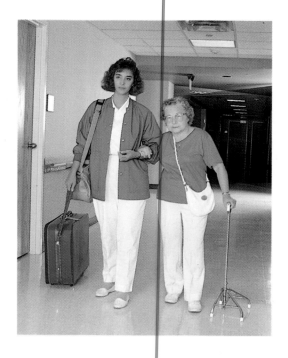

FIGURE 31–9

This elderly patient requires the assistance of the nursing assistant and a quad cane to ambulate safely.

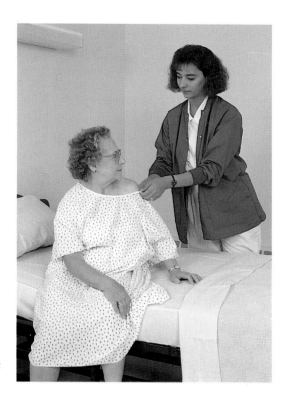

FIGURE 31–10
This nursing assistant is helping a patient who has morning stiffness dress herself.

CHANGES IN SLEEP PATTERN

A person's sleep habits often change with age, because the need for sleep decreases. Elderly persons may sleep for only 5 or 6 hours per night. Naps may be a daily habit. An early afternoon nap does not contribute to sleeplessness at night for most older adults. For some, a nap gives a person the extra energy required to maintain an evening social life. Help patients sleep by keeping to a bedtime routine as much as possible.

CHANGES IN NUTRITION AND METABOLISM

The older adult must have adequate **nutrition** in order to have an active and healthy life. Many factors can alter a person's nutritional intake as well as **metabolism:**

- The person's appetite may be reduced because of a decrease in the sense of taste and smell.
- The amount of **saliva** produced in the mouth decreases, making chewing and swallowing food more difficult. Be alert to the possibility that a patient may choke on food as a result of decreased saliva production.
- The need for calories decreases in the older adult. If elderly persons do not adjust their intake to correspond to their reduced need for calories, they may gain unwanted weight.
- The inability to open packages or pour liquids to prepare meals may result in a weight loss.
- Loose **dentures** affect chewing ability. Patients may not be able to chew nutritious food like apples or meats, so their intake of **calories, minerals,** and **vitamins** may decrease.
- Dietary intake may be affected by a person's finances and the inability to get to a store.

NUTRITION
the study of food's relationship to health; the act of providing food to nourish the body

METABOLISM
the process that produces energy in the body, allowing cells to grow and repair

SALIVA
watery substance secreted from the salivary glands; moistens food and makes it easier to swallow

DENTURES
artificial teeth

CALORIE
a measure of energy produced by the breakdown of food in the body

MINERAL
an inorganic (neither animal nor vegetable) substance needed for health

VITAMIN
an organic substance that is essential in small amounts to the body's health

CARING COMMENT

You can provide an environment that makes mealtime pleasant. Cut food and open wrappers for patients who are unable to do so. Stay with patients to provide company while they eat. In a nursing home, the dining room helps patients keep up with social interests.

ELIMINATION
the way the body rids itself of unusable food and fluid; the discharge of the waste products created by the body's metabolism

PERISTALSIS
alternate contraction and relaxation of the esophagus and intestines

DIGESTION
the mechanical and chemical breakdown of food into forms the body can use

CONSTIPATION
inability to have or difficulty in having a bowel movement

PROSTATE GLAND
the gland in males that surrounds the urethra and the neck of the bladder and secretes fluid that helps sperm move through the duct system

REMINISCE
to think or talk about events

SPOUSE
married person (husband or wife)

CHANGES IN DIGESTIVE AND ELIMINATION FUNCTIONS

With age, the passage of food from the esophagus to the stomach may be slowed because the **peristalsis** that helps move the food along slows down. Changes in the lining of the stomach and a decrease in the secretions necessary for the breakdown of food also reduce the efficiency of **digestion.**

Peristalsis in the intestine changes, resulting in **constipation** because fecal material is moved through the intestinal system too slowly.

The kidneys are still able to filter the blood to eliminate waste in old age, unless disease is present. The bladder has less capacity for holding urine so elderly persons may feel the need to void more frequently. In males, the **prostate gland** may enlarge and make emptying the bladder difficult.

Keep fluids within patients' reach and encourage activity and movement of extremities when possible. Encourage patients to eat the balanced diet provided by the institution because it includes foods that contain fiber. Fiber increases the bulk of the stool and makes it softer. These actions help the stool move faster through the intestinal tract and thus prevent constipation.

CHANGES IN PSYCHOLOGIC FUNCTION

One of the tasks of older adults is to **reminisce** about their life (Figure 31–11). It is normal for a person to discuss past life experiences; it is a retelling of life events. Reminiscing is also known as a "life review." Persons may verbalize that they have lived a good life and are satisfied. Persons who are not satisfied express regret and dissatisfaction with the way they lived their life.

The older person may become depressed for a number of reasons:

- loss of a **spouse**
- inability to live alone
- decreased financial resources
- separation from friends and family

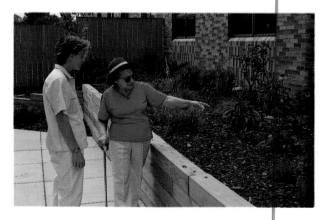

FIGURE 31–11

The older adult is reminiscing with the nursing assistant about the gardening awards she has received over the years. This gives the patient a sense of self-worth.

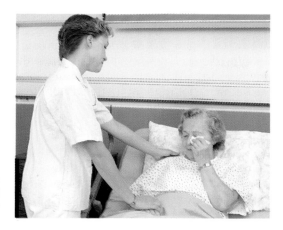

FIGURE 31–12
Use touch as part of the care you give to elderly patients. Touch conveys a sense of caring and keeps the lines of communication open.

- relocation to a new home or living quarters
- inability to accept changes in the body
- loss of usefulness to society (loss of a job or the ability to volunteer)

CARING COMMENT

You may need to spend more time talking with older patients. Use touch often to show that you care (Figure 31–12). Listening to patients' reminiscing is important to their sense of self-worth.

CHANGES IN COGNITIVE FUNCTION

Loss of Memory

Changes in the ability to remember events may occur. Changes are noticeable in short-term memory and long-term memory. Short-term memory (memory for events that happened in the recent past) is sometimes lost. Long-term memory (memory for events that happened long ago) is usually keen. The ability to learn remains, but learning may take longer because the brain may need more time to process information. You may need to remind patients about items or events such as mealtime or special activities that are scheduled.

Disorientation

An older adult may experience **disorientation.** A change in routine or environment, such as being hospitalized or admitted to a nursing home, may contribute to disorientation in older adults. Persons who are disoriented may not know

- their identity
- others' identity (such as family members and friends)
- where they are
- the time (year, month, date, and hour)

Disorientation is *not* a normal change due to aging. It may be due to a disease such as Alzheimer's disease, an infection, or medications. Medications can cause disorientation in the following ways:

- The wrong amount was taken by the patient.
- Multiple medications react with each other in the brain.
- A side effect of the medication occurs.
- A buildup of the medication occurs.

DISORIENTATION
not knowing self, time, or place

REALITY ORIENTATION

When you care for disoriented patients, you can use a technique known as reality orientation to help them know their name, the time, and the place. It involves the use of visual and auditory cues, for example, calendars, clocks, and name tags, to reorient patients to the environment. It is a way of bringing patients back to the present. For example, a patient may tell you, "I am going shopping today." You should reply honestly and truthfully and say, "You are in the hospital (or nursing home) now."

Use the following verbal and visual aids to help your patients become oriented to person, place, and time:

- Tell patients their name.
- Call patients by their name whenever you provide care.
- Tell patients what day and time it is.
- Tell patients your name and wear your name tag so they can see it.
- Place a calendar in the room. You can help patients cross off each date at the end of the day.
- Place a clock with large numerals in the room so that patients can read the time. Talking clocks are available for the patient with vision problems. The patient pushes a button on the top, and a voice announces the time.
- Tell patients where they are.

For patients in a long-term care institution, the following actions can be added:

REALITY ORIENTATION BOARD (Figure 31–13)   Show patients the reality orientation board. The board usually includes information such as

- the name of the institution
- the current date and day
- the expected weather

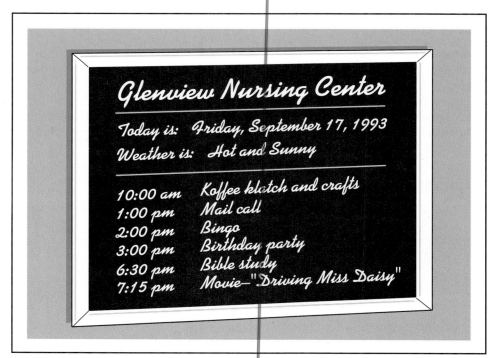

FIGURE 31–13

Show the reality orientation board to patients who are confused about where they are, the time, their own identity, or the identity of a family member. This board may be located in dining areas or in halls near the nurse's station.

- information on the day's activities
- the day's menu

PATIENT PARTICIPATION IN ACTIVITIES   Long-term care institutions usually have a separate department that organizes patient activities. Participation in the activities is extremely important to patients' well-being. These activities may be one-on-one discussions or games like checkers, reading, music, even just talking or group activities. Group activities usually include exercise, bingo, animal visits, games, and reminiscing. As already discussed, reminiscing can increase patients' feelings of well-being and worth. It can also help with reality orientation. Encourage your patients to participate in some of these activities.

FAMILY MEMBERS' INVOLVEMENT IN PATIENTS' REALITY ORIENTATION   Encourage family members to help keep patients oriented. By using many of the methods just discussed, they can help with reality orientation. This also helps the family to feel involved in patients' care.

FANTASY VALIDATION

In certain circumstances, reality orientation may not be appropriate, for example, when the patient becomes agitated and physically aggressive when reality orientation is attempted. In this case, fantasy validation is an alternative you may be able to use.

Fantasy validation is reinforcing the patient's fantasy (an unreal mental image) in order to decrease stress and prevent agitation. Fantasy validation allows the patient to have a fantasy that helps the patient maintain self-esteem. This use of an unreal image can also assist you to help patients overcome fear. For example, if the patients think they see a frightening object in the bathroom, fantasy validation allows you to "remove" it. This helps decrease patients' fear and stress.

Fantasy validation is not appropriate for all patients. The supervisor or nurse can direct you when you need to use fantasy validation. The patient's care plan can also be checked to be sure this is the appropriate way to proceed.

FANTASY VALIDATION
a technique that reinforces the patient's fantasy in order to decrease stress and prevent agitation

INSTITUTIONALIZATION

To institutionalize means to place an individual in the care of an institution. Contrary to popular belief, only a small percentage of older adults live in a long-term care institution such as a nursing home (Figure 31–14). An estimated 5–10% of individuals over the age of sixty-five are institutionalized. People who

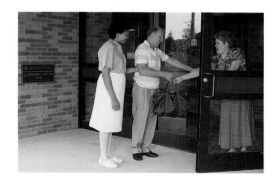

FIGURE 31–14
The patient who is entering the nursing home is often greeted at the door by staff. This helps the older adult feel welcome.

live in a nursing home often prefer to be called residents. Residents of a nursing home can be there for a variety of reasons:

- Their illness makes them unable to care for themselves at home.
- They do not have family or friends nearby who can help them with ADLs so they can remain in their home.
- They may be disoriented and require the constant supervision available in the nursing home.
- They are recovering from an illness or surgery for which they were hospitalized.
- They need physical therapy.

CARING COMMENT

Some people view a nursing home as a place to die. In fact, most of today's homes provide a worthwhile living environment for the older adult.

FAMILY SUPPORT

Family members or significant others are important to the resident in a long-term care institution because they

- Give the resident a sense of belonging and well-being.
- Provide the resident a vital link to the outside world that care givers cannot. Family news (such as a new grandchild or even the death of a relative) helps the resident to feel included in the family's activities and concerns.
- Give the resident emotional support.
- Contribute to the resident's care by telling the nursing staff about
    the resident's likes and dislikes and
    the resident's usual daily routine. (By using the family's information to care for the resident, you make the family feel useful as well as provide quality care.)
- Participate in care by
    joining in the scheduled activities (Figure 31–15).
    taking the resident home when permissible.

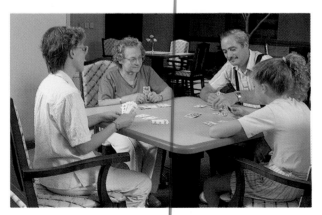

FIGURE 31–15
Family and friends provide emotional support and a link to the outside world.

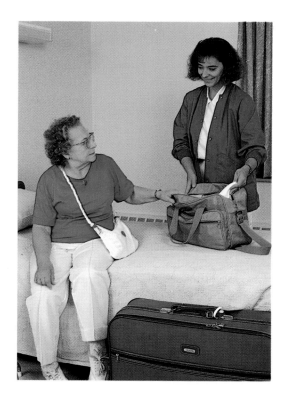

FIGURE 31-16
Relocation stress can occur when the patient moves from home to a long-term care institution. Stress may cause a patient to become withdrawn or temporarily confused.

You should provide the family with a comfortable visiting environment so that they are encouraged to continue to visit. You can make their visit comfortable by using courtesy when talking to them and showing genuine care and concern for the resident. Be certain the resident is neat and clean when the family comes to visit. Be sure to relay all concerns the family has to the supervisor or nurse. When family members or friends call the nursing unit to ask about a resident's condition, refer the call to the nurse in charge.

RELOCATION STRESS

Relocation stress is a form of **stress** that occurs when the patient is transferred from one place to another, for example

- from home to the nursing home or hospital (Figure 31-16)
- from the hospital to the nursing home
- from the nursing home to the hospital
- from room to room within the health care institution

Relocation stress can cause changes in the patient's personality and behavior:

- A usually happy person may become withdrawn.
- A patient may become confused and disoriented. Disoriented persons are unaware of their own identity, the time, or the identity of their environment.

These changes are temporary. Be aware that family and friends of the patient can become upset because of this change. They require special attention during this time. You should

- Help decrease the family's stress by listening.

STRESS
pressure caused by something in the internal or external environment

- Remind the family that the personality and behavior changes usually last 6–8 weeks.
- Be available so that the patient and family do not feel alone.
- Encourage the family to visit because a familiar person may help to decrease the patient's stress.
- Help by orienting the patient to the new environment.

ELDER ABUSE

Elder abuse is the mistreatment of an elderly person through physical, verbal, or psychologic means. Physical abuse may take the form of hurting the person's body; sexual abuse; or withholding food, clothing, or medical help. Restraining the person in a bed or locking the person in a room is also a form of abuse. Not cleaning and changing a person who has been incontinent is a form of abuse. Verbal abuse includes shouting or swearing at the person. Psychologic abuse includes threatening the person with punishment. For example, an abuser might withhold water if the person is incontinent of the bladder.

Older persons may be subject to abuse because their illness makes them dependent on others for care and help with personal affairs. There may be a history of poor family relationships or violence. The older person may feel isolated from others and suffer abuse silently because the abuser may also have the power to withhold food, clothing, and shelter.

Each person should be treated with respect. Report any observations of abuse to the nurse or supervisor. For a care giver to abuse an elderly person is a serious offense. The health care institution may fire any care giver who abuses any patient. Charges may be brought against the abuser in a court of law.

SELECTED DISRUPTIONS OF THE AGING PROCESS

ALZHEIMER'S DISEASE

ALZHEIMER'S DISEASE
an irreversible (cannot be changed or cured), progressive (patient continues to get worse) disease that affects brain function

Alzheimer's disease is an irreversible (cannot be changed or cured), progressive (continually worsening) disease that affects brain function. The messages in the brain become confused, and memory fails. The ability to perform ADLs declines. The changes that occur in the patient with Alzheimer's disease can be identified. They occur in the following three stages:

Stage 1: Early Stage

- Memory loss
- Forgetfulness
- Carelessness in dress
- Neglect of job and family responsibilities
- Lack of interest in life

Stage 2: Middle Stage

- Continued memory loss
- Speech problems (slurred words and difficulty in finding the right words)
- Inability to read
- Wandering and getting lost
- Decline in ability to care for self

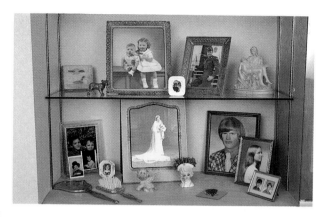

FIGURE 31-17

Memory cabinets are located outside the patient's room in a nursing unit for patients with Alzheimer's disease. Items from a patient's past can help jog memory.

Stage 3: Late Stage

- Complete disorientation
- Inability to speak
- Inability to move and walk
- Incontinence of bowel and bladder
- Complete dependency
- Death

Each person who has Alzheimer's disease progresses through the stages at different rates. For example, a patient may spend a few months or years in the early stage. The cause of Alzheimer's disease is unknown, and there is no cure.

Care of the patient with Alzheimer's disease is based on the degree to which the patient can interact with the environment, especially during the early stage. Your responsibilities as nursing assistant are to

- Use visual cues (clocks, pictures, and written messages) to keep the patient oriented.
- Mark the room with familiar items, such as old pictures of the patient (Figure 31-17).
- Keep routines flexible enough to meet the patient's needs.
- Post a reality orientation board.
- Help the patient reminisce about life events.
- Speak slowly and allow the patient time to answer.
- Help orient the patient to meals (for example, put the utensils in the patient's hands).
- Feed the patient who is unable to use utensils.
- Provide a calm environment when the patient becomes agitated.
- Protect the patient from danger (for example, stairways and medication carts) when the patient wanders.
- Provide an environment that protects the patient from injury. For example, keep the bed in a low position and put sturdy shoes on the patient for walking.
- Help the patient keep a bedtime routine.
- Listen to the family's concerns.
- Encourage family members and visitors to talk with the patient.
- Increase the amount of care you give as the patient's abilities decline.
- Be careful not to make loud, unexpected noises.
- Approach the patient from the front. Do not surprise the patient by touching his or her back.

Alzheimer's disease can be frightening and frustrating for the patient and family. Quality nursing care is the best treatment possible for the Alzheimer's patient.

CARING COMMENT

Encourage the family of the Alzheimer's patient to contact the Alzheimer's Disease Association. The association gives many useful tips and provides emotional support for all those who care for a person with Alzheimer's disease.

PARKINSON'S DISEASE

PARKINSON'S DISEASE
a disease that affects the brain and muscles and is characterized by a ·stooped posture, shuffling gait, and hand tremors

TREMOR
trembling or shaking

Parkinson's disease is a disease in which the muscles lose the ability to move. This disease can be traced to an imbalance in the chemicals of the brain. The patient's body movements become slower, **tremors** appear, and muscles become stiff and rigid. As the disease progresses, the patient usually walks with a stooped posture and a shuffling gait (Figure 31–18). Because the muscles of the mouth are rigid, the patient may drool and have difficulty swallowing. The

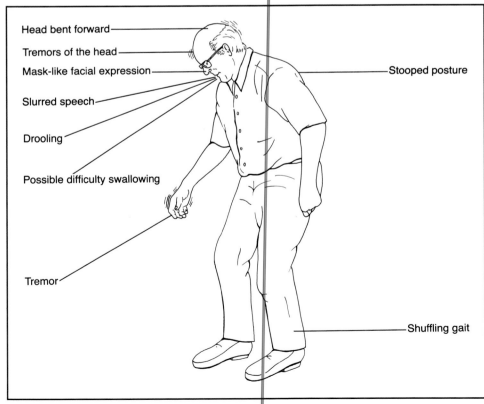

Head bent forward
Tremors of the head
Mask-like facial expression
Slurred speech
Drooling
Possible difficulty swallowing
Tremor
Stooped posture
Shuffling gait

FIGURE 31–18
Observations you can make of the patient with Parkinson's disease.

patient may have slurred and slowed speech and develop a mask-like expression on the face.

Your responsibilities in the care of patients with Parkinson's disease, are to

* Help patients perform exercises to decrease muscle stiffness, because their walking ability may be improved.
* Encourage patients to use specially designed adaptive instruments to help them complete ADLs. These instruments include scoop plates, large-handled silverware, and Velcro fasteners on clothing and shoes.
* Keep patients safe from falls by assisting them with ambulation. Their muscle stiffness and shuffling gait increases these patients' risk of falling.
* Place sturdy shoes on patients' feet before they walk. Shoes that fit well and have nonskid soles can be helpful. Also, the removal of throw rugs is advisable.
* Provide soft foods that are high in calories and protein (or the diet ordered by the physician). A diet may also be high in fiber and fluids if the patient experiences constipation.
* Because patients with Parkinson's disease have a risk of choking due to swallowing difficulties, place them in a semi- or high Fowler's position to eat. This reduces the risk of aspiration (food or fluid going into the lungs).
* Keep to the toileting routine listed in the care plan to promote bowel regularity.
* Listen closely when patients speak, because they may speak softly, have difficulty forming words, or garble their words.
* Follow through on the speech therapist's treatment program to help the patient communicate. This may include the use of word or picture boards to decrease frustration for the patient.

The physical changes that occur in patients with Parkinson's disease may affect patients' psychologic functioning. Patients may feel helpless or depressed. They may need counseling to help them deal with their illness.

As a nursing assistant, you need to be aware that although patients' physical condition **deteriorates,** their mental abilities do not. When you care for patients with Parkinson's disease, keep in mind that their intelligence is not affected.

DETERIORATE
worsen

CARING COMMENT

Patients with Parkinson's disease need help getting in and out of a bed or chair. Once they are up, they may propel themselves forward at a fast rate, because the motor center in the brain is affected by the disease. It is your responsibility to prevent injury by being ready to provide help.

CANCER

Cancer is a disease in which certain **cells** of the body change into nonfunctioning cells. They then grow and crowd out healthy, functioning cells. The nonfunctioning cells can spread out to other areas of the body. Cancer can affect any part or organ in the body.

Cancer is most frequently seen in patients over the age of 65 and is the second leading cause of death in older adults. The prevention of cancer is important. If a patient mentions any of the following warning signs to you, or

CANCER
a disease in which certain cells of the body change into nonfunctioning cells and grow and crowd out healthy, functioning cells
CELL
the basic unit of any living organism

you observe any of these signs in your patient, record them and report them to the supervisor or nurse (see Seven Warning Signs of Cancer chart).

SEVEN WARNING SIGNS OF CANCER

1. A persistent cough.
2. A sore that will not heal.
3. Any change in a wart or mole.
4. Any change in bowel or bladder habits.
5. **Indigestion** or a difficulty in swallowing.
6. Presence of a lump in the breast or elsewhere.
7. Unusual bleeding or discharge from a body opening.

INDIGESTION

difficulty in digesting something

Care of patients with cancer varies according to individual needs. One of the most important nursing concerns for the patient with cancer is pain control. You need to work closely with the supervisor or nurse to help keep the patient comfortable and pain-free. Communicate the patient's concerns about pain to the supervisor or nurse so that an adjustment in pain control and treatment can be discussed with the physician. The goal of care is to help the patient remain comfortable. The care of patients in pain is discussed in Chapter 15.

TERMINAL ILLNESS

TERMINAL ILLNESS

an illness in which the end result is death; the patient's life expectancy must be 6 months or less

A **terminal illness** is an illness in which the end result is death. The words *terminally ill* refer to the patient who is expected to die. The patient must be expected to live only 6 months or less. Dr. Elisabeth Kübler-Ross studied and talked to many patients who were dying. She identified five stages that dying individuals go through after learning they are terminally ill. (see Five Stages of Dying). Knowing these five stages can help you understand the emotional changes that occur in the dying patient. The five stages Kübler-Ross talked about are:

FIVE STAGES OF DYING

Denial

* Denial begins when the person learns about the life-threatening illness.
* Denial helps the person cope and provides time to come to grips with what is happening.

Anger

* The person vents feelings and frustrations about the changes and losses caused by the illness.
* Anger may take the form of rage, resentment, and blaming others for the illness.
* The person is easily upset by simple changes (such as changes in routine).

Bargaining

* The person bargains to be allowed to complete tasks or attend events deemed important.
* The person may promise to do something good in return for a cure.
* The person may bargain with God, family, and care givers.

DENIAL

refusal to admit the truth or reality

Depression

- Depression is a way of handling a great loss.
- The person realizes that death will occur and nothing can change that expectancy.
- The person appears sad.
- The person may begin to talk about impending death.

Acceptance

- The person acknowledges and accepts that death will occur.
- The person may make funeral arrangements.
- The person may say good-bye to family and friends.

DEPRESSION
sadness and a decrease in the usual behaviors associated with daily functioning

Dr. Kübler-Ross stated that these stages are only guidelines. Individuals progress through them at their own rate, and not all people reach the acceptance stage. Nor do all five stages occur in all patients. A patient may remain in any stage until death occurs. A patient may skip stages or return to a previous stage during an illness. The five stages may also be experienced by the patient's family, friends, and care givers.

CARING COMMENT

Terminally ill patients in the anger stage require special care. They may upset family and friends. Be sure to provide support to the family as well as the patient.

Care of the Terminally Ill Patient

Care of terminally ill patients requires a special kind of person. Special qualities include being a good listener. You need to listen to what patients say as well as what they do not say. When patients talk to you, be attentive and encourage them to talk. If you are not comfortable talking with the patient about death and dying, find a co-worker who feels comfortable talking about death. Terminally ill patients may also communicate needs nonverbally. You should practice observing and interpreting patients' nonverbal communication in order to determine their needs (Figure 31–19).

Their anger and depression may influence terminally ill patients' interac-

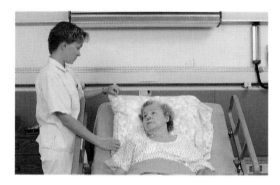

FIGURE 31–19
A terminally ill patient may use nonverbal communication. Note the patient's eye contact with the nursing assistant as well as the patient's position.

tions with you. You need to remember the stages of dying and not pass judgment on patients. Include patients' family and significant others in your caring and concern. Be sure to follow the nursing care plan for the patient who is terminally ill so that you help the patient remain pain-free and as comfortable as possible until death occurs.

Signs of Impending Death

Certain physical and mental changes can signal the approach of death. You may observe changes in vital signs, mental ability, the skin, the senses, nutritional intake, and elimination.

VITAL SIGNS Changes in vital signs include a decrease in blood pressure and a slowing and weakening of the pulse. Respirations often become irregular and shallow. Body temperature may be either lower or higher than its usual range.

MENTAL CHANGES Mental changes may include disorientation or unresponsiveness. Some patients may remain alert and oriented right up until the time of death, however.

MOTTLING
marked with spots or blotches

SKIN The skin may become pale and cool. You may notice **mottling.** Mottling of the skin occurs because the blood circulation is decreasing.

SENSES The senses are also affected by impending death. The eyes may appear unfocused and staring. Patients may not be aware of your touch even when you position them. Hearing may be present until death occurs. It is important to be aware of conversations that you hold around the patient. Be sure to talk to the patient during care. Tell the patient who you are, what day it is, and whatever else you are comfortable saying. Encourage the family and significant others to do the same when they are in the room with the patient.

NUTRITIONAL INTAKE The nutritional intake of the dying patient may change. The patient may be unable to take food or fluids by mouth and may be receiving nutrients and medication intravenously for comfort.

ELIMINATION The dying patient may become incontinent of both bowel and bladder. Be sure to provide hygienic care to keep the patient clean and comfortable.

CARING COMMENT

Conversations held between care givers outside the patient's room may be overhead by the patient or family. If you need to discuss confidential information with another care giver, be sure to communicate in an appropriate place away from the patient's room.

It is not your role to inform family members or visitors of a patient's death. The registered nurse has the education, experience, and responsibility to communicate such delicate information in the appropriate manner.

HOSPICE
a place for the care of persons (and their families) who are in the last stages of life

Hospice Care

Hospice care is a program that provides physical and psychologic support to the dying patient and the patient's family. The terminally ill patient may choose to die at home rather than in the hospital or nursing home. Hospice care is available for the dying patient of any age, not just the older adult. A hospice program can provide:

- the home health services of nurses, nursing assistants, home-maker helpers, etc.
- resources that are necessary to care for the patient in the home, such as hospital beds, bandages, and supplies.

Care of the patient who is dying at home is the same as for the person dying in a health care institution. The main focus is on comfort and cleanliness. Chapter 32 discusses the specific responsibilities of the nursing assistant in the care of a patient in the home.

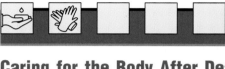

PROCEDURE

Caring for the Body After Death

GATHER EQUIPMENT

Wash basin	Disposable pads
Towels	Comb
Soap	Dentures
Disposable gloves	Artificial eyes and/or other **prostheses**
Identification tags	**Body bag** or **shroud**

ACTION	RATIONALE
Preparation	
1. Wash hands.	Prevents the spread of microorganisms.
2. Identify the patient.	Maintains patients' rights.
3. Provide privacy.	Maintains patients' rights.
4. Explain the procedure to the family, if present.	Informs family what is happening.
Procedural Steps	
5. Collect required equipment.	Check your institution's policy for the specific equipment required, because each institution has its own method of preparing the body after death.
6. Put on the disposable gloves.	Protects you from contamination.
7. Wash the body and comb the hair. Work quietly.	Shows respect for the patient.
8. Close the eyelids gently. Do not apply pressure.	Pressure can leave marks on the body.
9. Remove any tubes.	Follow your institution's policy on removing and discarding tubes.
10. Place a disposable pad beneath the body. Remove gloves and discard appropriately.	Collects body wastes.
11. If the family will be viewing the body, • Put a gown on the patient • Arrange bed linens neatly • Place the patient's hands on the abdomen, above the sheet • Minimize noise and allow for privacy	Provides a calm and peaceful environment.

Continued on following page

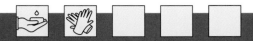

PROCEDURE

Caring for the Body After Death *Continued*

ACTION	RATIONALE
Preparation	
12. Place identification tags on the body (usually on the right toe) and on the patient's belongings.	Decreases the risk of body misidentification.
13. Place body in the shroud after the family leaves (Figure 31–20).	Preserves patient dignity.

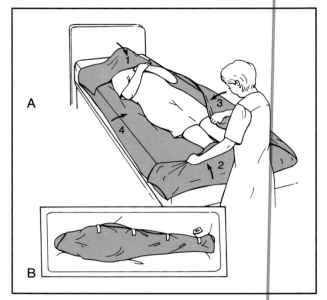

FIGURE 31–20

A, Place the body in the middle of the shroud, fold down the top to cover the face and neck, fold up the bottom to cover the feet and lower legs, and then fold both sides toward the middle. B, The shroud entirely covers the body. Secure the shroud with tape applied over the shoulders, waist, and legs. A second identification tag may be pinned to the outside of the shroud.

ACTION	RATIONALE
13. Collect all personal belongings and make a list.	Prepares for the return of personal effects to the family.
14. Ask another care giver to help you transfer the body onto a cart.	
15. Take the body to the **morgue.**	To await pickup by the funeral home personnel.
Follow-Through	
16. Wash your hands.	Prevents the spread of microorganisms.
17. Document the care given.	Provides a legal record.

MORGUE
the place where bodies are kept until they are identified and claimed by relatives

CHAPTER WRAP-UP

- The older adult faces many physical challenges. As a nursing assistant, you can help patients use their abilities to the fullest.
- You are responsible for helping to prevent injury in elderly patients.
- Reality orientation and fantasy validation are two techniques used for the patient experiencing disorientation.
- Common disruptions in function for the older adult include Alzheimer's disease, Parkinson's disease, and cancer.

- The terminally ill patient, who has a life expectancy of less than 6 months, may be cared for in a health care institution or in the home.
- Dr. Kübler-Ross identified five stages of dying. Patients progress at their own rate through the stages.

REVIEW QUESTIONS

1. List at least 10 changes that are a normal part of aging.
2. How can the normal changes of aging cause safety problems?
3. What can you do to increase patients' reality orientation?
4. What are the five stages of dying identified by Dr. Kübler-Ross?
5. What are the signs of impending death?
6. What is the procedure for caring for a body after death?

ACTIVITY CORNER

List things you can do to help increase an elderly person's self-esteem.

_____   _____

_____   _____

32 Caring for Patients in the Home

Objectives

AFTER YOU COMPLETE THIS .
CHAPTER, YOU WILL BE ABLE TO:

Give examples of the types of
    patients who may require
    home health care.
Plan and prepare meals for the
    patient in the home.
Make a safe environment for the
    patient in the home.
Give personal care to the patient
    in the home.
Complete light housekeeping
    duties in the patient's home.
List three examples of patient
    exploitation by a home health
    aide.

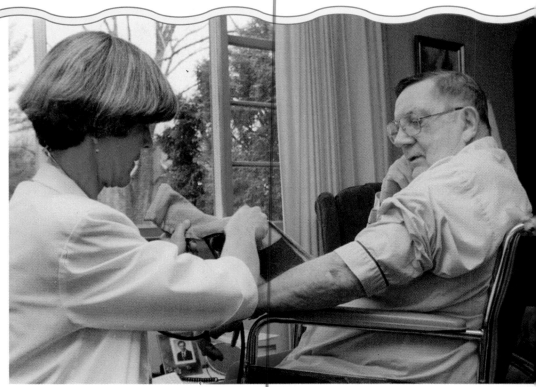

Overview Caring for the patient in the home requires certain skills and techniques in addition to those you have already learned. You need to learn about the personal needs of the patient, including safety needs. Knowledge of basic housekeeping and menu planning is also necessary to help you maintain a smooth running home.

Your responsibility in the home environment is great. Independence is a very important quality in home health care because you are expected to work without direct supervision. In addition, sensitivity is required because you interact with families on a very personal level. The patient as well as the family benefits a great deal from your assistance.

WHAT DO YOU KNOW ABOUT GIVING CARE IN THE HOME?

Here are five statements about caring for a patient in the home. Consider them to test your current ideas about home health care. If you think the statement is true, circle the T; if you think the statement is false, circle the F. Change the false statements to make them true.

1. T F Home care of a patient can include hygiene care, grocery shopping, and housecleaning.

2. T F The family is frequently not involved in care when the patient at home is ill.

3. T F Environmental safety for the patient is the responsibility of the patient, the family, and the nursing assistant.

4. T F Accommodating patients' cultural food preferences is an important part of providing home health care.

5. T F The nursing assistant uses organizational and problem-solving skills to provide home health care.

ANSWERS

1. **True.** Hygiene care, grocery shopping, and housecleaning all may be part of a home health care assignment.

2. **False.** Many families are very involved in caring for the family member who is ill at home.

3. **True.** All people are responsible for providing a safe environment in the home.

4. **True.** Honoring cultural food preferences is an important part of meeting the needs of the patient.

5. **True.** The organized nursing assistant who can problem-solve is able to provide quality patient care.

WHAT IS HOME HEALTH CARE?

HOSPITAL

an institution for the care and treatment of the acutely ill and injured

HOUSEKEEPING

keeping the home neat, clean, and free of safety hazards

In the past, people who were hospitalized for surgery or a medical condition stayed in the **hospital** for 7–14 days or longer. Today, patients may be discharged from the acute care institution in fewer than 7 days. Often, patients go home in a weakened physical state. They may be unable to care for themselves adequately. This is where home health care comes in. *Home health care* is the provision of basic nursing care and **housekeeping** duties for patients in their home. As a nursing assistant, you may be hired to provide home health care for a new mother and her infant, an elderly person, or the dying patient of any age. The care can be provided on a temporary (days or weeks) or permanent (months to years) basis.

Years ago, family members often took care of the patient in the home setting. In today's world, all family members may be working and unable to personally provide care 24 hours a day. As a nursing assistant, you can help fill in the gap in care.

THE ROLE OF THE NURSING ASSISTANT IN HOME HEALTH CARE

HYGIENE

the practice of cleanliness used to promote health

VITAL SIGNS

the signs of life: temperature, pulse, respirations, and blood pressure

Caring for a patient in the home can be a very rewarding experience. Your care allows the patient to remain at home where objects are familiar and routines are more comfortable. You must do many things in the home that are done in a hospital or nursing home setting. Giving a bath, feeding, and helping with activities of daily living (ADLs) are as important as keeping the home neat and clean and shopping for and preparing meals. Your duties may include

- Giving personal **hygiene** care
- Monitoring **vital signs** (Figure 32–1)
- Giving food and fluids

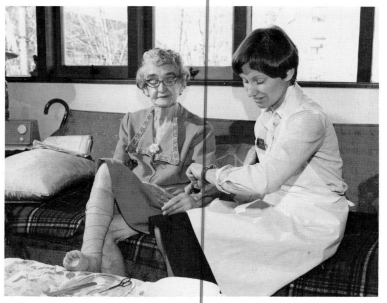

FIGURE 32–1

Measuring vital signs is part of the home health care routine. (From DuGas BW: Introduction to Patient Care: A Comprehensive Approach to Nursing, 4th ed. Philadelphia, W. B. Saunders Company, 1983.)

- Maintaining patient **safety** and comfort
- Planning meals
- Purchasing food and household supplies
- Cleaning the home environment
- Completing forms from the institution to record the patient's activities

You may be hired and supervised by an outside agency that specializes in home health care. Such agencies include

- The local Visiting Nurses Association
- The county public health department
- A private home health care agency

All agencies and the state in which they are located have very specific policies and procedures on what you can and cannot do in the home of the patient. Be sure to check with the home health care agency about what you are permitted and expected to do. Examples of what you *cannot* do include

- Give medications—As a nursing assistant you can remind patients to take their medications or you can read the label to them, but you *cannot* actually give the medication to patients.
- Perform any kind of heat treatment—You cannot apply hot water bottles, heating pads, or heat lamps.
- Perform sterile procedures—You cannot change dressings, insert a **catheter,** do irrigations, or provide **tracheostomy** care.
- Perform any task or procedure that you have not been taught.

Note: There may be exceptions, according to the laws of your state.

You are working as part of a team. The nurse in charge develops a nursing care plan that guides you in caring for the patient. The care plan is developed at the time of discharge and updated as the patient's **health** status changes. The physician, nurse, physical therapist, social worker, and clergy may all visit the patient in the home. The patient and family are also part of the **health care team.** They provide valuable information about the patient's needs and feelings. However, as a nursing assistant, you may be the care giver who is on the scene most often. Your observations of the patient are a very valuable contribution to planning the care of the patient in the home.

THE ROLE OF THE FAMILY IN HOME HEALTH CARE

Patients who require home health care often have a **family** who is involved in their care. The family members may include a spouse, brothers, sisters, sons, daughters, and other members of the patient's extended family (Figure 32–2). The health care worker can ask family members for information about the patient that can help in patient care. Family members can tell you the methods they have used to care for their loved one (Figure 32–3). They can tell you the activities the patient likes or dislikes. This information saves you time and prevents patient frustration. Be sure to check with your supervisor when procedures requested by the patient or family are not what you have been taught to do.

Families frequently want to be involved in care. You can help by being open and honest in your **communication** with them. At times, the family may be overwhelmed by the patient's illness or disability. You can assist by being caring, understanding, and open when you are giving care and communicating with the family.

PROVIDING CARE IN THE HOME

You must be very organized in order to provide patient care in the home. The wide range of responsibilities—patient care, light housekeeping, and meal

SAFETY
the status of being safe from experiencing or causing hurt, injury, or loss

CATHETER
a flexible tube passed into body openings to allow fluids to enter or exit the body
TRACHEOSTOMY
an artificial opening in the windpipe
HEALTH
any state of physical, emotional, and social well-being felt by an individual
HEALTH CARE TEAM
the group of people who have the education necessary to provide care to patients

FAMILY
a group of people (not necessarily related) having a relationship

COMMUNICATION
an exchange of information

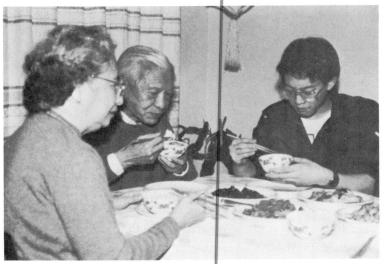

FIGURE 32–2

The elderly person who receives home health care should be included in daily activities. (From Foster RLR, Hunsberger MM, Anderson JJT: Family-Centered Nursing Care of Children. Philadelphia, W. B. Saunders Company, 1989.)

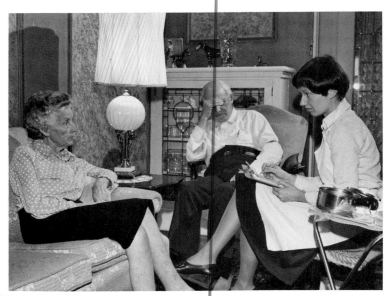

FIGURE 32–3

The family is an important source of information about the patient who needs home health care. (From DuGas BW: Introduction to Patient Care: A Comprehensive Approach to Nursing, 4th ed. Philadelphia, W. B. Saunders Company, 1983.)

planning and preparation—can be overwhelming sometimes. Use your organizational skills to assist you in meeting the patient's needs. Organizational skills that are helpful include

- Knowing the patient's and family's preferences
- Writing out a daily or weekly plan for care
- Seeking **feedback** from your supervisor about care

TAKING CARE OF THE PATIENT'S PHYSICAL NEEDS

Using the **problem-solving process** (see Chapter 4) can assist you in setting up a schedule for meeting all of the patient's physical needs. When making your schedule, include the days and times to accomplish the following:

- Bathing
- Dressing
- Grooming
- **Ambulation**
- Performing passive **range of motion exercises** if indicated
- Measuring vital signs
- Preparing meals
- Assisting the patient with eating
- Providing **incontinent** care
- Positioning the patient if indicated
- Checking for safety in the home **environment**

FEEDBACK
when the receiver in the communication process repeats the information the sender sent or otherwise acknowledges it to make sure the message is understood
PROBLEM-SOLVING PROCESS
the systematic method used to resolve problems

AMBULATION
walking
RANGE OF MOTION
the range, measured in degrees like a circle, through which a joint can be extended and flexed (bent)
INCONTINENT
unable to respond to the urge to eliminate the waste products of the body
ENVIRONMENT
the conditions, circumstances, or objects that surround a person

CARING COMMENT

Include patient and family preferences when you develop the schedule. Remember that each household requires an individualized schedule.

Review the following sample schedule to give you some ideas.

SAMPLE SCHEDULE FOR A MORNING'S CARE

Time	Activity
0700	Get a verbal report from the 11:00 PM–7:00 AM shift care giver. Check on the patient and attend to immediate needs (for example, toileting).
0720	Begin breakfast by referring to the weekly meal plan. While the meal is cooking, wash the patient's face and hands. Assist the patient to a table or roll up the head of the bed and place the over-bed table within reach of the patient.
0735	Serve breakfast and assist the patient with eating as needed.
0800	Clean up breakfast dishes and assist the patient with morning care.
0900	Check with the patient for preference in watching television, listening to the radio, or reading. Change the patient's position if the patient cannot do so independently. Release **protective devices**

PROTECTIVE DEVICE
a piece of equipment designed to prevent patients from harming themselves or others; formerly called a restraint

Continued on following page

SAMPLE SCHEDULE FOR A MORNING'S CARE *Continued*

	if they are in use and reapply them when you leave the bedside.
0930	Offer the patient a midmorning snack if permitted and desired.
0940	Work on the weekly meal plan, checking the newspaper for coupons.
1000	Check on the patient and begin to take care of housekeeping duties. (For example, put a load of clothing into the washer, dust, and run the vacuum cleaner.)
1030–1100	Check with the patient for needs, **positioning**, and release of the protective device. Reapply the protective device when you leave the bedside. Begin to prepare lunch.
1200	Assist the patient to the table or set up the over-bed table. Assist the patient with eating as necessary.

POSITIONING

placing a body in a certain posture

FULFILLING THE PATIENT'S PSYCHOLOGIC NEEDS

Remember to meet the patient's psychologic needs. Encourage visits by family members and friends. Help the patient with grooming and personal hygiene so that the patient appears neat and well rested for visitors. Read greeting cards to the patient who cannot do so independently (only if the patient or family requests that you open the mail), give phone messages, and assist the patient in placing phone calls. You can also provide companionship to the patient by talking with and touching the patient and making the home environment comfortable. All of these things help the patient feel better inside.

OTHER RESPONSIBILITIES

You need to be resourceful to help the patient in the home. Equipment that you are accustomed to using in the health care institution may not be available or may be made by a different manufacturer. You may have to improvise, that is, use things in the home to replace hospital equipment. Below are some very useful tips and suggestions:

- To wash a patient's hair without getting the patient or the chair wet, place a plastic bag over a pillow. Use this pillow to support the patient's head and neck while tilting the head toward the sink. You can use a plastic pitcher to wet and rinse the hair. This keeps the patient comfortable and dry.
- Cut plastic bags up the long sides and use these bags as substitute waterproof pads for the mattress or chair cushions. Large trash bags work well.
- Always find out from the family and your supervisor what has been done in the past to perform a particular procedure. This can save you a lot of time and wasted energy.
- Keep emergency phone numbers for police, fire, and ambulance squads near the phone. Place a list by every phone in the house, because during an emergency you might forget where the list is located.
- Whenever possible, ask the patient about food preferences. Family members can help with this too. In addition, keep in mind how the

patient likes food prepared and remember to provide only food that is allowed by dietary restrictions.

SAFETY IN THE HOME

During your first visit to the home, do a safety survey (Figure 32–4). Check for any safety **hazards** such as frayed electrical cords and loose carpeting. After you do your safety survey, inform the family and your supervisor about your concerns and any changes you think need to be made. You should work with everyone to provide a safe environment. Make sure all emergency phone numbers are readily available (fire department, police, and ambulance). In the event of a life-threatening emergency, follow these steps:

1. Take the patient to safety.
2. Call for necessary help.
3. Tell the help you are calling your exact location.

HAZARD
a source of danger

CARING COMMENT

You may want to write down the patient's address and telephone number along with the emergency numbers. It is easy to forget such basic information when under stress. You should fill out an emergency information card and place it in a convenient place (near each phone) so the information is accessible when needed (Figure 32–5).

PROVISION OF MEALS

As mentioned earlier, your role in the home may include grocery shopping, menu planning, and meal preparation.

Menu Planning

Menu planning includes budgeting money, planning what meals will be cooked during the week, and purchasing groceries and other household supplies. When planning the menu for the patient, you must keep in mind dietary restrictions and cost. Whenever possible, try to provide meals that include cultural favorites. **Prescription diets** are very important to a patient's overall health (see Chapter 19). Include the patient in meal planning whenever possible (Figure 32–6). When making a meal plan, consider

- Personal food preferences
- Cultural food preferences
- Efficient use of grocery store specials
- How to avoid costly errors

PRESCRIPTION
an order for a procedure, medication, diet, or other service written by a physician
DIET
the total amount of food eaten by an individual

Cost is very important, especially for the patient who is on a fixed income. If you are responsible for shopping for the patient's food, make every attempt to cut costs without cutting quality. You can help reduce food costs by:

- Checking grocery store ads for coupons and weekly specials.
- Checking magazines and newspapers for manufacturer's coupons.
- Buying food in bulk when it is appropriate to do so and the patient has storage space in cupboards or refrigerator.

When you are asked to shop for food and other supplies, you should account for all the money you spend:

- Check for overcharges as you go through the checkout line.

CARING HOME HEALTH SERVICES
HOME SAFETY SURVEY

FIRE SAFETY
   Smoke detectors: Present _____ Absent _____ Working _____
                            Non-working _____
   Electrical cords: Frayed _____ Location: _____
                     Multiple cords in one outlet _____
                     Location: _____
   Natural gas odors _____ Location: _____
   Flammable materials in the home _____ Location: _____
   _____
   Inappropriate use of heating devices _____
   Specify type: Electric _____ Gas _____ Kerosene _____ Wood burning _____
   Describe the safety problem: _____
   Smoking _____ Specify who and where permitted: _____
   Fire extinguishers _____ Charged _____ Not charged _____
   Locations and types: _____
   Other potential hazards _____ Specify: _____
   _____
   _____

HEALTH
   Medications not put away _____ Location: _____
   Cleaning solutions not put away _____ Location: _____
   Hallways cluttered _____ Location: _____
   Loose carpeting _____ Location: _____
   Throw rugs _____ Location: _____
   Slippery floors _____ Location: _____
   Stairways: Loose boards _____ Loose carpeting _____
   Handrails present _____ Absent _____ Loose _____ Location: _____
   _____
   Lighting: Adequate _____ Dim _____ Location: _____
   Bathrooms: Handgrips present _____ Seat by sink _____
              Seat in tub or shower _____
              Nonskid strips in tub or shower _____
              High rise toilet seat _____
   Unwashed dishes _____ Home temperature _____ Specify: _____
   _____
   Other potential hazards _____ Specify: _____
   _____

FIGURE 32–4
A sample home safety survey form.

CARING HOME HEALTH SERVICES

Emergency Call Card

Fire: _____   Police: _____

Ambulance: _____   Physician: _____

Family member: _____   Agency supervisor: _____

Address: _____   Home phone: _____

Others to notify in case of emergency: _____

Steps to follow when making a call:

1. Take the patient to safety.
2. Place the call.
3. Identify yourself.
4. Describe the problem (be brief).
5. Give address and phone number of your location.
6. Listen to the person answering your call, follow directions, and stay on the phone line to answer questions.
7. Wait until the emergency phone answerer hangs up first.

FIGURE 32–5

A sample emergency call card.

- Keep receipts for all items you purchase.
- Give the correct change to the patient or other responsible person.

Meal Preparation

Meal preparation is an important part of your home health care duties. You may be asked to make meals for the time you are present in the home. You may also be asked to make a sandwich or other quick meal that the patient can eat when you are not there. Place prepared food in a covered container or plastic wrapping in the refrigerator. Remember that the patient may want a

---

Menu Plan for a Regular Diet

Monday:
Breakfast: Coffee with milk, apple, juice, oatmeal with milk and teaspoon of sugar
Mid-morning snack: Orange
Lunch: Chicken noodle soup and grilled cheese sandwich, tea
Afternoon snack: 2 peanut butter cookies and a glass of milk
Supper: Lasagna, tossed salad, garlic bread, coffee with milk, and chocolate cake

Tuesday:
Breakfast: Pancakes, maple syrup, coffee with milk, orange juice
Mid-morning snack: Bagel with cream cheese and milk
Lunch: Hamburger on roll and fries, can of soda pop
Afternoon snack: Apple and glass of juice
Supper: Turkey, stuffing, sweet potato pie, green beans, celery and carrot sticks, coffee with milk, glass of milk

FIGURE 32–6

A sample meal plan.

snack during the day or at bedtime. Be sure to plan for a snack if this is part of your patient's routine. A snack might include foods or fluids such as tea and crackers, cookies, a piece of fruit, or a glass of juice.

Be sure to familiarize yourself with the equipment in the patient's kitchen. If you are not sure how to use the stove, dishwasher, or any other appliance, ask the patient or a family member to show you the correct procedure. You should write down any instructions until you have become familiar with the equipment.

HOUSEKEEPING

Organization is also the key to performing the housekeeping duties you may be assigned to perform. You and the responsible family member may work together to set up a schedule of cleaning activities. You may be asked to

- Vacuum and dust twice a week.
- Clean up after yourself and the patient on a ongoing basis.
- Clean the bathroom and kitchen every week.

Your duties are limited by most agencies to what is considered light housekeeping. Light housekeeping includes keeping the home clean, neat, and free of safety hazards. Light housekeeping does *not* include

- Moving heavy furniture
- Painting
- Mowing the lawn
- Washing the windows
- Any other activities not permitted by the agency

Discuss with the patient and family which cleaning products they prefer to be used in the home. If you choose cleaning products, be sure to choose products that offer the best buy, are convenient to use, and leave a pleasant scent.

CARING COMMENT

Never mix cleaning products, such as ammonia and bleach. Such a mixture may produce toxic fumes.

SPECIAL SITUATIONS

Certain situations may arise when you are employed as a care giver in the home, such as

- Offering of gifts
- Use of patient and family resources
- Elder **abuse**

ABUSE
improper use; mistreatment

Gifts

You should not accept any gifts from the patient or family. Accepting gifts changes the relationship from one of care giver to friend. Your role as care giver implies (means) that you do certain things for the good of the patient. As a friend, you may become too relaxed and fail to observe something important or fail to complete a procedure as you have been taught.

It may be very difficult to refuse a gift; however, it can be done graciously and firmly. You will gain the respect of the patient and family when you display these qualities as you refuse a gift. If a patient offers you a gift such as money, jewelry, or other object, you should respond in one of the following ways:

"Thank you, but I cannot accept any gifts."

"Thank you for thinking of me, but I prefer not to accept gifts from my patients."

"I appreciate the thought you put into selecting this gift. Thank you, but my practice is not to accept gifts."

The patient or family may offer you candy or a piece of fruit. You may choose to accept such a token gift according to the rules of your health care institution. Always follow the rules of your institution about accepting gifts from patients and families.

Using the Patient's and Family's Resources

Do not **exploit** the patient or family for your own purposes. Examples include eating the patient's food, using the patient's telephone for long-distance calls, or using any of the patient's personal or household supplies for your own needs. To exploit the patient and family is dishonest and can be considered a form of patient abuse.

EXPLOIT
take advantage of unfairly

You should not ask the patient or family for privileges such as money, food, or use of special equipment, because the request may put the person on the spot. Finances may not allow a request to be granted. Such requests may lead to embarrassment for you and the patient or family. They interfere with the care giver–patient trust that should be maintained.

You may be present in the home during mealtimes; in fact, you may be shopping for groceries and preparing meals. Never use the patient's food to provide yourself with a meal. The patient and family are not obligated to offer you a meal. Bring a meal from home or from a take-out restaurant.

Elder Abuse

Please refer to Chapter 31 for information on elder abuse. The spouse or children of the elderly person may be abusers. If you observe any indication that your home health care patient is a victim of abuse, report it to the nurse or supervisor. In many communities, a person called a home health ombudsman or community ombudsman is available for help. The **ombudsman** works to find a solution to problems such as elder abuse. Your only responsibility is to report your observations.

OMBUDSMAN
person who receives reports and investigates situations that need outside assistance

KEEPING NOTES

Many agencies keep very specific records on the patient receiving home care (Figure 32–7). You must know what information you are required to chart and on what forms. Keep accurate notes for your employing agency. They may be consulted by insurance companies to determine payment for patient care services. Complete all records in a timely manner. Make sure you know when reports are expected to be completed. These notes also help you and other health care givers moniter any changes in the patient's health. Some areas that may be included in daily charting include

- Unusual occurrences, such as falls
- Unusual observations, such as a change in the patient's status
- The care provided (for example, hygiene, positioning, use of protective devices, range of motion exercise, meals, and housekeeping activities)
- Patient status (orientation, vital signs, reaction to visitors, appetite, and fluid intake and output)

```
┌─────────────────────────────────────────────────────────────────────┐
│ Daily Flow Sheet                               Shift:* _____     │
│ Patient name: _____  Date: _____      │
│ Check one:                                                            │
│ Knows self    Yes _____ No _____                                      │
│ Knows date    Yes _____ No _____                                      │
│ Knows place   Yes _____ No _____                                      │
│ Temperature _____ Pulse _____ Respirations_____                 │
│ Blood pressure _____ Time _____    Weight _____                 │
│ Key: I   - Independent                                                │
│      A1 - Assisted with help of one                                   │
│      A2 - Assisted with help of two                                   │
│      NA - Not applicable                                              │
│ Breakfast _____ Lunch _____ Dinner _____                        │
│ Taking fluids _____ Snack _____ Bathing _____                   │
│ Toileting _____ Voiding _____ Bowel movement _____              │
│ Dresses self _____ Grooms self _____ Out of bed _____           │
│ Moves and turns _____ Walks _____                                 │
│                                                                       │
│ Check one:                                                            │
│ Menu planned     Yes _____ No _____                                   │
│ Meal prepared    Yes _____ No _____                                   │
│ Meal(s) served   Breakfast _____ Lunch _____ Dinner _____       │
│ Housekeeping completed Yes _____ No _____                             │
│ Personal care completed  Yes _____ No _____                           │
│ Complete bath given      Yes _____ No _____                           │
│ Partial bath given       Yes _____ No _____                           │
│ Passive range of motion exercises  Yes _____ No _____                 │
│ Incontinent  Yes _____ No _____ Urine _____ Bowels _____              │
│ Sleep  Yes _____ No _____                                             │
│ Out of bed  Yes _____ No _____ Chair _____ Walk _____                 │
│ Visitor(s)  Yes _____ No _____ If yes, name _____         │
│                                                                       │
│ Notes _____        │
│ _____        │
│ _____        │
│ _____        │
│ _____        │
│ _____        │
│                                                                       │
│ Signature _____  Date _____         │
│ * Fill out one flow sheet each shift.                                 │
└─────────────────────────────────────────────────────────────────────┘
```

FIGURE 32–7

A sample record that an agency might require from a nursing assistant in a home health care setting.

Be sure to be as complete as possible. Write comments about patient care and patient reactions on the record sheet.

CARING COMMENT

The family may ask you for a report of the day's activities. You should include the highlights of the patient's day. Respond to questions as honestly as you can. Such information can help with the family's psychologic acceptance of the patient's condition.

CHAPTER WRAP-UP

- Care of the patient in the home requires you to be independent enough to work with minimal supervision.
- The keys to providing quality care in the home environment are
    Caring
    Organizational skills
    Problem-solving abilities
- Home health care can provide comfort and security for ill or disabled individuals. Their family can continue to work and feel secure in knowing that the patient is being cared for.
- Your responsibilities in home health care can include
    Patient care
    Planning, preparing, and serving meals
    Light housekeeping tasks completed in an organized, safe, and efficient manner
- The family is an excellent source for specific information about the patient. Ask for information and use it in the care you give. Include family members in both planning and carrying out patient care.
- Keep accurate records for your employing agency.

REVIEW QUESTIONS

1. What three qualities are important for you to have when giving care to patients in their home?
2. What observations should you make when doing a safety survey in the home?
3. When grocery shopping for the patient, what are three cost-saving measures you can use?
4. Which procedures or nursing skills are *not* part of your responsibilities in home health care?
5. What is the role of the family in home health care?
6. Give three examples of patient exploitation.

ACTIVITY CORNER

All persons should live in a safe environment. Use the Home Safety Survey on page 850 to do a survey of your own home.

What did you find that is unsafe? _____

What can you do to correct unsafe conditions in your environment? _____

An emergency call card is a good idea for any home. Use the emergency call card on page 851 as a guide to make one for yourself. Keep this valuable information near your telephone.

33

Providing Emergency Care

Objectives

AFTER YOU COMPLETE THIS CHAPTER, YOU WILL BE ABLE TO:

Identify at least five types of injuries that require emergency care.

Describe the purpose of a Good Samaritan law.

List initial observations to make at an accident scene.

Explain what the Heimlich maneuver is used for and how to perform it.

Provide care for the patient with a wound, hemorrhage, burn, no respirations, or no heartbeat.

Explain how to perform cardiopulmonary resuscitation and when to use it.

Apply a nonsterile dressing.

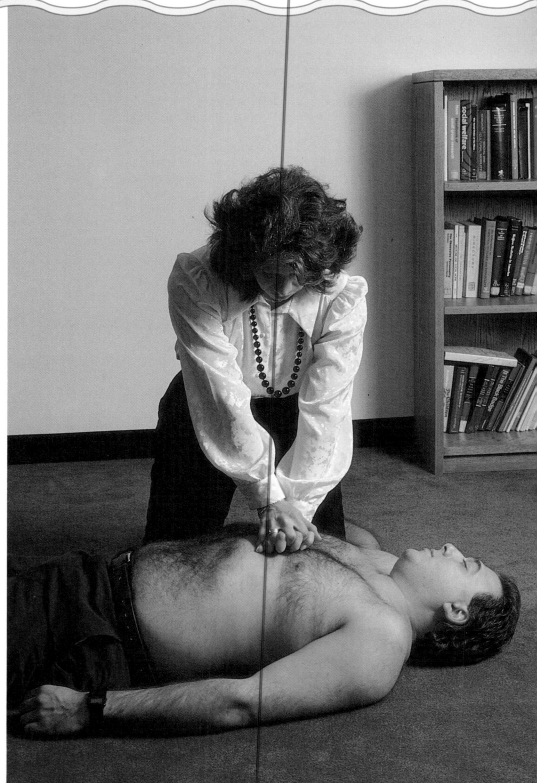

Illustration from Henry M, Stapleton E: EMT: Prehospital Care. Philadelphia, W. B. Saunders Company, 1992.

Overview The care of a patient in an emergency requires specialized knowledge. In this chapter, you will learn the basic skills required to assist in an emergency. As a nursing assistant you may be one of the first persons on the scene of an accident. It is important for you to know your responsibilities. Your help can make a life-or-death difference to an individual.

WHAT DO YOU KNOW ABOUT EMERGENCY CARE?

Here are five statements about emergency care. Consider them to test your current knowledge of emergency care. If you think the statement is true, circle the T; if you think the statement is false, circle the F. Change the false statements to make them true.

1. T F Ambulance attendants are the only ones allowed to give basic emergency care.
2. T F Never move the patient at the accident scene.
3. T F A nursing assistant can provide cardiopulmonary resuscitation.
4. T F Hemorrhage is uncontrolled bleeding.
5. T F The best way to help a choking child is to pull the arms straight up.

ANSWERS

1. **False.** Emergency care is given by all types of people. Many individuals attend first-aid classes given in their communities.

2. **False.** Although it is usually best not to move the patient, in situations such as potential fire or explosion, the patient must be moved.

3. **True.** With the training provided by organizations such as the American Heart Association and the American Red Cross, you can learn to provide cardiopulmonary resuscitation.

4. **True.** Hemorrhage is uncontrolled bleeding.

5. **False.** Holding the child's arms up in the air does not stop choking. In fact, this may delay the treatment needed to stop choking (the Heimlich maneuver).

EMERGENCY CARE

EMERGENCY

a situation that calls for immediate action

FIRST AID

health care treatment provided to a person injured in an emergency situation

An **emergency** is a situation that calls for immediate action. Your role in caring for patients who are hurt in an accident or who suddenly become ill is to be a good observer and know when to contact professional assistance. You may be the first person on the accident scene or in the home who provides health care to the patient. The first person on the scene to provide care is known as a *first responder*. You need to learn how to perform basic **first-aid** procedures for the times these skills are needed. Your initial observations of the patient are crucial to other health care professionals who will also be providing care.

For you to be able to care for the patient in an emergency, it is necessary for you to know certain procedures. These include:

- Cardiopulmonary resuscitation (CPR)
- The Heimlich maneuver
- Application of pressure to stop bleeding
- Application of a dressing (bandage)

GOOD SAMARITAN LAWS

GOOD SAMARITAN LAW

law that protects you from being sued by the person you assist in an emergency; this law varies from state to state

In many states, you will be covered by what are known as **Good Samaritan laws.** These laws are designed to protect you from being sued by the patient that you assist in an emergency. You are protected if you act in "good faith," that is, doing your best and trying not to do something that can cause harm. Each state has different Good Samaritan laws, so it is a good idea for you to discuss them with your instructor or supervisor so you can make sure you are working within the limits of the law.

USING BASIC UNIVERSAL PRECAUTIONS

UNIVERSAL PRECAUTIONS

measures taken in advance by all health care workers to prevent the spread of infection and disease

VICTIM

term used to refer to the injured person at the site of an accident

CARDIOPULMONARY RESUSCITATION

CPR; a method to reestablish heart and lung action

When you provide care to the patient in the hospital or the nursing home, you know that person's medical history. You know whether the person has an illness or disease that you could contract. When caring for a stranger in an emergency situation, it is most important to follow **universal precautions** to protect yourself because you do not know what disease the person might have. For example, diseases such as acquired immune deficiency syndrome (AIDS) and hepatitis B can be contracted from the body fluids of an accident **victim** if universal precautions are not practiced.

Devices such as personal masks, gloves, and goggles should be worn whenever you may come in contact with the victim's body fluids. For example, when you are performing **cardiopulmonary resuscitation** (CPR) or bandaging a wound. It is a good idea to carry these supplies in your car if you would stop at an accident scene. Remember that your own health is very important.

The patient in extreme pain or confusion may become combative. You need to protect yourself in these situations much the same as you do when providing care in the nursing home or hospital.

CARING COMMENT

If you choose to keep disposable gloves and disposable face masks in your car be sure to replace them frequently. The intense temperatures that can be reached in an automobile or in your wallet can destroy protective equipment.

INITIAL ACTIONS IN AN EMERGENCY SITUATION

INITIAL OBSERVATIONS

When you approach an emergency situation, you immediately begin to make observations. As a nursing assistant, your observations are more skilled than those of a bystander who has not had any health care education.

Begin your observations with a visual overview. This means that you observe the entire scene of the accident as well as the injured person. For example, you are driving along and see a car in a ditch next to a tree. Your first observations would be

- the position of the car
- whether there are people in the car
- whether the environment is safe for both you and the victim

Use your senses to make further observations.

- Look

    Is smoke visible?

    What position is the patient in?

    Is an arm or a leg bent at an awkward angle?

    Is there bleeding?

    Is the patient's chest moving up and down?

    Is the patient breathing?

    How many people are injured?

- Listen

    Is the patient saying anything?

    Do you hear a crackling sound that could indicate a fire?

    Is the patient talking, crying, or silent?

- Smell

    Is there an odor of gasoline in the air?

    Is there an odor of smoke?

After making these beginning observations, you determine whether you and the patient are safe from further harm. If it is safe for you to approach the accident, begin your next observations—checking the patient's vital signs.

VITAL SIGNS

The vital signs reveal the patient's condition. You should begin with checking respirations and pulse.

- Respirations

    Is the patient breathing?

    What are the rate and rhythm of the respirations?

    Is the patient having any difficulty breathing?

- Pulse

    Does the patient have a pulse?

    What is the pulse rate?

    Is the rhythm regular or irregular?

    Is the pulse difficult to find? Is it weak or thready?

CALMING THE PATIENT

The patient in an accident may be very anxious and fearful. Part of your responsibility is to reassure the person. You can begin to do this by telling the person who you are and that you are a nursing assistant. If other people are involved in the accident, the patient may be concerned about them. Let the patient know that emergency care is on the way and that you will stay as long as you are needed.

OBSERVATIONS ABOUT PAIN

You also need to determine how much pain the patient has. This involves both subjective and objective observations. You can ask where the pain is located and what type of pain it is (for example, achy, stabbing, dull, etc.).

Observe the patient closely for any obvious reason for the pain, such as a broken bone, as well as facial expression. The patient may grimace instead of telling you something hurts. The patient may also do what is known as *guarding*. Guarding is protecting the area that is painful by putting the hands over the area or pulling away from you when you try to touch a painful area.

MOVING THE PATIENT

The patient in immediate danger from fire or explosion needs to be moved quickly. If you decide to do this, be sure that the danger from the accident itself outweighs any danger to the patient caused by moving.

If you do not have to move the injured person, don't. When the person has obvious broken bones or when there is the possibility of neck or back injuries, it is advisable not to move the person except in extreme emergencies. Moving the person may increase the severity of the injury or cause other injuries.

GETTING ASSISTANCE

In many communities, a call for help in an emergency is made by dialing 911. If this system is not available in your community, you need to know the emergency phone numbers to use. It is a good idea to have these numbers written down, because even the most calm person can forget in an actual emergency.

When you call 911, be sure to give the following information:

- location of the accident
- number of people involved
- the kinds of injuries present (fractures, burns, etc.)
- any other information requested by the emergency phone operator

The emergency phone operator should hang up before you do. This allows you to be sure that no additional information is needed. If a patient is seriously injured and there are people just standing around the scene, one of them can make the call with your directions. Make use of any bystanders. Ask if anyone is skilled in first aid or CPR and ask for that person's assistance.

CARING COMMENT

Be sure to request help when dealing with an emergency. The help that others can provide can be very valuable to the patient and to you.

PATIENT WITHOUT RESPIRATIONS

When a patient stops breathing, it is known as respiratory arrest. There are many causes of respiratory arrest, including obstruction of the airway by the

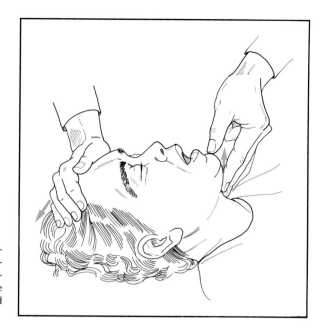

FIGURE 33–1
Opening the airway of the patient without a pulse or respirations. Press down on the forehead with one hand and use three fingers of your other hand to lift the chin.

tongue and epiglottis. It is important to open the airway as soon as possible so that oxygen can get to the body's tissues, especially the brain (Figure 33–1). Remember that damage to the brain can occur in as little as 4 minutes.

AIRWAY OBSTRUCTION

Airway obstruction can occur in the unconscious patient because the tongue and epiglottis fall backwards into the throat and close off the air going into the lungs. Obstruction can also occur when someone is eating. For adults, the most common cause of an obstructed airway when eating is a piece of meat. In the small child, the cause is usually a foreign object, such as the small part of a toy.

When the airway is completely obstructed, the person is unable to talk, breathe, or cough. You may see the patient grasping the neck with the hands. This is known as the **universal distress signal** (Figure 33–2). Ask the person if he or she is choking—most people will nod the head up and down to indicate "yes."

AIRWAY
passageway for air to go into and out of the lungs
OBSTRUCTION
blockage

UNIVERSAL DISTRESS SIGNAL
hands grasping the neck to indicate the airway is blocked

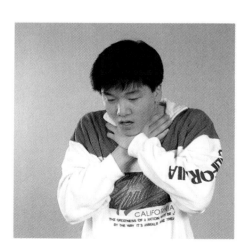

FIGURE 33–2
Universal distress signal. (From Henry M, Stapleton E: EMT: Prehospital Care. Philadelphia, W. B. Saunders Company, 1992.)

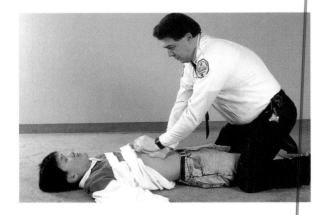

FIGURE 33-3

Your position for performing the Heimlich maneuver on a person lying on the floor. (From Henry M, Stapleton E: EMT: Prehospital Care. Philadelphia, W. B. Saunders Company, 1992.)

HEIMLICH MANEUVER

HEIMLICH MANEUVER
procedure to clear the airway of a person who is choking

To assist the individual with an obstructed airway due to a foreign object, you need to know how to perform the **Heimlich maneuver.** The Heimlich maneuver is a special technique used to dislodge or loosen foreign objects from the airway of a choking person. This technique is also called "abdominal thrusts." The thrusts that are given to the individual increase the pressure inside the chest; the pressure forces the foreign object out of the airway.

Clearing the Airway

UNCONSCIOUS
unaware of the environment and not responsive to stimuli; unconsciousness occurs during sleep, fainting, and coma

First, make sure the tongue is not obstructing the airway. If it is not, position yourself according to the patient's current position. If the patient has become **unconscious** and fallen to the floor, place the patient flat on the back. Straddle the patient at the thighs (Figure 33–3). If the person choking is sitting or standing, stand behind the person and put your arms around the body at waist level (Figure 33–4).

Abdominal Thrusts

To perform the abdominal thrusts, you need to know where to place your hands. Feel for the lower edge of the patient's rib cage. Next locate the navel.

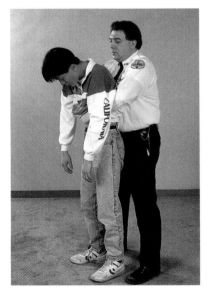

FIGURE 33-4

Your position for performing the Heimlich maneuver on a person who is sitting or standing. (From Henry M, Stapleton E: EMT: Prehospital Care. Philadelphia, W. B. Saunders Company, 1992.)

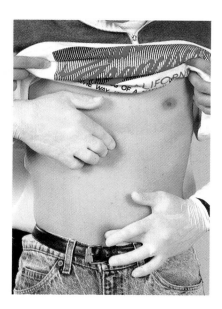

FIGURE 33-5

Feeling for the lower edge of the rib cage and the umbilicus in performing the Heimlich maneuver. Place your hands midway between these two points. (From Henry M, Stapleton E: EMT: Prehospital Care. Philadelphia, W. B. Saunders Company, 1992.)

Place your hands midway between the bottom edge of the rib cage and the navel (Figure 33-5). If the patient is lying on the floor, use the flat part of your hand. Lace your fingers together so that one of your hands is directly below the other (Figure 33-6). If the patient is sitting or standing, make a fist with one hand. Place the thumb side toward the patient's abdomen in the area described above (Figure 33-7). Grab the fist with the other hand (Figure 33-8).

To perform the abdominal thrust, push quickly upward toward the patient's ribs (Figure 33-9). Continue these thrusts until the foreign object is pushed out. When the foreign object is removed, the patient will breathe easier and be able to respond to your questions.

CARING COMMENTS

Take extra care when choosing children's toys. Look for small parts that can break off or fit into a child's mouth. These parts can easily be swallowed by a child and obstruct the airway.

When performing abdominal thrusts on a child who is choking, use less force. To clear the airway of an infant, use blows to the back combined with abdominal thrusts.

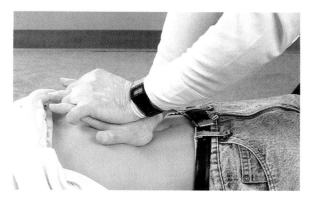

FIGURE 33-6

Lacing your fingers together with one hand under the other in performing the Heimlich maneuver on a patient who is lying on the floor. (From Henry M, Stapleton E: EMT: Prehospital Care. Philadelphia, W. B. Saunders Company, 1992.)

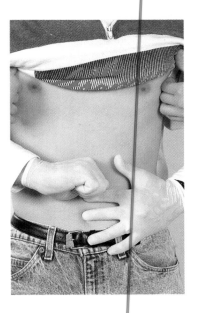

FIGURE 33-7

Placing the thumb side toward the abdomen above the umbilicus and below the ribs in performing the Heimlich maneuver on a patient who is sitting or standing. (From Henry M, Stapleton E: EMT: Prehospital Care. Philadelphia, W. B. Saunders Company, 1992.)

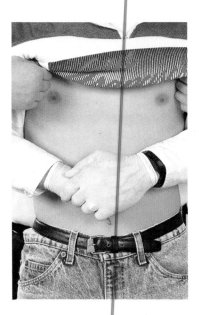

FIGURE 33-8

Grabbing your fist with your other hand in performing the Heimlich maneuver on a patient who is sitting or standing. (From Henry M, Stapleton E: EMT: Prehospital Care. Philadelphia, W. B. Saunders Company, 1992.)

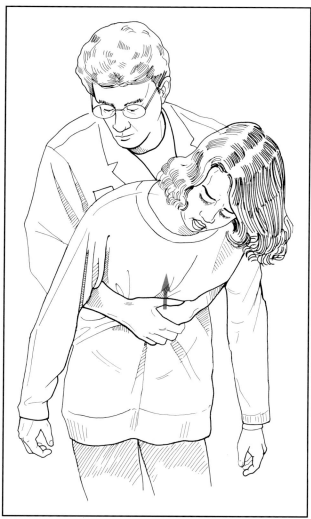

FIGURE 33–9
Thrusting up toward the ribs in performing the Heimlich maneuver.

CARING FOR A PATIENT WITHOUT RESPIRATIONS

1. **Open the airway**—Press down on the forehead with the palm of one hand and place three fingers of the other hand below the patient's chin (Figure 33–10).
2. **Straighten the airway**—With your hand in place on patient's forehead, lift upward with the fingers under the patient's chin. This straightens the airway and allows air to get in.
3. **Decrease the risk of injury**—Place your fingers only on the bony part of the chin to decrease the risk of further injury to the patient.
4. **Clear the mouth**—Use two fingers to sweep any debris out of the mouth. Make sure you put on disposable gloves to do this (Figure 33–11).
5. **Observe for respirations**—Watch for the rise and fall of the chest. You may also want to place your hand on the chest and feel it rise and fall. Another alternative is to place you ear next to the patient's mouth and feel the air moving in and out.
6. **Position the patient's head**—If the patient does not begin breathing after you reposition the head for the second or third time following steps 1 and 2, you must begin breathing for the patient.

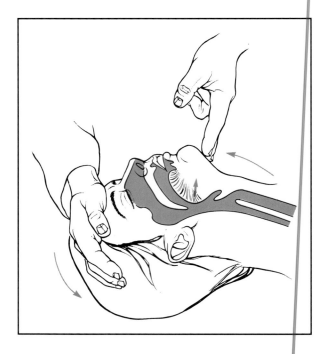

FIGURE 33–10

Opening the airway of the patient who has stopped breathing. (From Henry M, Stapleton E: EMT: Prehospital Care. Philadelphia, W. B. Saunders Company, 1992.)

RESUSCITATION

bringing an individual whose heart or lungs have stopped functioning back to life

7. **Position the patient to receive respiratory resuscitation**—Place one of your palms on the patient's forehead. With the same hand, reach down and pinch the nose using your thumb and forefinger. Place your mouth over the patient's mouth (Figure 33–12). Be sure no air can escape the patient's mouth. You may wish to use a disposable face shield to provide a barrier between you and the patient for protection (see Caring Comment at the end of this section).

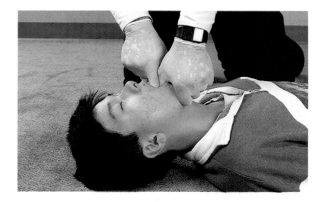

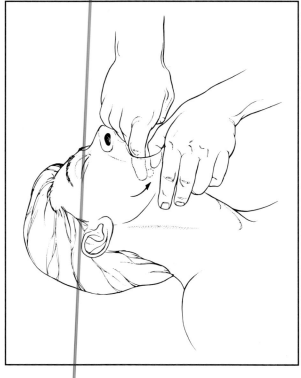

FIGURE 33–11

Removing a foreign object from the mouth of a patient who has stopped breathing. (From Henry M, Stapleton E: EMT: Prehospital Care. Philadelphia, W. B. Saunders Company, 1992.)

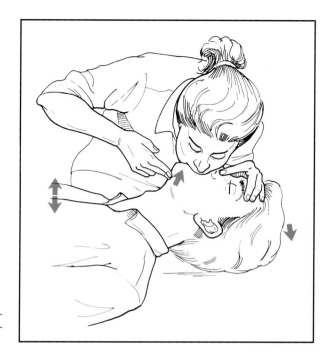

FIGURE 33–12

Placing your mouth over the patient's mouth to provide respiratory resuscitation.

8. **Provide oxygen to the patient**—Blow into the patient's mouth. Watch and listen. Watch for the rise and fall of the patient's chest. Listen and feel the air coming from the patient's mouth after each breath you give.

9. **Continue to provide oxygen**—If the patient does not begin to breathe independently, continue breathing for him or her. Twelve breaths per minute is the rate at which you give breaths to the patient. This amounts to one breath every 5 seconds. Remember that unless the airway is open, you cannot provide oxygen to the patient.

CARING COMMENT

If you notice the patient's abdomen getting larger when giving cardiopulmonary resuscitation, it can mean that air is going to the stomach instead of the lungs. Reposition the patient's head and begin giving breaths again.

In the event you cannot use the patient's mouth to provide oxygen because it has been severely injured, use the patient's nose to get oxygen into the lungs. If the patient has an artificial airway, commonly known as a stoma or tracheostomy, this opening can be used to provide the needed oxygen. This artificial opening is located on the patient's neck.

CARING COMMENT

Use a face shield to protect yourself from disease when performing respiratory resuscitation on patients. This thin, plastic shield is placed between your mouth and the patient. It allows you to breathe for the patient without coming into contact with blood or saliva.

Note: At this time, there is no indication that the human immunodeficiency virus, the virus that causes AIDS, can be transmitted by saliva.

CARDIOPULMONARY RESUSCITATION

Cardiopulmonary resuscitation is a method of reestablishing heart and lung action. It is abbreviated CPR. The meaning of the word *cardiopulmonary resuscitation* becomes clear when you take the word apart:

> **Cardio** means heart.
> **Pulmonary** means lungs.
> **Resuscitation** means to restore life.

With CPR, you can give life back to a patient who is not breathing and whose heart has stopped beating. CPR is a useful and worthwhile skill for all people to have, not just those involved in the health care field. You may be able to save the life of a family member, friend, or patient if you can perform CPR correctly.

CPR is taught by organizations such as the American Heart Association and the American Red Cross. The course includes instruction, practice on a manikin, and a certified teacher to guide you. It is highly recommended that you take a CPR course from one of these organizations, because the following information is not intended to substitute for such a course.

DETERMINING THE NEED FOR CPR

Your first observations help you determine whether CPR is needed.

- Is the patient unconscious? Shake the patient and speak loudly.
- Check the vital signs. Is the patient breathing? Is there a pulse?
- What position is the patient in—lying on the back, side, or stomach?

PERFORMING CPR

1. Position the patient. Once you have observed that the patient is not breathing and the heart is not beating, position the patient so you can begin the procedure. For CPR to be the most effective, the patient should be on his or her back. If you must reposition the patient, be sure

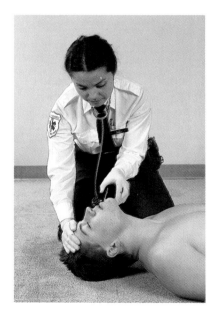

FIGURE 33–13

Checking for an obstructed airway in the patient whose heart has stopped beating. (From Henry M, Stapleton E: EMT: Prehospital Care. Philadelphia, W. B. Saunders Company, 1992.)

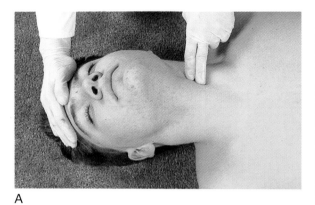

A

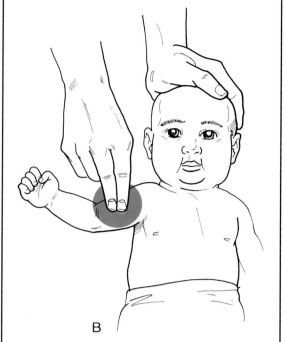

B

FIGURE 33-14
A, Checking the pulse at the carotid artery in the adult patient to determine the need for cardiopulmonary resuscitation. (From Henry M, Stapleton E: EMT: Prehospital Care. Philadelphia, W. B. Saunders Company, 1992.) B, Use the brachial artery to find the pulse in an infant.

to do so carefully. The patient should be lying on a hard surface in order for you to give the most effective chest compressions (pressing down to move the blood out of the heart into the body).

2. Perform rescue breathing. As with any patient who is not breathing, check for an obstructed airway. Do this by looking for a foreign object or the tongue obstructing the airway. Position the head to open the airway (Figure 33-13). If the patient does not begin to breathe after you reposition the head, *give two quick breaths* using the same hand position as for the patient with respiratory arrest (see Figure 33-12).

3. Check the patient's pulse. For the adult, check the pulse at the carotid artery (Figure 33-14). The patient's pulse may be very weak or slow, so be sure to take at least a full 5 seconds to check.

4. Perform chest compressions. When no pulse is felt, you must help the patient's heart move oxygenated blood throughout the body. This is done by doing chest compressions. Chest compressions squeeze the heart between the ribs and the back to push the blood through the body. As you breathe for the patient and provide chest compressions, you are giving oxygen to the blood (by breathing into the lungs) and moving the blood (by compressing the chest). To perform chest compressions,

• Position yourself to the right or the left of the patient's chest in a kneeling position.

• Place your hands on the patient in the following manner: Trace the patient's rib cage with one hand, beginning with the side nearest you. Locate the xiphoid process (the breastbone) in the middle of the sternum. Mark this spot by putting one finger on it. Place the heel of your other hand above the spot. Once you have the heel of your hand in place, bring the first hand up on top of the hand on the patient's chest. Lace your fingers together while you keep your hands on top of each other on that spot on the patient's chest (Figure 33-15).

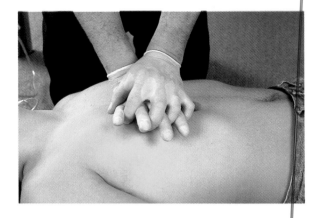

FIGURE 33–15

Positioning your hands to give chest compressions. (From Henry M, Stapleton E: EMT: Prehospital Care. Philadelphia, W. B. Saunders Company, 1992.)

- Push down on the patient's chest. Be sure to press down directly on the chest, not to either the right or left side. This correct positioning and compressing will prevent injury to the patient. Do not bend your elbows during compressions (Figure 33–16). Allow the patient's chest to move upward after you compress it. But always keep your hands on the chest so that you do not lose the correct spot. Compressions should be smooth and even (this requires practice on a manikin).
- When compressing the chest of an adult, the breastbone must be compressed 1½–2 inches to be effective. The chest must be compressed at least 100 times per minute. You need to give the patient two breaths for every 15 compressions. At the end of four sets of compressions and breaths, check the patient for breathing and a pulse. Continue CPR if there is no pulse and wait for emergency personnel.

PREVENTING THE NEED FOR CPR

Frequent causes of **respiratory arrest** and **cardiac arrest** in children are

Automobile accidents
Smoke inhalation
Choking/aspiration
Near drowning

RESPIRATORY ARREST
sudden stop in breathing

CARDIAC ARREST
a sudden stop in the beating of the heart

CHOKING
a feeling of strangulation that occurs when an airway obstruction interferes with breathing

ASPIRATION
the act of inhaling vomitus, mucus, or a small object into the respiratory system; may occur in persons who are unconscious, under the effects of anesthesia, or having difficulty swallowing

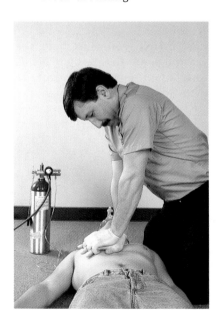

FIGURE 33–16

Correct positioning of your body for giving chest compressions. (From Henry M, Stapleton E: EMT: Prehospital Care. Philadelphia, W. B. Saunders Company, 1992.)

In each of these situations, simple measures may prevent the need for CPR in the child or infant.

Automobile Accidents

In many states, the use of infant/child car seats is required by law. Be sure that the car seat meets safety guidelines. When buying a used car seat, make sure all latches and belts are in good working order and not frayed. Adult seatbelts should be used on children who weigh more than 40 pounds.

Smoke Inhalation

Smoke inhalation can result from fires, often started by children playing with matches. Be sure to put matches and lighters out of a child's reach. Practice different ways of escaping from the home in case of actual fire. Teach children that they should stay below the level of the smoke by crawling. A meeting place for all members of the house should also be designated so that all can meet outside safely.

Choking and Aspiration

Small toys or parts of toys often cause choking, a potentially fatal problem. Objects such as parts of toys or large pieces of food can block the airway and stop the flow of oxygen to the brain. Be sure that the toys children play with are appropriate for their age. Be sure the child's age is within the age range printed on the packaging. Look for small parts that may become loose that a child might swallow. This is particularly important when children are in a stage in which they put everything in their mouth (infancy through early preschool age). Children should be discouraged from running with toys or food in their mouths. When feeding children, be sure to cut up food such as hot dogs or marshmallows into small pieces. Do not give peanuts to children who do not chew them before swallowing.

Near Drowning

Think of scenes from television—a child floating face down in a swimming pool and no adult in sight. It takes only seconds for a water accident to occur. Adult supervision is a must when children are in or near water. In a near-drowning accident, the victim can often be resuscitated after being removed from the water. Brain damage may occur from the lack of oxygen that occurs in a near-drowning accident. If precautions fail and an accident occurs, CPR is useful to know.

PERFORMING CPR ON AN INFANT OR CHILD

Physical differences between adults and children require some changes in how CPR is performed on children. However, there are some basic similarities also:

- Observe for responsiveness.
- Call for help.
- Observe and change the patient's position, if necessary.
- Check for respirations and a pulse.
- Begin chest compressions and breathing if there are no pulse and respirations.

Because of the physical differences between adults and children (e.g., size and weight), there are different rules for performing CPR on adults and children (see Differences Between Adult and Infant/Child CPR Chart).

DIFFERENCES BETWEEN ADULT AND INFANT/CHILD CPR

	Adult	Child (1–8 Years)	Infant (0–1 Year)
Pulse site	Carotid artery	Carotid artery	Brachial artery
Compress chest using	2 hands	1 hand	2 or 3 fingers
Depth of compressions	1½–2 inches	1–1½ inches	½–1 inch
Compressions per minute	80–100	80–100	At least 100
Number of compressions to breaths	15:2	5:1	5:1
Two-person CPR	Yes	No	No

Adult CPR is generally used for children over 8 years of age. This is only a guideline, however. Your decision should be based on the child's size and physical development.

There is a procedure known as two-person CPR. With this method, one person gives breaths and a second person gives chest compressions. The persons may take turns and switch jobs while reviving the patient. Switching from breathing to chest compressions periodically helps decrease rescuers' fatigue. Two-person CPR can only be used on patients whose size allows it. A child's body is too small for two people to perform CPR.

CARING COMMENT

You should complete an approved CPR course to become capable of performing this procedure.

WOUNDS AND HEMORRHAGE

WOUNDS

When caring for a victim involved in an accident, you may see wounds and bleeding. A **wound** is a break in the skin. Wounds can be caused by surgery or injury/trauma. The following are specific types of wounds:

- **Abrasion**—An abrasion is a wound in which the outer layer of skin is rubbed or scraped off (Figure 33–17). An abrasion may bleed because the smaller blood vessels (the capillaries) are injured.
- **Laceration**—A laceration is a cut in the skin caused by a sharp object (Figure 33–18). The edges of a laceration may be straight or jagged.
- **Puncture Wound**—A puncture wound extends beneath the first layer of skin. It is caused by a sharp object that pierces the skin. A puncture wound can be the result of a knife or a bullet from a gun. Often there is very little bleeding from a puncture wound. This does not mean that the patient is not bleeding; rather, it may mean that the blood is collecting inside the body.

WOUND
an injury to the body usually caused by physical means
ABRASION
a wound that results from rubbing or scraping the skin
LACERATION
cut in the skin caused by a sharp object
PUNCTURE WOUND
wound that goes beneath the first layer of skin, caused by a sharp, usually pointed object

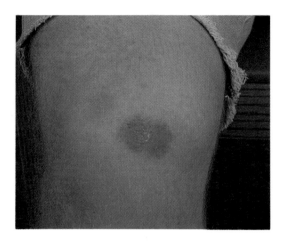

FIGURE 33–17
A partially healed abrasion.

HEMORRHAGE

A **hemorrhage** is defined as uncontrolled bleeding. It is caused when blood vessels are cut or ruptured. To care for a patient with uncontrolled bleeding, do the following:

HEMORRHAGE

the escape of blood from a ruptured blood vessel; uncontrolled bleeding

- Wear gloves to prevent contact with body fluids.
- Place a sterile gauze pad over the wound. If unavailable, use a clean cloth.
- Apply pressure directly on the wound.
- **Caution:** Do not pick up the gauze to check if the bleeding has stopped. Instead, simply look at the gauze to see if there is an increase in the amount of blood on it. If you keep lifting the gauze, you are releasing pressure.

Controlling Bleeding

If the bleeding is not controlled by direct pressure on the wound, you need to apply pressure to the nearest artery *above* the wound. By applying pressure above the wound (between the wound and the heart), you decrease blood flow to the wound. You need to be familiar with the pulse sites so you know where to apply pressure to stop bleeding. The pulse sites are named after arteries. For example, if someone has a wound in the forearm that is hemorrhaging, you would put firm, even pressure on the brachial artery, which is located on the inner part of the arm at the elbow (the antecubital space). See Chapter 10 for a discussion on pulse sites.

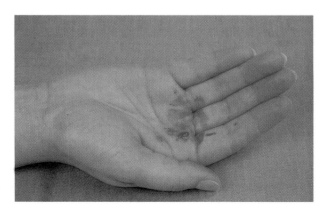

FIGURE 33–18
A lacerated hand.

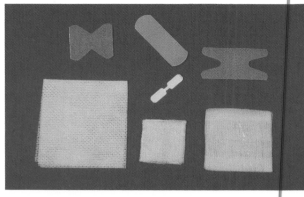

FIGURE 33-19
A wide variety of dressings are available.

Remember that patients who are hemorrhaging may have changes in their vital signs. The pulse and respirations may increase in the beginning as the heart and lungs work faster to get oxygenated blood to the blood and other body organs. Notify the nurse if you are in a health care setting. In an emergency situation, continue to control bleeding and wait for emergency medical services.

Dressing a Wound

If a wound is bleeding, you should apply a dressing. The gauze absorbs the blood and protects the wound from further injury (Figure 33-19).

PROCEDURE

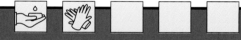

Applying a Dressing

GATHER EQUIPMENT

Sterile 4 × 4s   Tape
Two pairs of disposable gloves   Waste bag

ACTION	RATIONALE
Preparation	
1. Wash your hands if possible.	Prevents the spread of microorganisms.
2. Identify the patient.	Maintains patients' rights.
3. Provide privacy.	Maintains patients' rights.
4. Explain what you are going to do.	Informs patients what is happening.
Procedural Steps	
5. Damp-dust the over-bed stand if you are in a health care setting.	Provides a clean work area.
6. Make a cuff on the top edge of the waste bag and place it away from the wound but within your reach.	Allows you to close the bag when finished without touching contaminated equipment.
7. Cut pieces of tape long enough to secure the dressing and hang cut tape within your reach. (Use the edge of the over-bed table if you are in a health care setting.)	Allows for easy placement of tape after dressings are placed on the wound.
8. Open the 4 × 4 packages *without touching* the gauze (Figure 33-20).	Keeps the gauze sterile.

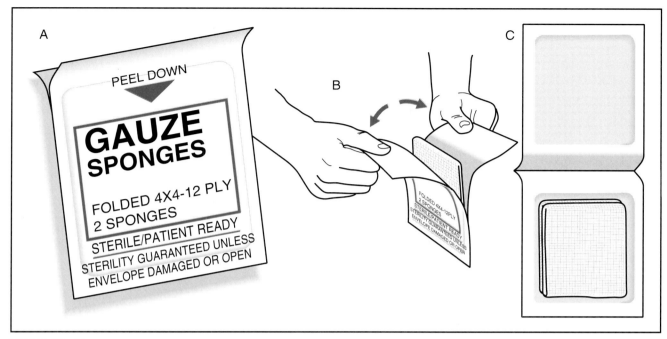

FIGURE 33-20

Opening a packaged 4 × 4 gauze. A, Read the directions on the package. B, Use your fingers to open the package and peel down. C, Lay the package on a clean, flat surface until you pick up the gauze. (Redrawn from Sorensen RC, Luckmann J: Basic Nursing: A Psychological Approach, 2nd ed. Philadelphia, W. B. Saunders Company, 1986.)

9. Place opened packages of 4 × 4s on a clean, flat surface.	Prevents packages falling to the floor and becoming contaminated.
10. Put on disposable gloves.	Prevents the spread of microorganisms.
11. Remove the old dressing if present.	
• Pull tape gently toward the wound.	Avoids pulling on the wound.
• Remove the soiled dressing by lifting it off the wound. *Do not* drag it across the wound.	Prevents further damage to the wound.
• Observe the soiled dressing for odor and amount and color of drainage.	Allows you to check progress or lack of it in the healing process.
• Place the soiled dressings in the waste bag.	
• Remove the gloves and place them in waste bag.	
• Put on clean gloves.	Decreases the transfer of microorganisms from the old dressing.
12. Apply the new 4 × 4s. Touch only the outer edges of the dressing.	Decreases the risk of contaminating the new dressing and causing a wound infection.
13. Apply the tape to the edges of the dressing.	Secures the dressing in place.
• Place the tape around all four edges of the dressing or as directed by the nurse.	Keeps microorganisms away from the wound.
• The tape should be half on the dressing and half on the skin.	Secures the dressing and prevents leaking of drainage.

Follow-Through

14. Wash hands.	Prevents the spread of microorganisms.
15. Report your observations and the time of the dressing change to the nurse.	Keeps the nurse informed about the wound.

THE PATIENT IN SHOCK

Shock is a condition in which the blood supply to the heart is decreased. It is a life-threatening medical emergency. The decreased blood supply to the heart causes less blood to go to the lungs, where it needs to pick up oxygen. Therefore, a decreased amount of oxygen is delivered to the whole body. The lack of oxygen results in shock.

Observations of the patient in shock include

- pale skin
- cyanosis (blue color of the skin)
- staring eyes
- increased pulse and respirations
- decreased blood pressure (may be difficult to measure)
- extreme thirst

Shock may be caused by a variety of conditions. There are different names for shock caused by different things.

- **Anaphylactic shock**—Anaphylactic shock results from an allergic response. It can be the result of an allergy to a medication or food.
- **Cardiogenic shock**—The heart is unable to pump out enough blood to supply the body's tissues.
- **Electric shock**—Electric shock results when the body contacts a high-voltage electric current. This type of shock can be treated with CPR.
- **Septic shock**—Septic shock results from a bacterial infection in the body.
- **Traumatic shock**—Injury or surgery can cause traumatic shock. The severity of shock depends on the severity of the injury to the body.

CARE OF THE PATIENT IN SHOCK

When your patient is in shock, quick action is necessary. Follow these basic guidelines:

- Place the patient in a supine (back-lying) position with the head lower than the body. This helps keep blood flowing to the brain.
- Keep the patient warm. You can cover the patient with a blanket.
- If the patient is thirsty, offer small sips of water.
- Keep the environment calm and quiet.
- Get medical help as soon as possible. Emergency treatment is necessary to save the patient's life.

BURNS

Burns are an emergency situation that a nursing assistant may encounter at work or while off duty. As a care giver, you need to know how to provide basic first aid to a burn victim.

CAUSES OF BURNS

Burns can be caused by many different things.

HEAT Burns from fire, hot liquids, or a hot object or surface such as hot metal on the stove are examples of burns caused by heat.

CHEMICALS Substances such as acid from a car battery can cause chemical burns.

INHALATION   Substances such as smoke or steam can cause burns in the respiratory system.

ELECTRICAL   Burns can result when an electric current passes through the body.

CLASSIFICATION OF BURNS

The classification of burns is intended to let the care giver know how severe the burn is and how much tissue has been destroyed. There are three basic layers to the skin:

- **Epidermis**—the thin outer layer that has no blood vessels.
- **Dermis**—the layer below the epidermis that is thicker and contains blood vessels, nerve endings, sweat glands, and hair follicles.
- **Subcutaneous**—The lowest layer, which contains fatty tissue, nerves, and large blood vessels.

You may have heard burns referred to as first, second, and third degree. (Some books also mention fourth-degree burns.) These classifications are not used as much now as they had been in the past. Currently burns are classified as follows:

- **Partial-thickness burns**—There are two types of partial-thickness burns: superficial (epidermis) and deep (dermis).
- **Full-thickness burns**—All three layers and bone may be destroyed.

OBSERVATIONS OF THE PATIENT WITH A BURN

You should be aware of the different observations associated with each category of burns.

SUPERFICIAL PARTIAL-THICKNESS BURNS   Observe for redness, pain, or swelling. There are no blisters in this kind of burn. Sunburn is a superficial partial-thickness burn.

DEEP PARTIAL-THICKNESS BURNS   Observe for blistering of skin, pain, and swelling (Figure 33–21).

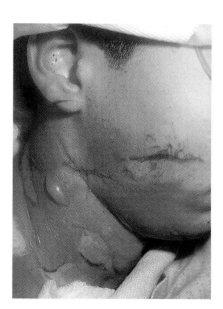

FIGURE 33–21

Observations for deep partial-thickness burns: blistering skin, pain, and swelling. (From Henry M, Stapleton E: EMT: Prehospital Care. Philadelphia, W. B. Saunders Company, 1992.)

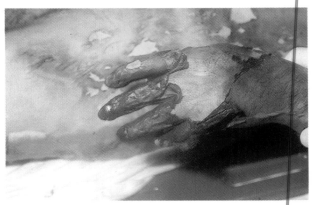

FIGURE 33–22

Observations for full-thickness burns: shiny, hard-appearing skin and skin that may be white in color. (From Henry M, Stapleton E: EMT: Prehospital Care. Philadelphia, W. B. Saunders Company, 1992.)

FULL-THICKNESS BURNS   Observe for shiny, hard-appearing skin and skin that may be white in color (Figure 33–22). There is no pain because nerves are destroyed. You may be able to see bone and muscle tissue. You may smell a charred odor.

CARING FOR THE PATIENT WITH A BURN

The most important action you can take is to remove the victim from the source of the burn (flames, smoke, etc.). Be cautious if the burn is from an electrical current so that you do not harm yourself. An electrical current can travel from the patient to you. Follow the ABCs—Airway, Breathing, and Circulation—just as you do with other emergencies. Call for help immediately.

For small burns use clean water to decrease heat and prevent further injury. You can place a clean towel that has been dampened with cool water over the burned area.

For larger, more severe burns, remove as much of the patient's clothing as possible. Do *not place ice on the burn* area, because this causes further damage to tissues instead of helping. Wrap the patient (or the burned part) loosely in a clean, dry sheet. This protects the patient from infection and further injury. Do not rub the patient's skin because you can further damage skin that is affected by the burn. Poor healing results.

CARING COMMENT

Stay with the patient until specially trained personnel arrive to help.

CHAPTER WRAP-UP

- An emergency is a situation that calls for immediate action.
- The Good Samaritan laws in many states protect you when you help others. You need to be aware of your state's specific law.

- When you help at the scene of an accident, you should
  Make observations of the person and the scene of the accident.
  Measure respirations and pulse.
  Provide reassurance to the patient.
- Threats to the life of a person include:
  Choking
  Respiratory arrest
  Cardiac arrest
  Hemorrhage
  Shock
  Burns
- The knowledge you have gained in this chapter is only a beginning for you. Many organizations offer CPR and first aid courses. Attend these courses for the benefit of your patients, family, friends, and yourself.

REVIEW QUESTIONS

1. What is a first responder?
2. List the steps to take if a person is choking.
3. What is cardiopulmonary resuscitation?
4. Identify the pressure points to use when a person is bleeding heavily from injury to the following: the hand, the foot, the upper arm, the upper thigh.
5. List the steps to take to help a person in shock.
6. Identify the three classifications of burns.

ACTIVITY CORNER

Locate two people who have assisted at the scene of an accident. Ask them the following questions about their feelings.

	First Person	Second Person
Did you stay calm?	Yes _____ No _____	Yes _____ No _____
Were you excited?	Yes _____ No _____	Yes _____ No _____
Did you know what to do?	Yes _____ No _____	Yes _____ No _____
What did you say to the victim?	_____	_____
How did you feel about helping an accident victim?	_____	_____

Glossary

Abbreviation: shortened form of a word or phrase used in place of the word or phrase

Abdominal: pertaining to the abdomen

Abduction: the act of taking away from a center or middle line

Abrasion: a wound that results from rubbing or scraping the skin

Absorption: the way the body makes use of the end products of digestion (nutrients); the passage of fluids and other substances into the bloodstream

Abuse: improper use; mistreatment

Accident: unforeseen or unplanned event

Accident/incident report: facts written on a report to describe the event that caused an accident or injury

Accountability: taking responsibility for your actions

Ace bandage: an elasticized material that provides support and even pressure when wrapped over the site of injury; same as elastic bandage

Acetone: a by-product of a certain acid; produced in abnormal amounts by persons with diabetes mellitus

Acidity: having extra acid

Acquired immune deficiency syndrome (AIDS): the advanced stage of an infection by the human immunodeficiency virus, which destroys the cells of the immune system

Active range of motion exercise: exercise performed by the patient without assistance

Activities of daily living: actions used to accomplish tasks such as toileting and grooming on a daily basis

Activity: an action or function

Acute illness: illness in which the symptoms may be severe but do not last very long

Adduction: the act of bringing back to a center or middle line

Admission: letting someone or something into someplace; the process by which the patient enters the health care system

Admission kit: a package containing disposable equipment such as a basin, water pitcher and glass, emesis basin, soap dish, tissues, and other items the patient might need

Admission process: the process by which the patient enters the health care system

Adolescence: a time of transition from childhood to adulthood (age 13 to 18) 21

Adolescent: the child who is maturing; teenager

Advance directive: a notice of the patient's wishes about what should be done if the patient's heart and lungs stop functioning

Advertisements: public notices, usually placed in a newspaper

Advocate: to speak or act for persons who are unable to speak or act for themselves

Aerobic: needing oxygen to live and grow

Aging: the physical and psychologic changes that occur as life continues

AIDS: See **Acquired immune deficiency syndrome.**

Airborne transmission: sending or transferring something through the air

Airway: passageway for air to go into and out of the lungs

Alignment: proper positioning of body parts

Allergy: an abnormal response caused by exposure to an allergen (for example, dust or food); hypersensitivity

Alveoli: tiny air sacs in the lungs

Alzheimer's disease: an irreversible (cannot be changed or cured), progressive (patient continues to get worse) disease that affects brain function

Ambulate: walk

Ambulation: walking

Amniotic fluid: fluid in the uterus that surrounds the fetus, protecting it from injury, allowing it to move, and maintaining its temperature

Amputation: removal, either surgical or accidental

Anerobic: able to live and grow without oxygen

Anal area: the skin that surrounds the anus

Anal canal: final portion of the large intestine

Analgesic: a medication that relieves pain

Anatomic position: the human body standing erect with palms and toes facing forward

Anatomic: pertaining to body structure

Anatomy: the science of body structure

Ancestor: one from whom a person is descended

Anecdotal: concerning a brief story about something that happened

Anemia: reduced number of red blood cells

Anesthesia: the loss of sensation in one part of or all of the body caused by an anesthetic medication

Anesthesiologist: a physician who specializes in giving anesthetic medication

Anesthetist: a registered nurse who is certified to administer anesthetic medication under the direction of a physician

Anorexia: loss of appetite

Antecubital: the inner part of the elbow

Anterior: located toward the front

Antibiotic: a substance that kills or stops the growth of certain microorganisms

Antibody: a substance that helps protect the body; part of the body's immune system

Antiembolic stockings: elastic stockings worn to prevent the formation of an embolus

Antimicrobial: a substance that kills or slows down the multiplication of a microorganism

Antiperspirant: a preparation that reduces excessive perspiration

Antiseptic: a substance that inhibits the growth of bacteria

Antiviral: an agent effective against viruses

Anuria: without urinary output

Anus: the posterior opening of the body through which waste materials are expelled

Anxiety: an uneasy feeling that comes from something that is going to happen or an individual believes might happen

Aorta: the largest artery in the body; it arises from the left ventricle

Apathy: lack of interest

Apical pulse: pulse counted by listening through a stethoscope over the apex (tip) of the heart

Apical–radial pulse: pulse counted by two persons to determine whether a pulse deficit exists (one person counts the apical pulse, and the second person counts the radial [wrist] pulse at the same time)

Apnea: the absence of respirations

Apparatus: equipment designed for a particular use

Appendix: a slender growth located where the small intestine meets the large intestine

Application: a form used to request something, such as employment

Aqueous humor: watery fluid that fills the anterior chamber of the eye

Arabian, Arab: person who comes from a Middle Eastern country, such as Saudi Arabia, Iran, Iraq, or Kuwait

Arteriole: smallest part of the artery

Arteriosclerosis: thickening and stiffening of the walls of the blood vessels; also called "hardening of the arteries"

Artery: a blood vessel that carries blood away from the heart to the body's organs

Arthritis: inflammation of a joint

Articular: pertaining to a joint

Asepsis: the absence of harmful microorganisms; free from infection or infectious material

Ashen: gray skin color

Asian: person who comes from the continent of Asia

Aspiration: the act of inhaling vomitus, mucus, or a small object into the respiratory system; may occur in persons who are unconscious, under the effects of general anesthesia, or having difficulty swallowing

Assault: the intentional attempt to touch or threat to touch another person's body without that person's consent

Assessment: gathering information through the use of subjective and objective observations

Assistive device: an item a person uses to accomplish a task

Asthma: a disease of the bronchi characterized by difficult, wheezing respiration

Atheist: person who denies the existence of a god

Atherosclerosis: bumpiness of the walls of the blood vessels due to fat deposited there

Atrium: one of the two upper chambers of the heart (together called the atria)

Atrophy: to waste away or decrease in size

Attitude: a pattern of mental views based on previous experience that was gathered over time

Auditory: relating to the sense of hearing

Auditory canal: the tube in the ear through which sound waves travel

Aura: an odd feeling, such as numbness or dizziness, just before a seizure or migraine headache starts

Autoclave: device that sterilizes reusable objects through steam pressure

Axilla: the armpit

Bacteria: microorganisms that reproduce by cell division; also called germs

Baptism: a Christian ritual marked by the use of water

Barrier: a way of blocking something; an obstruction

Battery: the act of touching another person's body without that person's consent

Bed rest: the physician's order that the patient stay in bed

Behavior: the manner of conducting oneself

Benefit: something extra, such as a service provided by an employer

Benign prostatic hyperplasia: enlargement of the prostate gland

Bile: substance secreted by the liver that breaks down fat in the duodenum

Biopsy: removal of living tissue and examination of it under a microscope

Bisexual: person who shows sexual attraction to persons of either sex

Black: person belonging to a dark-skinned race

Bladder: the elastic muscular sac that collects urine before it leaves the body

Bladder elimination: discharge of the body's waste from the bladder; also called urination and voiding

Blindness: inability to see

Blood glucose (blood sugar): a term used to describe the level of glucose in the circulating blood

Blood pressure: pressure caused by the blood circulating against the arteries

Body alignment: the body's correct, straight position

Body bag: a large plastic bag in which a body is placed after death

Body image: the feelings and thoughts individuals have about their body

Body language: the posture, gestures, and facial expressions that a person uses in communicating with others

Body mechanics: the use of the body to push, pull, or lift objects

Body system: a group of organs that work together to complete a certain function (for example, in the urinary system the kidneys produce urine and the bladder stores urine)

Body temperature: the degree of body heat or coldness measured by a clinical thermometer

Bonding: creating an emotional tie with a mate or a newborn

Bone: the hard, rigid connective tissue that makes up most of the skeleton

Bony prominence: any area of the body where bone lies close to the skin (such as the elbow or ankle)

Bowel: the intestine

Bowel elimination: the way the body gets rid of its solid waste, produced in the bowel

Bowel movement: the waste material that forms as food moves from the digestive tract through the intestinal tract; also called feces and stool

Brace: a metal or plastic appliance that supports or protects a weakened body part

Bradycardia: a heart rate less than 60 beats per minute

Bradypnea: respiration rate less than 12 breaths per minute

Braille: a system of writing/reading used by persons who are blind

Bronchi: the air passageways in the lungs

Burp: to help a baby expel gas from the stomach through the mouth by patting the back

Caffeine: a substance in coffee, tea, colas, and chocolate that acts as a stimulant and diuretic

Calcium: the chemical element that is important to bone and tooth formation

Calculi: stones in the body made up of mineral salts

Call signal: a communication tool used by patients who must remain in bed or in a chair; also called a call light or call bell

Callus: thickening

Calorie: a measure of the energy produced by the breakdown of food in the body

Calorie count: a record of the amount of calories eaten

Cancer: a disease in which certain cells of the body change into nonfunctioning cells and grow and crowd out healthy, functioning cells

Canthus: the angle created by the eyelids in either corner of the eye; the inner canthus is the corner near the nose; the outer canthus is the outer corner

Capillary: the very small vessel that connects arterioles and venules

Carbohydrate: a source of energy in the body; found in sugar and starches

Carbon dioxide: an odorless, colorless gas that is expelled from the lungs

Cardiac arrest: a sudden stop in the beating of the heart

Cardiopulmonary: pertaining to the heart and lungs

Cardiopulmonary resuscitation: CPR; a method to reestablish heart and lung action

Care giver: a member of the health care team who is involved in giving care to patients

Care plan: a written tool developed by a registered nurse to communicate and document a plan for the care of a patient

Caring: an attitude of interest in and concern about helping others

Cartilage: fibrous, semi-rigid tissue found in adults

Cataract: a milky cloudy spot on the lens or capsule of the eye

Category-specific isolation: the infection control measures practiced for a group of infectious diseases that have similar characteristics

Catheter: a flexible tube passed into body openings to allow fluids to enter or exit the body

Cavity: a hollow or a space

Cell: the basic unit of any living organism

Celsius scale: a temperature scale with the freezing point at 0° and the boiling point of water at 100°; abbreviated as C

Cerebrovascular accident: when the blood stops going to the brain, causing brain tissue to die; a stroke

Certification: being certified that one has met requirements and may practice to the level indicated on the certificate

Certified nursing assistant: a person who is certified to give care to patients under the direct supervision of a registered nurse or a licensed practical/vocational nurse

Cerumen: earwax

Cervix: birth canal; opens to allow passage of the fetus from the uterus to the vagina during childbirth

Cesarean section: the delivery of the fetus through an abdominal incision

Chamber: an enclosed space

Change of shift report: a report of a patient's condition and needs, given when care givers change shift, to ensure continuity of care

Chemotherapy: the use of chemical agents to treat disease and illness

Cheyne-Stokes: periods of deep breaths followed by very short or no breaths, repeated in a cycle

Chickenpox: a communicable disease caused by a virus spread by contact with a blister or by droplet infection

Child: a young person from toddlerhood through school age

Choking: a feeling of strangulation that occurs when an airway obstruction interferes with breathing

Cholesterol: fatty substance that attaches to the lining of arteries; comes from animal fats and oils

Christianity: religion based on the teachings of Jesus Christ

Chromosome: the part of the cell that contains genetic information

Chronic: lasting for a long time

Chronic illness: illness in which the symptoms last a long time

Chronological charting: a method of charting in which events are recorded according to the sequence in which they happened

Cilia: tiny hairs that protect the respiratory tract by making a wave-like upward motion to carry mucus up and out of the body

Circadian: occurring about every 24 hours

Circulation: the movement of blood through the body caused by the heart's pumping action

Circumcision: removal of the male foreskin

Circumduction: circular movement of a limb or eye

Civil law: the law governing relationships between people

Clammy: damp, sticky, and usually cool feeling

Classified: divided into sections or special parts

Clean-catch urine specimen: a urine specimen collected after the urinary meatus and surrounding tissue have been cleansed

Cliché: a very familiar phrase people use automatically without thinking about what they are saying

Clitoris: small organ that has nerve endings that make it sensitive to sexual arousal in females

Coccyx: tailbone

Cochlea: the essential organ for hearing; a snail-shaped tube that forms part of the inner ear

Code: a system of principles and rules

Code of ethics: a system of principles and rules that a group or person follows as a guide for what is good and bad and morally obligated

Cognition: one's awareness and judgment of something

Cognitive: pertaining to cognition, one's awareness and judgment of something

Colon: the large intestine; extends from the end of the small intestine to the rectum

Colostomy: an opening (stoma) made in the abdomen that permits the large intestine to be brought to the surface to provide a route for the evacuation of stool

Comfort: a sense of contented well-being

Commode: portable toilet

Communicable disease: an illness that can be transmitted to another person

Communication: an exchange of information

Communication board: a board that helps persons express their needs by pointing at specific words that are printed on it

Communication process: a method of communicating that uses a sender of a message and a receiver who responds with feedback

Communion: an act of sharing; in the context of bread and wine

Complication: the occurrence of another disease or problem in addition to the original disease or problem

Computer: a device that electronically stores, retrieves, and processes information

Conception: the joining of the ovum and the sperm; fertilization

Condom: a sheath worn over the penis that decreases the risk of transmitting or contracting sexually transmitted diseases and has limited value in preventing pregnancy

Condom catheter: a sheath with a tube at the bottom that allows urine from the penis to flow into a collection bag

Conduct: to act or behave in a particular way; escort

Conduction: a mechanism of heat loss in which body heat is carried away through contact with an object

Confidentiality: the act of keeping information private

Conflict: a struggle; a disagreement between what is happening to the individual and what is expected

Confused: not oriented to time, place, or person; disoriented

Congestion: excessive fullness of a body organ; the fullness interferes with the function of the body organ (heart or lung)

Conjunctiva: the delicate membrane that covers the inner eyelids and the eyeball

Connective tissue: tissue that connects and holds parts of the body together (for example, tendons)

Conscious: awake, alert; not sleeping

Consciousness: state of being awake, alert; not sleeping

Consistency: the degree of thickness

Constipation: inability to have or difficulty in having a bowel movement

Constrict: to make narrow; to close off

Contact lenses: prescription lenses that float on the cornea to help correct a defect in vision

Contaminate: to soil or infect by contact

Contamination: soiled or infected by contact

Continuity: condition of having no breaks or interruptions

Continuum: a way to show how you feel about something; a range

Contraction: shortening or tightening of a muscle fiber

Contracture: a shortening of muscle that causes the permanent disability of an extremity; the extremity loses flexibility and freezes in position

Convalesce: to recover health and grow stronger gradually after an illness

Convection: a mechanism of heat loss in which heat is moved away from the body on currents of air

Copulation: sexual union

Cornea: the clear, transparent anterior (front) of the eye

Cough: sudden expulsion of air from the lungs

Coughing and deep breathing: exercises that help the patient expand the lungs; included in preoperative teaching, the patient performs the exercises after a surgical procedure in which general anesthesia was given

Cramp: the feeling that results from a muscle spasm

Cranial: inside the skull

Crime: a wrong committed against a person or the person's property; the wrong may be a crime under criminal or civil law

Crisis: a sudden change; a turning point in an illness; a period of overwhelming disorganization

Criticize: to find fault

Culture: the beliefs, social expectations, and characteristics of a racial, religious, or social group

Cytoplasm: the substance surrounding the nucleus, contains smaller bodies that do the work of the cell

Dander: small particles from the hair or feathers of animals that may cause an allergy

Deafness: complete or partial lack or loss of the sense of hearing

Debris: dirt

Deciduous: subject to falling or being shed

Decubitus ulcer: a bedsore; a sore caused by continual pressure on the body parts of a patient who must stay in one place

Deduction: taking something away

Deep: below or away from the surface

Deep breathing: the intake of air deep into the lungs, followed by a slow release of air from the lungs

Defamation: harming the reputation of another by words you write (libel) and say (slander) about another individual

Deformity: abnormal part

Degenerate: deteriorate; decline

Dehydrate: to remove or lose water

Dehydration: condition resulting from a loss of body fluid

Dementia: changes in the ability to think and remember; changes in personality

Demineralize: to lose minerals or organic salts

Denial: refusal to admit the truth or reality

Dental floss: a special string used to clean between the teeth

Dentures: artificial teeth

Deodorant: a preparation that destroys unpleasant odors

Dependable: reliable; when people know they can count on you

Depression: sadness and a decrease in the usual behaviors associated with daily functioning

Deprivation: lack of something

Dermis: the inner layer of the skin; the layer below the epidermis

Deteriorate: worsen

Development: growth from a lower to a higher state of functioning

Developmental stage: stage during which certain behaviors are expected of an individual

Developmental task: an expected accomplishment that helps a person develop as an individual

Diabetes mellitus: a disorder that affects the body's ability to use glucose (sugar) because the body cannot use or produce insulin

Diabetic coma: a coma (unconscious state) that results when the diabetic patient lacks insulin

Diagnosis: determination of the nature of a disease

Diagnostic study: a procedure or examination that helps the physician diagnose a disease or illness

Dialysis: an artificial method of removing liquid waste products from the body when the kidneys produce little or no urine

Diaphoresis: perspiration; sweating

Diaphragm: the muscular membrane that separates the thoracic and abdominal cavities

Diarrhea: frequent, watery stools

Diarthrosis: a moveable joint

Diastolic pressure: pressure resulting when the heart rests between beats

Diet: the total amount of food eaten by an individual

Dietician: professional who promotes good health through proper diet

Digest: to break down chemically and mechanically

Digestion: the mechanical and chemical breakdown of food into forms the body can use

Digital: an electronic number display

Dilation: widening

Diphtheria: an infection of the tonsils, pharynx, larynx, or nose

Disadvantaged: handicapped; a person who lacks resources that are needed to function as an equal in society

Disaster: a sudden extraordinary event that brings great damage, loss, or destruction

Discharge: the process that prepares a patient to leave a health care institution

Discharge plan: a written plan of teaching that prepares a person to perform self-care after discharge from the health care institution

Discomfort: distress; mental or physical uneasiness

Disease: sickness; a condition of the body or one of its parts that causes a change in the body's functioning

Disease prevention: actions taken to prevent disease

Disinfectant: a chemical that destroys or disables microorganisms

Disinfection: the process of destroying or disabling harmful microorganisms

Disorientation: not knowing self, time, or place

Disoriented: in a state of disorientation; unaware of self, time, or place; confused

Disruption: an interruption of normal function or activity

Distal: the farthest point of reference

Distention: the act of being expanded

Diuretic: a substance that causes an increase in urination

Document: to write to communicate information

Doppler: an instrument that measures the wave movement of blood in the arteries

Dorsal: toward the back

Dorsiflexion: bending backwards

Double-bagging: placing a bag of contaminated waste inside a clean bag to prevent the escape of microorganisms

Douche: the introduction of a fluid into the vagina for the purpose of cleansing or medical treatment

Draw sheet: a piece of linen about half the size of a regular sheet, placed over a protector pad (rubber or plastic) for patient comfort; when edges are loosened from under the mattress, it can be used by two people to move a patient up in bed

Dress code: guidelines for dressing

Duct system: small tubes that connect the testicles with the urethra in the male reproductive system and provide the route for sperm to reach the outside of the male's body

Duodenum: the first part of the small intestine; where bile breaks down fat in the body

Dyspnea: difficult or labored breathing

Dysuria: difficult or painful urination

Ear: organ of hearing and balance

Ecchymosis: skin that is black and blue or purplish

Edema: an abnormal accumulation of fluid between cells

Ego: the self

Elderly: a term frequently used to refer to older adults, usually individuals over age 65

Elective surgery: optional; surgery that is not urgent

Electrocardiogram: a recording of the heart's electrical activity

Elimination: the way the body rids itself of unusable food and fluid; the discharge of the waste products created by the body's metabolism

Elongated: lengthened

Embolism: the sudden blocking of an artery by an embolus

Embolus: a clot that moves from a larger blood vessel to a smaller one and obstructs (stops) the flow of blood

Embryo: the development of the baby in the uterus from fertilization to the second month

Emergency: a situation that calls for immediate action

Emesis: stomach contents brought up and expelled from the mouth; vomitus

Empathy: understanding or being aware of another person's feelings, thoughts, or experiences

Emphysema: destruction of the alveoli (tiny air sacs in the lungs) and enlargement of air spaces so oxygen and carbon dioxide cannot move in and out of the lungs

Employment: an activity usually done for pay

Endometrium: the inner layer of the uterus; it sheds once a month and causes menstruation

Enema: a solution that loosens fecal material and stimulates peristalsis of the intestines

Enteric: pertaining to the small intestine

Environment: the conditions, circumstances, or objects that surround a person

Enzyme: a protein substance made by the body that helps break down chemicals in the body

Epidermis: the outer layer of the skin

Epistaxis: nosebleed; rupture of small blood vessels in the nose

Epithelial tissue: tissue that covers the internal and external surfaces of the body (for example, the skin)

Erection: when erectile tissue fills with blood and becomes rigid

Erotic: pertaining to sexual desire

Escherichia coli: a bacteria found in the large intestine of humans

Esophagus: a muscular tube from the pharynx to the top of the stomach

Estrogen: female sex hormone

Ethical: acting or behaving within the rules of good and moral conduct

Ethics: rules that govern right conduct (see code of ethics)

Ethnic: referring to the customs, language, and values of a group, especially a minority group

Ethnicity: certain qualities associated with a member of an ethnic group

Etiology: cause

Eustachian tube: the auditory tube; the narrow channel between the tympanum and the nasopharynx

Evacuate: to empty or remove something or someone

Evaluation: a critical assessment of value, worth, character, or effectiveness

Evaporation: a mechanism of heat loss in which body heat is converted into a vapor (beads of sweat)

Eversion: a turning outward

Exacerbation: making more severe; a flare-up

Excess: too much

Excoriation: a scratch or abraded (rubbed off) area of the skin

Excruciating: very intense

Exercise: the performance of physical activity to improve health

Expiration: breathing out

Exploit: to take advantage of unfairly

Extend: to stretch out to fullest length

Extension: straightening of a flexed (bent) limb

External: outside

Extinguish: to put an end to

Extremity: a limb of the body; an arm or leg

Eye: organ of vision

Fahrenheit scale: a temperature scale with the freezing point at 32° and the boiling point of water at 212°; abbreviated as F

Failure to thrive: the failure of an infant or child to gain weight

Fallopian tubes: tubes located on each side of the uterus that help move the ovum from ovary to uterus

Family: a group of people (not necessarily related) having a relationship

Fantasy validation: a technique that reinforces the patient's fantasy in order to decrease stress and prevent agitation

Farsightedness: the ability to see distant objects clearly and the inability to focus clearly on objects that are near; hyperopia

Fat: source of energy in the body; adipose tissue

Fatigue: tiredness; weariness

Fat-soluble: able to dissolve in fat

Feces: waste eliminated from the body through the anus

Feedback: when the receiver in the communication process repeats the information the sender sent (or otherwise acknowledges it) to make sure the message is understood

Fertilization: joining of the ovum and sperm; conception

Fetal alcohol syndrome: a wide range of abnormalities of the fetus caused by alcohol consumption by the pregnant woman

Fetus: the developing human in the uterus, from the second month of pregnancy to birth

Fever: above-normal body temperature; also called pyrexia

Fiber: the portion of food that passes through the intestine and colon undigested; it increases the bulk of the stool and makes it softer

Finger stick: drop of blood is produced by piercing the finger with a special instrument (lancet)

First aid: health care treatment provided to a person injured in an emergency situation

Flatulence: presence of too much gas in the stomach or intestine

Flatus: the expulsion of gas from the gastrointestinal tract

Flex: bend

Flexible: bendable

Flexion: bending

Flossing: using a special string to clean between the teeth

Flow sheet: a record of a series of measurements and observations made at frequent intervals during a specific time period

Fluid deficit: condition in which the body loses fluid and fluid is not replaced in the amount needed by the body

Fluid excess: condition in which the body's tissues hold extra fluid

Fluids: liquids

Folk healer: nonprofessional person who is consulted about health care and healing

Folk medicine: a tradition of medicine practiced by non-professionals, using parts of plants for treatment

Fontanelle: soft spot on the infant's skull where the bones do not meet; closes up as the infant grows

Footboard: a device that keeps feet in a correct anatomical position

Foreskin: a fold of skin that covers the tip of the penis in males who are not circumcised

Formula: milk mixture that is fed to babies

Fractional: relatively small

Fracture: a break in the bone at any point or place

    closed f.: a break in the bone that does not result in an open wound

    comminuted f.: three or more bone fragments are present

    compression f.: the bone is crushed

    depressed f.: fragments of bone are pushed inward (usually occurs in the skull)

    impacted f.: the bone ends are pushed or shoved into each other

    longitudinal f.: the break runs across the length of the bone rather than across the bone

    oblique f.: the break slants in the direction of the bone

    open f.: the bone or bone fragments pierce the protective skin covering the body

    segmented f.: a piece of the bone is broken off the bone

    spiral f.: the break goes around the bone

    transverse f.: the break travels across the bone

Fracture bedpan: a small bedpan that slides easily under the hips, generally used for patients with a hip fracture

Friction: the rubbing of one object against another

Fulcrum: a support for a lever

Function: the normal or proper action of any part or organ

Functional nursing: the type of nursing wherein patient care is divided into certain functions (for example, one nursing assistant might be assigned to weigh all patients)

Fungus: a microorganism that uses spores to reproduce

Fuse: to blend or join together

Gallbladder: small, pear-shaped sac under the liver that concentrates and stores bile

Gangrene: death of body tissue caused by lack of blood supply

Gastric: pertaining to the stomach

Gastrointestinal: pertaining to the stomach and intestines

Gastrointestinal tract: the small and large intestines

Gene: biologic unit of heredity located in the chromosome

General anesthesia: loss of sensation in the entire body caused by an anesthetic medication introduced into the blood

Genital: pertaining to the genitalia

Genitalia: the external organs of the reproductive system

Gestation: the period that starts with fertilization of the ovum and ends at birth

Gesture: motioning of the limbs or body as a means of expression

Glans penis: the head of the penis; may be covered with a hood of skin known as the foreskin

Glaucoma: a group of eye diseases that result in increased intraocular pressure

Globulin: a protein

Glucose: sugar

Goal: aim

Gonorrhea: bacterial infection of the organs of reproduction and the organs of the urinary system; a sexually transmitted disease

Good Samaritan law: law that protects you from being sued by the person you assist in an emergency; this law varies from state to state

Gram: unit of weight used in the metric system

Graphic: a drawing or word display that makes information more clear and understandable

Groin: the area from the lower abdomen to the inner part of the thighs

Grooming: making one's appearance neat and attractive

Growth spurt: when a child gains weight and adds inches in a short period of time

Gurney: stretcher on wheels; a cart used to transfer patients

Gustatory: associated with the sense of taste

Handicap: disability

Handroll: a device placed in the palm of the hand to prevent contracture of the hand and fingers

Hazard: a source of danger

Health: any state of physical, emotional, and social well-being felt by an individual

Health care team: the group of people who have the education necessary to provide care to patients

Health–illness continuum: a way to show how you feel about your own state of health or illness

Health promotion: actions taken to promote the quality of life

Hearing aid: a device that makes sounds louder for persons who are hard of hearing

Heart: the hollow muscular organ located in the left side of the chest that is an electrical pump that controls the flow of blood

Heartburn: a burning sensation in the area of the heart or the esophagus

Heart rate: number of heartbeats per minute

Heimlich maneuver: procedure to clear the airway of a person who is choking

Hematoma: a collection of clotted blood

Hemiplegia: paralysis of one side of the body

Hemorrhage: the escape of blood from a ruptured blood vessel; uncontrolled bleeding

Hemorrhoid: an enlarged (swollen) vein located inside or just outside the rectum

Hemovac drain: a drain placed in the body during surgery that allows secretions to flow out of the body into a collection container

Hepatitis: inflammation of the liver

Hepatitis A: an inflammation of the liver caused by the type of virus that is primarily transmitted by the oral–fecal route

Hepatitis B: inflammation of the liver caused by the type of virus that is transmitted only through blood and blood products

Heredity: the physical and mental traits you receive from your ancestors; inheritance

Herpes simplex: a virus that causes genital redness, swelling, itching, pain, and pimple-like lesions that open and crust over in the genitals

Heterosexual: person who shows an attraction for persons of the opposite sex

Hispanic: of Spanish, Mexican, or Puerto Rican heritage

Home health care: nursing care and personal services (housekeeping, shopping, etc.) provided for patients who live at home and cannot perform activities of daily living for themselves

Homeostasis: a state of balance

Homosexual: person who shows an attraction to persons of the same sex; male homosexuals are referred to as gays, and female homosexuals are called lesbians

Horizontal: the state of being flat; the flat or even view one sees when looking at a bed or the horizon

Hormone: a substance that endocrine glands secrete directly into the blood; the hormone travels to a designated place in the body where it is used in a chemical action

Hospice: a place for the care of persons (and their families) in the last stages of life

Hospital: an institution for the care and treatment of the acutely ill and injured

Household: those who live under one roof and make up a family

Housekeeping: keeping the home neat, clean, and free of safety hazards

Humidifier: a device (run by electricity) that produces a fine mist of water particles

Humidity: moisture

Hydrate: to add water to

Hygiene: the practice of cleanliness to promote health

Hymen: a thin piece of tissue found in the vaginal opening of the female

Hyperalimentation: delivery of proteins, carbohydrates, vitamins, and minerals through a large vein

Hyperextension: overextension of a limb or part

Hyperglycemia: the presence of an abnormally high amount of glucose (sugar) in the blood

Hyperopia: farsightedness

Hypertension: persistently high blood pressure

Hypervolemia: an increase in the amount of fluid in the circulation

Hypoglycemia: the presence of an abnormally low amount of glucose (sugar) in the blood

Hypostatic pneumonia: infection of the lung that occurs as a result of lying on the back for a long period of time

Hypotension: low blood pressure

Hypothalamus: an area of the brain that controls body temperature

Hypothermia: lower than normal body temperature

Hypothyroidism: a disease of the thyroid gland

Hysteria: extreme emotional agitation

Ileum: the last part of the small intestine

Illness: sickness; a condition different from the normal health state; any change, temporary or long-lasting, in a person's physical, emotional, or spiritual health and well-being

Immigrant: a person who arrives in a country with the intent of living there

Immobility: the inability to move; loss of freedom of movement

Immobilizer: a device that keeps someone or something from moving

Immune system: the body's defense system against harmful microorganisms

Immunization: a procedure that helps the body develop an antibody against a specific harmful microorganism

Impaction: the lodging of hard fecal material in the rectum

Implantation: the attachment of the fertilized egg to the uterine wall

Impotence: inability of the male to achieve and maintain the rigid erection needed for successful sexual intercourse

Impregnate: to make pregnant

Incident: an event; an unusual event that is likely to cause an accident

Incision: a cut or wound made by a sharp instrument

Incontinent: unable to respond to the urge to eliminate the waste products of the body

Intricate: complex

Incus: the middle ossicle of the ear; also called the anvil

Indelible: can't be erased or washed out

Indigestion: difficulty in digesting something

Indwelling catheter: a tube inserted into a body opening and secured in place

Infancy: the time from birth to 1½ years, during which all needs must be met for a person

Infant: the person at the beginning of life (from birth to 1½ years), for whom all needs are met by others

Infarction: an area of dead or dying tissue due to a lack of blood supply

Infection: the body's response to invasion by harmful microorganisms and their multiplication in the body

Infection control: procedures enacted to control the spread of infection, particularly nosocomial (originating in the hospital) infections

Infectious agent: a harmful microorganism that takes its nourishment from healthy tissue

Inferior: located at a point closer to the soles of the feet; downward

Inflammation: a painful red swelling; the body's response to illness or injury

Influenza: a communicable disease caused by a virus; "the flu"

Informed consent: when a person is informed of (told about) a procedure or treatment and agrees (gives consent) to having the procedure or treatment done

Ingestion: taking in food and fluid by mouth

Insomnia: the inability to fall asleep easily or remain asleep throughout the night

Inspiration: breathing in

Institution: an establishment; something or someone associated with a place or thing

Institutionalize: the process of placing an individual in the care of an institution

Insulin: a hormone produced by cells in the pancreas that helps the body use glucose (sugar) for energy

Insulin shock: low blood sugar caused by the presence of too much insulin

Intact: complete, whole, no breaks

Intact skin: having no injury or breaks of the skin

Integument: a covering, such as skin

Interact: to communicate with

Interaction: communication between two or more people

Intercourse: sexual contact between individuals

Internal: inside

Intervention: action taken to help a patient; carrying out the patient's plan of care

Interview: a formal meeting to obtain information

Intestine: the tube that extends from the stomach to the anus

Intimacy: closeness

Intraocular pressure: increased pressure inside the eyeball

Intravenous: through the vein

Intricate: complex

Inventory: a list of, for example, personal preferences, attitude, interests, or items

Inversion: a turning inward

Iris: the circular pigmented (colored) membrane of the eye

Iron: a dietary substance that is necessary for the replacement of red blood cells

Iron deficiency anemia: low level of iron in the blood; a common nutritional disorder

Ischemia: lack of blood supply in a body part due to a blockage of a blood vessel

Islam: religion based on the teachings of Allah and his prophet, Muhammad

Isolation: being separated

IV: abbreviation for intravenous

Jackson-Pratt drain: a drain placed in the body during surgery that allows secretions to flow out of the body into a collection container

Jaundice: yellowness of the skin, sclerae, mucous membranes, and body excretions caused by an accumulation of bile pigments (substances that provide color) in the blood

Jejunum: the part of the small intestine between the duodenum and the ileum

Job description: a statement of the behaviors expected of a person who performs a specific job

Joint: the place where two or more bones meet

Judaism: religion developed by ancient Hebrews

Kaposi's sarcoma: a rare form of skin cancer, associated with acquired immune deficiency syndrome

Ketone: an acetone-like compound

Kidney: one of two organs that filter waste products out of the blood to be eliminated by the body

Kilogram: a unit of weight in the metric system

Knead: to press down with the hands

Knee gatch: equipment that helps raise the lower part of the bed so the legs are elevated

Knowledge base: the basis of one's information and understanding

Labia: folds of skin surrounding the urinary meatus (opening) and vagina in females

Labia majora: long outside folds of skin surrounding the urinary meatus and vagina in females

Labia minora: small folds of skin inside the labia majora surrounding the vaginal opening in females

Labor: a series of muscle contractions that expel the fetus from the body

Laceration: cut in the skin caused by a sharp object

Lactose: a sugar present in milk; many persons lack the enzyme that breaks down lactose for use by the body

Lactose intolerance: inability to digest milk because of the lack of the enzyme that breaks down lactose (a sugar found in milk) for use by the body

Lateral: toward the side; away from the middle of a body part

Law: a rule or regulation; a binding custom or practice of a community; a rule of conduct formally recognized

Laxative: a medication that loosens the stool and makes it easier to pass out of the body

Legal: conforming to rules and the law

Legume: plant source of fiber; found in dried beans and peas

Lens: glass or other transparent material that bends or scatters light rays

Lesion: a break in the skin caused by a sore or any other tissue damage

Lethargy: abnormal drowsiness and indifference

Lever: an object that moves or raises another object

Leverage: mechanical advantage gained by using a lever

Liability: the state of being liable (responsible by law)

Libel: writing something that harms an individual's reputation

Licensed practical nurse/licensed vocational nurse: a graduate of a school of practical nursing who is licensed by a state authority and practices under the supervision of a registered nurse

Listening: paying attention; hearing a message with thoughtful attention

Liver: the largest organ in the body; stores red blood cells and secretes bile

Living Will: a form patients sign when they do not wish to have their life prolonged by any means

Local anesthesia: loss of sensation in the part of the body in which an anesthetic medication has been injected or applied on the skin

Log-rolling: moving a patient's body as one unit

Lubricant: a substance that reduces friction

Lumpectomy: removal of a lump from body tissue, commonly the female breast

Lungs: the two main organs of respiration

Malleus: largest of the three ossicles of the ear; also called the hammer

Malnutrition: a condition that results from poor nutrition

Malpractice: failure to give a service for which one is trained

Mammogram: x-ray of the breast

Mastectomy: surgical removal of the breast

Maturity: state of full development

Measles: a communicable disease caused by a virus

Measurement: an extent or amount determined by measuring

Medial: located in the middle

Medical asepsis: clean technique; the performance of cleanliness procedures to destroy or limit the spread of harmful microorganisms

Medical diagnosis: the decision a physician makes about a patient's illness based on information gained through a physical examination, an interview with the patient or family, a medical history of the patient, and results of laboratory and radiologic testing

Medical terminology: the group of special terms used in the medical field

Medication: a drug

Medulla oblongata: the respiratory control center in the brain

Membrane: a layer of tissue that acts as a covering or lining

Menopause: the changes that end the female's ability to bear children; also called climacteric and change of life

Menstrual: pertaining to menstruation

Menstruation: the discharge through the vagina of blood and tissue from the uterus of the nonpregnant female; also called monthly flow, menses, and period

Mental health: emotional wellness

Mental illness: disruption in psychologic functioning

Menu planning: budgeting money, purchasing groceries, and planning the meals for the week

Mercury: a chemical agent that expands with heat

Metabolism: the process that produces energy in the body, allowing cells to grow and repair

Meticulous: careful attention to detail

Microorganism: an organism so tiny it can be seen only under a microscope; capable of helping the body as well as causing disease

Milestone: a significant point in development

Mineral: an inorganic (neither animal nor vegetable) substance needed for health

Mitral valve: the valve between the left atrium and the left ventricle of the heart

Mobility: ability to move or be moved

Modesty: being shy, humble, or moderate

Morgue: the place where bodies are kept until they are identified and claimed by relatives

Mottling: marked with spots or blotches

Mucous membranes: the covering of skin that lines the organs of the gastrointestinal organs (from lips to anus)

Mumps: a communicable disease caused by a virus

Muscle: fibrous tissue that expands and contracts to allow the body to move

Musculoskeletal: referring to muscle and skeleton

Mutilation: destroying or crippling a part of the body

Myocardial infarction: death of cells of the heart due to obstruction of the blood supply to the heart

Myopia: nearsightedness; shortsightedness

Nares: the nostrils; the external (outside) openings of the nasal cavity

Narrative charting: a written description of information observed and patients' statements about themselves

Nasal drainage: secretions from the nasopharynx that exit through the nares

Nasogastric tube: tube inserted through a nostril into the stomach

Nasopharynx: the part of the pharynx located above the soft palate

Native American: descendant of persons who lived in North America before it was settled by people from other countries

Nausea: an unpleasant, uncomfortable feeling in the stomach; may be experienced with vomiting

Navel: umbilicus; a scar that marks the connection of the umbilical cord to the fetus

Nearsightedness: the ability to see near objects more clearly than distant ones; myopia

Necrosis: death of tissue

Negligence: an unintentional act that results when your actions harm a person or his or her property

Nervous tissue: tissue that sends and receives messages

Nonjudgmental: not passing judgment on someone whose beliefs are not the same as yours

nonREM sleep: the deep, restful stage of sleep, in which eyeball movement is slow and rolling

Nonverbal: using a method to communicate that is other than verbal

Nonverbal communication: the exchange of information without using words, for example, shrugging the shoulders to express "I don't know"

Normal flora: microorganisms that belong in a specific body site

Nose: the organ of smell and the means of bringing air into the lungs

Nosocomial: pertaining to or beginning in the hospital

Nosocomial infection: any infection acquired in a health care institution

Nostrils: the two external openings of the nasal cavity

Nourishment: a food or fluid that adds carbohydrates, proteins, and/or fats to the diet

Noxious: foul

NPO: abbreviation for nothing by mouth

Nuclear family: family group consisting of parents and children

Nucleus: a small body inside the cell that acts as the control center; also contains chromosomes

Nulliparity: never having experienced pregnancy

Nursing: the art and science of caring for others

Nursing diagnosis: a description of actual or potential health changes that a nurse is legally allowed and professionally prepared to treat

Nursing process: a systematic problem-solving method used by registered nurses to care for patients

Nutrient: a chemical substance that helps the body break down, absorb, and use foods and fluids

Nutrition: the study of food's relationship to health; the act of providing food to nourish the body

Obese: very fat

Obesity: overweight; the presence of too much fat in the body

Objective observation: information gathered by using the five senses; sight, hearing, smell, taste, and touch

Obliterate: erase

Observation: noting a fact or occurrence about something or someone

Obstruction: blockage

Occult: hidden; unseen

Occupational therapist: professional who helps patients relearn self-care, work, or leisure activities when illness or injury has made them incapable of performing these activities

Occupied bed: type of bedmaking in which the patient remains in the bed while linens are changed

Ointment: a preparation that is applied to the body's surface and contains a medication

Olfactory: associated with the sense of smell

Oliguria: decreased urinary output

Ombudsman: person who receives reports and investigates situations that need outside assistance

Opacity: a condition in which light rays cannot penetrate a normally transparent object

Optic nerve: the nerve in the eye that carries impulses for the sense of sight

Oral: pertaining to the mouth

Oral cavity: the opening in the body that consists of the mouth, salivary glands, tongue, and teeth

Organ: a body part that performs a specific function or functions

Orientation: special time set aside to tell you about something, such as a new job

Orthopneic position: an upright position supported by pillows; relieves difficulty in breathing

Orthostatic hypotension: a dizzy feeling caused by a fall in blood pressure; occurs when a person sits or stands too quickly

Ossicle: a small bone, especially of the middle ear

Osteoblast: a special cell associated with bone production

Osteoporosis: disease in which calcium leaves the bones and enters the bloodstream

Ostomy: an artificial opening

Otitis media: inflammation of the middle ear; occurs most often in infants and children

Otoscope: an instrument used to inspect the ear

Ovaries: egg-shaped organs located on each side of the uterus in females; produce the ovum and hormones

Overview: a summary

Ovulating: the releasing of an ovum at intervals of about 28 days

Ovum: the egg needed for reproduction

Oxygen: a colorless, tasteless, odorless gas; the air we breathe is about 20% oxygen

Oxygenated: carrying oxygen

Oxygenation: putting oxygen into something or someone

Oxygen flow-meter: a meter that regulates the amount of oxygen prescribed for delivery to a patient

Pacifier: a nipple-shaped device used by babies to satisfy sucking needs

Pain: a feeling of discomfort, suffering, or agony

Pallor: paleness; the loss of color from one's face

Pancreas: organ behind the stomach that secretes insulin

Panic: acute or extreme anxiety

Paralysis: loss of feeling in a body part and the inability to move that body part

Paraplegia: paralysis of the legs or the lower part of the body

Parasite: one who depends on another for support without giving anything back

Parkinson's disease: a disease that affects the brain and muscles and is characterized by a stooped posture, shuffling gait, and hand tremors

Passive range of motion exercise: range of motion exercise that is done for the patient by the care giver

Pathogen: any agent or microorganism that causes disease

Pathogenic: relating to any disease-producing agent or microorganism

Patient abuse: verbal, emotional, or physical mistreatment of a patient

Patient record: patient chart; a document that contains information about a patient and the patient's condition

Patient's Bill of Rights: statement written of the rights patients are entitled to when receiving health care

Peer: an equal; one who belongs to the same group (age, school, etc.)

Pelvic: pertaining to the pelvis

Pelvic inflammatory disease: disease of the female reproductive organs

Pelvis: the lowest part of the trunk; the area between the hip bones and the lower spine

Penetration: passing into or through

Penile drainage: drainage or secretions coming from the penis

Penis: external organ of urination and copulation in males

Penrose drain: a drain placed in the body during surgery that allows secretions to flow out of the body into an absorbent pad

Performance: an action; how you do something

Perianal area: area around the anus

Perineal area: the area between the legs, including the genitals and anus

Perineum: the pelvic floor, extending from the pubic bones at the front of the body to the coccyx (tailbone) at the back

Perioperative: the period before, during, and after a surgical procedure

Periorbital edema: swelling surrounding the eye

Peripheral: outer edge

Peripheral neuropathy: loss of sensation (feeling) in the lower limbs

Peripheral vascular disease: a disease caused by decreased blood supply to the extremities

Peristalsis: alternate contraction and relaxation of the esophagus and the intestines

Peritoneum: the membrane that lines the abdominal and pelvic cavities

Personnel: the people employed in an organization

Perspiration: sweat; moisture excreted through the pores of the skin

Pertussis: a communicable disease, also known as whooping cough

Pharynx: the throat; a muscular tube located at the top of the esophagus

Physiatrist: a physician who specializes in physical therapy

Physical abuse: mistreatment that causes harm to the body

Physical examination: an examination of a person's state of health by a physician

Physical therapist: professional who helps ease the pain of muscle, bone, nerve, or joint injury or disease

Physician: a medical doctor or doctor of osteopathy

Physiology: the study of body function

Pigment: a substance that gives color to something

Pincer grasp: movement of the thumb and fingers to pick up objects

Pinna: the part of the ear that projects outside the head; also known as the auricle

Pivot: turn

Placenta: the organ that forms at the site where the fertilized egg implants; provides the fetus with essential nutrients and oxygen and carries away the fetus's waste products

Planning: developing a program of how to go about doing something; also a step in the nursing process that is like a blueprint for action

Plantar flexion: the act of bending the sole of the foot

Pneumocystis pneumonia: a lung infection, associated with acquired immune deficiency syndrome

Pneumonia: acute inflammation or infection of lung tissue

Podiatrist: a doctor who treats diseases and conditions of the foot

Poisoning: a condition produced by swallowing, touching, or breathing in a harmful substance; may also be produced by injection by a stinging insect

Polio: a viral disease that can result in paralysis

Pollen: the substance that fertilizes flowering plants

Polydipsia: excessive thirst

Polyphagia: excessive food intake

Polyuria: increased urine production and output

Port: an opening

Portal: an opening

Positioning: placing the body in a certain posture

Posterior: located toward the back

Postoperative: after surgery; used to refer to the period of recovery

Postpartum: the first 6–10 weeks after the birth of the infant in reference to the mother

Posture: the natural and comfortable bearing of the body in healthy persons

Potassium: a chemical element required for cell function

Precaution: care taken in advance to prevent or reduce harm

Prefix: a word element placed before a root word to help describe the root word

Pregnancy: the presence of a developing embryo or fetus within a woman's body

Premature birth: an infant born before 38 to 40 weeks of gestation

Premenstrual syndrome: symptoms including irritability, water weight gain, breast enlargement and tenderness that occur in many females before menstruation

Preoperative period: the period of time between the decision for surgery and surgery

Preoperative checklist: a record that shows that the activities required to prepare the patient for surgery have been completed

Preoperative routine: activities that are performed to prepare the patient for surgery; usually the 24-hour period before surgery

Presbyopia: a visual condition in which the eye is unable to focus on near objects

Preschool age: the child from 3 to 6 years of age

Prescription: an order for a procedure, medication, diet, or other service written by a physician

Pressure points: certain parts on the body where bone is located close to the skin, such as the elbow; also, various areas of the body where pressure is applied to control hemorrhage

Prevention: stopping a problem or situation before it occurs

Primary nursing: the nurse's 24-hour accountability for the patient's care

Probe: a slender instrument used to explore and send back information

Problem-solving process: the systematic method used to resolve problems

Progesterone: hormone that plays a major part in menstruation

Prognosis: a forecast about the way a disease or illness may progress

Pronation: turning the palm downward

Prostatectomy: surgical removal of the prostate gland

Prostate enlargement: an overgrowth of prostate tissue that can block the urethra

Prostate gland: the gland in males that surrounds the urethra and the neck of the bladder and secretes fluid that helps sperm move through the duct system

Prosthesis: an artificial replacement for a missing part of the body

Protective device: a piece of equipment designed to prevent patients from harming themselves or others; formerly called a restraint

Protein: a material needed for cell growth; used in muscles

Protozoa: microscopic single-celled organisms

Proximal: the nearest point of reference

Psychiatrist: a physician who helps people with mental, emotional, and behavioral disorders

Psychologic: relating to psychology; mental

Psychologic abuse: mistreatment that causes a person to feel threatened

Psychologist: a professional who helps people with mental, emotional, and behavioral problems

Psychology: the study of mental development, mental processes, and behavior

Psychosocial: referring to the influence of society on mental development and behavior

Puberty: the developmental and physical changes that result in adult sexual characteristics and the ability to reproduce

Pubic area: the area of the lower abdomen covered by hair in the adult

Pubic lice: small insects that live in pubic hair

Pulmonary artery: large artery that carries blood from the right ventricle to the lungs

Pulmonary vein: the large vein that carries oxygenated blood from the lungs to the left atrium of the heart

Pulse: the beat of the heart as felt through the walls of the arteries

Pulse deficit: the numerical difference between the radial pulse and the apical pulse

Pulse rate: the number of heartbeats per minute felt at a pulse site; same as the heart rate

Puncture wound: wound that goes beneath the first layer of the skin, caused by a sharp, usually pointed object

Pupil: the opening in the center of the iris that helps control the amount of light entering the eye

Puree: strained food

Purulent: containing pus

Pyrexia: fever; elevated body temperature

Quadriceps exercise: a leg exercise patients perform in bed to help the circulation of blood

Quadriplegia: paralysis of all four limbs

Qualifications: special abilities or skills

Radiation: a mechanism of heat loss in which heat is given off or thrown off by the body

Random: unplanned and unexpected

Rales: an abnormal lung sound that indicates air is moving through fluid in the lungs

Puncture wound: wound that goes beneath the first layer of skin, caused by a sharp object

Range of motion: the range, measured in degrees like a circle, through which a joint can be extended and flexed (bent)

Rape: the criminal act of having sex with someone without that person's consent

Rapid eye movement (REM) sleep: the active stage of sleep, in which the eyeballs move rapidly

Rash: reddened spots close together on the skin; spots can be flat or raised

Rationale: an underlying reason

Reality orientation: a technique used to help patients know their name, time, and location; involves the use of visual and auditory cues such as calendars, clocks, and name tags

Reception: the act of receiving

Recording: writing down information about a patient or an occurrence

Recovery room: a room near the operating room where the patient is observed immediately after surgery

Rectal: pertaining to the rectum

Rectum: the last part of the large intestine that ends at the anal canal

References: people you name on an employment application as being able to provide a statement of your qualifications

Reflex: an automatic response to a stimulus

Registered nurse: a graduate nurse registered and licensed to practice by a state authority

Rehabilitation: a program that helps a patient return to as normal a life as possible

Reinforce: to strengthen by giving extra support

Rejection: not wanted by or not satisfied with someone or something

Relaxation: easing of tension; resting

Religion: an organized set of beliefs about a high power

Relocation stress: a form of stress that occurs when the patient is transferred from one place to another

Reminisce: to think or talk about past events

Remission: a time during which a patient does not feel the symptoms of a disease

Reporting: giving a verbal account of a patient or an occurrence

Reproduce: to produce again in the same image

Reproduction: the process by which a new individual is produced

Reservoir: a holding place

Residue: a layer of particles

Respiration: the exchange of oxygen and carbon dioxide between air and the body's cells

Respiratory arrest: sudden stop in breathing

Responsibility: reliability; trustworthiness

Rest: freedom from activity and labor

Resuscitate: to bring back to life from unconsciousness or apparent death

Resuscitation: bringing an individual whose heart or lungs have stopped functioning back to life

Retina: the inner light-sensitive layer of the eye

Retract: to pull back

Retraining program: a program designed to help a person relearn a skill or activity

Rhonchi: a coarse dry lung sound that indicates disease is present

Right: something to which a person has a just claim

Role: a socially accepted behavior pattern

Root: origin

Root word: the part of a word that indicates the disease or condition

Rotation: the process of turning on an axis, for example, turning the head from side to side

Rubella: a communicable disease caused by a virus; German measles

Sacrum: triangular shaped bone at the lower end of the spine

Safety: the status of being safe from experiencing or causing hurt, injury, or loss

Saliva: watery substance secreted from the salivary glands; moistens food and makes it easier to swallow

Scabies: a contagious disease that causes itching in folds of skin, such as the groin and under the breasts

School age: the child from 6 to 12 years of age (the years before adolescence)

Sclera: the tough, white outer covering of the eyeball

Scrotum: the pouch (sac) that contains the testicles and their accessory organs in males

Secondary sexual characteristics: changes in males and females that occur with puberty

Secretion: discharge; drainage material that leaves the body through an opening

Seizure: a change in body function caused by abnormal electrical activity in the brain; a convulsion

Self-esteem: how confident and satisfied a person feels

Self-image: your idea of who you are and what your role in life is

Semen: the fluid that helps sperm move through the duct system in males

Semicircular canal: the passage shaped like a half-circle in the inner ear that controls the sense of balance

Semilunar valves: one valve that is located in the right ventricle and guards the entrance into the pulmonary trunk; one valve that is located in the left ventricle and guards the entrance into the aorta

Senses: the ways we receive and interpret the stimuli; sight, sound, touch, taste, and smell

Sensitivity: awareness of others' physical and emotional needs

Sensory deficit: a condition in which a person is unable to respond to stimulation

Sensory deprivation: a condition in which a person receives less than normal sensory input; there is inadequate quality or quantity of stimuli

Sensory organs: the organs that control or regulate vision, hearing, touch, taste, or smell; eyes, ears, nerve endings in the skin, taste buds, nose

Sensory overload: a condition in which a person's senses receive too much stimuli

Sensory stimuli: something that stimulates the sensory organs

Sexuality: the sense of being male or female; the intimacy that exists between two people

Sexually transmitted disease: a disease that is transmitted (passed on) during the sexual act between partners

Sheath: a case or cover

Shock: a life-threatening condition in which the blood supply to the heart is decreased

Shroud: a piece of linen or other material in which the body is wrapped after death

Sigmoid colon: the final part of the colon; shaped like a C or S

Sign language: a formal language that uses hand and matching mouth gestures to communicate words and meanings to people who cannot hear

Sitz bath: placing the hips and buttocks in water to relieve pain and discomfort of organs in the perineal area

Skin: the body's protective outer covering

Slander: to say something that harms an individual's reputation

Sleep: the natural periodic suspension of consciousness during which the body's mental and physical powers are restored

Sleep deprivation: a prolonged loss of sleep that occurs when rapid eye movement sleep is interrupted over a long period of time

Sleepwalk: to rise from bed and walk in an apparent state of sleep

Sling: a hanging bandage from the neck that supports an injured arm or hand

Socialization: participation in a social group

Social worker: a professional who helps patients and their families deal with psychosocial problems

Sodium: a chemical element found in the body's fluids

Soft palate: the part that separates the mouth and the pharynx (the upper throat cavity)

Sonogram: a test that uses sound waves to make a picture of an organ

Spasm: a sudden contraction (tightening) of a muscle or group of muscles

Specimen: sample; a small piece of body tissue or a secretion used for examination

Sperm: the male cell that joins with the female ovum to produce a new individual

Sphygmomanometer: the instrument used to measure the arterial blood pressure

Spinal: pertaining to the spine (backbone)

Spinal anesthesia: loss of feeling or sensation in the body parts below the area of the back where anesthetic medication was injected

Spirituality: belief in or sensitivity to religious values

Spleen: an abdominal organ that stores red blood cells and helps keep the blood free of waste material

Splint: a device that supports a body part

Spouse: married person (husband or wife)

Sputum: a mucous secretion from the lungs, bronchi, and trachea that is ejected (brought up) through the mouth

Standard: a rule, principle, or measure established by an authority

Stapes: the innermost ossicles of the ear; also called the stirrup

Staphylococcus: a harmful microorganism that looks like grape clusters when seen through a microscope

Stereotype: an image one holds of members of a group

Sterilization: the process of killing all harmful microorganisms on an object by placing it in an autoclave or in boiling water

Sterilize: to kill all harmful microorganisms on an object by placing it in an autoclave or in boiling water

Stertorous: noisy breaths that sound like snoring

Stethoscope: an instrument used to hear and amplify the sounds of an internal organ (heart, lungs, or bowels)

Stimuli: something that causes an activity to start

Stomach: pouch-like organ located on the left side of the abdomen; the widest part of the gastrointestinal system

Stool softener: a medication that softens the stool and makes it easier to pass out of the body

Straight catheter: a tube inserted one time to drain urine from the bladder, after which it is removed

Strainer: a device that collects particles but permits fluid to pass through

Stranger anxiety: a fear of strangers in which the infant may cry, hide, and refuse to go to an unfamiliar person

Streptococcus: a harmful microorganism that looks like pairs or chains when seen through a microscope

Stress: pressure caused by something in the internal or external environment

Stress incontinence: the leakage of urine when abdominal pressure is increased, such as during a cough, sneeze, or laugh

Stridor: a shrill, harsh breathing sound that may be heard without a stethoscope

Stroke: cerebrovascular accident; when blood stops going to a part of the brain

Structure: the arrangement of parts in the body

Stupor: lethargy; partial or nearly complete loss of consciousness

Subcutaneous fat: an inner layer of skin that insulates the body

Subjective observation: information gathered through the statements of another person, for example, "I'm cold"

Suffix: a word element that, when placed after a root word, creates a new word

Suffocation: a stop in breathing due to a lack of oxygen

Summary: brief repetition of the main points of a discussion

Superficial: near the surface

Superior: located at a point closer to the head; upward

Supination: turning the palm upward

Supine: lying with the face up; lying on one's back

Supplement: to complete or add to

Supportive device: a device used to hold up or serve as a support for a patient

Support system: the individuals a person can turn to for help

Suppository: a capsule of medication administered into a body cavity such as the rectum, vagina, or urethra

Surgery: operation

Surgical bed: a bed prepared especially for the patient who is returning from the recovery room; also called an OR (operating room) bed

Susceptible: unable to resist

Symmetry: balance

Sympathy: feeling pity for another person

Synarthrosis: an immovable joint

Syncope: fainting

Synovial fluid: a fluid that lubricates joints to reduce friction when they move

Syphilis: a contagious sexually transmitted disease (STD)

Syringe: instrument used to inject fluids into or remove fluids from the body

Systolic pressure: pressure caused by the blood circulating through the body when the heart contracts and ejects (pushes) the blood from the left ventricle

Tachycardia: a heart rate over 100 beats per minute

Tachypnea: more than 24 breaths per minute

Tactile: pertaining to touch

Taste buds: cells on the tongue that distinguish salty, sweet, sour, and bitter tastes; organ of taste

Teaching/discharge plan: a written plan of teaching that prepares persons to care for themselves after discharge from the health care institution

Team nursing: a team of care givers caring for a group of patients

Temperature: the degree of heat or cold, expressed in terms of a specific scale

Temper tantrum: display of behavior in which children may throw themselves on the floor and kick and scream

Terminal illness: an illness in which the end result is death; the patient's life expectancy must be 6 months or less

Terminology: a group of special terms

Testicle: organ of the male reproductive tract that is located in the scrotum and produces sperm

Testosterone: an important male sex hormone

Tetanus: lockjaw

Therapeutic diet: diet that helps meet a patient's particular nutritional need; also called special, modified, or restricted diet

Thermometer: the instrument used to measure temperature

Thoracic: pertaining to the chest

Thrive: to grow vigorously; flourish

Thrombophlebitis: inflammation of a vein where a clot is formed

Thrombosis: formation or presence of a thrombus

Thrombus: blood clot

Tinnitus: noise in the ears (ringing, buzzing, or roaring)

Tissue: a group or layer of cells that all perform the same task

Toddler: the child from 1½ to 3 years of age

Toileting: assisting a patient to the toilet or commode, or onto a bedpan, for the purpose of emptying the bowel or bladder

Tongue: organ of taste; also aids in chewing, swallowing, and speaking

Toothette: sponge on a stick; brand name

Tort: a crime that breaks a civil law

Trachea: the air passage from the mouth to the lungs; the windpipe

Tracheostomy: an artificial opening in the windpipe

Traction: application of a pulling force to a fractured bone or a dislocated joint

Tradition: a practice that is handed down from generation to generation

Transfer: moving a patient from one room to another in the same institution or from one institution to another

Transient ischemic attack: temporary lack of oxygen to brain tissue

Transverse colon: the part of the large intestine that goes across the body from side to side

Trauma: injury

Treatment: a procedure, such as a dressing change or application of ointment, which can be done by a doctor or a nurse, or performing eye surgery, which can only be done by a surgeon

Tremor: trembling or shaking

Trichomoniasis: a sexually transmitted disease caused by a protozoa

Tricuspid valve: the valve between the right atrium and the right ventricle

Tube feeding: giving fluids or nutritional supplements through a tube inserted into the stomach

Tuberculosis: an infectious, inflammatory lung disease

Tumor: growth of tissue

Turbinates: thin membranes over bony cartilage that support the walls of the nasal chambers

Turgor: fullness or elasticity of the skin

Tympanic: pertaining to the eardrum

Tympanic membrane: the thin membrane that stretches across the ear canal, separating the middle ear from the outer ear; eardrum

Umbilical cord: the cord that connects the growing fetus to the mother's uterus through which oxygen, carbon dioxide, fluids, and other nutrients are exchanged

Umbilicus: navel; a scar that marks the connection of the umbilical cord to the fetus

Unconscious: unaware of the environment and not responsive to stimuli; unconsciousness occurs during sleep, fainting, and coma

Universal distress signal: hands grasping the neck to indicate the airway is blocked

Universal precautions: measures taken in advance by all health care workers to prevent the spread of infection and disease

Unoccupied bed: type of bedmaking in which no one is in the bed while the linens are changed

Ureter: tube through which urine passes from the kidney to the bladder

Urethra: tube that carries urine from the bladder to the outside of the body

Urinal: a container into which a person urinates

Urinalysis: a laboratory test of urine that helps the physician form a diagnosis

Urinary: pertaining to urine

Urinary incontinence: inability to control the elimination of urine

Urinary meatus: the opening of the urethra through which urine flows to the outside of the body

Urinary retention: accumulation of urine in the bladder because of inability to urinate

Urinary tract: the kidneys, ureters, bladder, and urethra

Urinary tract infection: infection of the urinary tract, especially the bladder and urethra

Urination: discharge of urine; voiding

Urine: fluid that contains water and the waste products of the body

Urine glucose: a test of the urine in which dipsticks indicate whether glucose (sugar) is present in the urine

Urine retention: accumulation of urine in the bladder due to the inability to urinate

Urostomy: an opening in the abdomen that provides a route for the evacuation of urine from the ureters or bladder

Uterus: the womb; pear-shaped organ located above the cervix in the pelvic region of females; expands and contracts during pregnancy

Vaccine: a preparation administered to produce or artificially increase immunity to a particular disease

Vagina: the canal from the cervix to the vaginal opening that stretches during intercourse and childbirth in females

Vaginal opening: opening located between the urinary meatus and the anus in females

Vaginitis: inflammation of the vagina; a vaginal infection

Validate: to confirm; make sure

Value: something or someone of importance or worth

Vasectomy: cutting or tying of the duct system of the male to prevent the sperm from getting to the urethra, renders the male infertile

Vector: a carrying agent

Vein: a blood vessel that carries blood from the body's organs to the heart

Vena cava: the large vein that returns blood to the right atrium of the heart

Ventral: toward the front

Ventricle: a small chamber or cavity located in the heart or brain; the heart has two lower chambers (together called the ventricles)

Venule: smallest part of a vein

Verbal: the use of words to communicate

Verbal abuse: any use of words that are not considerate and respectful of the patient's rights

Verbal communication: the use of words or other sounds, such as music or groans, to exchange information

Vertigo: dizziness; a feeling that one's body or one's surroundings are moving

Victim: term used to refer to the injured person at the site of an accident

Virus: a microorganism that needs living tissue in order to reproduce

Visual: pertaining to the ability to see

Vital signs: the signs of life: temperature, pulse, respirations, and blood pressure

Vitamin: an organic substance that is essential in small amounts to the body's health

Vitreous humor: the transparent substance that fills the part of the eyeball between the lens and the retina

Vocabulary: the collection of words or phrases used by a person

Void: to empty the bladder

Vomit: to eject material from the stomach through the mouth

Vomitus: results of vomiting; material ejected from the stomach through the mouth

Wages: payment for services

Water: clear, odorless, tasteless fluid necessary for life

Water-soluble: able to dissolve in water

Water-soluble lubricant: a substance that reduces friction and dissolves in water

Well-being: a healthy, happy life; living a full life

Wheeze: a whistling sound associated with breathing

White: a person belonging to the Caucasian race

Word elements: parts of words

Workplace: the place (such as a factory or office) where work is done

Wound: an injury to the body usually caused by physical means

Answers to Review Questions

CHAPTER 1

1. A healthy person is one who is in a state of physical, emotional, and social well-being. When a person becomes ill, he or she experiences a change in physical and emotional health and social well-being. Physical changes may include pain or loss of a body part. Emotional changes may include the inability to cope with stress and anxiety. Changes in social well-being may include an inability to participate in social activities.

2. Health care institutions include acute care and long-term care institutions. Other institutions include those that provide hospice care, rehabilitation care, mental health and home health care. The acute care institution provides services needed by persons who are acutely ill: nursing care, nutrition, radiology (x-ray), laboratories, operating rooms, emergency room, and delivery room and newborn nursery. The long-term care institution provides nursing care, nutrition, recreation and activities, and may provide physical therapy and beautician services.

3. The registered nurse assesses, plans, intervenes, and evaluates patient care. Other duties include coordinating and managing patient care, teaching patients, and supervising other nursing care personnel.

   The practical/vocational nurse gives direct care to patients and performs treatments under the supervision of a registered nurse.

   The certified nursing assistant gives patient care under the supervision of the registered nurse or the practical/vocational nurse.

   The physician directs care. Social workers and nutritional therapists are among the many people who are health care team members.

CHAPTER 2

1. The hiring process includes: filling out an application for employment, being interviewed for a position, and completing a physical examination.

2. Information a prospective employer needs includes your name, address, telephone number, Social Security number, education history, and work experience. Also, include the names, addresses, and telephone numbers of people who agree to give you a reference.

3. To keep your job, you should: report to work on time, follow the rules and regulations of the health care institution that hires you, dress according to the dress code, keep your patients comfortable and safe, treat all people you meet with courtesy and kindness, complete all of your job assignments on time, complete only the tasks for which you have been trained, ask questions whenever you are unsure of what you should do, work as a member of the health care team, and accept responsibility for your own actions.

4. A job description is important because it is a statement of the behaviors expected of a person who does a specific job. It acts as a guideline for you.

CHAPTER 3

1. A tort is a crime that occurs when a wrong is committed against an individual or his or her property. Examples of intentional torts include:
   - Defamation—saying untruthful things about another person
   - Assault and battery—moving a patient to a stretcher when he or she has refused to leave his or her bed
   - False imprisonment—keeping a person in a place against his or her will

   Examples of unintentional torts include:
   - Negligence—failing to open food cartons when the patient is too weak to do so by him or herself
   - Malpractice—you may be assigned to give an enema to your patient who is scheduled for surgery. The patient may be at risk for complications if you do not give the enema as you were taught

2. The Patient's Bill of Rights is a document that tells about the expectations a patient has when he or she is receiving health care. It is important because it helps ensure effective care and satisfaction for the individual patient.

3. Personal qualities for nursing personnel include caring about others, a desire to help others, sensitivity and gentleness, empathy, respect, and honesty.

CHAPTER 4

1. Steps of the nursing process are: assessment, planning, intervention, and evaluation.

2. A nursing assistant may observe the patient's ability to use all extremities, the color and odor of urine, and the condition of the patient's skin.

3. Nursing diagnosis describes actual or potential health changes that a nurse is legally allowed and professionally prepared to treat.

4. The problem-solving technique is a systematic way to solve a problem. An example problem is studying about the layer of skin: (1) Gather textbook and class notes. (2) Review the information on skin layers. (3) Problem is lack of knowledge of terms related to the skin. (4) Look up words in the glossary of the textbook or a dictionary. (5) Read the assignment with a list of definitions nearby. (6) Read and understand the assignment about the layers of the skin.

CHAPTER 5

1. The essential parts of communication are the sender, message, receiver, and feedback.

2. Communication helpers keep open the lines of communication and help build a sense of trust between health care team members and patients. General leads such as "Oh?"—broad opening statements such as "Tell me about your pain"—and the use of silence are all examples of communication helpers.

3. Examples of communication barriers include clichés; clichés can be replaced by listening to the patient and reflecting an important concern back to the patient. Using "why" questions is a barrier; instead, try to use clarification by telling the patient you are uncertain of what he or she is saying and requesting that information be made more clear. Changing the subject is another barrier that can be corrected by using a general lead such as "Go on."

4. To communicate with a visually impaired person, make sure the room is light, the patient has on clear glasses, and stand where you can be seen by the patient.

For a hearing-impaired patient, make sure the hearing aid (if the patient has one) is working and inserted correctly, stand in front of the patient when talking, and repeat what you are saying if necessary. Writing can also be used to communicate.

For the handicapped, speak directly to him or her, not to the person who is a companion.

For children, position yourself for good eye contact and use simple terms they can understand.

For the elderly, make sure assistive devices are being used correctly (glasses, hearing aids, etc.) and allow time for the patient to respond.

CHAPTER 6

1. Patient statements about anxiety, pain, sadness, or fatigue are examples of subjective observations.

2. Examples include: the rise and fall of the chest (seeing), the pulse through a stethoscope (hearing), warmth of a patient's skin (touching), fruity odor on the breath (smelling), flavor of chocolate (tasting).

3. Reporting occurs when you tell someone about your observations; recording occurs when you write down your observations.

4. When subjective observations are reported and recorded, use the statement "The patient said" in front of the observation(s). When objective observations are reported and recorded, use terms that describe what you observed so that another person who hears or reads your work can interpret it the way you intended.

5. A written change of shift report may include the patient's name and room number, the physician's name and patient's admitting diagnosis, age, allergies, and agency number.

CHAPTER 7

1. Medical terminology consists of terms used by people who are in the medical field. Health care workers use it for clearer communication about their patients.

2. Pathology is made up of the root *path(o)*, meaning disease, and the suffix *ology*, meaning study of. Pathology is the study of disease. Urinalysis is from the root *urin(o)*, meaning urine, and the suffix *lysis*, meaning breakdown of. Urinalysis is the breakdown of urine (for testing purposes). Hysterectomy is from *hyster(o)*, meaning uterus, and *ectomy*, meaning removal of. Hysterectomy means the removal of the uterus. Gastroenteritis is from the roots *gastr(o)* (meaning stomach) and *enter(o)* (intestines) and the suffix *itis* (meaning inflammation). Gastroenteritis means the inflammation of the stomach and intestines. Ophthalmologist is made up of the root *ophthalm(o)*, meaning the eye, and *ologist*, meaning specialist. Ophthalmologist means a physician who specializes in care of the eye.

3. With = c, without = s, before = a, after = p, head of bed = HOB, nothing by mouth = NPO, hour of sleep = HS.

CHAPTER 8

1. Vital signs = VS; temperature, pulse, and respirations = TPR; blood pressure = BP.

2. Age, sex, environment, food and fluid intake, exercise, life-style, fear and anxiety, disease, and medications all affect the vital signs.

3. Take vital signs according to the routine of the health care institution, any time the patient's condition changes, and whenever the patient tells you he feels different.

CHAPTER 9

1. Sites to measure body temperature are the mouth, rectum, axilla, and the eardrum.

2. Thermometers are used to measure body temperature. They may be glass, electronic, or disposable.

3. A patient with a fever may have hot, dry skin; flushed face; loss of appetite; thirst; sweating; and generalized weakness.

CHAPTER 10

1. Peripheral pulse sites are in the following areas: temporal, carotid, brachial, radial, femoral, popliteal, posterior tibial, and dorsalis pedis.

2. Place stethoscope on the left side of the chest at the nipple line.

3. To help a patient breathe more comfortably, you can place him or her in a sitting position, give fluids if permitted, keep air moving in the room, loosen clothing, check the setting on the oxygen flow-meter when oxygen is ordered, and monitor humidity when it is ordered.

4. The cuff of the sphygmomanometer is filled with air by the pumping action of the handheld bulb. The cuff becomes tight and flattens the artery over which it is placed. When the pressure is released, one can hear the rush of blood returning to the arteries through a stethoscope. When sound is heard, the number observed on the dial (or the mercury in the column) is the systolic pressure. When the last sound is heard, that number (dial or column) is the diastolic pressure.

5. In most health care institutions, the patient can be told what his or her pressure is. The nurse or supervisor will direct you in special situations.

6. Refer to the chart "Problems with Blood Pressure Measurement and Ways to Avoid Them."

7. The patient may need assistance with personal care, safety, reducing stress, exercise, teaching about sitting and standing up slowly, following through on instructions from other therapists, and observing for medication side-effects as instructed by the nurse.

CHAPTER 11

1. Microorganisms are recognized by shape, size, and method of reproduction.

2. Steps are presence of an infectious agent, a reservoir, a portal of exit from the reservoir, a method of transmission, a portal of entry to the host, and a susceptible host. Infection can occur at any point if the conditions are suitable to the growth of harmful microorganisms.

3. Transmission occurs by contact, by carrier, through the air, and/or from a vector.

4. A person acquires a nosocomial infection when he or she is in a health care institution.

5. The most common technique used is hand washing.

6. Universal precautions are measures taken in advance to prevent the spread of infection. Wear clean disposable gloves whenever you contact blood and body fluids, the patient's mucous membranes, and skin with breaks in it.

7. Clean with a solution of 1 part household bleach to 10 parts water.

8. Category-specific isolation procedures are guidelines that are used when the patient is diagnosed with a specific illness.

CHAPTER 12

1. Raise side rails for infants, toddlers, and preschoolers; elderly patients who are confused; as well as any patient who is sedated, confused, or disoriented. Be certain to cool foods like soups or beverages so that no patient burns the mucous membranes of the mouth.

2. Protective devices are used to protect a patient from harm or from harming others. You need to check for tightness, remove the device and exercise the body part, check skin condition under the device every two hours, and document the above actions as well as what kind of protective device is being used.

3. A health care worker cannot put on protective devices without a physician's order.

4. In case of fire, know the procedure in the procedure book of the agency. This includes sounding the alarm, notifying appropriate personnel of the location of the fire, taking patients to safety, extinguishing the fire if it is small, turning off electrical equipment and oxygen, and closing windows and doors.

5. During a disaster, patients need to be evacuated to a safe place after which air, food, and water must be supplied. Medical treatment should be available for those who are injured.

CHAPTER 13

1. The skin is the body's first line of defense against infection.

2. Observe for the following characteristics: color, texture, temperature, and intactness. Observe skin every time a patient contact is made.

3. For a.m. care, position the patient; offer assistance with toileting; offer glasses, hearing aids, and dentures; offer a warm wash cloth to freshen up the skin; straighten the bed linens; ask if he or she has any special needs; and offer a beverage.

    For p.m. and HS care, provide articles for oral care, a clean gown or personal night clothes, give a back rub, offer an extra blanket, and assist in any routine that helps the patient prepare for the night.

4. Before starting any procedure, you should wash your hands, identify the patient and yourself, provide privacy, and explain what you are going to do.

5. Clean disposable gloves are worn to provide a barrier in case of contact with blood and body fluids when you are giving care to patients.

CHAPTER 14

1. A closed bed has linens pulled up to the top of the bed with the pillow placed over the linens. In an open bed, the linens are fanfolded down to the foot of the bed, and in a surgical bed, the linens are folded over to the side of the bed.

2. Linens are changed according to the policy of the health care institution, whenever they are soiled, and whenever they are dampened by perspiration.

3. A patient who is on bed rest must remain in bed while linens are changed; this bed is called an occupied bed.

CHAPTER 15

1. Listen to what the patient is saying (subjective observation) and observe for any patient behavior that indicates pain or discomfort (crying, moaning, grimacing, refusing to move, etc.).

2. The patient in pain needs a calm, quiet environment; a darkened room; a stress-free environment; a gentle touch by the care giver; help in changing position; and elevation of the affected body part as directed by the nurse.

3. Sleep restores the body physically and refreshes and restores one's mental processes.

4. Factors that affect sleep are age, eating and exercising prior to going to bed, environment, hormonal changes, illness, medications, and sleep patterns.

CHAPTER 16

1. Proper use of body mechanics prevents injury to the care giver's back. It keeps the care giver as well as the patient safe from injury.

2. To maintain activity and mobility, you can offer fluids, encourage coughing and deep breathing, encourage movement of extremities, perform passive range of motion, and help with turning and positioning.

3. Complications such as the following occur: hypostatic pneumonia (lungs), thrombophlebitis (veins), orthostatic hypotension (decreased blood supply to the brain), weight loss (stomach and intestines), urinary tract infection and calculi formation (kidneys, ureters, and bladder), constipation (intestines), atrophy and contracture of muscles (musculoskeletal), decubitus ulcer (skin), and depression (psychologic functioning).

4. Preventive actions include offering fluids, keeping pressure off the skin, encouraging and performing range of motion exercises, and encouraging dietary intake.

5. Cast care includes keeping the cast clean and dry; elevating the extremity as directed; checking for swelling, skin discoloration, odor, and loss of sensation; and asking about pain or itching.

6. The patient on bed rest may need help with any combination of bathing, eating, toileting, and grooming. Follow the directions of the nurse, who will tell you what the patient should be encouraged to do for him or herself.

CHAPTER 17

1. Anatomy is learning how the body is built. Physiology is the study of how parts of the body work.

2. Cells need food, water, and oxygen for survival.

3. The ankles are inferior to the knees. The elbows are superior to the hands. The nose is in the anterior, medial part of the head.

CHAPTER 18

1. Sensory organs include the eyes, ears, nose, tongue, and nerve endings in the skin.

2. The eyes see a person's mouth move when he or she is talking, and the ears hear what the person is saying. The tongue tastes the chili one is eating, and the nerve endings in the tongue sense how hot the food is. The nose smells the chili during cooking.

3. Disruptions in senses include: in sight, decreased vision or blindness; in hearing, decreased hearing or deafness; loss of the sense of touch or smell; and a decrease or loss of the sense of taste.

4. A sensory deficit is a condition in which a person is unable to respond to stimuli— for example, when hearing is affected, one cannot respond to sound. Sensory overload is a condition in which the person receives an excessive amount (too much) of stimuli to the senses.

5. For the patient with impaired vision, you can offer glasses or a magnifier for reading and keep the person safe from injury. For the person with impaired hearing, you can assist with insertion of a hearing aid if the patient has one; if the patient is able to hear a little without a hearing aid, stand in front of him or her, speak slowly, and repeat what you are saying when necessary.

6. For patients with a history of seizure disorder, you should listen for reports of an aura; sudden stiffening or jerking of the limbs; change in the level of consciousness; eye changes; and possible increased saliva, tongue or lip biting, incontinence, and changes in breathing patterns.

CHAPTER 19

1. Nutrients include carbohydrates, proteins, fats, vitamins, minerals, and water.

2. Food is converted through the processes of ingestion, digestion, absorption, and elimination.

3. Carbohydrate foods include cereals and grains as well as fruits and vegetables. Protein is found in meats, fish, poultry, eggs, and dairy products. Foods that include fat are meats, dairy products, nuts, and eggs.

4. The fat-soluble vitamins are A, D, E, and K.

5. Vitamins are needed for good body (cell) function; minerals are needed for good bones and teeth and for nerve function.

6. Fats, oils, and sweets are found in oils used for cooking, cakes, and candy bars. Ice cream, yogurt, and cheese are milk-containing (dairy) products. Any food source from meat, fish, poultry, dry beans, eggs, and nuts contributes to this food group. Vegetables and fruits (beets, lettuce, and apples, pears, etc.) are part of this food group.

7. Clear liquid diet foods are fluids clear enough to see through such as broth and ginger ale. Full liquid diet foods include ice cream and custard. Soft diet foods include puréed foods (usually fruits or vegetables) and ground-up meats. A regular diet consists of all foods one normally eats.

8. The diabetic patient needs to monitor intake of foods with carbohydrates. The patient with excess fluids may have fluid restrictions, need special skin care, and have extremities elevated. The patient with fluid deficit may need fluids to be offered frequently and may be given intravenous fluids (IV). The patient who is obese will be placed on a reduced calorie diet, asked to increase exercise, and need emotional support. The patient with anorexia needs a pleasant mealtime environment, frequent small meals, and emotional support. The anorectic may also receive nutrition through tube feedings. The person who is unable to feed him or herself needs to be fed all foods and fluids.

CHAPTER 20

1. Constipation is inability or difficulty in having a bowel movement. Diarrhea is frequent passage of watery stools. Impaction is a condition that results when hard fecal material remains in the rectum. Flatulence is too much gas formation in the stomach or intestines.

2. Causes of constipation include aging (decreased peristalsis), disease, medication, changes in dietary intake, lack of exercise, the postoperative period, a decrease in fluid intake, and ignoring the urge to have a bowel movement.

3. Usual observations include information about the time of the last bowel movement, and if pain was present; looking at the color, consistency, frequency, and amount of the bowel movement. Unusual observations include any changes in the above.

4. To collect a stool specimen, gather equipment, put on gloves, and use a wooden tongue blade to take a specimen from the bedpan or "hat" that catches a specimen when the patient uses the toilet. Put the specimen in a container labeled with the patient's name, room number, date, and time, and take the specimen to the laboratory.

CHAPTER 21

1. Table 21–1 lists the usual and unusual observations you will make when the patient empties his or her bladder.

2. Care for a person who is incontinent includes changing incontinent pants or pads, applying a condom catheter, giving good skin care, and helping with a bowel and bladder retraining program.

3. For the female, wash with strokes that go from front to back; for the male, work in a circular motion from the meatus out to the glans penis.

4. To collect a clean-catch urine specimen, gather the equipment needed and ask the patient to cleanse the perineal area (females should spread the labia and keep them spread while voiding) before voiding into the container.

CHAPTER 22

1. External organs of the female are the labia majora and minora, clitoris, and vaginal opening; internal organs are the vagina, cervix, uterus, fallopian tubes, and ovaries. External organs of the male are the penis and scrotum; internal organs are the testicles and duct system.

2. Appearance of secondary sex characteristics: in the female—broadening of hips, enlargement of breasts, and appearance of pubic and axillary hair. Male secondary sex characteristics include the growth of facial, axillary, and pubic hair; enlargement of the penis and scrotum; sperm and testosterone production; and the ability to have and maintain an erection.

3. The enlarging abdomen caused by the fetus growing in the enlarging uterus, breast enlargement, urinary frequency and urgency, and an increased pulse are physical changes that occur during pregnancy. Psychologic changes relate to the knowledge that a new life is forming as well as the acceptance and preparation for the role of mother. After delivery, the mother may have feelings of depression.

4. Three ways to prevent sexually transmitted disease are: not having multiple sexual partners, not engaging in risky sexual acts such as oral or anal sex, and using condoms during intercourse.

5. A douche provides for a cleansing action of the female vagina.

6. The male with prostate enlargement may have a decrease in the flow of urine, dribbling instead of a steady stream, and difficulty in starting the stream of urine.

7. Diseases that can be sexually transmitted include genital herpes simplex, syphilis, pelvic inflammatory disease, pubic lice, gonorrhea, and acquired immune deficiency syndrome (AIDS).

CHAPTER 23

1. To prepare a room for a newly admitted patient, fanfold the linens to the foot of the bed, fold the hospital gown and place at the foot of the bed, unpack and store the admission package, prepare the equipment for measuring vital signs, and lower the bed to the lowest position if the patient is walking in or coming in a wheelchair (keep in the high position if the patient is arriving on a stretcher).

2. People admitted to a health care institution may have feelings of fear, anxiety, anger, unhappiness, and loss of control.

3. Reasons for a patient transfer can include a request by the patient and/or family, change in patient condition, and transfer to another health care institution.

CHAPTER 24

1. To help with the discharge procedure, you should take a wheelchair or a cart to the room, help the patient pack belongings, retrieve valuables from the safe, make sure the patient has the discharge instructions, help the patient dress and help him or her into the wheelchair, and take the patient and the discharge slip to the designated place (cashier, discharge desk, etc.). Wheel the patient to the car or other vehicle and say good-bye. Clean and store the wheelchair after return to the unit, return forms appropriately, and return to the patient's room to remove linens from the bed. Report observations made during the discharge to the nurse or supervisor.

2. The discharge plans include information on diet, activity, medications, treatments, restrictions, follow-up appointments, and any other instructions that make the transition to another environment safe.

CHAPTER 25

1. Refer to preoperative checklist for duties that are to be completed before the patient leaves the unit for the operating room.

2. A completed preoperative checklist ensures that the activities required for preparation of the patient have been done.

3. Gather equipment for shaving and tell the patient what you are going to do. Put on gloves and moisten the skin, apply shaving solution and work up a lather, stretch

the skin taut, and shave the skin with the razor at a 45-degree angle. Wash, rinse, and dry shaved skin, then check closely to be sure no hair remains. Discard equipment appropriately and report to the nurse that the procedure has been completed. Complete the preoperative checklist in the space that addresses shaving.

4. An enema cleans out the bowel prior to surgery and prevents constipation after surgery.

5. Makeup and nail polish are removed so that care givers can observe for changes that might signal a problem during or after surgery.

6. Three types of anesthesia are general, local, and spinal anesthesia.

CHAPTER 26

1. To prepare for a patient's return from surgery, you should make a surgical bed, place an IV pole near the bed, move all furniture out of the way so that the cart can be placed next to the bed, and place needed supplies on the overbed table and bedside stand.

2. Postoperatively, you will measure vital signs, remind the patient to cough and deep breathe, keep the patient safe, orient the patient, provide fluids, assist with elimination, help the patient move and turn, and provide for patient comfort.

3. General anesthesia works to slow down all body functions—for example, there is decreased awareness, decreased rate of respirations, decreased output (bowel and bladder), and decreased motor activity.

4. Patients at risk for complications are those who do not move and turn, ambulate early, take fluids, and cough and deep breathe.

CHAPTER 27

1. The best way to help a person meet his or her developmental needs is to know what the needs are and be able to attend to those needs in your patients.

2. Observe for changes in the patient's behavior such as changes in physical functioning (lack of sleep, loss of appetite, etc.) and/or psychologic behaviors (sadness, worthlessness, helplessness, etc.).

3. The person with mild anxiety might have a heightened awareness and be very interested in what is going on in the environment. The person with moderate anxiety pays less attention to what is going on and may need help in directing his or her energy.

4. The person who is depressed may have changes in appetite, sleep patterns, elimination patterns, and energy; there may also be feelings of hopelessness, lack of concern for self, poor self-esteem, and rejection of family and friends.

5. When you care for the anxious patient, remain calm, be aware of your body language, use simple terms to communicate, provide a quiet atmosphere, and support the patient by spending time with him or her.

   When you care for the depressed patient, encourage the patient to eat, exercise, and participate in daytime activities. Keep a record of food and fluid intake. Spend time and listen to what the patient is saying. If the patient is deeply depressed, he or she may need assistance with activities of daily living and praise and encouragement when performing with activities of daily living. Spend time with the patient and encourage communication.

CHAPTER 28

1. Socialization is the ability to participate actively in a social group; culture includes beliefs, social expectations, and characteristics of a racial, religious, or social group; ethnicity refers to a certain ethnic quality associated with a member of a group; spirituality is a belief or sensitivity to religious values; and stereotyping is judging a person according to an image one holds of members of a group.

2. Socialization in infancy consists of the family members' interaction with the infant. If socialization is positive, the infant will grow up trusting that the world is a good

place and be able to socialize positively with others. Negative interaction may result in a person who is not trusting, fearful, and anxious.

3. The adolescent learns to interact and develop peer relationships. The positive interactions allow the adolescent to grow and extend relationships to people other than peers.

4. Socialization helps the older person by developing self-esteem and giving a feeling of self-worth.

5. Allowing a stereotype (of an ethnic group or religious group, for example) may cause you to make poor judgments or interfere with care because you feel the person deserves less than the usual amount of care.

6. Blacks seek health care from health care professionals but may use folk medicine practices; Hispanics may employ a folk healer before seeking professional health care; whites desire professional health care; Asians employ professionals but may also use herbs; Native Americans may seek a medicine man and professional health services when available.

7. To help a patient meet spiritual needs, provide time to observe religious practices, ask if a visit from clergy is desired, and report patient requests to the nurse.

CHAPTER 29

1. Factors that may affect development of sexuality are religious beliefs, cultural behaviors, ethnic background, physical attributes, age, and health.

2. A heterosexual is a person who has an attraction for persons of the opposite sex; a homosexual is a person who has an attraction for a person of the same sex; a bisexual is a person who has attraction for persons of both sexes.

3. The person who is a rape victim should be observed for discharge from the vagina or anus; bruises or lacerations around the outside of the external genital area; discomfort or pain; and the presence of blood, hair, or semen. Psychologically, the victim may be angry; disbelieving; crying; hysterical; and fearful of the rapist's return, the possibility of pregnancy, and/or contracting a sexually transmitted disease.

CHAPTER 30

1. During the first year of life, pulse and respirations are rapid while blood pressure is low. The toddler's pulse and respirations are still rapid but are beginning to slow down, and the blood pressure is a little higher than the infant's; the preschooler's pulse and respirations are still slowing down, and the blood pressure is becoming higher; the school-age child's vital signs are similar to the preschooler's range; during adolescence, pulse, respirations, and blood pressure stabilize to the normal ranges of an adult.

2. Play helps the infant learn to socialize with the family group; explore surroundings; and develop control of the head, hands, and feet. Play helps the preschool-aged child learn to interact with others and prepare to function in the outside world.

3. The infant's length increases by 50% and the weight triples during the first year of life. During adolescence, a growth spurt occurs and may add 25% to the height; boys gain between 15 and 60 pounds, while girls gain from 15 to 50 pounds.

4. When fluids are lost because of vomiting and/or diarrhea, dehydration occurs.

5. Observe level of activity, appearance, body temperature, level of comfort or pain, weight, and amount of nourishment taken in for the patient who is experiencing vomiting or diarrhea. Give fluids as ordered, encourage dietary intake, give meticulous skin care, clean the mouth out after each bout of vomiting, and remove waste products so air is fresh. Be sure to change diapers as often as needed to keep the patient dry if the patient having diarrhea is incontinent.

6. Communicable diseases associated with childhood include diphtheria, pertussis (whooping cough), measles, mumps, rubella, influenza, and chicken pox. Many of these diseases can be prevented by immunization against any disease for which a vaccine is available.

7. Failure to thrive may result from physical defects, lack of parent's knowledge of good nutrition, and/or emotional deprivation.

CHAPTER 31

1. Changes associated with aging include decreased efficiency of blood vessels; decreased lung expansion; drier and more fragile skin; less hair; a less efficient immune system; decreased ability to see, hear, smell, taste, and touch; a shorter stature; higher risk of bone fracture; decreased strength of muscles; decreased need to sleep; changes in metabolism and decreased need for calories; slowed function in the intestines; decreased bladder capacity; changes in memory; and the need for more time to respond to stimuli.

2. The changes of aging usually occur slowly over a period of time, and the person often feels he or she has adjusted well to them. Because the person may feel that he or she still responds as well as when younger, accidents resulting in injuries may occur.

3. Use visual (calendars, orientation boards, etc.) and auditory cues (tell the patient his or her name, the date, and where he or she is) to help your patient be oriented.

4. The five stages of death are denial, anger, bargaining, depression, and acceptance.

5. Impending death may be signaled by the following: decreased blood pressure and pulse; irregular, shallow respirations; disorientation or unresponsiveness; pale, cool skin that may be mottled; unfocused or staring eyes; inability to take in food or fluids; and incontinence of bowel and/or bladder. The ability to hear may remain until death.

6. After death occurs, bathe the body if that is your institution's procedure, close the eyelids gently, put a hospital gown on the body, comb hair, place the hands across the abdomen, straighten the linens, and provide privacy if the family wishes to view the body. Identification tags are placed on the toes, and the body is placed in a shroud or body bag. The body may be taken to the morgue or kept in the room until funeral personnel arrive, depending on the procedure followed in your agency.

CHAPTER 32

1. Qualities for the nursing assistant working in the home include being able to work without direct supervision, being organized and reliable, and caring about others.

2. Refer to the safety checklist in the chapter. Use it as a basis for doing a safety check in the patient's home.

3. When grocery shopping, use coupons, take advantage of weekly specials, and buy food in bulk to help the patient save money.

4. Nursing assistants **cannot** give medications, give any kind of a heat treatment, perform any sterile procedure such as a dressing change or catheterization, or perform any procedure for which they have not been trained.

5. The family is an excellent source of information about the patient, may assist in the care of the patient, and is a support system for the patient.

6. Three examples of patient exploitation are eating the patient's food, using the patient's money for your own purposes, and not completing care the way you were taught.

CHAPTER 33

1. The first person on the scene of an accident is known as a first responder.

2. Use the Heimlich technique if a person is choking. Make sure you know how to position your hands correctly on the victim's abdomen and do abdominal thrusts.

3. Cardiopulmonary resuscitation is a technique that reestablishes heart and lung function and may revive the person on whom it is performed.

4. The pressure point above the hand is over the radial artery; the pressure point above the foot is the posterior tibial artery; the pressure point in the upper arm is

located in the axilla; the pressure point for injury to the thigh is the femoral artery in the groin.

5. To care for the patient in shock, you should place the patient in a back-lying position with the head lower than the body, keep the patient warm, offer sips of water if the patient is thirsty, make a calm environment, and get help as soon as possible.

6. Burns are classified as superficial, deep partial thickness, and full-thickness burns.

Index

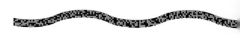

Page numbers in *italics* refer to illustrations; numbers followed by t indicate tables.